MW00379085

MACNAB'S BACKACHE

FOURTH EDITION

FOURTH EDITION

MACNAB'S BACKACHE

David A. Wong, MD, MSc, FRCS(C)
Past President North American Spine Society
Director Advance Center for Spinal Microsurgery
Presbyterian St. Luke's Medical Center
Denver, Colorado

Ensor Transfeldt, MD, FRCS(C)
Associate Professor
Department of Orthopaedic Surgery
Twin Cities Spine Center
Minneapolis, Minnesota

Lippincott Williams & Wilkins
a Wolters Kluwer business
Philadelphia • Baltimore • New York • London
Buenos Aires • Hong Kong • Sydney • Tokyo

Acquisitions Editor: Robert Hurley
Managing Editor: Jenny Koleth/Michelle La Plante
Production Manager: Fran Gunning
Manufacturing Coordinator: Kathleen Brown
Director of Marketing: Sharon Zinner
Design Coordinator: Stephen Druding
Production Services: Nesbitt Graphics, Inc.
Printer: Edwards Brothers

530 Walnut Street
Philadelphia, PA 19106 USA
LWW.com

Printed in the USA

Library of Congress Cataloging-in-Publication Data

Wong, David A.
Macnab's backache / David A. Wong, Ensor Transfeldt. -- 4th ed.
p. ; cm.
Rev. ed. of: Macnab's backache / John McCulloch, Ensor Transfeldt.
Includes bibliographical references and index.
ISBN 13: 978-0-7817-6085-0
ISBN 10: 0-7817-6085-2
1. Backache. I. Transfeldt, Ensor. II. Macnab, Ian. III. McCulloch, John A. Macnab's backache. IV. Title. V. Title: Backache.
[DNLM: 1. Low Back Pain. WE 755 W872m 2007]
RD771.B217M33 2007
617.5'64--dc22
2006029187

Care has been taken to confirm the accuracy of the information presented and to describe generally accepted practices. However, the authors and publisher are not responsible for errors or omissions or for any consequences from application of the information in this book and make no warranty, expressed or implied, with respect to the currency, completeness, or accuracy of the contents of the publication. Application of this information in a particular situation remains the professional responsibility of the practitioner.

The authors and publisher have exerted every effort to ensure that drug selection and dosage set forth in this text are in accordance with current recommendations and practice at the time of publication. However, in view of ongoing research, changes in government regulations, and the constant flow of information relating to drug therapy and drug reactions, the reader is urged to check the package insert for each drug for any change in indications and dosage and for added warnings and precautions. This is particularly important when the recommended agent is a new or infrequently employed drug.

Some drugs and medical devices presented in this publication have Food and Drug Administration (FDA) clearance for limited use in restricted research settings. It is the responsibility of the health care provider to ascertain the FDA status of each drug or device planned for use in their clinical practice.

To purchase additional copies of this book, call our customer service department at (800) 638-3030 or fax orders to (301) 223-2320. International customers should call (301) 223-2300.

Visit Lippincott Williams & Wilkins on the Internet: at LWW.com. Lippincott Williams & Wilkins customer service representatives are available from 8:30 am to 6pm, EST.

10 9 8 7 6 5 4 3 2

To Ian and Gillian
To John and his hero Conor

Dedication

This Textbook is dedicated to the memory of:

The late Ian Macnab, MB, ChB, FRCS
Former Chief, Division of Orthopaedic Surgery
The Wellesley Hospital
Former Emeritus Professor of Surgery
University of Toronto
Toronto, Ontario, Canada

The late John A. McCulloch, MD, FRCS(C)
Former Professor of Orthopaedics
Northeastern Ohio Universities
College of Medicine
Rootstown, Ohio USA
Former Director
Advanced Center for Spinal Microsurgery
Presbyterian St. Luke's Medical Center
Denver, Colorado USA

Preface to the Fourth Edition

The fourth edition of *Macnab's Backache* is an enhancement and update of the concepts Ian committed to paper 30 years ago. Today, those concepts are even more relevant to the serious scholar of clinical back pain.

The diagnosis of patients with spinal complaints has always been a complex affair. The key to accurate evaluation and treatment of patients is a thorough understanding of pathoanatomy. This area was Ian's forte. It is notable that the "Macnab concepts" were formulated in an era before magnetic resonance imaging (MRI), computerized axial tomography (CAT scans), and many other present-day tools of investigation and analysis. These modern technologies have only served to confirm the descriptions published in the first edition of *Backache*. Macnab's basic concepts are, therefore, timeless. As the authors of the fourth edition, our responsibility lies in allowing readers of this edition to embrace these key concepts in a contemporary context. To accomplish this goal, we have shaped the fourth edition in a "back-to-basics" format supplemented by more current imaging and references.

The previous third edition was a wide-ranging expansion of the original *Backache* monograph into a comprehensive reference directed toward the spine surgeon. It remains a valuable tool for that group and for subspecialist physicians. For the fourth edition, part of the governing "back-to-basics" principle includes a return to the core audience that Macnab envisioned for the original work. The first *Backache* monograph was written as a primer for orthopedic residents, fellows, interns, and medical students. The high incidence of back pain in our society today and the diverse clinical settings for spine evaluation and treatment suggest that this edition would also be pertinent to the education of practitioners in a variety of physician subspecialties such as neurosurgery, neurology, physical medicine, and rehabilitation, occupational medicine, radiology, emergency medicine, general internal medicine and family practice. In addition, the book is appropriate for physician's assistants (PAs), nurse practitioners, nurses, workers' compensation case managers, administrative law judges, and industry sales representatives wanting a clearer understanding of the spinal conditions present in patients they encounter and help care for.

The scope of this new fourth edition has been deliberately constructed to emphasize the initial evaluation of the patient with back pain and/or sciatica. There is no detailed description of surgical procedures. With knowledge of Macnab's well-organized thoughts on pathophysiology and its correlation to clinical symptoms, we hope to uniquely empower the reader in the accurate evaluation and effective initial treatment of the spine patient.

David Wong
Ensor Transfeldt

Preface to the Fourth Edition

Preface to the First Edition

"In seeking absolute truth we aim at the unattainable and must be content with finding broken portions."

—Sir William Osler

Low back pain is a remarkably common disability. Hirsch stated that 65% of the Swedish population was affected by low back pain at some time during their working lives. Rowe stated that, at Eastman Kodak, back pain was second only to upper respiratory tract infections as the reason for absence from work. In 1967, the US National Safety Council reported that 4,000,000 workers were disabled by back pain each year and, in Ontario, Canada, 20,000 claims for disability resulting from backache are received annually by the Workmen's Compensation Board. However, despite its frequency, backache is not a dramatic disease that arouses the scientific curiosity and interest of medical practitioners. Physicians are understandably disenchanted by the frequently obscure etiology of this irksome syndrome and the commonly disappointing response to treatment.

In an attempt to dispel some of the clouds of confusion that obscure the problem, this book has been designed to present a working classification of the common causes of low back pain and to act as a guide to the examination and management of a few commonly seen syndromes.

Some readers may have no intention of entering into the field of spinal surgery. Surgeons in training always find that a surgical textbook is a poor substitute for experience in the operating room. Because of the rapid changes in the minutiae of surgical technique, a textbook is "dated" as soon as it is written, and a description of surgical techniques is of little value to the practicing surgeon who must depend on articles published in medical journals to modify the surgical procedures employed. However, one has to accept the fact that, on occasion, a patient suffering from discogenic backache comes to the end of the road as far as conservative treatment is concerned. The back becomes a malevolent dictator determining what the patient can do at work and play. The physician directing treatment must then decide whether surgical intervention is indicated. In order that he/she can give intelligent and informed advice to patients, he/she must have some knowledge of the operative procedures, including the preoperative investigation that must be undertaken, factors involved in the postoperative investigations that must be undertaken, and factors involved in postoperative care. The surgeon in training also needs to know the indications for considering operative intervention and, in addition, must have some knowledge of the general principles of operative technique. The practicing surgeon will understandably skip over the descriptions of operative technique but may find value in a detailed description of the preoperative investigation of obscure lesions.

For these reasons, chapters have been devoted to the preoperative evaluation and operative technique of laminectomy and fusion, and space has been devoted to discussion of that bête noire of orthopedic surgeons and neurosurgeons alike, the failure of spinal surgery.

Because this book is designed to discuss only the principles of diagnosis and treatment, it has been illustrated by simple line drawings. No attempt has been undertaken to make this text into an authoritative atlas of clinical syndromes, radiological changes, or operative techniques.

Although diagnosis and treatment are presented with unmitigated dogmatism, it must be remembered that, with the frequent absence of scientific facts, and treatise on the management of back pain must, perforce, be regarded as a philosophy and, moreover, a philosophy that must be modified to fit the needs of the physician's community.

It is almost impossible to acknowledge all of the people who have played a role in the preparation of this book and to thank them adequately. To Mr. Philip Newman, I owe special thanks or initiating my interest in the problem of low back pain while I was still a Registrar at the Royal

National Orthopaedic Hospital in London, England. The late R.I. Harris made it possible for me to investigate the pathological and mechanical changes associated with disc degeneration, and his contagious enthusiasm encouraged me to study the clinical aspects of the problem in greater depth.

It was with considerable reluctance that I later accepted the offer made by Dr. A.W. M. White to study a group of patients under the care of the Workmen's Compensation Board of Ontario, Canada, who continued to be disabled by back pain despite all forms of treatment, including only too often, several surgical assaults. I shall be eternally grateful for Bill White's persistent insistence that I should take on this unenviable task, because it was from this study that I learned of the vital necessity to know as much about the patient who has the backache as about the backache the patient has. Dr. Allan Walters led the world on his observation on pain syndromes, and it was from him that I learned of the varying and variable relationship of the disability complained of to the pain experienced.

For the preparation of the manuscript, I would like to pay my special thanks to: Margot McKay for illustrations; Kathleen Lipnicki for photographic prints; and Jennifer Widger for typing, retyping, and retyping the script without complaint.

Finally, I would like to express my gratitude to Sara Finnegan of Williams & Wilkins, who patiently and gently guided me through the task of transforming my handwritten notes and sketches into a form more suitable for publication.

I sincerely hope that our combined efforts have produced a text that the reader can use as a basis on which he/she can build a personal philosophy of the management of this commonplace syndrome.

Ian Macnab

Acknowledgments

On the Denver end of the paper trail, my wife Lynn filled the primary role of editor, researcher, typist, photographer, and critic. Daughters Katherine and Caroline also provided support for literature searches and general research. The assistance of my medical assistant Marty Goff and physician assistant Ken Gartzke is also much appreciated.

Dr. Ron Hattin provided several images of interventional procedures for the new injections chapter. The staff of the Denver Medical Library assisted in providing full literature articles.

The Lippincott Williams & Wilkins team was particularly helpful and considerate. Bob Hurley and Eileen Wolfberg at the Philadelphia office kept the project on track with their unique brand of support and enthusiasm. Our editors, Martha Cushman and Jenny Koleth and project manager Maria McColligan helped enormously in the final organization and presentation of the material.

Particular thanks to Rita Macnab and Barb McCulloch, the wives of Ian and John. Their encouragement was key in our decision to take on the project of developing a new edition of *Backache*. The support of the members of the Macnab Orthopedic Research Society (The Macnab Club) was also heartening and very much appreciated.

Contents

CHAPTER 1

Musculoskeletal Anatomy, Neuroanatomy, and Biomechanics of the Lumbar Spine

"You will have to learn many tedious things which you will forget the moment you have passed your final examination, but in anatomy it is better to have learned and lost than never to have learned at all."

—Authors

It is a convention observed by most authors of medical texts to start the book with a chapter devoted to the anatomy of the subject covered. In many instances, this is a form of brownian movement having very little purposive significance. Having skipped through many such essays with ill-concealed impatience, it was with considerable trepidation that we continued to follow this well-established precedent. The purpose of this introductory chapter is to remind the reader of anatomic terminology and to correlate the gross anatomic features of the lumbar vertebrae with normal biomechanics and pathologic changes of clinical significance. Remember, the key to understanding disease and completing exacting surgical techniques is an intimate knowledge of anatomy.

FUNCTIONAL MUSCULOSKELETAL ANATOMY

There are five lumbar vertebrae and the sacrum making up the lumbar spine. We can consider each vertebra as having three functional components: the vertebral bodies, designed to bear weight; the neural arches, designed to protect the neural elements; and the bony processes (spinous and transverse), designed as outriggers to increase the efficiency of muscle action.

The vertebral bodies are connected together by the intervertebral discs, and the neural arches are joined by the facet (zygapophyseal) joints (Fig. 1-1). The discal surface of an adult vertebral body demonstrates on its periphery a ring of cortical bone. This ring, the epiphysial ring, acts as a growth zone in the young and in the adult as an anchoring ring for the attachment of the fibers of the annulus. The hyaline cartilage plate lies within the confines of this ring (Fig. 1-2). The size of the vertebral body increases from L1 to L5, which is indicative of the increasing loads that each lower lumbar vertebral level has to absorb.

The neural arch is composed of two pedicles and two laminae (Fig. 1-1). The pedicles are anchored to the cephalad half of the vertebral body and form a protective cover for the cauda equina contents of the lumbar spinal canal. The ligamentum flavum (yellow ligament) fills in the interlaminar space at each level.

The outriggers for muscle attachment are the transverse processes and spinous process.

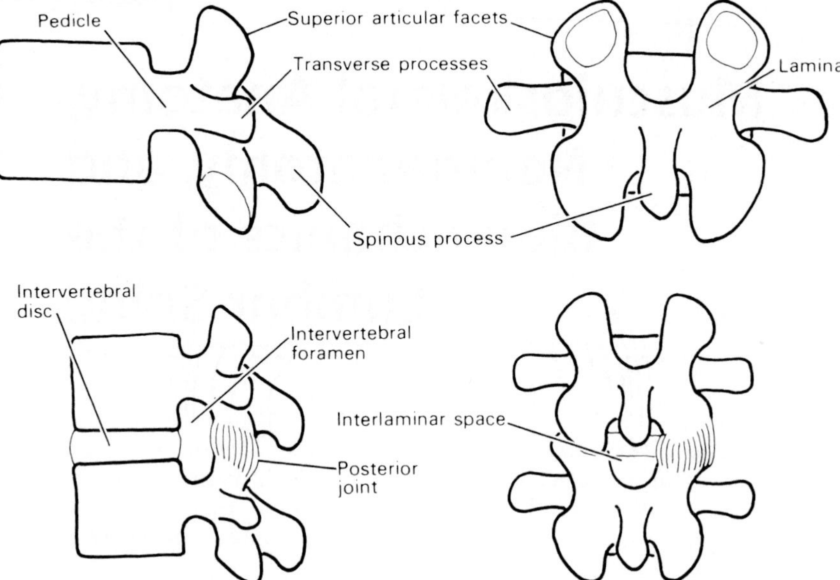

FIGURE 1-1 ● The components of a lumbar vertebra: the body, the pedicle, the superior and inferior facets, the transverse and spinous processes, and the intervertebral foramen and its relationship to the intervertebral disc and the posterior joint.

THE INTERVERTEBRAL DISC

The intervertebral discs (Fig. 1-3) are complicated structures, both anatomically and physiologically. Anatomically, they are constructed in a manner similar to that of a car tire, with a fibrous outer casing, the annulus, containing a gelatinous inner tube, the nucleus pulposus. The fibers of the annulus can be divided into three main groups: the outermost fibers attaching between the vertebral bodies and the undersurface of the epiphysial ring; the middle fibers passing from the epiphysial ring on one vertebral body to the epiphysial ring of the vertebral body below; and the innermost fibers passing from one cartilage endplate to the other. The anterior fibers are strengthened by the powerful anterior longitudinal ligament. The posterior longitudinal ligament affords

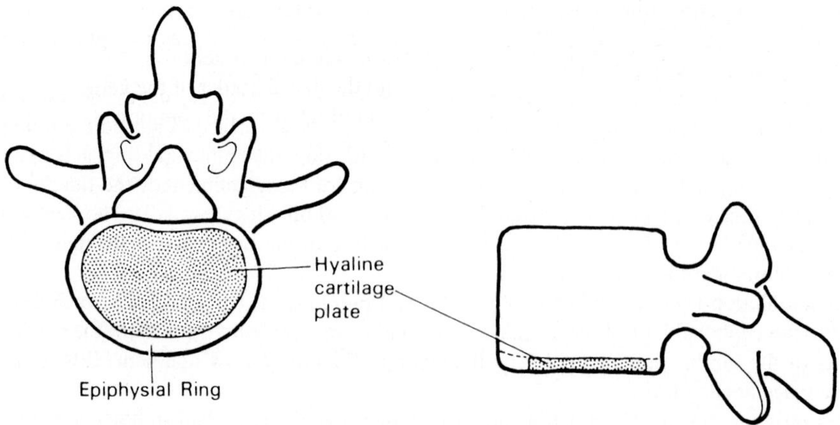

FIGURE 1-2 ● The epiphysial ring is wider anteriorly and surrounds the hyaline cartilaginous plate.

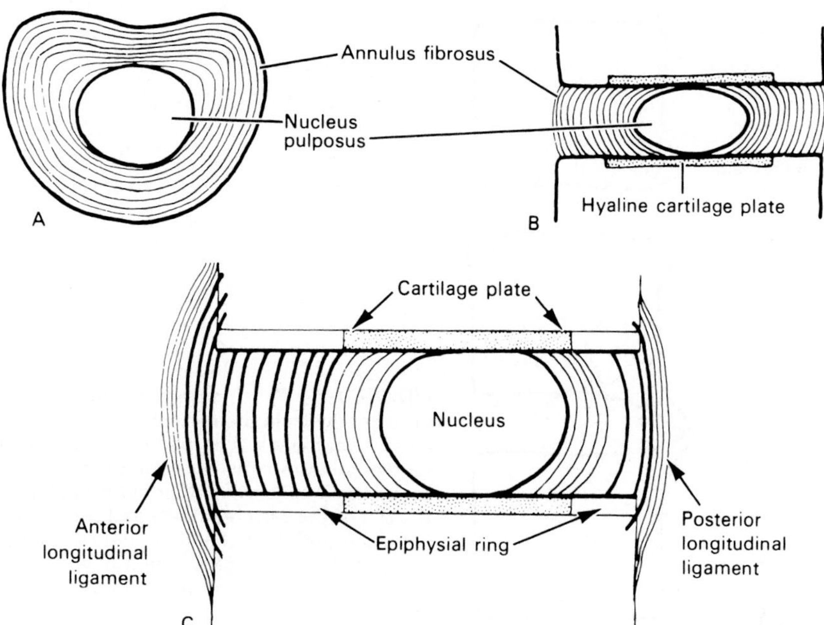

FIGURE 1-3 ● The annulus fibrosus is composed of concentric fibrous rings that surround the nucleus pulposus **(A).** The nucleus pulposus abuts against the hyaline cartilage plate **(B).** The outermost annulus fibers are most numerous anteriorly and are attached to the vertebral body immediately deep to the epiphysial ring. **C:** The epiphysial fibers run from one epiphysial ring to the other. The cartilaginous fibers run from one cartilage plate to the other cartilage plate. These comprise 90% of the annulus fibers posteriorly. The anterior fibers of the annulus are strongly reinforced by the powerful anterior longitudinal ligament, but the posterior longitudinal ligament only gives weak reinforcement to the posterior fibers of the annulus.

only weak reinforcement, especially at L4-5 and L5–S1, where it is a midline, narrow, unimportant structure attached to the annulus. The anterior and middle fibers of the annulus are most numerous anteriorly and laterally but are deficient posteriorly, where most of the fibers are attached to the cartilage plate (Fig. 1-3).

With the onset of degenerative changes in the disc, abnormal movements occur between adjacent vertebral bodies. These abnormal movements apply a considerable traction strain on the outermost fibers of the annulus, resulting in the development of a spur of bone, the so-called traction spur (Macnab spur) (6). Because the outermost fibers attach to the vertebral body beneath the epiphysial ring, this spur develops about 1 mm away from the discal border of the vertebral body and projects horizontally. This differs in its radiologic morphology from the common claw-type osteophyte, which develops at the edge of the vertebral body and curves over the outer fibers of the intervertebral disc (Fig. 1-4). The clinical significance of a traction spur lies in the fact that it indicates the presence of a vertebral segment in the early stage of instability.

The first stage of a disc rupture would appear to be detachment of a segment of the hyaline cartilage plate. The integrity of the confining ring of the annulus is then disrupted. Nuclear material can escape between the vertebral body and the displaced portion of the cartilage plate. On occasion, as a result of a compression force, a whole segment of the annulus may be displaced posteriorly, carrying with it the nucleus pulposus and displaced portion of the hyaline plate (Fig. 1-5A). This pathology is more common in younger patients (Fig. 1-5B).

The fibers of the annulus are firmly attached to the vertebral bodies and arranged in lamellae, with the fibers of one layer running at an angle to those of the deeper layer (Fig. 1-6). This anatomic arrangement permits the annulus to limit vertebral movements. This important function is reinforced by the investing vertebral ligaments.

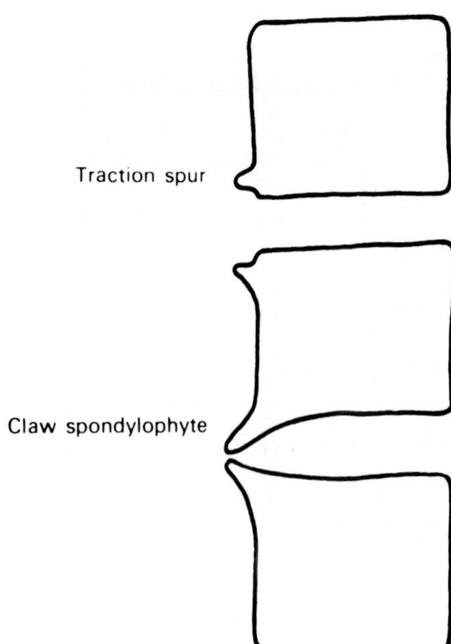

FIGURE 1-4 ● The traction spur projects horizontally from the vertebral body about 1 mm away from the discal border. It is indicative of segmental instability. The common claw spondylophyte, on the other hand, extends from the rim of the vertebral body and curves as it grows around the bulging intervertebral disc. It is associated with disc degeneration. It does not represent the radiologic manifestation of osteoarthritis.

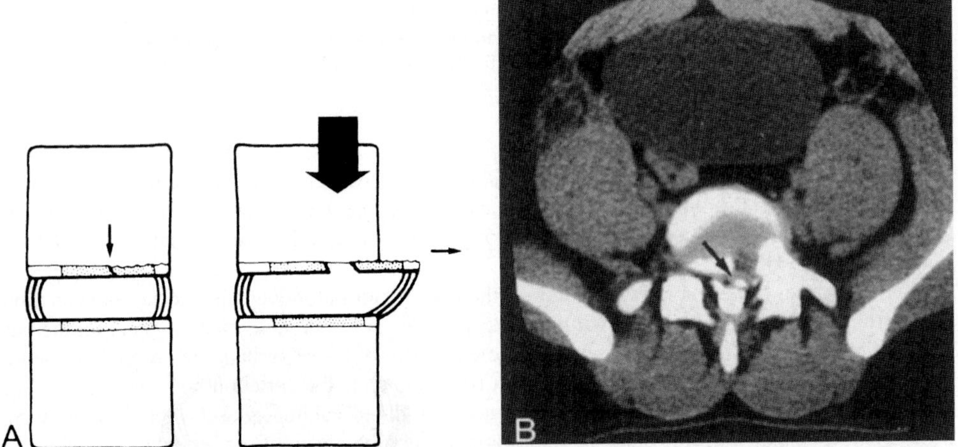

FIGURE 1-5 ● **A:** The first morphologic change to occur in a disc rupture is a separation of a segment of the cartilage plate from the adjacent vertebral body. Fissures run through the annulus on each side of the detached portion of the cartilage. When a vertical compression force is then applied, the detached portion of the cartilage plate is displaced posteriorly, and the nucleus exudes through the torn fibers of the annulus. **B:** Computed tomography (CT) of young patient with end-plate fracture *(arrow)* and herniated nucleus pulposus.

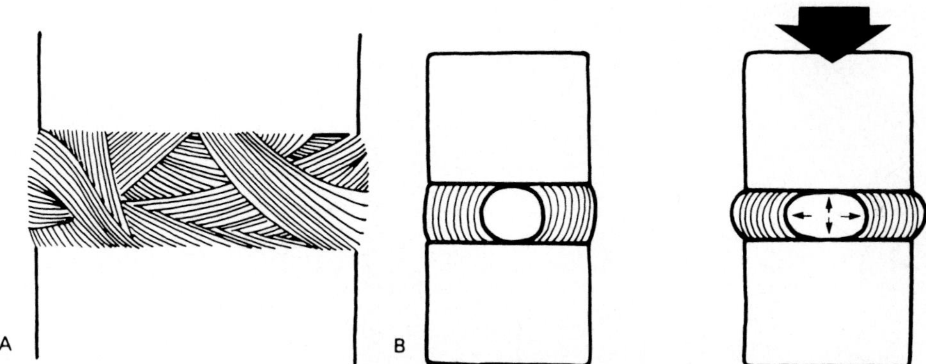

FIGURE 1-6 • **A:** The annulus is a laminated structure with the fibrous lamellae running obliquely. This disposition of the fibers permits resistance of torsional strains. **B:** The nucleus pulposus is constrained by the fibers of the annulus. When a vertical load is applied to the vertebral column, the force is dissipated radially by the gelatinous nucleus pulposus. Distortion and disruption of the nucleus pulposus are resisted by the annulus.

Because the nucleus pulposus is gelatinous, the load of axial compression is distributed not only vertically but also radially throughout the nucleus (5,8). This radial distribution of the vertical load (tangential loading of the disc) is absorbed by the fibers of the annulus and can be compared with the hoops around a barrel (Fig. 1-7).

Weight is transmitted to the nucleus through the hyaline cartilage plate. The hyaline cartilage is ideally suited to this function because it is avascular. If weight were transmitted through a vascularized structure, such as bone, the local pressure would shut off blood supply, and progressive areas of bone would die. This phenomenon is seen when the cartilage plate presents congenital defects and the nucleus is in direct contact with the spongiosa of bone. The pressure occludes the blood supply, a small zone of bone dies, and the nucleus progressively intrudes into the vertebral body. This phenomenon was first described by Schmorl and Junghanns (9), and the resulting lesion bears the name Schmorl's node (Fig. 1-8).

The annulus acts like a coiled spring, pulling the vertebral bodies together against the elastic resistance of the nucleus pulposus, with the result that when a spine is sectioned sagittally, the unopposed pull of the annulus makes the nucleus bulge. This has been referred to as "turgor" of the

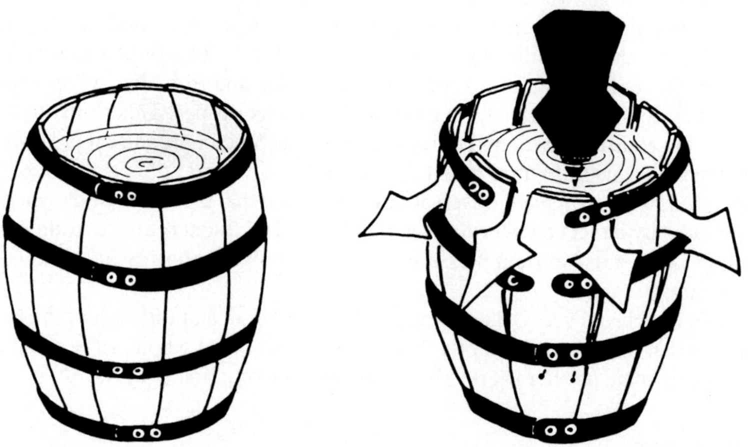

FIGURE 1-7 • Hoop stress. This diagram shows how the load of water in a barrel is resisted by the hoops around the barrel. When too great a load is applied, the hoops will break. The annulus functions in a manner similar to that of the hoops around a water barrel.

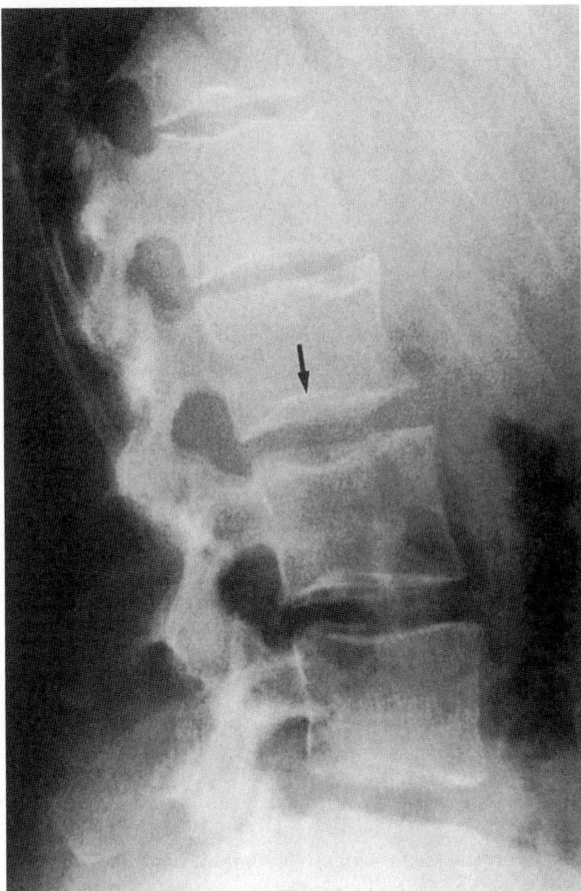

FIGURE 1-8 ● A Schmorl's node (L2–3) *(arrow)*, likely of no clinical significance. Have you ever seen a herniated nucleus pulposus at the same disc space as a Schmorl's node?

nucleus, but it is the manifestation of a springlike action, the compressing action of the annulus fibrosus. This makes for a very good coupling unit, provided that all of the structures remain intact. The nucleus pulposus acts like a ball bearing, and in flexion and extension the vertebral bodies roll over this incompressible gel while the posterior joints guide and steady the movements (Fig. 1-9).

The intervertebral discs of a person up to the age of 8 years have a blood supply, but thereafter they are dependent for their nutrition on diffusion of tissue fluids. This fluid transfer is through two routes: (a) the bidirectional flow from vertebral body to disc and from disc to vertebral body and (b) the diffusion through the annulus from blood vessels on its surface. This ability to transfer fluid from the disc to the adjacent vertebral bodies minimizes the rise in intradiscal pressure on sudden compression loading. This fluid transfer acts like a safety valve and protects the disc. Clinical experience supported by experimental observations has shown that the fibers of the annulus are less commonly ruptured by direct compression loading (Fig. 1-10). Sudden severe loading of the spine, however, may produce a rise in fluid pressure within the vertebral body great enough to produce a "bursting" fracture.

Although this has been a very cursory review of the structure and function of the intervertebral disc, one can see that the components of a disc act as an integrated whole, subserving many functions, in addition to being a roller bearing between adjacent vertebral bodies.

THE FACET JOINTS

The zygapophyseal joints are synovial joints that permit simple gliding movements. Although the lax capsule of the zygapophyseal joints is reinforced to some extent by the ligamentum flavum anteriorly and the supraspinous ligament posteriorly (Fig. 1-11), the major structures restraining

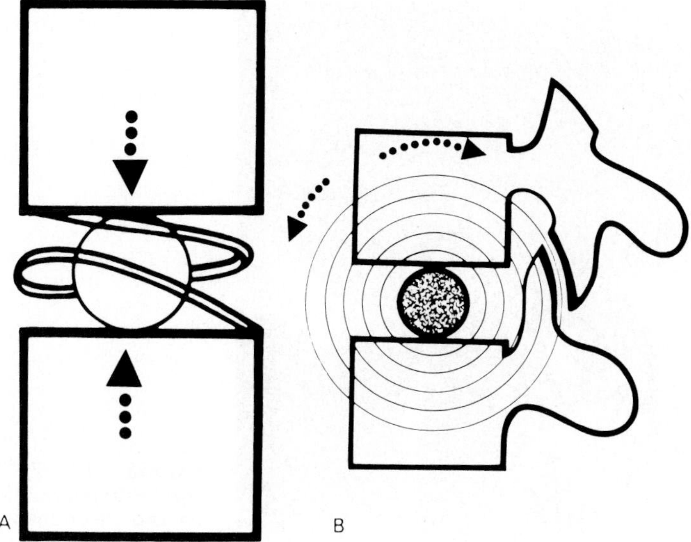

FIGURE 1-9 ● **A:** The annulus acts like a coiled spring, pulling the vertebral bodies together against the elastic resistance of the nucleus pulposus. **B:** The nucleus pulposus acts as a ball bearing, with the vertebral bodies rolling over this incompressible gel in flexion and extension while the posterior joints guide and steady the movement.

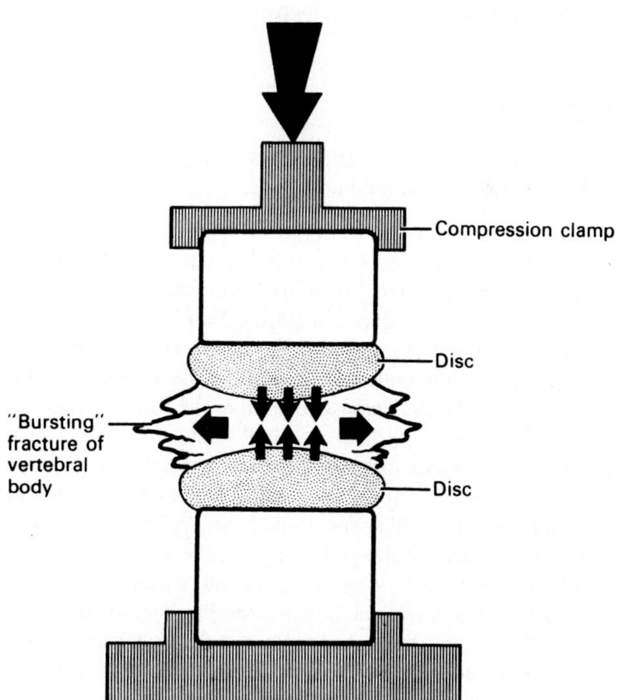

FIGURE 1-10 ● Diagram shows the experimental testing of vertical loading of the spine. When a very high compressive force is applied, the discs will remain intact, but the vertebral body shatters.

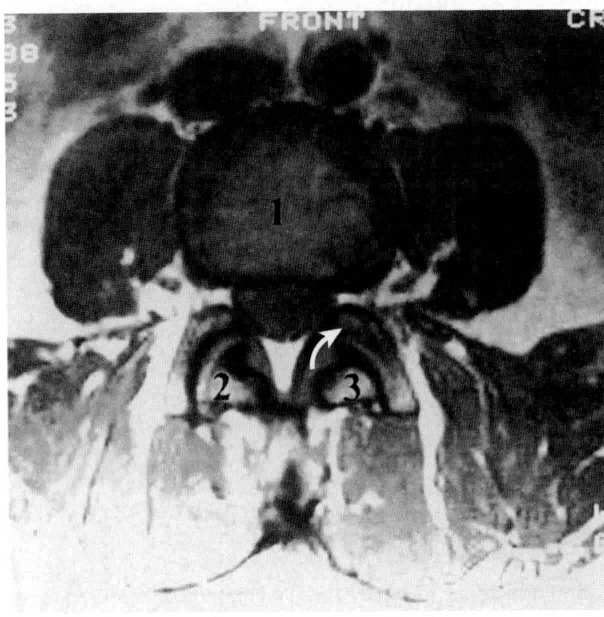

FIGURE 1-11 ● The ligamentum flavum inserts into the capsule on the superior facet *(arrow)*. The three-joint complex is composed of the disc space *(1)* and two facet joints (*2* and *3*).

movement in these joints are the outermost fibers of the annulus. When these annular fibers exhibit degenerative changes, excessive joint play is permitted. This is the reason why degenerative changes within the discs render the related posterior joints vulnerable to strain. The intimate relationship between the disc and its two facet joints has led to Kirkaldy-Willis et al. (4) labeling the unit "the three joint complex" (Fig. 1-11).

THE LIGAMENTS

Although the ligaments of the lumbar spine are no more important than the muscles, their names and functions are required knowledge.

Anterior longitudinal ligament (ALL). Obviously, this ligament runs the length of the anterior aspect of the spine (Fig. 1-12). It is intimately attached to the anterior annular fibers of each disc and is a fairly strong ligament useful in fracture reduction.

Posterior longitudinal ligament (PLL). This is the posterior mate to the anterior longitudinal ligament (Fig. 1-13). It is a significant ligament in all areas of the spine except the lower lumbar region. Although frequently mentioned in the discussion of lumbar disc disease, the ligament itself is rather flimsy and inconsequential in the lower lumbar spine where lumbar disc problems are most common.

Interspinous/supraspinous ligament complex. Although most authors draw these two ligaments backward and as separate structures, it does not take a rocket scientist to figure out that if you want to flex the lumbar spine, the ligaments have to be structured as depicted in Figure 1-14.

Ligamentum flavum (the yellow ligament). This ligament is so named because of the yellowish color that is given to it by the high content of the elastin fibers. The ligamentum flavum bridges the interlaminar interval, attaching to the interspinous ligament medially and the facet capsule laterally. It has a broad attachment to the undersurface of the superior lamina and inserts onto the leading edge of the inferior lamina at each segment. Normally, the ligamentum maintains a taut configuration, stretching for flexion and contracting its elastin fibers in neutral or extension. In this way, it always covers but never infringes on the epidural space. With aging, the ligamentum flavum loses its elastin fibers and the collagen hypertrophies, which results in buckling of the ligamentum flavum and encroachment on the thecal sac, potentially contributing to spinal stenosis.

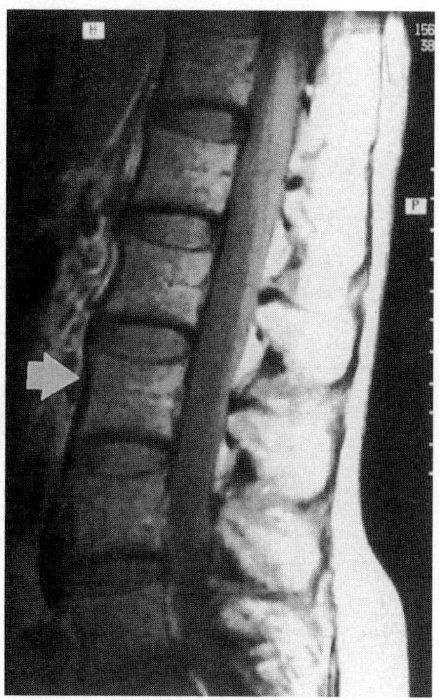

FIGURE 1-12 ● The anterior longitudinal ligament *(arrow)* on proton density magnetic resonance imaging (MRI).

ANOMALIES OF THE LUMBAR VERTEBRAL COLUMN

Normally, there are five vertebrae in the lumbar spine. But approximately 10% of the adult patients seen with symptomatic degenerative conditions of the low back have a congenital lumbosacral anomaly (2). These anomalies are mainly failures of segmentation, which may be symmetrical or asymmetrical. Our involvement with percutaneous spinal surgical procedures led to early recognition of the many traps these congenital lumbosacral anomalies present to the surgeon. These are two potential technical pitfalls for the surgeon operating on a patient with these anomalies. First, when using an image intensifier for identification of level, the surgeon has available a very limited image intensifier field. If the surgeon is unaware of congenital lumbosacral anomalies, it is easy to perform a percutaneous procedure at the wrong segment. Second, when operating through the midline microsurgical approach, the limited exposure available to the surgeon makes it very easy to enter the wrong level surgically.

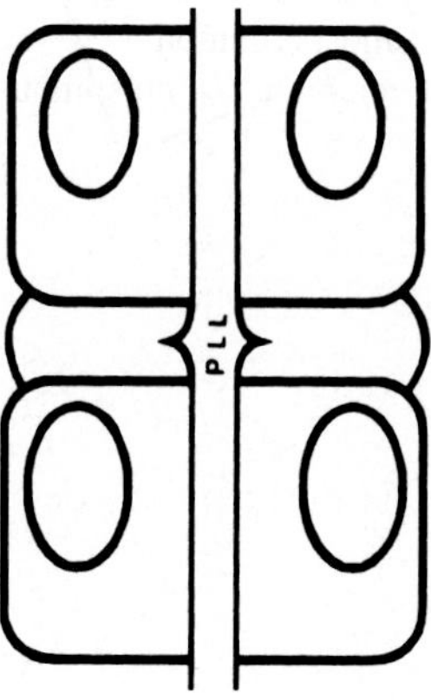

FIGURE 1-13 ● The posterior longitudinal ligament (PLL), which at L4-5 and L5–S1 is very thin and narrow.

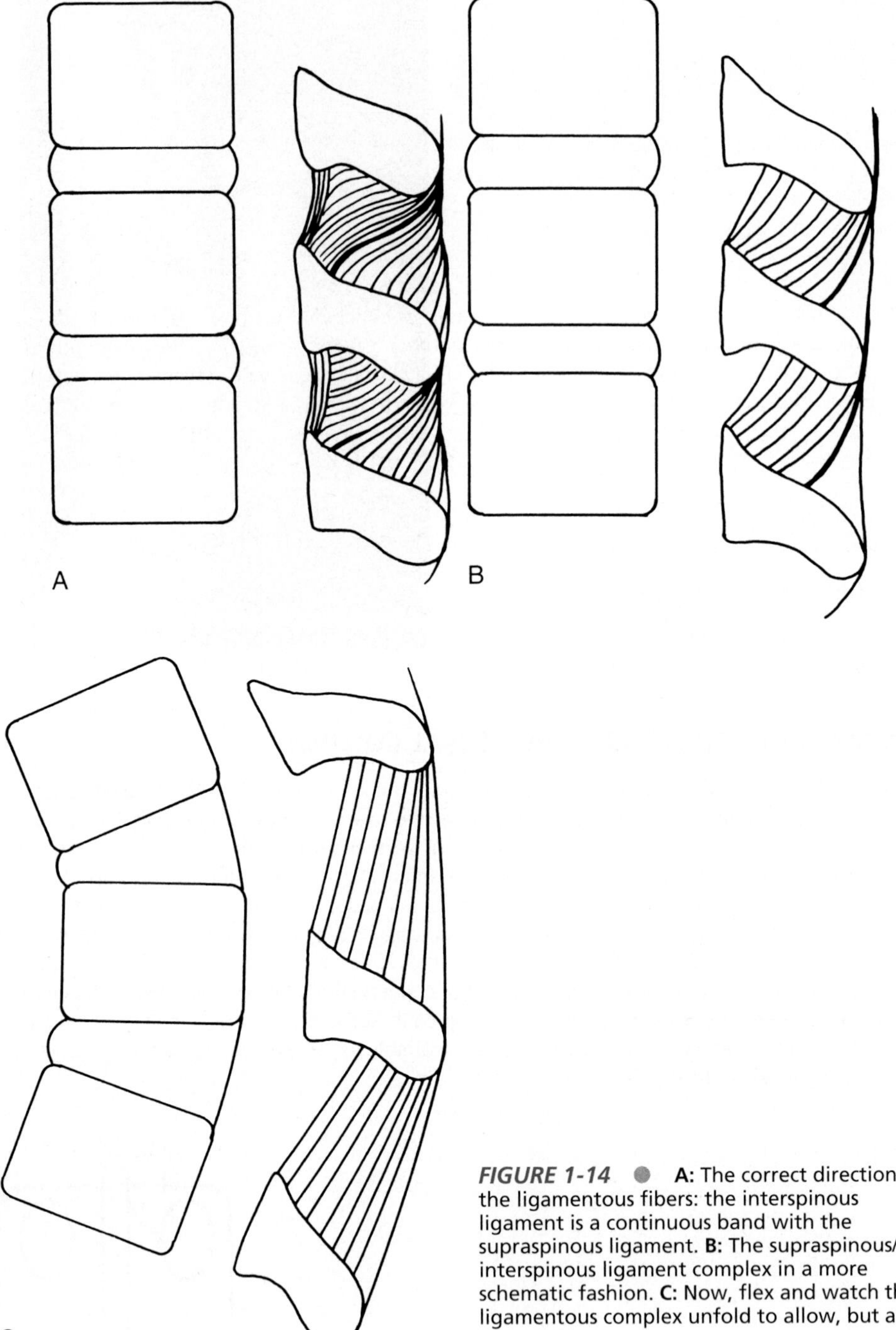

FIGURE 1-14 ● **A:** The correct direction of the ligamentous fibers: the interspinous ligament is a continuous band with the supraspinous ligament. **B:** The supraspinous/interspinous ligament complex in a more schematic fashion. **C:** Now, flex and watch the ligamentous complex unfold to allow, but also limit, flexion.

DEFINITIONS

It is best to designate a disc-space level as an interspace between two vertebral bodies; that is, the disc space between the fifth lumbar vertebral body and the first sacral vertebral body is the L5–S1 disc space. Further, it is best to designate a nerve root according to the pedicle beneath which it passes. Thus, the fifth lumbar nerve root passes beneath the fifth lumbar pedicle and is also described as the *exiting nerve root* at the L5–S1 segment. Proximal to this, the L5 root passes across the L4-5 disc space. The L5 nerve root is the *traversing* root at the L4-5 disc space, where it can be encroached on by an L4-5 disc herniation in the common posterolateral position. Distal to the L5 pedicle, the fifth lumbar nerve root lies just lateral to the L5–S1 disc space, and a lateral disc herniation at L5–S1 can encroach on the fifth lumbar nerve root at this level (Fig. 1-15).

It is not uncommon to see radiologic designations of congenital lumbosacral anomalies such as L4-S1 and L6-S. In addition, the terms *sacralization* and *lumbarization* are very common in reporting radiographs with lumbosacral anomalies (11,12). The frequent disagreement between radiologists and clinicians as to designation of levels is due to the fact that radiologists generally have an anteroposterior (AP) and a lateral radiograph to view and invariably count down from the last rib to number the lumbar vertebrae. On the other hand, spinal surgeons, who often count vertebrae in the operating room, have only a spot lateral radiograph and count from the sacrum up. If the patient has a normal lumbar spine, the radiologist and the surgeon will meet at the same L4-5 level. If the patient has six lumbar vertebrae, the radiologist and the surgeon will be at different levels and a wrong level exposure may result.

It is proposed that we use the terms *formed levels* and *mobile levels* to designate levels in congenital lumbosacral anomalies. A formed level is described as any level of the lumbar spine that has an interlaminar space and a disc space. The extent of interlaminar space formation usually parallels disc-space formation (Fig. 1-16). In a normal fully formed lumbar level, there is a transverse process that is free of any attachments to the pelvis or sacrum, and there are two facet joints.

A normally formed level such as the level usually between L5 and S1 should be a fully mobile level. Failure of complete segmentation may result in the transverse process being fixed to the pelvis or to the sacrum. This fixed level is called the *transitional segment.* This takes away mobility from that level but still leaves an interlaminar space and a disc space with various degrees of formation of transverse processes and facet joints. In this situation, the *lowest mobile level* (LML) is the level above the fixed transitional level and is designated the last mobile level (Fig. 1-17). Thus, the *last formed level* (LFL) is any level that has an interlaminar space (and usually a disc space, however rudimentary), with or without facet joints, and transverse processes that may or

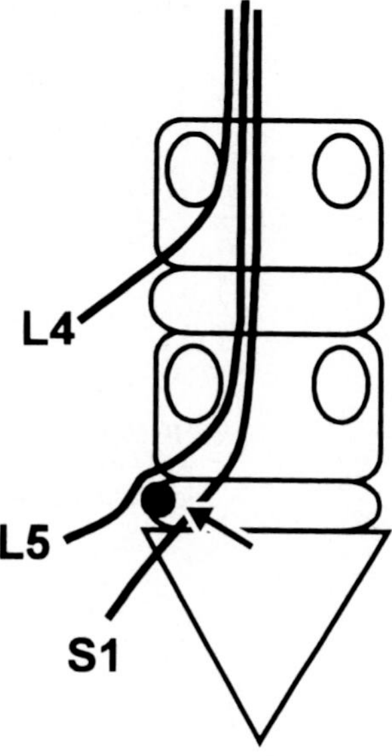

FIGURE 1-15 • A foraminal disc at L5–S1 will compress the L5 nerve root *(arrow).*

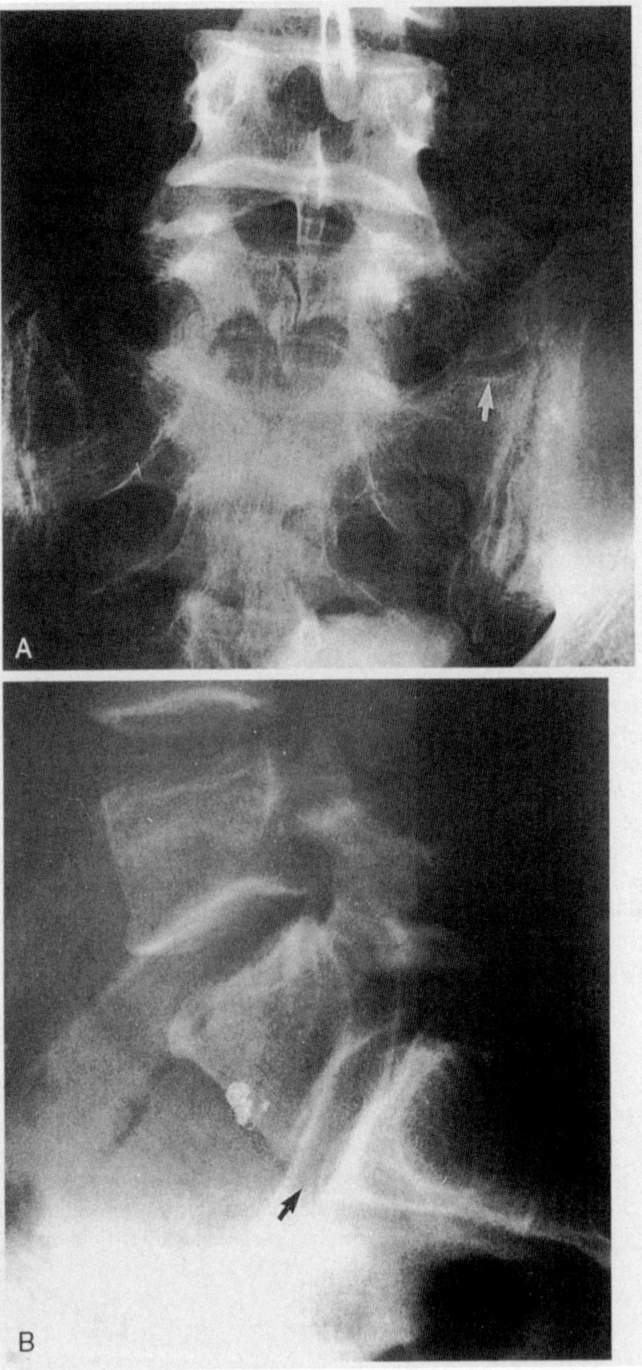

FIGURE 1-16 ● **A:** A fixed last formed level *(arrow)*, with a wide interlaminar space. **B:** Note a well-formed disc space on lateral radiograph *(arrow)*.

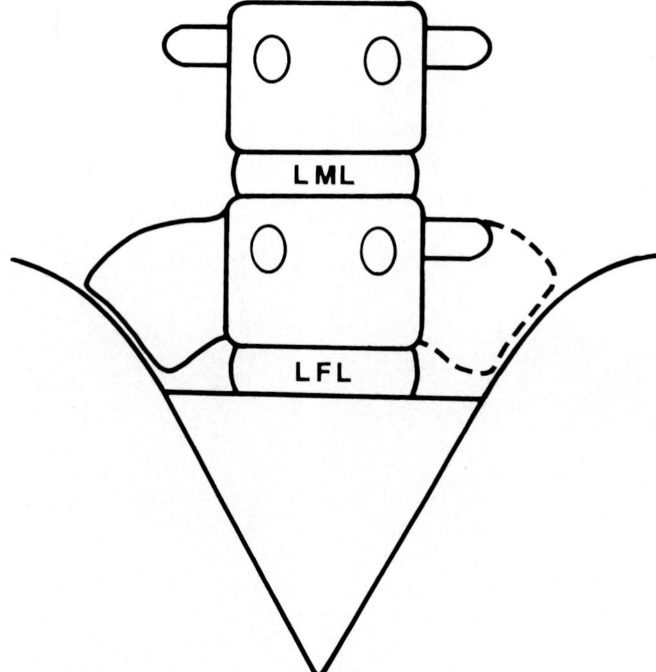

FIGURE 1-17 ● The fixed level (on the left of the spine and shown dotted in on the right) takes mobility away from the last formed level (LFL). The level above becomes the last mobile level (LML).

may not be attached to the pelvis. The *lowest mobile level* is the last formed level that is free of all bony attachments to the pelvis and is a fully mobile level. In a normal lumbar spine, the L5–S1 level is both the last formed level and the last mobile level.

DISCUSSION

The first anomaly that is of concern has already been mentioned; that is, the presence of six lumbar vertebrae with a pathologic condition reported by the radiologist at the L4-5 level. Figure 1-18 demonstrates this problem.

The second problem is the partially fixed last formed level, with five vertebrae above that are free of rib attachments. A radiologist may report a pathologic condition at the L5–S1 level. Figure 1-19 demonstrates this problem. If one is doing an image intensifier procedure with the patient in the lateral position, it is very easy, with the limited image intensifier field, to try to enter the last disc space level (last formed level). In fact, one should be entering the second-to-last formed level, which is the last mobile level, the level that the radiologist may have designated as L5–S1.

The third congenital anomaly of concern is demonstrated in Figure 1-20. Here, the patient had five lumbar vertebrae, with the last formed level being fixed and, to a certain extent, rudimentary. The pathologic condition was reported to be at the L4-5 level, and it would have been very easy to enter the third last formed, second last mobile level to perform discolysis.

Figure 1-21 demonstrates the newest problem that has arisen with congenital lumbosacral anomalies. Here, the patient had plain radiographs done in one radiography unit and a CT scan done in a separate radiography unit. Different numbering was used at the two units, which led to confusion as to designation of the level of the pathologic condition.

In congenital lumbosacral anomalies (with the various degrees of fixation between the last formed level and the pelvis), the last formed disc space is always narrow (3). A rudimentary level is narrowed in a parallel fashion but does not have any of the reaction of degenerative disc disease

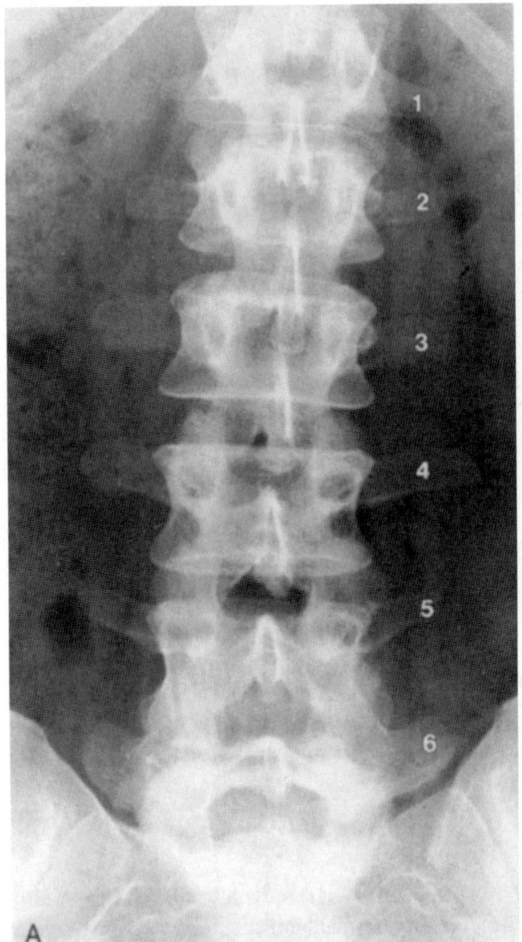

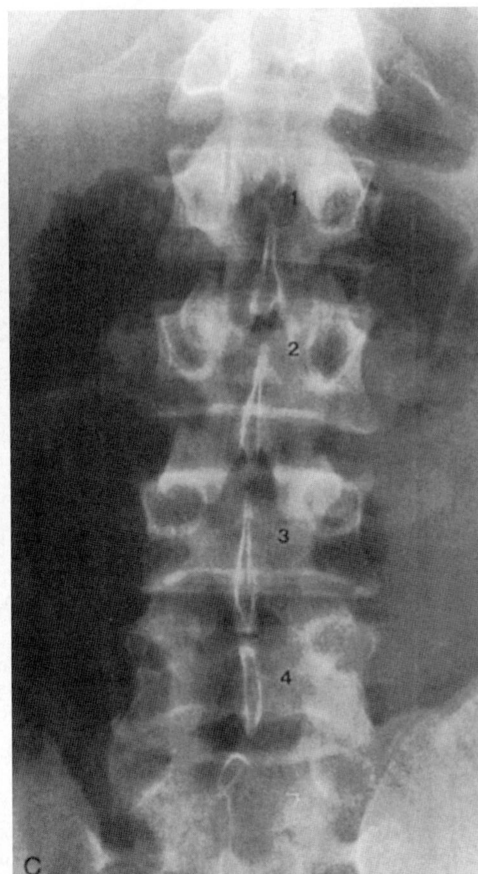

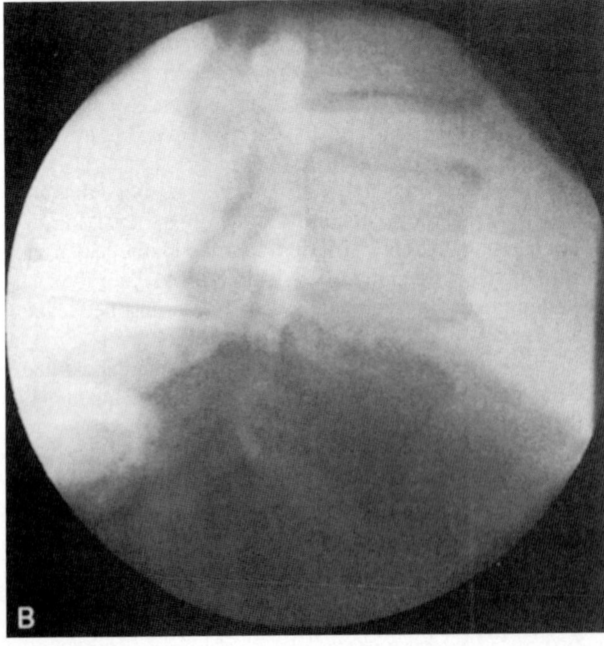

FIGURE 1-18 ● Six lumbar vertebrae numbered from the top down. Now, number them from the bottom up, designating the last formed level (LFL)/lowest mobile level (LML) L5–S1 as in most normal spines. You will be at a different L4–5 space.

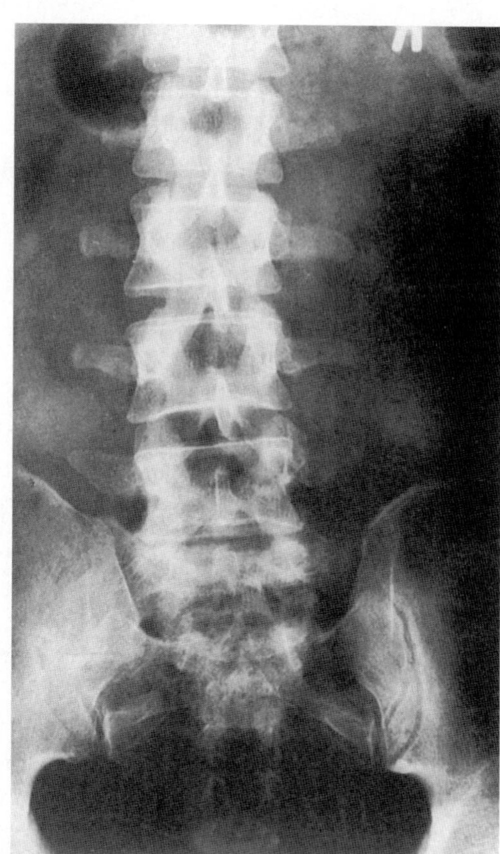

FIGURE 1-19 ● A fixed last formed level (fixed on the left side by "bat-wing" transverse processes), with five lumbar vertebrae above.

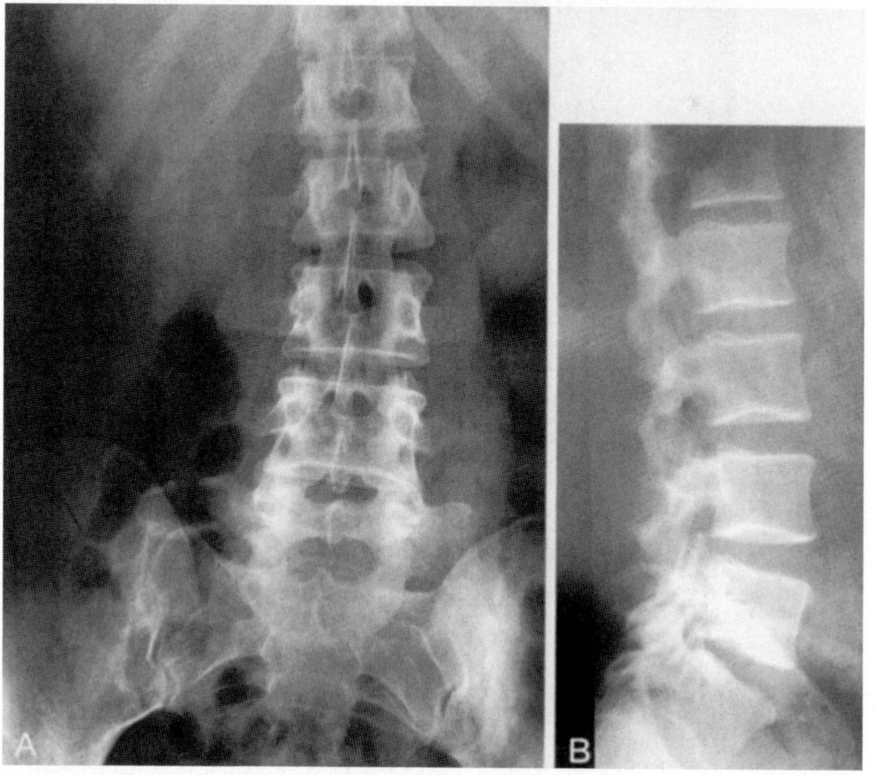

FIGURE 1-20 ● **A:** Five lumbar vertebrae with the last level fixed to the pelvis and nonmobile. Some radiologists might try to label the last mobile level (L5–S1), which would present serious problems to the surgeon looking at Figure 1-20B. **B:** Sacro-transverse articulations fixing the lowest formed level are not visible on the lateral. Different numbering of the segments may be the result.

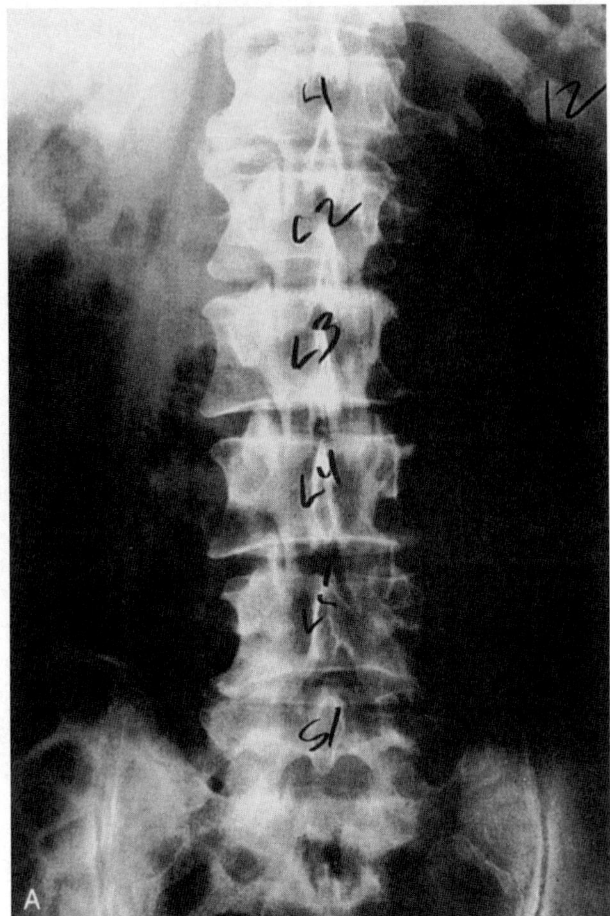

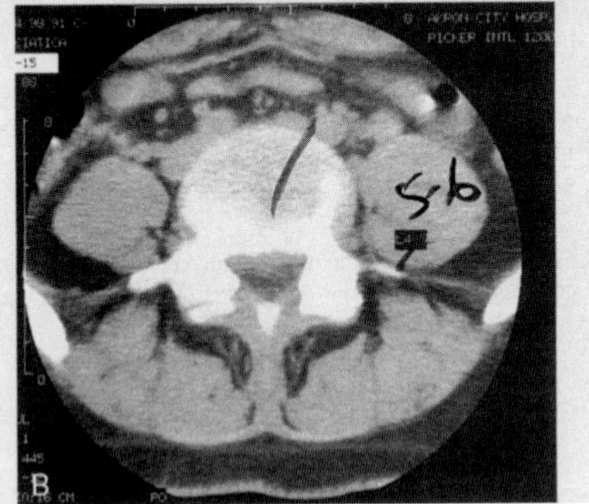

FIGURE 1-21 ● **A:** Anteroposterior (AP) radiograph numbered by a radiologist (he/she was kind enough to write the numbers very large so there would be no misunderstanding as to their position!). **B:** At another unit, patient underwent a computed tomography (CT) scan, which showed a disc herniation at a level labeled L4–5 by the technologist but changed to L5–6 by the radiologist. (Does anybody know who's on first?)

such as sclerosis, osteophyte formation, wedging of the disc space, retrospondylolisthesis, or air in the disc space (Fig. 1-16B).

CONCLUSION

With the advent of less invasive spinal surgery such as microdiscectomy, the surgeon must be very aware of congenital lumbosacral anomalies that might lead to injection or exposure of the wrong disc-space level. The high percentage of these anomalies puts 10% of patients at risk. In the past, rib counts and identification of the interiliac crest line and the longest and broadest transverse processes have been used to help localize levels. These clinical and radiologic parameters have been adequate, but we think that it is time to introduce the terminology *last mobile level* and *last formed level.*

NORMAL BIOMECHANICS OF THE LUMBAR VERTEBRAL COLUMN

LOAD BEARING

In lateral and posterior shear, axial compression, and flexion, the disc appears to be the major load-bearing element. In anterior shear and axial torque, the facets play a major role in dissipating the forces. The ability to absorb and dissipate these forces is significantly reduced by lumbar disc degeneration.

The Facet Joints

The facet joints are not major load bearers except in the lower lumbar spine, where they can accept up to 20% of a compressive load. This role is highest in extension movements. Rather, the normal facet joints guide the motion of the functional spinal unit (FSU). Viewing the orientation of the facet joints in the lumbar spine supports the concept that the facet joints facilitate movements in the sagittal plane (flexion/extension) and limit movements in rotation (torsion) and bending.

Biomechanics of Ligaments

The ligaments of the lumbar spine act like rubber bands. They have an elastic physical property that allows the ligament to stretch and resist tensile forces. Under compression, the ligaments buckle and serve little function. In resisting tensile forces, ligaments allow just enough movement without injury to vital structures. Passively, they maintain tension in a segment so that muscles do not have to work as hard.

Ligament Load Bearing

The strongest ligaments in the spine are the anterior longitudinal ligament and the facet joint capsules. The interspinous-supraspinous ligament complex is of intermediate strength, and weakest of all is the posterior longitudinal ligament. The ligamentum flavum contains significant amounts of elastin fiber, which indicates that its function is one of stretching rather than restraining.

Role of the Abdominal Cavity

There is some controversy as to what role the abdominal cavity plays in sharing the load on the lumbar spine. Farfan (1) has theorized that an increase in intra-abdominal pressure serves to protect the lumbar spine, but Schultz et al. (10) have concluded just the opposite. For now let us accept the fact that the abdominal cavity and its surrounding muscles stabilize the spine for activities such as lifting.

INTRADISCAL PRESSURE

Regardless of both the loads on the spine and the support of the muscles and ligaments, the final determining factor in biomechanical injury to the spine is the intradiscal pressure. Nachemson (7) and coworkers are leaders in this field. They designed a special transducer that measured pressures within the L3–4 disc space under various conditions of load (Fig. 1-22). These authors examined

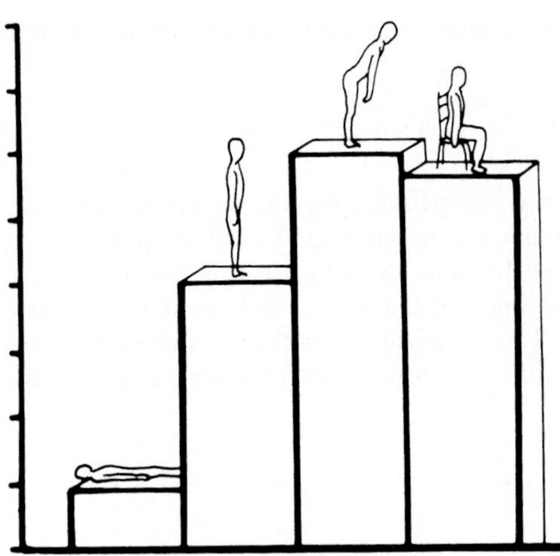

FIGURE 1-22 ● Dr. Nachemson's very famous study that measured pressures in the L3–4 disc in varying positions. The lowest pressure occurs when laying down, the highest pressure when bending forward.

normal discs only and showed that in various postures and loading positions, there are different forces across the disc space. If these forces exceed what the disc space can absorb, then injury to the motion segment occurs, and pathologic changes occur in the three-joint complex.

REFERENCES

1. Farfan HF. A reorientation in the surgical approach to capital degenerative lumbar intervertebral joint disease. *Orthop Clin North Am.* 1977;8:9–21.
2. Gibson ES, Martin RH, Terry CW. Incidence of low back pain and pre-employment x-ray screening. *J Occup Med.* 1980;22:515–519.
3. Hasner E, Jacobsen HH, Schalimtzek M, Snorrason E. Lumbosacral transitional vertebrae. A clinical and roentgenological study of 400 cases of low back pain. *Acta Radiol.* 1953;39:325–335.
4. Kirkaldy-Willis WH, Wedge JH, Yong-Hing K, Reilly J. Pathology and pathogenesis of lumbar spondylosis and stenosis. *Spine.* 1978;3:319–328.
5. Lucas DB, Bresler B. *Stability of the ligamentous spine.* Biomechanics Lab, University of California, Berkeley, Report No. 40; 1961.
6. Macnab I. The traction spur. *J Bone Joint Surg Am.* 1971;53:663–670.
7. Nachemson A. The load of lumbar discs in different positions of the body. *Clin Orthop.* 1966;45:107–122.
8. Nachemson A, Elfstrom G. Intravital dynamic pressure measurements in the lumbar discs. A study of common movements, maneuvers and exercises. *Scand J Rehab Med.* 1970;2(suppl 1):1–40.
9. Schmorl G, Junghanns H. *The human spine in health and disease.* New York: Grune & Stratton; 1971. Besemann EF, translator.
10. Schultz AB, Haderspeck-Grib K, Sinkora G, et al. Quantitative studies of the flexion-relaxation phenomenon in the back muscles. *J Orthop Res.* 1985;3:189–197.
11. Southworth JD, Borsack SR. Anomalies of the lumbosacral vertebrae in five hundred and fifty individuals without symptoms referral to the low back. *AJR.* 1950;64:624–634.
12. Timi PG, Wieser C, Zinn WM. The transitional vertebrae of the lumbosacral spine: its radiological classification, incidence, prevalence and clinical significance. *Rheum Rehab.* 1977;16:80–187.

CHAPTER 2

Classification of Low Back Pain and Alerts for Different Age Groups

"Seek facts and classify them and you will be the workmen of science."

—Nicholas Maurice Arthus

Low back pain, like abdominal pain, is a symptom, not a disease. The pathologic basis for the pain may be something within the spine or a lesion outside of the spine. The causes are many but may be broadly classified as spondylogenic or neurogenic and viscerogenic, vascular, or psychogenic.

SPONDYLOGENIC BACK PAIN

Spondylogenic back pain may be defined as pain derived from the spinal column and its associated structures. The pain is aggravated by general and specific activities and is relieved, to some extent, by rest.

The pain may be derived from lesions involving the bony components of the spinal column, changes in the sacroiliac joints, or, most commonly, changes occurring in the soft tissues (discs, ligaments, and muscles).

Because these lesions constitute the most common source of low back pain seen in clinical practice, the pathologic changes and the pathogenesis of symptoms are discussed in detail in the chapters that follow.

NEUROGENIC PAIN

Tension, irritation, or compression of a lumbar nerve root or roots will usually cause referral of pain symptoms down one or both legs. Although this interference with root function constitutes the most common cause of neurogenic pain, it is prudent to remember there are other causes. Lesions of the central nervous system such as thalamic tumors may present or develop a causalgic type of leg pain, and arachnoid irritation from any cause as well as tumors of the spinal dura may produce back pain. The pathologic lesions most likely to give rise to confusion in diagnosis are neurofibroma, neurilemmoma, ependymoma, and other cysts and tumors involving the nerve roots. These lesions usually occur in the upper lumbar spine outside of the field of view of many computed tomography scans and are missed on sagittal magnetic resonance image scanning if not looked for. The history may be indistinguishable from nerve root pressure due to a disc herniation. Frequently, however, patients report a history of having to get out of bed at night to walk around to obtain relief of their symptoms.

The difficulties that may arise in diagnosis are best exemplified by a patient who presented with severe sciatic pain associated with paresthesia involving the lateral border of the foot and the lateral two toes. His symptoms were aggravated by provocative activity and relieved to some extent by recumbency. Examination revealed an impairment of first sacral root conduction, as evidenced by weakness of the plantar flexors of the ankle, a markedly diminished ankle jerk, and diminution of

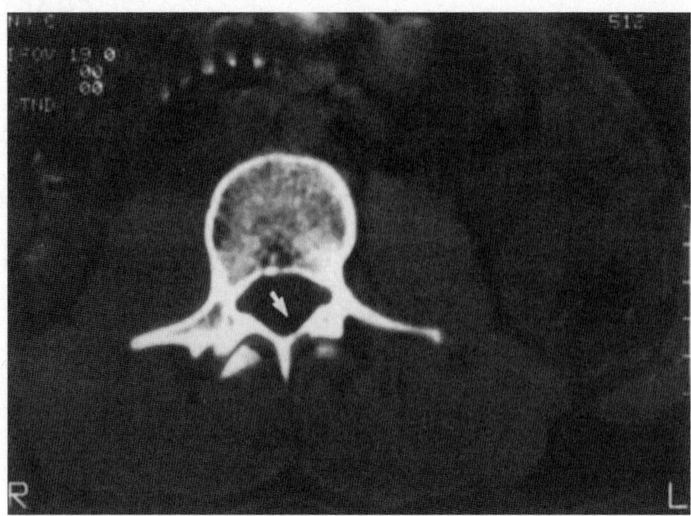

FIGURE 2-1 ● Conus lipoma, as depicted on computed tomography (CT) scan *(arrow)*. The patient presented with sciatica and first lumbar nerve root symptoms. Notice posteriorly on the left in the cauda equina, a lesion with the density of fat. This was a lipoma extending up to the conus.

appreciation of pinprick over the lateral border of the foot. The patient's history and clinical findings resembled the classic picture of a herniated lumbosacral disc with first sacral root compression. Myelographic examination was performed and demonstrated a gross defect opposite the body of L2. At surgery, a lipoma involving the first sacral root was found at the point where the root emerged from the conus (Fig. 2-1).

This case emphasizes not only the fact that nerve root tumors can mimic disc herniation but also the importance of looking at the conus region as an essential preoperative investigation in the surgical management of patients apparently suffering from discogenic root compression.

VISCEROGENIC BACK PAIN

Viscerogenic back pain may be derived from disorders of the kidneys or the pelvic viscera, lesions of the lesser sac, and retroperitoneal tumors (Fig. 2-2). Backache is rarely the sole symptom of visceral disease. Careful questioning will usually elicit description of other symptoms, depending on organ involved. The history of viscerogenic back pain can be differentiated from back pain derived from a disorder of the spinal column by one important feature. The pain is not aggravated by activity, and it is not relieved by rest. Indeed, with severe pain, the patient whose symptoms are visceral in origin will writhe around to get relief, whereas the patient suffering from the tortures of a septic discitis will lie perfectly still.

VASCULAR BACK PAIN

Abdominal aortic aneurysms or peripheral vascular disease (PVD) may give rise to backache or symptoms resembling sciatica. Abdominal aneurysms may present as a boring type of deep-seated lumbar pain unrelated to activity (Fig. 2-3). Insufficiency of the superior gluteal artery may give rise to buttock pain of a claudicant character, which is aggravated by walking and relieved by standing still. The pain may radiate down the leg in a sciatic distribution. However, the pain is not precipitated or aggravated by other activities that put a specific stress on the spine (e.g., bending, stooping, lifting, and so forth).

Intermittent claudication—intermittent pain in the calf—associated with PVD may on occasion mimic sciatic pain produced by root irritation, but the history of specific aggravation

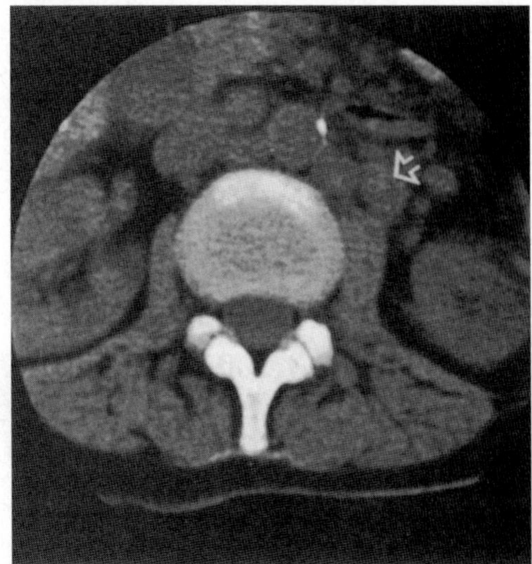

FIGURE 2-2 ● Axial computed tomography (CT) of a patient who presented with back pain. Note the extensive retroperitoneal nodes *(arrow)*. The patient had Hodgkin disease.

by walking and relief by standing still will make the clinician look for signs of peripheral vascular insufficiency.

The symptoms associated with PVD may be mimicked by spinal stenosis. A patient suffering from PVD frequently complains of pain and weakness in the legs, which is initiated and aggravated by the act of walking a short distance. In spinal stenosis, one distinguishing feature, however, is that the pain is not relieved by standing still. For a more detailed discussion of neurogenic claudication, the reader is referred to Chapter 17.

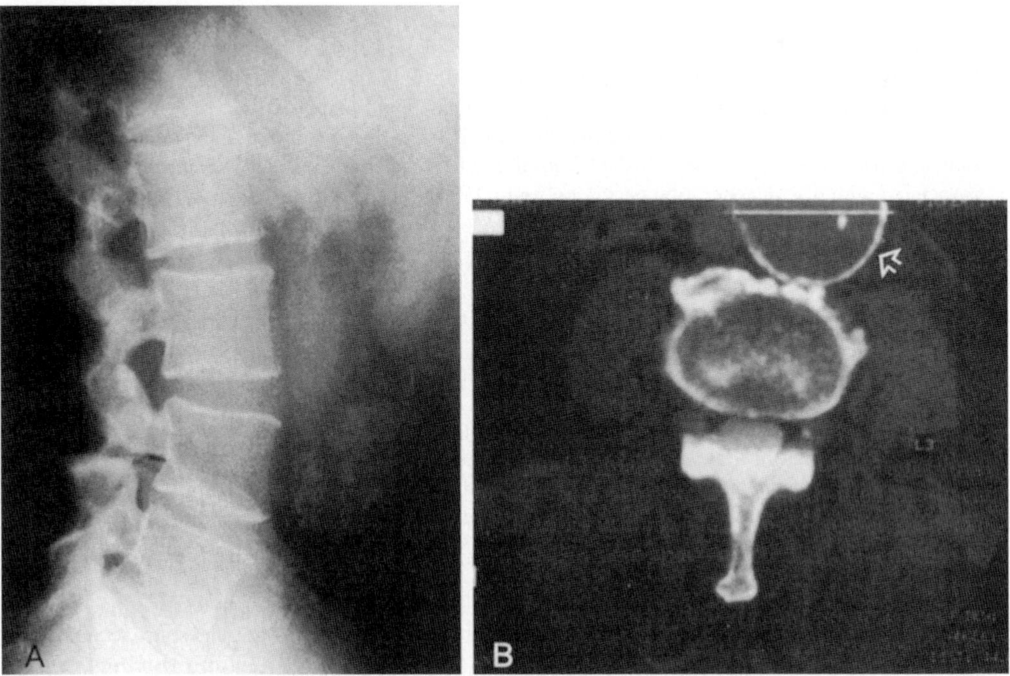

FIGURE 2-3 ● **A:** Plain lateral lumbosacral radiograph showing calcified aortic aneurysm. **B:** Computed tomography (CT) scan (axial) showing degenerative changes. Note the aortic aneurysm (*arrow*), a condition that may cause back pain.

PSYCHOGENIC BACK PAIN

Pure psychogenic back pain is rarely seen in clinical (civilian) practice. Clouding and confusion of the clinical picture by emotional overtones are more commonly seen. Although the physician must learn to recognize the presence of an emotional breakdown, he or she must never forget that emotional illnesses do not protect a patient against organic diseases. In such patients, although the task may be difficult, the physician must be prepared to accept the possibility of an underlying significant pathologic process and investigate its probability thoroughly. Because this is such an important aspect of proper decision making in lumbar spine surgery, Chapter 12 covers the topic in extensive detail.

DIAGNOSIS AND RECOGNITION OF PAIN PATTERNS BASED ON UNDERLYING PATHOLOGY AND AGE

The major symptom of spine-related problems is pain. It is a high-frequency complaint and often causes impaired function. It has a high impact on income and disability and has a high cost of treatment. Although disc degeneration is by far the most common source of low back pain, there are many other more serious causes of back pain and other causes that are more elusive in diagnosis and thus result in failure of treatment. Disc degeneration may be present in patients of all ages, and in the absence of any clearcut diagnosis, disc degeneration is frequently attributed as the major source of the back pain. The clinician needs to have a high index of suspicion for other underlying causes to rule out those possibilities.

TYPICAL BACK PAIN PATTERNS

Many conditions are characterized by typical patterns of pain and should alert the clinician to the possibility of a diagnosis.

Structural Spinal Disorders

Structural spinal disorders such as disc degeneration frequently result in pain that is aggravated by activities or staying in one position for prolonged periods. Pain relief may be partial with rest or may even be associated with changing position. If the pain is predominantly discogenic in origin, the pain is frequently worse with sitting, bending, lifting, and straining activities. Facet type pain is usually worse with extension type activities and associated with abnormalities of spinal movement rhythm. The pain of disc degeneration may be associated with radicular pain and symptoms. True radicular pain needs to be distinguished from nonradicular pain. The peak incidence of back pain associated with disc degeneration occurs between 35 and 55 years of age (Fig. 2-4).

Inflammatory Spine Pain

Inflammatory spine pain is usually worse in the morning and improves with activity. It is generally worse with any degree of inactivity during the course of the day. It is frequently associated with increased stiffness. The pain may radiate to the knees and be insidious in onset. The pain may also involve other joints, including the hips and shoulders. There may also be associated asymmetric peripheral arthritis.

Common pathologic and clinical features include spinal joint inflammation and injury and fusion, sacroiliac joint inflammation or fusion, peripheral joint arthritis and oligoarthritis, enthesitis, or other extra-articular manifestations. Spondyloarthropathies (SPA) frequently have strong genetic associations. There are common associated diseases, including Ankylosing Spondylitis, psoriatic arthritis, reactive arthritis, and enteropathic SPA: arthritis associated with inflammatory bowel diseases.

Distinctive x-ray changes include squared vertebral bodies, syndesmophytes, bamboo spine, sacroiliac pseudowidening erosions, sclerosis of the sacroiliac joint, periostitis, and spurs at enthuses.

Tumors

Patients with malignant tumors frequently will have night and rest pain or pain associated with inactivity if there is vertebral destruction and instability. They may also have associated mechanical

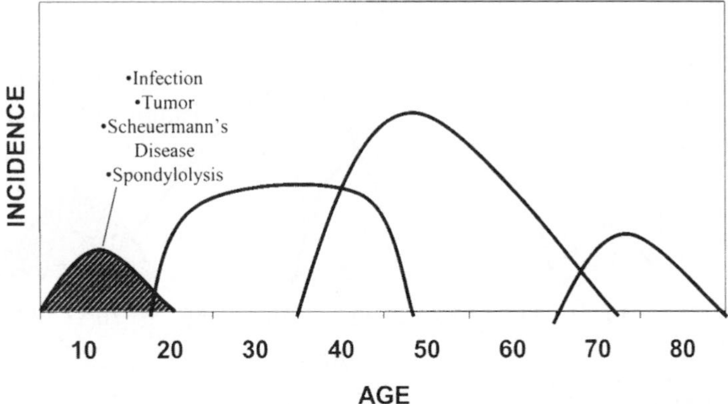

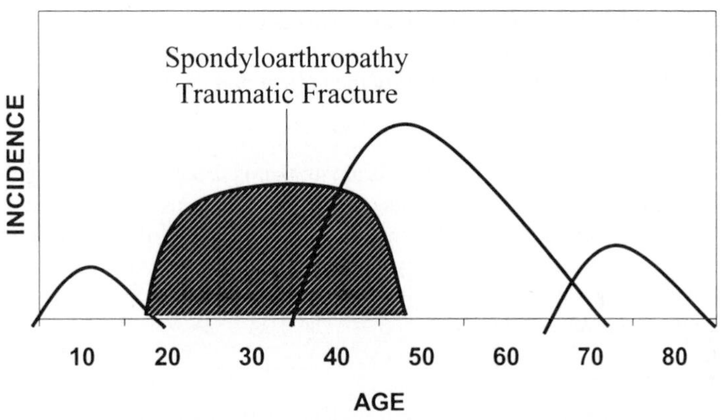

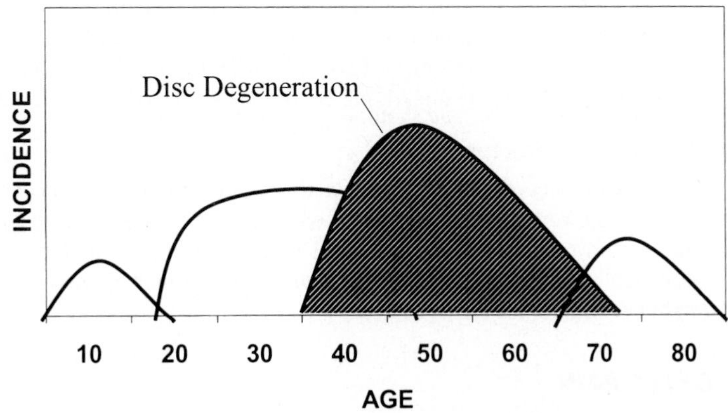

FIGURE 2-4 ● Alerts for different age groups. **A:** Alerts for juveniles and adolescents. **B:** Alerts for young adults. **C:** Alerts for middle-aged adults. *(continues)*

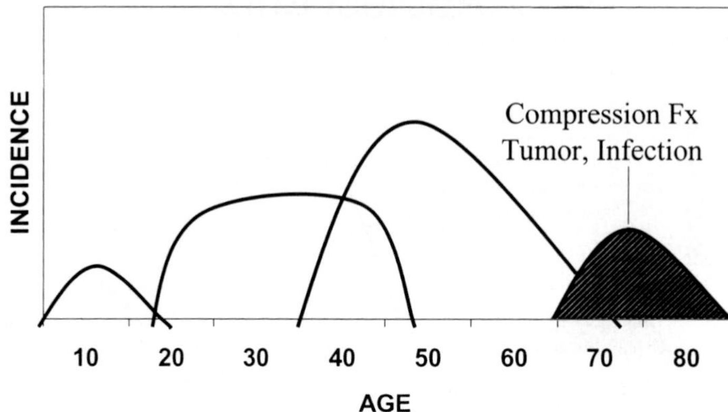

FIGURE 2-4 ● **D:** Alerts for the elderly. *(Continued)*

pain that is worse with activity. Patents will give a history of weight loss, malaise, loss of appetite, and other constitutional symptoms. It is important for the clinician to follow up this pain pattern with questions related to a history of cancer in the patient and the family.

Infections

The pattern of pain in patients with infection is a pain that is usually worse at night and at rest, and the pain may be associated with night sweats as well as chills. Onset of the pain may be preceded by an infection elsewhere in the body, in particular, bladder infections or respiratory tract infections. Patients frequently have a history of being immunocompromised, for example, diabetes or human immunodeficiency virus (HIV). In general, primary infections of the spine are seen more commonly in juveniles and the elderly.

Trauma

Etiology of the pain in these situations is self-evident. A traumatic event results in onset of severe pain. Minor injuries with soft tissue involvement following motor vehicle accidents may exhibit a delayed onset of pain. There may be initial discomfort at the time of the injury with a worsening of the symptoms in the next few days. In the majority of fairly major injuries, however, the onset of severe pain immediately follows the injury. Hereafter, pain may continue to diminish. In some instances, patients may have fairly minor injuries that result in the onset of back pain for the first time, and this may be the trigger for intermittent back pain in the future. The continuation of chronic pain is most likely interrelated to some underlying conditions such as disc degeneration.

Osteoporotic Compression Fractures

In elderly individuals with osteoporosis, multiple small repeated traumas may occur, resulting in a compression fracture of the vertebrae. There may be one single event, however, that results in fairly severe compression or a fracture. This type of pain is immediate in onset and may be severe. The pattern is that of constant severe pain that is unrelenting and further aggravated by movement, activity, and weight bearing.

PATTERNS OF LEG PAIN

Leg pain may be due to nerve root irritation or nonradicular in etiology. Radicular leg pain involves nerve root irritation and compression due to spinal stenosis (central spinal stenosis, subarticular stenosis, and foraminal stenosis). Nonradicular leg pain may be vascular or result from arthritis. It may affect soft tissue (tumor, infection, injury) or bony tissues (injury, infection, inflammation, tumor).

ALERTS TO ONSET OF PAIN IN DIFFERENT AGE GROUPS

The acute onset of severe and disabling pain, especially if associated with constitutional symptoms, should always alert the clinician about a serious underlying pathology. The peak incidence of spine pain associated with disc degeneration occurs between the ages of 35 and 55 years, but patients may have pain associated with disc degeneration throughout the spectrum of life. There are conditions, however, that tend to occur more frequently within age groups and the clinician should be aware of these and evaluate patients for those specific conditions.

Infancy and Adolescence

Onset of persistent pain in this age group should alert one to the possibility of an infection and tumor. Vertebral osteomyelitis is prone to occur in infancy and there is a predilection for osteomyelitis in infants to occur in the spine as opposed to nonspinal locations. Malignant bone tumors are rare in this age group and osteoid osteoma would be a more common, benign tumor. Other benign conditions that may present with back pain, particularly in adolescence, include spondylolysis and Scheuermann disease (juvenile disc degeneration).

Young and Middle Aged Adults

During this time period, patients may be undergoing premature disc degeneration, and this would still be a fairly common cause. However, this is also the age when, more commonly, the onset of pain due to spondyloarthropathies is seen. Young and active adults are more prone to trauma and injury.

Younger and Older Adults

This is the phase of disc degeneration and by far the most common cause of back pain. Ninety percent of patients presenting with an onset of back pain will have disc degeneration. Evaluating the pattern of pain will be useful in excluding other more serious causes of back pain.

Older Age Group

If patients have had persistent pain for many years they may continue to experience back pain in their late 60s and beyond. However, acute onset of back pain in patients of this age group without a history of any significant prior pain should alert one to the possibility of tumor. The most common tumor would be a metastasis and this does require a careful workup. Infections also occur in the older individual. Patients with osteoporosis may also undergo compression fractures.

CHAPTER 3

Spondylogenic Back Pain: Osseous and Intervertebral Lesions

"The spine is a series of bones running down your back. You sit on one end of it and your head sits on the other."

—Anonymous

Patients with severe pathologic processes involving the vertebrae (and the intervertebral joints), such as infections, neoplasms, and metabolic disorders, frequently present with pain in the back. Although there may be minor aggravation by activity, the significant distinguishing feature of these conditions is the fact that the pain is not relieved by rest. Major trauma resulting in fracture and fracture dislocations is not the thrust of this book. Low impact fractures are covered briefly as they can be a diagnostic dilemma with entities such as tumor and/or resulting in back pain as a tiresome sequel. The diagnosis of all of these conditions is largely dependent on radiographic findings, and treatment is along well-established lines. New computed tomography (CT) scanning and magnetic resonance imaging (MRI) techniques are giving us a better understanding of these various conditions and allowing, in some cases, for a more aggressive surgical treatment option.

Although these lesions constitute a relatively small percentage of the backaches seen in clinical practice, some aspects of each group are discussed very briefly.

LOW IMPACT TRAUMATIC EVENTS AFFECTING THE LUMBAR SPINE

THE OSTEOPOROTIC COMPRESSION FRACTURE

The most common spine fracture you will see in the emergency department is the compression fracture in osteoporotic bone. Your patient will usually (but not always) be a woman and will describe the sudden onset of midback pain brought on by a simple maneuver such as a cough or lifting of a bag of groceries. In approximately 20% of the patients, the compression fracture will be asymptomatic and unrecognized until a radiograph is done for some other purpose.

Most patients will experience the sudden onset of pain so severe they will appear in the emergency department. Even though the fracture may be affecting a single vertebral level, the pain will be described as a diffuse discomfort; for example, a fracture of T9 will radiate widely, even to the lower lumbar region.

Careful palpation or percussion of the spinous processes will usually reveal the level of fracture. Rarely will there be evidence of radicular or cord involvement in simple compression fractures.

Plain radiographs will reveal one of three fracture patterns (Fig. 3-1). The anterior wedge is the fracture pattern most commonly seen in the thoracic vertebrae, with the biconcave endplate fracture being more common in the lumbar region. If there is any question that the middle column of the vertebrae is involved, a CT scan should be obtained to rule out a more serious, potentially unstable burst fracture. Measure the distance between the pedicles and the height of the posterior

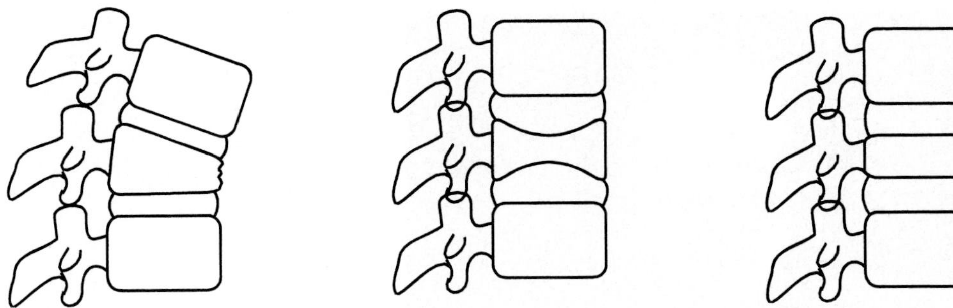

FIGURE 3-1 • The three varieties of compression fracture: **left**—wedge; **middle**—"codfish"; **right**—uniform compression, anterior and posterior.

vertebral body on the plain x-rays. If the interpedicular distance is wider than the average of the levels above or below, or the posterior body height is less than the average of the adjacent levels, then the middle column of the vertebral segment may have been fractured and compressed. A thin cut CT scan through the area will answer this question.

Most patients with benign compression fractures can be treated outside of the hospital. Occasionally the pain is so severe that admission becomes a necessity. The rare complications of ileus, urinary retention, and neurologic complications will require hospital admission. In this older population, excessive narcotic use (e.g., oxycodone and hydrocodone) will cause more problems than solutions. Often strong analgesia is needed in the first couple of days, but this should be quickly reduced as the patient is ambulated in corset support (Fig. 3-2). Bracing is especially important in ambulating these patients, but the design has to be simple to accommodate frailty and the often accompanying arthritic hands. Obviously, severe osteoporosis or osteoporosis in the younger patient

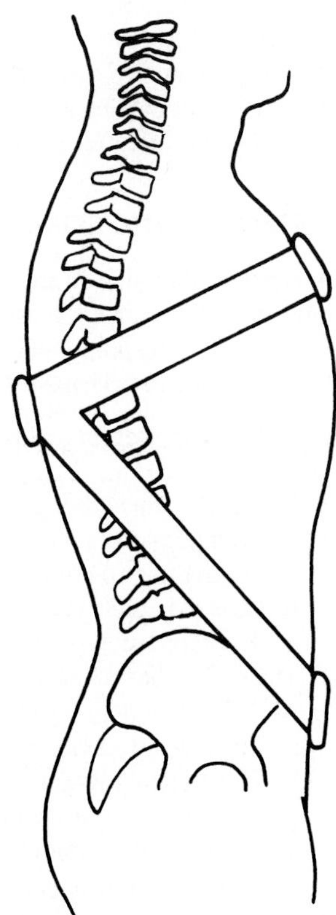

FIGURE 3-2 • Brace support: Three points of support—one posterior below fracture, one on sternum, and one on the symphysis pubis.

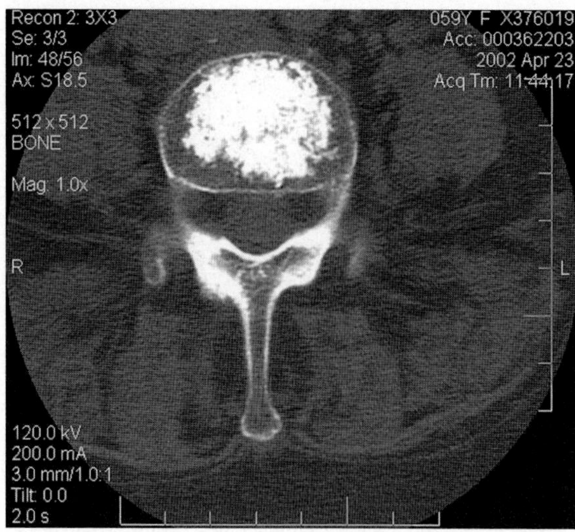

FIGURE 3-3 ● Cement injection into a thoracic vertebral body for osteoporotic compression fracture. Ideal cement pattern with spread throughout the body and no leakage.

(younger than 65 years) requires redress. The 2004 U.S. Surgeon General's Report on Osteoporosis (4) suggests that a patient sustaining a fragility fracture (such as a vertebral compression fracture) should have a bone densitometry performed and appropriate treatment instituted if necessary.

Healing is best followed by the patient's symptoms, although serial radiographs will show any progressive collapse. It will take 6 to 12 weeks before patients are comfortable enough to shed their brace and increase their activities. Once a comfort level is achieved, the institution of an extension exercise program and low impact aerobics is important.

In patients who continue to have significant pain beyond a few weeks, stabilization by injection of bone cement into the vertebral body may be an option (Fig. 3-3) (6,7,11,14). There have been reports of reduction of the fracture and improvement in alignment with these injections (11,14).

Repeated compression fractures will lead to an increasing kyphotic deformity of the chest, with the ribs eventually settling on the pelvis. This causes discomfort and is associated with poor posture, a protuberant abdomen, respiratory compromise, and a very unhappy patient. There is little the physician can offer in this situation; thus, prevention is an important goal.

OSTEOPOROTIC COMPRESSION FRACTURE VERSUS TUMOR

A constant dilemma in the emergency room is to decide whether the thoracic fracture you are looking at is occurring in osteoporotic bone or bone weakened by a tumor.

The following points suggest that you are dealing with a secondary malignant lesion (or primary hematopoietic neoplasm such as multiple myeloma):

1. The patient presents with severe pain, and any attempt to roll or sit up becomes a moment of agony.
2. Radicular pain and/or cord symptoms and signs are present.
3. Plain radiographs reveal:
   a. Destruction of cortex.
   b. Loss of pedicle (Fig. 3-4).
   c. A compression fracture above T7 or below L2.
4. The patient has a history of a past malignancy.
5. An MRI (Fig. 3-4) reveals:
   a. The marrow cavity is completely obliterated, with no fatty marrow left.
   b. The cortical margins are gray and mottled, rather than black and distinct.
   c. There is a soft tissue mass outside of the vertebral body such as cord effacement (Fig. 3-5).
   d. There are skip lesions (Fig. 3-6).
   e. Gadolinium injection on MRI is not a reliable way to sort out malignancy from benignity.
6. A bone scan is often helpful in distinguishing malignant from benign lesions (Fig. 3-7).

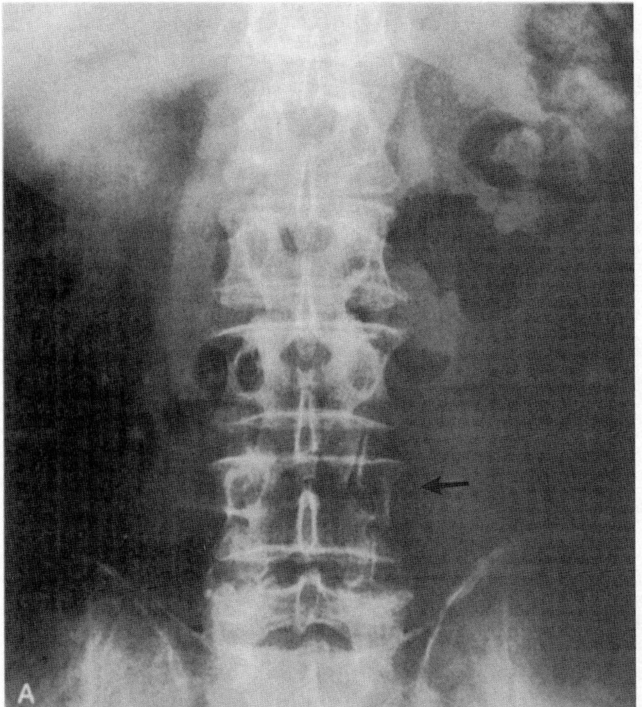

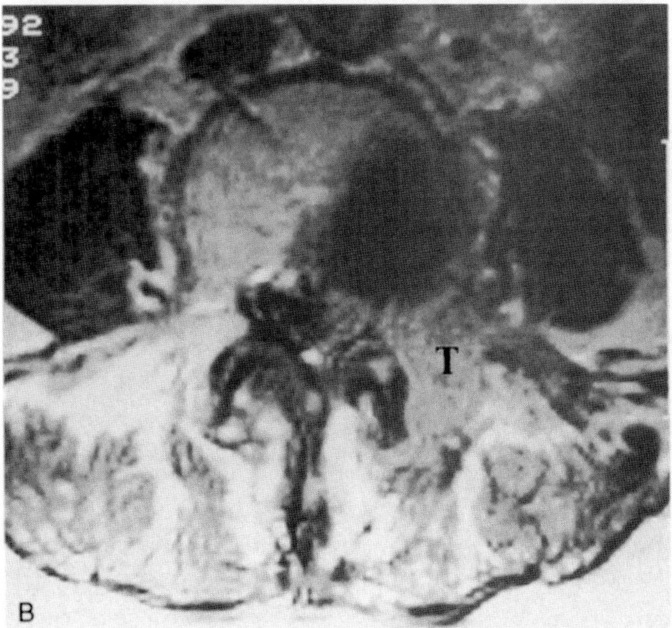

FIGURE 3-4 ● **A:** Note the loss of pedicle of L4 *(left)*; the patient had metastatic lung cancer. **B:** An axial (T1) magnetic resonance imaging (MRI) in same patient showing tumor replacing the left pedicle (T).

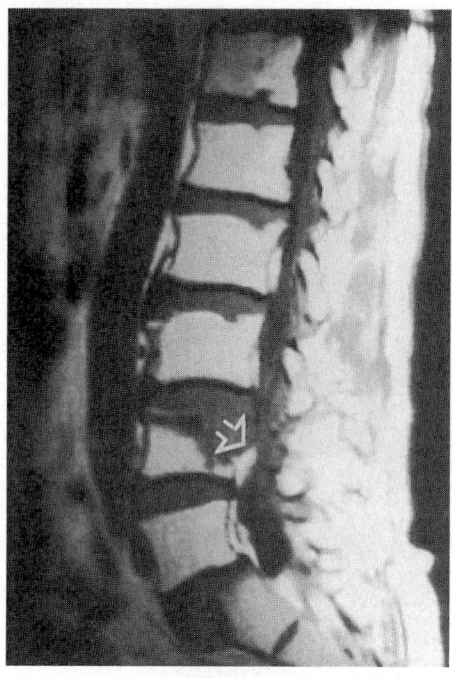

FIGURE 3-5 ● The soft tissue mass of tumor on MRI (sagittal T1) is pressing on the cauda equina *(arrow).*

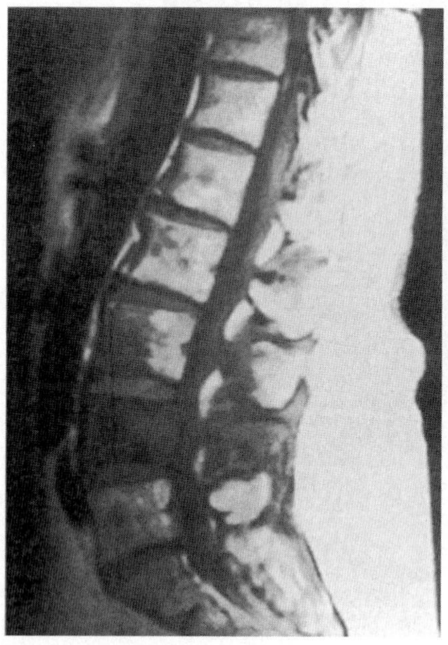

FIGURE 3-6 ● Metastatic skip lesions on magnetic resonance imaging (MRI) (T1 sagittal): the main tumor mass (black or low signal intensity) is in L4. Note the additional "skip" lesions in L5, L3, L2, and L1, with preservation (skipping) of the disc spaces.

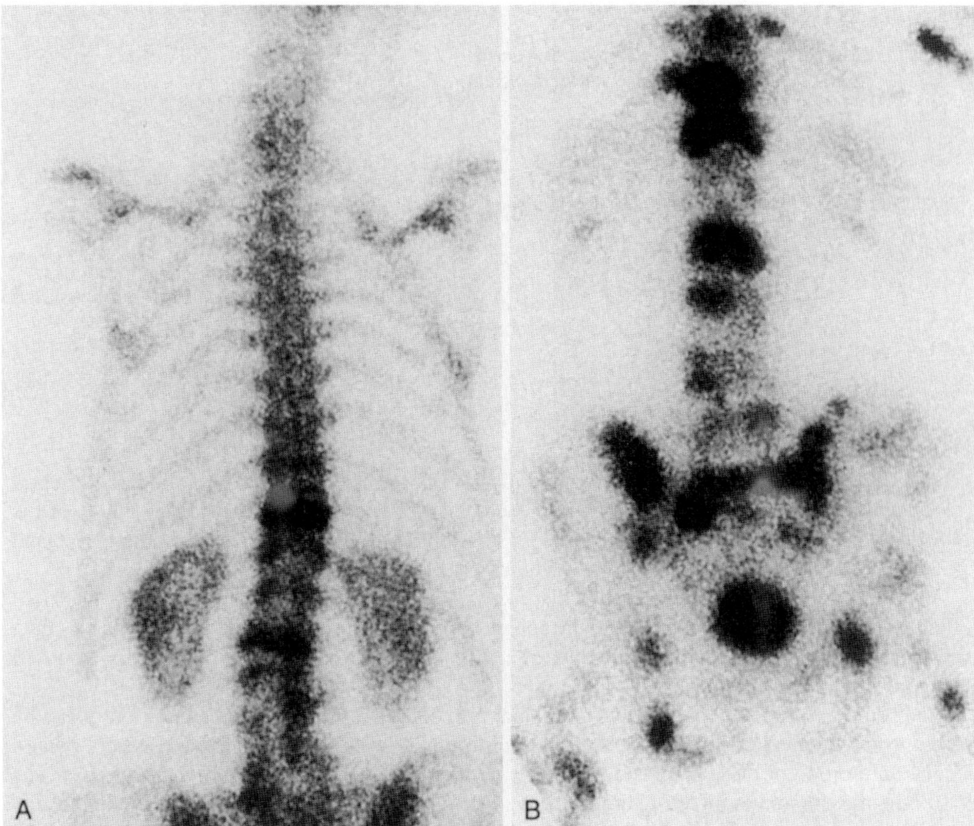

FIGURE 3-7 • Bone scans in a fracture **(A)** and tumor **(B).** There is no difference in the intensity of the hot spot, but there are multiple "hot spots" in **(B)** indicative of metastatic tumor.

If, after all of the considerations just mentioned, you have still not pinned down the diagnosis, a CT-guided biopsy will be required.

INFECTION

Spinal infections, despite their relative rarity, must be remembered as a potential source of back pain. For convenience of discussion, infections involving the vertebral column may be considered under the following clinicopathologic syndromes:

1. Vertebral osteomyelitis
   a. Pyogenic
   b. Granulomatous (tubercle bacillus)
   c. Miscellaneous
2. Epidural abscess
3. Intervertebral disc "infection"

Pyogenic vertebral osteomyelitis and epidural abscess will be discussed together as they are often closely associated in clinical practice.

PYOGENIC VERTEBRAL OSTEOMYELITIS

Although pyogenic spinal lesions may result from discography, discectomy, and open wounds, most vertebral osteomyelitis results from hematogenous spread through an arterial or venous route. Probably the most common source of infection is from a pelvic inflammatory lesion (e.g., bladder infection), with spread occurring through Batson's (1) plexus (Fig. 3-8) sometimes after a surgical procedure such as cystoscopy.

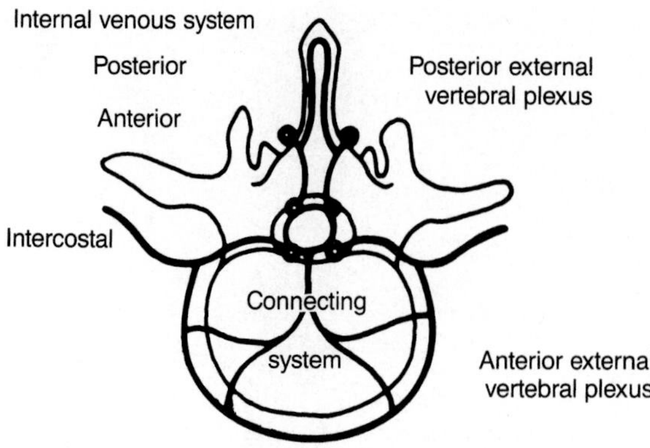

FIGURE 3-8 ● Batson's plexus is a network of veins that connects the abdominal and thoracic cavities (via the vena cava) to the vertebral body and epidural space. The components of the plexus around the spinal column are shown and include the external vertebral veins, the internal (epidural) veins, and the connecting veins.

The clinical features of vertebral osteomyelitis have altered from the preantibiotic era. Vertebral osteomyelitis used to be a disease of adolescence and was very acute in onset. The source of the infection was rarely known. *Staphylococcus* was by far the most common organism involved, and the disease had a dreadful mortality of approximately 60%.

Vertebral osteomyelitis is presently a disease of adults. The onset may still be acute, but more often than not the onset is insidious, and the course is chronic. This leads to more misdiagnoses than you can imagine; in fact, the first time you meet a patient with vertebral osteomyelitis, you will likely miss the diagnosis!

The source of infection can be localized in approximately 50% of patients and usually can be linked to infection or instrumentation of the genitourinary system. It is interesting to note that a significant portion of these patients are elderly, debilitated, or diabetic. Although *Staphylococcus* is still the most common infecting organism, *Escherichia coli* and other gram-negative organisms are increasing in frequency. *Streptococcus* can be seen in diabetics. The drug subculture has added a new dimension, with its own group of gram-negative organisms (*Pseudomonas*).

The lumbar spine is more commonly affected than the thoracic or cervical spine. Because the vertebral body has a richer vascular network than the posterior elements, the majority of infections involve the body. Commonly, two adjacent vertebrae and the intervening disc space are involved (Fig. 3-9). Varying degrees of vertebral body destruction and collapse occur. With the spread of the infection, an abscess may develop and extend either anteriorly or posteriorly.

Neurologic damage may result from the development of an angulatory kyphosis, an epidural abscess, or a sequestrated disc or bone fragments. Occasionally, the spinal cord may be destroyed by obliteration of its vascular supply.

Clinical Presentation

Backache is the most common presenting symptom: indeed, early in its course, the disease may be indistinguishable symptomatically from a mechanical backache. The insidious onset and the lack of radiographic changes account for the usual delay of often weeks in diagnosis. With progression of the disease, the back pain increases in intensity, becoming constant, and is particularly noticeable in bed at night. More often than not, the back pain has reached severe proportions before the diagnosis is made. On occasion, pain will be referred to the abdomen, leading to a search for intra-abdominal disease.

The patient may appear sick and will have a variable temperature elevation. The findings at examination vary with the stage and severity of the disease. All spinal movements and especially weight-bearing (sitting, standing, jarring) intensify the pain. Paravertebral muscle and hamstring spasms are sometimes severe. The patient may stand with a marked list of the spine to one side. Gross spinal rigidity is a characteristic feature. The spinous processes are usually tender on pressure. The back pain is intensified by percussion of the involved area. Straight leg raising (SLR) is restricted because of hamstring spasm. If the infection has spread to involve the meninges, SLR may be markedly reduced from the meningismus. On the rare occasion, neurologic findings of root compression will be detected, but every so often a delay in diagnosis will be followed by epidural

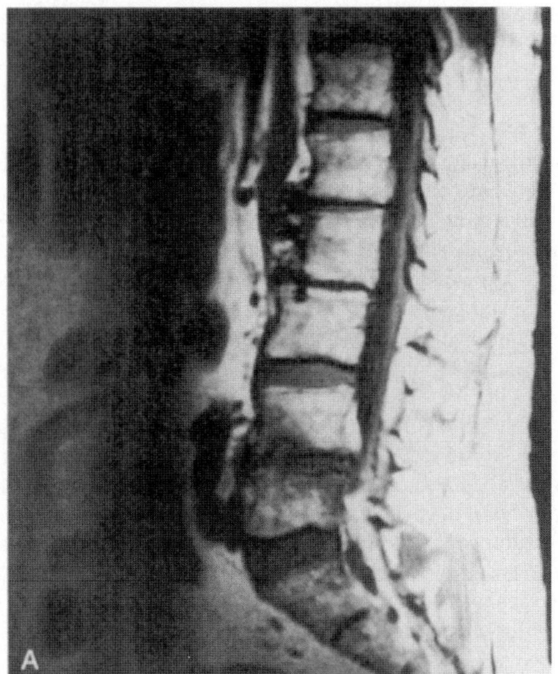

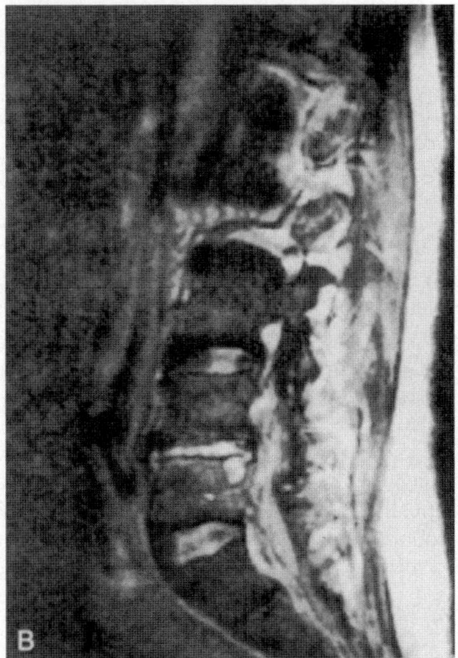

FIGURE 3-9 ● Magnetic resonance imaging (MRI) of osteomyelitis: **A:** Sagittal (T1) showing decreased signal intensity on either side of L4–5 disc space. **B:** Sagittal (T2) showing increased signal intensity in same area: this is the typical MRI picture of the edema of inflammation.

abscess formation, and either direct compression or a vascular lesion will damage the lower cord or cauda equina. If paralysis is the outcome, there is little chance for recovery from this tragic sequence of events.

Laboratory

In half of the patients, the white blood count (WBC) will be within normal limits, and even when elevated, the WBC rarely rises above 15,000/mm^3. The erythrocyte sedimentation rate (ESR) and particularly the C-reactive protein (CRP), however, will be consistently elevated and are the most useful tests for monitoring disease activity and the efficacy of treatment. On occasion, a very debilitated patient will show no signs of fever, no elevated WBC, or no increased ESR. The CRP is the most sensitive test and usually is elevated. Blood cultures may be positive in up to 50% of patients, particularly in those who present with a markedly febrile clinical course.

Radiology

Radiologic evidence of the spinal disease lags 4 weeks or more behind the clinical manifestations. The earliest changes are localized rarefaction of the vertebral endplates (Fig. 3-10), followed rapidly by involvement of the adjacent vertebrae and narrowing of the disc spaces. With the increasing recognition of disc degeneration as a source of spondylogenic pain, there is an inherent danger of misinterpretation of the radiologic changes. The early specific radiologic features that distinguish the disc narrowing that is the result of infection from the disc narrowing that is associated with degenerative changes are very subtle and include fuzziness of the cortical endplate and a "divot" out of the anterior-superior or anterior-inferior portion of the vertebral body (Fig. 3-10).

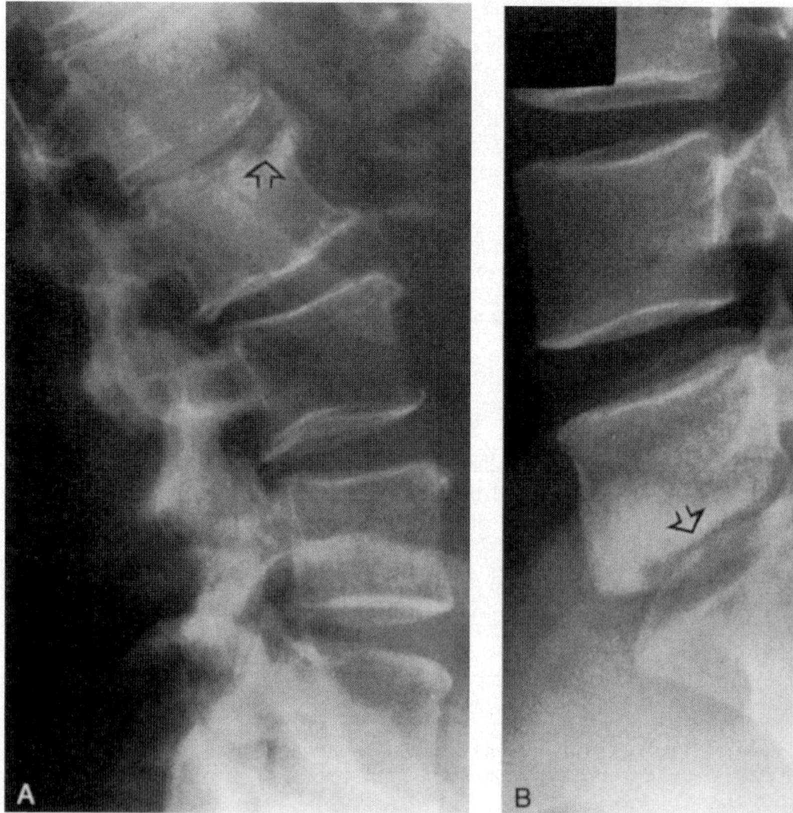

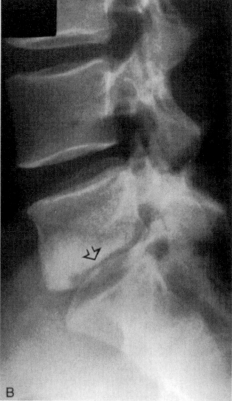

FIGURE 3-10 ● Plain radiograph of the stages of discitis/osteomyelitis. **A:** Early: a small "divot" out of the anterior aspect of L2 *(arrow)*. **B:** Midphase: irregularities of vertebral endplate of L5 *(arrow)* and disc space narrowing L5-S1.

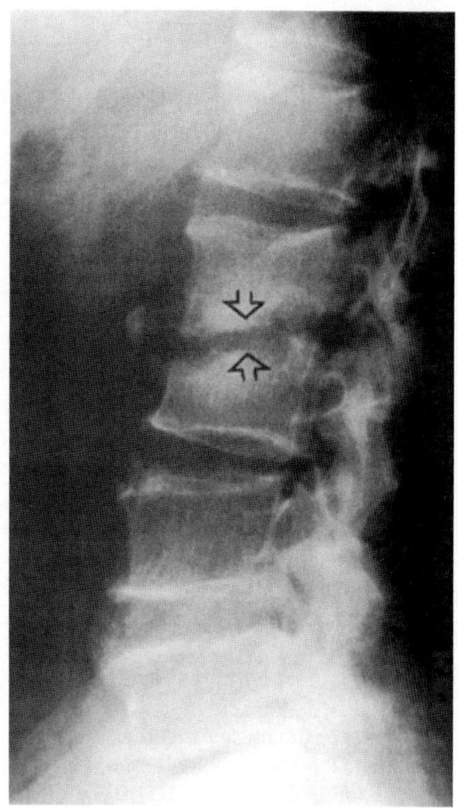

FIGURE 3-11 • The late stage: total destruction of disc space and adjacent vertebral bodies *(arrows).*

This raises another distinguishing feature of infection versus tumor: early radiologic changes reflective of infection affect the endplate region and are anterior, whereas tumors affect the medullary/marrow space and tend to be posterior in the vertebral body.

The radiologist frequently is not provided with enough clinical information, and there is no reason why the minimal radiologic changes should make him or her suspicious of an infective lesion. So the diagnosis is suggested by the clinical findings: a sick patient with severe pain, a rigid back, fever, and an elevated WBC and ESR. Early plain radiologic changes are minimal but may give an indication of the site of the lesion. At this stage, the diagnosis is best made by an MRI (Fig. 3-9) (13). But even with these sophisticated tests, the diagnosis can be missed because of nonspecific changes.

Later in the course of infective disease, the plain radiographs reveal destructive erosion of the contiguous vertebral bodies, starting first and usually most extensive anteriorly (Fig. 3-11). Subsequently, there is sclerosis and the development of reactive bone. Evidence of soft tissue reaction is revealed on radiograph by distortion of the psoas shadow or by a localized paravertebral mass.

There may be some difficulty in distinguishing the radiologic changes of an infective lesion from those produced by a neoplasm, but as a general rule it may be said that with infection the disc space is the first structure to be destroyed, whereas with secondary metastatic tumor deposits in the vertebral body the disc space is spared (Fig. 3-12).

Diagnosis

It is essential to search for the causative organism. The triad of cultures—blood, infection site, and potential source—are to be completed before institution of antimicrobial therapy. The blood culture and source culture (e.g., urine or sputum) are readily obtained. A culture of the infection site often requires a percutaneous biopsy (Fig. 3-13) Securing tissue for culture is preferred because of the occasional case of blood cultures revealing organisms different from the actual organism cultured from the infected site.

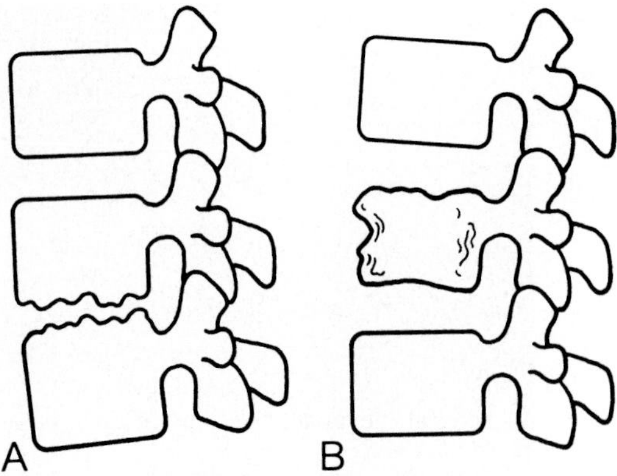

FIGURE 3-12 ● **A:** Pyogenic infections attack and narrow the disc space early. **B:** Tuberculosis and neoplasms spare the disc space.

Antibiotic treatment is absolutely dependent on the isolation of the organism and on the stage of the disease. No longer is it safe to presume that the infection is staphylococcal. Because of the increasing incidence of gram-negative infections and infections by more than one organism, the offending organism must be identified by blood culture and/or a vertebral biopsy and culture, in order that its sensitivity may be determined. If needle biopsy fails to obtain enough material to permit isolation of the organism, then an open biopsy is necessary.

Treatment

Intravenous antibiotics and bed rest to start are followed by bracing, oral antibiotics, and activity limitation. Treatment should be continued until the ESR has returned to normal. The brace should be worn for an arbitrary period of 3 months, and antibiotic coverage should be continued at least 6 weeks during this period of time, providing the clinical course allows. Serial ESRs and CRPs that return toward normal should be included in this regimen. Routine radiologic assessment should be carried out at 4- to 6-week intervals for at least 3 months. Fusion occurs in 50% of pyogenic disc space infections in approximately 1 year, and the majority of the remainder show bony obliteration of the disc space in 2 years. Routine radiologic reassessment is of importance to evaluate effectiveness of antibiotic treatment as measured by no ongoing bone destruction.

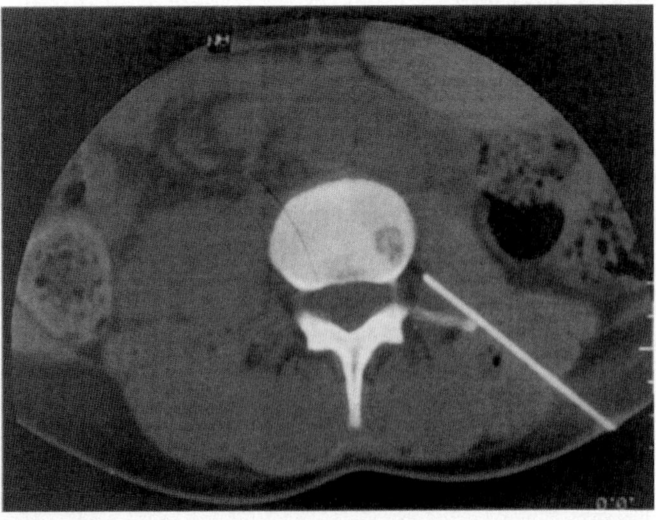

FIGURE 3-13 ● A computed tomography (CT) guided biopsy of a lytic lesion in L4.

The endpoint in medical treatment has been reached when the patient's pain and fever have resolved, there is radiographic evidence of fusion, and the ESR and CRP are back to normal for that patient. Remember, in a lot of elderly debilitated patients there is no such occurrence as "normal" ESR. When you have met these four criteria, administration of antibiotics can be stopped, the brace can be shed, and rehabilitation for lost function can start.

Surgery

The indications for surgical intervention are as follows:

1. Failure of medical management: Despite rest and massive intravenous antibiotics, the patient's fever and pain persist.
2. A large abscess forms. Small abscesses, providing they are not in the epidural space, may be successfully treated with medical management. In general, never let the sun set on a large paraspinal or any size epidural abscess.
3. Progressive neurologic deficit. If the patient arrives on your service paraplegic, you must intervene on an emergency basis, but there is little likelihood of salvage. If on your watch (a neurologic examination every 2–4 hours), you detect an increasing deficit despite medical treatment, take the patient to the operating room without delay.
4. Biomechanical instability is a likely outcome (e.g., anticipated or actual kyphosis of >15 degrees).
5. Failure to obtain an adequate biopsy specimen sufficient to make a definitive diagnosis.

Type of surgery. The basic rule in spine infection (and almost any other spinal problem) is to go directly to the problem. Because these infections are in the vertebral body and disc space, the surgical approach is anteriorly. The only exception to this rule is an epidural abscess, which should be approached posteriorly (laminectomy).

The surgical goals anteriorly are adequate debridement, decompression of any material in the spinal canal, and stabilization of the interspace with rib strut grafts or tricortical iliac crest grafts. A satisfactory fusion rate with this approach, along with antibiotics and rest, is a very high likelihood.

TUBERCULOUS VERTEBRAL OSTEOMYELITIS

Tuberculous infections of the lumbar spine usually have a clinical course that distinguishes them from pyogenic infections (Table 3-2). Skeletal tuberculosis is almost always secondary to a focus elsewhere, particularly the pulmonary and urinary tracts. The most frequent site of vertebral involvement is the lower thoracic and upper lumbar region. The vertebral body, as in pyogenic osteomyelitis, is the site of localization. The intervertebral disc is relatively resistant to tuberculous destruction and the infection simply migrates under the anterior longitudinal ligament to the adjacent vertebral body.

The disease is very insidious, and the time that elapses from the onset of symptoms to hospital admission is often well more than 6 months. This is further complicated by the fact that, in North America, tuberculosis is now a much rarer condition and is frequently overlooked in differential diagnosis. However, over the past decade, there has been an increase in the incidence of pulmonary tuberculosis, and it is reasonable to assume there will be a subsequent increase in tuberculous osteomyelitis.

In the younger child, irritability and refusal to sit or walk are presenting features. Older children and adults present with simple backache. The symptoms do not have the dramatic disability characteristic of the later stages of a pyogenic vertebral osteomyelitis.

A careful history will reveal the association of constitutional symptoms of intermittent fever, sweats, anorexia, weight loss, and easy fatigability. At examination, marked splinting of the spine can usually be demonstrated. Although the gross tenderness associated with pyogenic osteomyelitis is rarely apparent, localized bony deformity associated with vertebral collapse, presenting as gibbus, is common.

Because of the insidious nature of the disease and the consequent delay in seeking advice, the patient may present with evidence of neurologic impairment even when seen for the first time.

Laboratory and Radiograph

As in pyogenic lesions, the CRP and ESR are elevated. The WBC is variable, however, and may even be depressed. The plain radiographic features that distinguish the lesion from pyogenic osteomyelitis are as follows: (a) there may be multiple vertebral bodies affected and (b) there may be scalloping of the anterior surface of the vertebral bodies by the tuberculous abscess (Fig. 3-15) (3). The disc space is usually spared until late in the disease, when it may rupture into the tuberculous cavities within the vertebral bodies or paraspinal abscesses. In fact, the vertebral body destruction in tuberculosis is not unlike that caused by neoplasm, except that tuberculous lesions tend to be anterior in the vertebral body, and neoplasms, especially secondaries, are more posterior in the vertebral body and invade the posterior elements.

As noted earlier, tuberculous infections of the lumbar spine are rarely primary. They are commonly secondary to foci either in the lungs or the genitourinary tract. Radiographs of the chest and bacteriologic examination of the urine must always be carried out in routine clinical assessment. The Mantoux test, when positive, can be regarded as suggestive but never diagnostic. As with pyogenic vertebral osteomyelitis, vertebral biopsy is essential for diagnosis.

Treatment

It is possible to treat the patient with antituberculous drugs and immobilization. However, anterior debridement of the lesion with immediate grafting is probably the treatment of choice, especially if there is neurologic involvement. Surgical ablation of the tuberculous lesion significantly shortens the course of the disease process, and the incidence of deformity and residual neurologic complications is markedly reduced. It must be emphasized once again that, unlike pyogenic osteomyelitis, tuberculous lesions of the vertebral column are commonly associated with neurologic lesions. In such instances, the prognosis after decompression is carried out early is excellent. In contrast, in neglected cases, paraplegia caused by penetration of the dura and involvement of the cord by tuberculous granulation tissue produces irreversible changes.

EPIDURAL ABSCESS

Introduction

It is highly unlikely that you will ever see a lumbar epidural abscess. If you happen upon it when it appears in the emergency department, you will probably miss it, something that happens most of the time. It does not sound very promising, does it?

Demography

Epidural abscess is predominantly an adult disease, affecting the thoracic and lumbar spinal canal more than the cervical region. As a spontaneous hematogenous event in a normal adult, it is highly unlikely. Most often it occurs after spine surgery, and more frequently it appears in debilitated (diabetic or alcoholic) or immunocompromised patients. If you work in an area with high drug abuse, you will see epidural abscesses more frequently.

Bacteriology

The majority of patients will have cultures that reveal *Staphylococcus aureus*; drug abusers have a higher incidence of gram-negative infections such as *Pseudomonas,* but the majority of patients will have cultures that grow *S. aureus.*

Pathogenesis and Clinical Presentation

The mass of infective cells in the epidural space may be either granulation tissue or pus. Both occupy space needed for neurologic structures. Initially, the patient will have local pain (especially nonmechanical night-time pain). As the mass expands, radicular pain will appear, followed by weakness and, in the end, paralysis. How fast this clinical progression occurs is variable, but the pain to paralysis stage may take but a few hours, making the diagnosis and treatment of epidural abscess an emergency.

At the stage of radicular pain and early in the stage of neurologic changes, the patient is usually unable to move in bed because of the severity of pain. The meningismus will be evident by a profound reduction in SLR due to back pain.

In the thoracic and lumbar spine, there is a posterior epidural space filled with fat. Because of this anatomy, it is easy to understand why epidural abscesses tend to occur posteriorly in the thoracic and lumbar regions. If abscesses occur after anterior spine surgery or discography, then obviously most epidural collections will be anterior. They may be confined to one segment, but more often the pus or granulation tissue collection spreads over multiple segments.

TABLE 3-1

MRI Epidural Abscess (Granulation Tissue) Appearance

MRI Sequence	Compared with Spinal Cord	Compared with CSF
T1-weighted spin echo	Most often isointense[b]; sometimes hypointense	Hyperintense
T2-weighted spin echo	Almost always hyperintense	Hyperintense
Gradient echo T2[a]	Same as T2 SE	Same as T2 SE
Gadolinium enhancement	Hyperintense periphery (granulation tissue) Hypointense core (abscess)	Not routinely done

CSF, cerebrospinal fluid.
[a]T2 is a fast imaging technique that appears somewhat like a T2 spin echo but requires much less time in the machine.
[b]Isointense: same signal intensity. Hyperintense: higher (whiter) signal intensity. Hypointense: lower (grayer) signal intensity.

Diagnosis

The quickest path to diagnosis is a high index of suspicion in any adult, especially those debilitated by drugs, disease, or decay, and in whom there is presentation of night-time back pain and stiffness with fever. Sometimes, because of immunosuppression, the fever, CRP, ESR, and WBC will show minimal change.

Any suspected infectious disease needs immediate identification of the underlying organism through direct abscess culture, blood culture, or culture of a remote but more accessible source, such as an infected skin lesion, kidney, or lung.

Unless there is associated discitis/osteomyelitis, plain radiographs are likely to be negative. Until the advent of MRI, myelography with CT scanning was needed for diagnosis. MRI is now the investigative modality of choice, which avoids all the dangers of subarachnoid puncture in a patient with a spinal infection (Table 3-1) (Fig. 3-14).

TABLE 3-2

Comparison of Pyogenic Vertebral Osteomyelitis (PVO) and Tuberculous Spondylitis (TS)[a]

Comparison Factors	PVO	TS
Onset	Some insidious; some acute	Always insidious
Average interval to diagnosis	3 mo +	8 mo +
Apparent antecedent infection or surgery	50%	100%
Back pain	Can be severe	Rarely severe
Neurologic involvement	Unusual	Usual
Paralysis	More common	Less common
Levels	Single segment; lumbar most common	Multiple segments possible Equally lower thoracic and lumbar
ESR	Very high (more than 100 mm/hr not unusual)	Rarely more than 50 mm/hr
Radiograph	Disc space narrowing occurs early	Disc space preserved
Requirement for surgery	Not usual	More common
Residual deformity	Unusual	Common

ESR, erythrocyte sedimentation rate.
[a]The only surefire way to distinguish between these two diseases is histologic and culture examination of a direct biopsy.

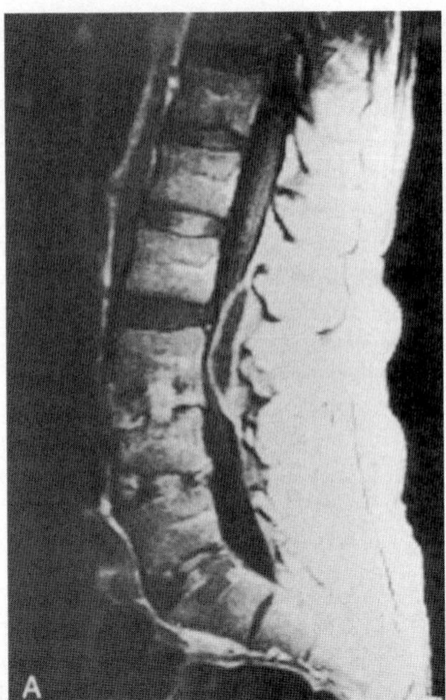

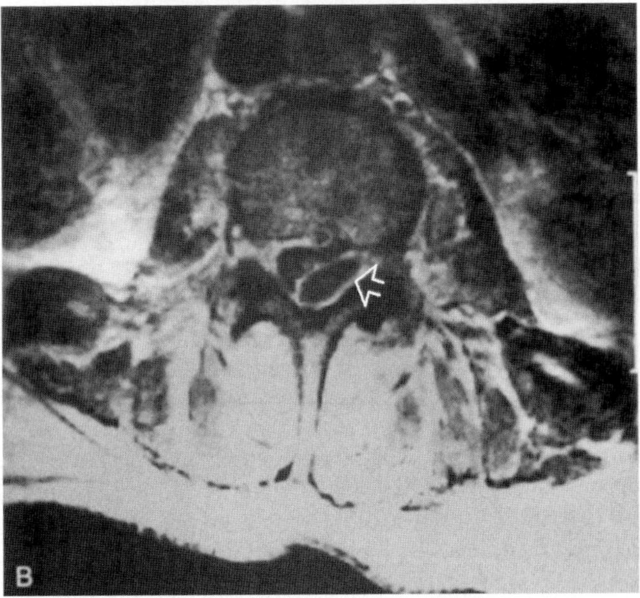

FIGURE 3-14 ● Magnetic resonance imaging (MRI) of epidural abscess after gadolinium injection. **A:** Sagittal. **B:** Axial *(arrow).*

Treatment

An epidural abscess is an urgent medical situation. If you are fortunate enough to catch it early, before weakness has occurred, conservative care with the appropriate antibiotic is a choice. Most cases of epidural abscesses require surgical drainage because:

1. The disease is diagnosed late, and radicular pain and weakness are present.
2. The time interval between weakness and paralysis can be measured in hours. Some surgeons think this is because of venous or arterial thrombosis in the vascular tree of the spinal cord and/or cauda equina.

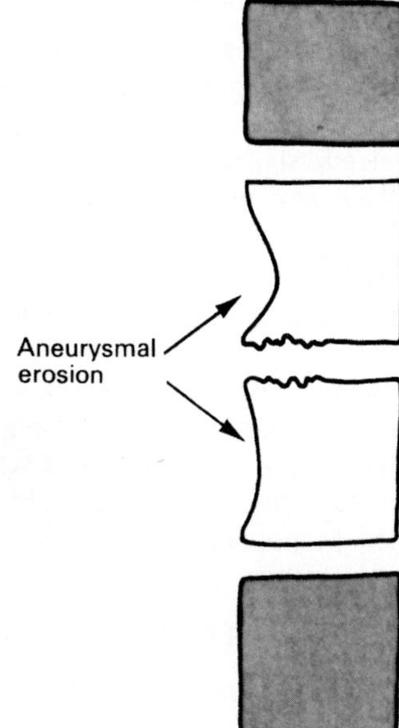

FIGURE 3-15 • When an abscess forms on the anterior surface of the vertebral column, the x-ray shows scalloping of the vertebral bodies. Because a similar type of scalloping is seen with abdominal aneurysms, this radiologic lesion is sometimes referred to as "aneurysmal erosion." (From Macnab I. *Backache.* Baltimore: Williams & Wilkins; 1977:27 with permission.)

3. The lesion is not only a space-occupying lesion in neurologic territory, but it is an abscess with a necrotic center that may not be reached by antibiotics.
4. The presence of paralysis for more than 36 hours usually results in either no functional recovery or death.

Surgery should proceed under appropriate antibiotic coverage once an organism is identified. Obviously, the goal of surgery is to evacuate the pus. As with any other spinal condition, the approach is dictated by the location of the pathology. If the pus is posterior, go posteriorly (laminectomy); if it is anterior, and confined to one segment in the conus or cord region, go anteriorly. If the pus is anterior in the cauda equina region (L2 and caudally), it is best to use a laminectomy approach. Pus spread over many segments will require a multisegmental decompression and/or catheter lavage of the site.

There is always the possibility that anterior destruction of the vertebral elements will lead to a deformity that will have to be corrected at a later date.

MISCELLANEOUS INFECTIONS OF THE SPINE

Uncommon Pyogenic Lesions

The spine may be involved by actinomycosis, typhoid, or brucellosis. Unlike other pyogenic infections, the vertebral body frequently shows a reactive sclerosis appearing like a white block on radiograph.

Fungal Infections

Fungi can establish growth within body tissue: mycotic osteomyelitis. The most common fungal infections seen are coccidioidomycosis and blastomycosis. The skeleton, however, is rarely involved except as part of a disseminated disease. From a clinical standpoint, it must be remembered that each one of these mycotic infections can mimic tuberculosis radiologically, again emphasizing the need for vertebral biopsy as an essential part of establishing the diagnosis and initiating appropriate treatment. Vertebral osteomyelitis may also rarely occur due to *Candida* species as a complication of candidemia, which is increasing as a nosocomial occurrence.

Parasitic Infections

Hydatid disease has been known as a clinical entity from ancient times. When bone involvement is present, the spine is also involved in approximately one fifth of patients. Diagnosis is difficult. Radiographs reveal lytic lesions in the vertebral body. Neurologic involvement occurs early and relentlessly progresses to an irreversible paraplegia. To date, it would appear that treatment fails to obtain any significant response.

Syphilis

The incidence of syphilitic bone and joint involvement decreased from 36% in 1900 to less than 0.5% in 1936, and this decline has been maintained. Charcot's arthropathy is the most common manifestation of syphilitic involvement of the vertebral column and is seen most frequently at the thoracolumbar junction. Although the lesion may be symptomless and detected solely by incidental radiographs, pain may arise when destructive and hypertrophic changes are marked. Similar changes may be seen with diabetes, although this is rare. Complete collapse of the vertebral column may occur with transection of the cord or cauda equina.

INTERVERTEBRAL DISC SPACE INFECTION

Disc space infections in adults most commonly occur following disc puncture, either at open surgery or closed percutaneous procedures, such as chemonucleolysis, discography, or percutaneous discectomy. The clinical picture is fairly characteristic. There is an initial relief of the preoperative sciatic pain after the procedure. Approximately 1 to 8 weeks later, severe backache occurs, with marked cramps of pain. The pain is described as being "excruciating" and is out of proportion to the objective findings.

There are very few constitutional symptoms, except in those patients who run a febrile course. If the ESR or CRP is elevated, it is useful in following the subsequent treatment program.

Radiographs do not show abnormality for approximately 4 or 6 weeks when, for the first time, narrowing of the disc space is revealed. This narrowing occurs much earlier than the anticipated narrowing subsequent to the physical act of discectomy and, of course, is much more marked. Later, irregularity and loss of definition of the vertebral endplates are noted, with subsequent vertebral destruction. More than half of the patients progress to disc space obliteration and interbody fusion. As with vertebral osteomyelitis, early diagnosis is facilitated by bone scanning (Fig. 3-16) and imaging with either CT or MRI.

Aspiration by needle biopsy is essential to establish a bacteriologic diagnosis in order that the lesion may be treated with appropriate antibiotics. The treatment, in essence, is the same as the treatment of pyogenic vertebral osteomyelitis.

TUMORS (NEOPLASMS)

The diagnosis of neoplasms of the vertebral column is largely dependent on radiographic examinations. This text is not intended as an atlas of lesions of the vertebral column, and no attempt is made here to describe the specific radiologic and histologic characteristics of the tumors that occur. An attempt is made to outline the principles of diagnosis and treatment. Benign neoplasms and primary malignancies in the vertebral column are rare. Secondary deposits are common.

BENIGN TUMORS

Benign tumors predominantly affect the generation younger than 30 years (8). Backache at the site of the lesion is the dominant symptom, and this may be associated with a painful scoliosis. Idiopathic scoliosis is rarely painful. When a patient presenting with a scoliosis complains of severe backache, remember the possibility of a benign tumor and examine its likelihood with detailed radiologic assessment.

Benign lesions usually occur in the posterior elements or accessory processes (except for giant cell tumor, eosinophilic granuloma, and hemangioma) and present two specific difficulties in

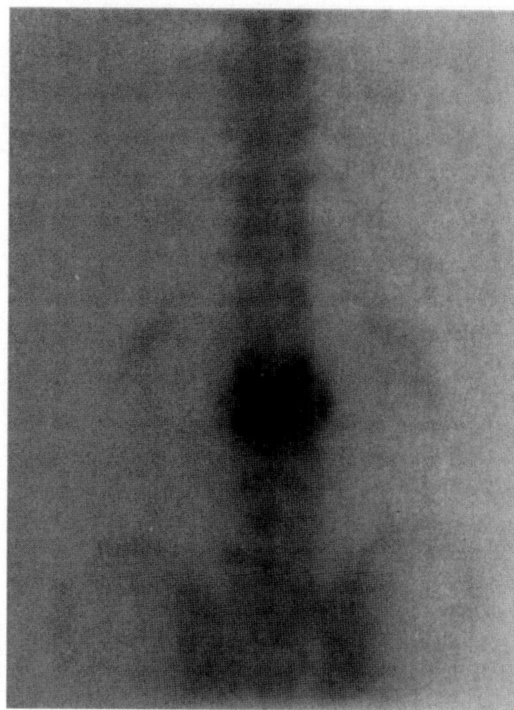

FIGURE 3-16 • A bone scan of an L2–3 discitis after surgery. Note how the increased tracer uptake is in adjacent portions of the L2 and L3 vertebral bodies.

evaluation and treatment. First, there is the difficulty in demonstrating the lesion on regular radiograph. When clinical suspicion is high but radiologic findings are equivocal, a technetium bone scan is useful. If the scan can localize the tumor and confirm a lesion, CT or MR imaging may be used to further define its exact site and characteristics. When the scan is negative, plain radiographs and the scan should be repeated after a 3-month interval if the clinical problem persists. Eventually, plain radiographs will show all benign lesions.

Second, benign lesions may be inaccessible for surgical removal. Fortunately, incomplete removal may be all that is necessary (except for giant cell tumor).

The following is a summary of the clinical features of the more commonly seen benign lesions.

Osteoid Osteoma

The classic clinical presentation is a gradual progressive backache, which is nonmechanical in nature and relieved by aspirin. The majority of the patients are men (2:1) and between 15 and 25 years of age. It can be said that backache in adolescents or young adults associated with marked paravertebral muscle spasm and the sudden onset of scoliosis warrants consideration of an osteoid osteoma. On radiograph, the small-sized lesion is most frequently seen to involve the posterior elements and is typically an area of dense sclerosis surrounding a central nidus (Fig. 3-17). On occasion, symptoms occur before it is possible to demonstrate the lesion on radiograph, at which time a single photon emission computed tomography scan or CT is necessary to establish the diagnosis. The rarity of the lesion and its elusive radiographic diagnosis often lead to erroneous diagnoses, such as psychogenic pain.

The pain from an osteoid osteoma may resolve spontaneously with symptomatic treatment. If this does not happen, treatment is a local excision of the tumor.

Pathology will show a nidus of immature osteoblasts, osteoid, and some blood with a surrounding margin of dense mature, lamellar bone.

Osteoblastoma

In contrast to all other primary neoplasms of bone, osteoblastoma manifests a most distinct predilection for the spine. Forty percent of all osteoblastomata are found in the spine, almost

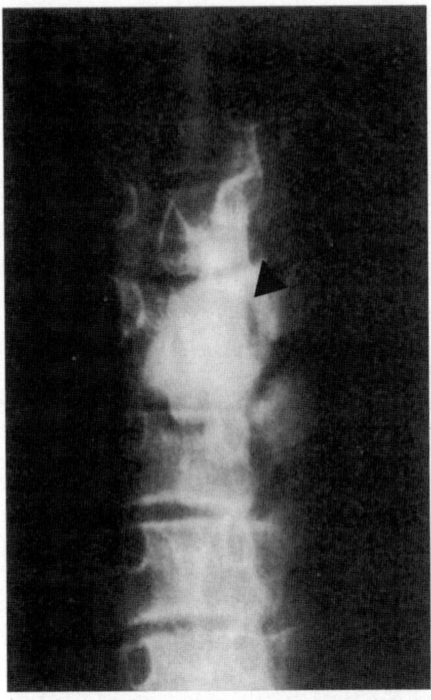

FIGURE 3-17 ● Osteoid osteoma *(arrow)* in a thoracic vertebral body.

invariably in the posterior elements of the lumbar spine and sacrum. The tumor is seen most commonly in boys and men, and 80% of the patients are younger than 30 years.

Insidious, low-grade back pain is always the presenting symptom, with some scoliosis being demonstrated in more than half of the patients. Because of the expansile nature of the tumor, many of the patients will present at examination some evidence of a neurologic irritation or compression. The tumor is larger than an osteoid osteoma and is often seen on plain radiograph (Fig. 3-18); if not, CT will make the diagnosis.

Treatment is by surgical excision, and even incomplete removal is compatible with complete symptomatic relief. The histology is often identical to osteoid osteoma, but at times the cells are atypical enough to confuse the lesion with osteogenic sarcoma, thus requiring an experienced pathologist for interpretation of the slide.

Medullary Bone Island

These radiologically demonstrated discrete osteosclerotic foci seen on radiographs (Fig. 3-19) are composed of normal compact bone. They have no clinical significance, but care must be taken not to confuse them with osteoblastic metastases.

Aneurysmal Bone Cyst

This tumor generally is first seen as a solitary expansile lesion involving the vertebra (8). Although the tumor is seen in all age groups, 90% of the patients are younger than 20 years. The clinical presentation is one of back pain with or without neurologic symptoms that develop as a result of the expansile nature of the tumor.

Radiographs reveal a destructive expansile lesion, usually in the posterior elements (Fig. 3-20). Cortical bone is destroyed, but the periosteum is able to maintain a reactive rim of bone surrounding the lesion. It is the only benign lesion that may extend across a disc space to involve an adjacent vertebral element.

Treatment is by excision, with spinal fusion often unnecessary because posterior element excision may be limited. The operative procedure can be associated with a significant blood loss for which the surgical team should be prepared.

Histology reveals vascular lakes surrounded by reactive fibrous tissue with numerous giant cells and hemosiderin pigmentation.

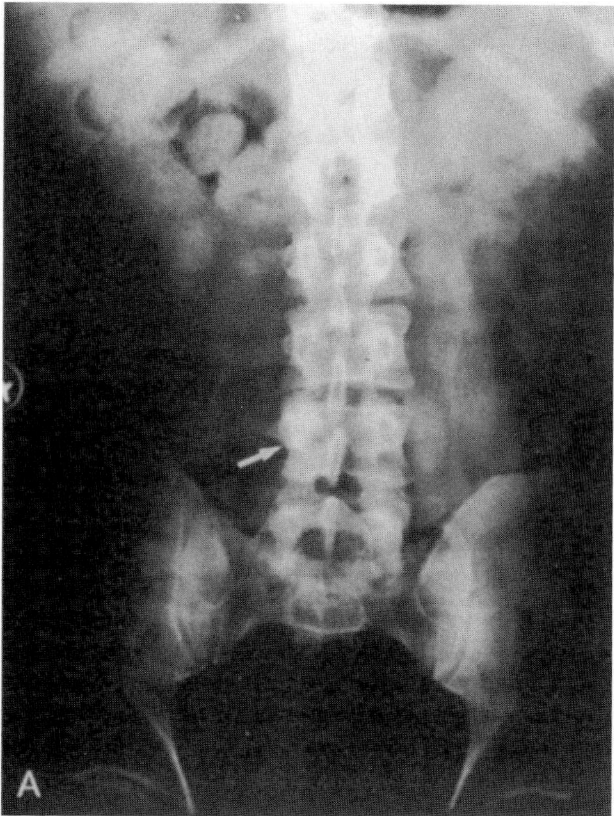

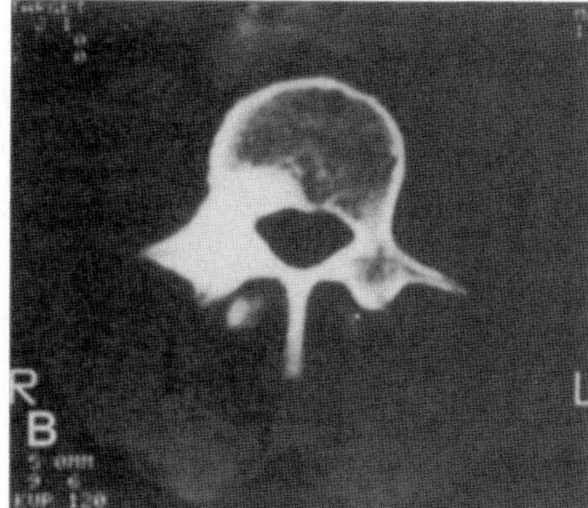

FIGURE 3-18 • Osteoblastoma. **A:** Plain anteroposterior (AP) x-ray showing a sclerotic pedicle, L4, right *(arrow)*. **B:** Axial computed tomography (CT) showing lesion in pedicle.

Hemangioma

Characteristically, on radiograph, the affected vertebra demonstrates linear striations that give rise to a corduroy cloth or honeycomb appearance (Fig. 3-21). This radiologic finding can be demonstrated in nearly 12% of all vertebral columns, with the incidence increasing with age (8). The incidence in the backache population is no greater, which emphasizes the fact that the mere demonstration of a hemangioma of a vertebral body on radiograph does not indicate that the source of the patient's backache has been found.

Treatment is simply observation. In a few patients with constant disabling pain, local radiotherapy may sometimes relieve the symptoms, but the risk of malignant degeneration makes this treatment less desirable. On the rare occasion that neurologic compromise necessitates surgical intervention, embolization, followed by surgical excision, may be done. Surgery, and its attendant bleeding, carries with it a high morbidity, and even mortality, and should not be undertaken lightly.

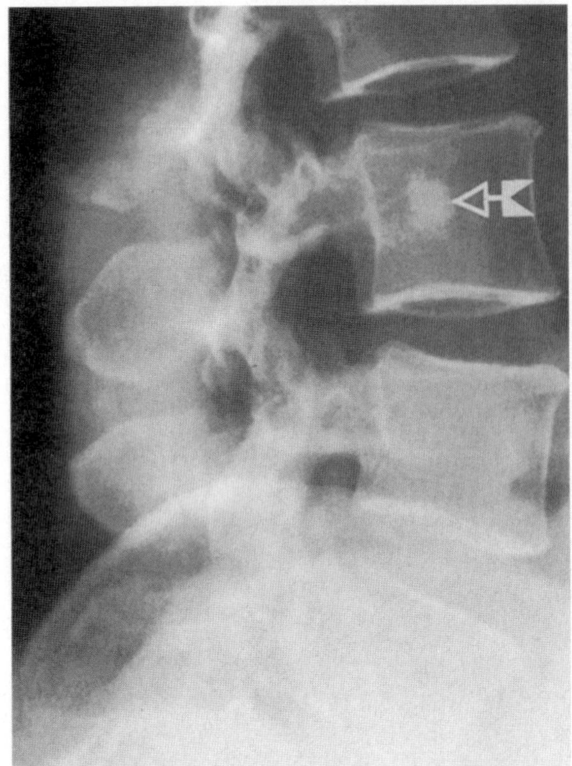

FIGURE 3-19 ● A medullary bone island in the body of L3 *(arrow).*

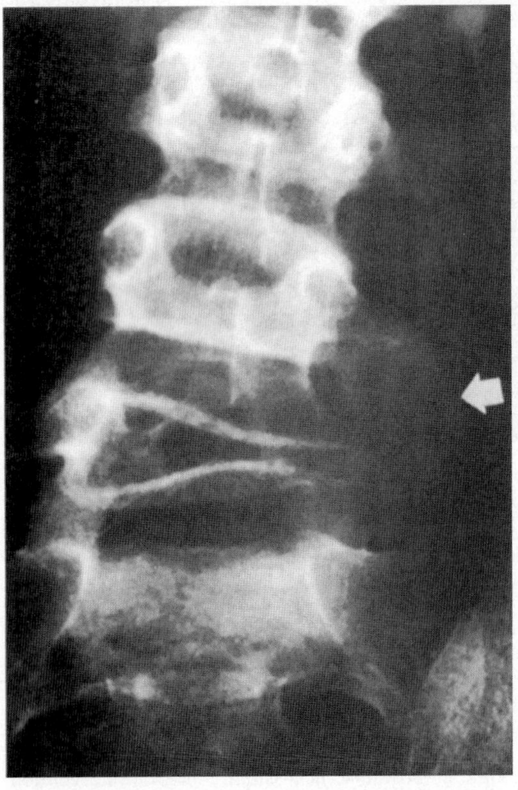

FIGURE 3-20 ● Aneurysmal bone cyst (ABC) in the body of L5. The *arrow* points to the expanding margin of the lesion.

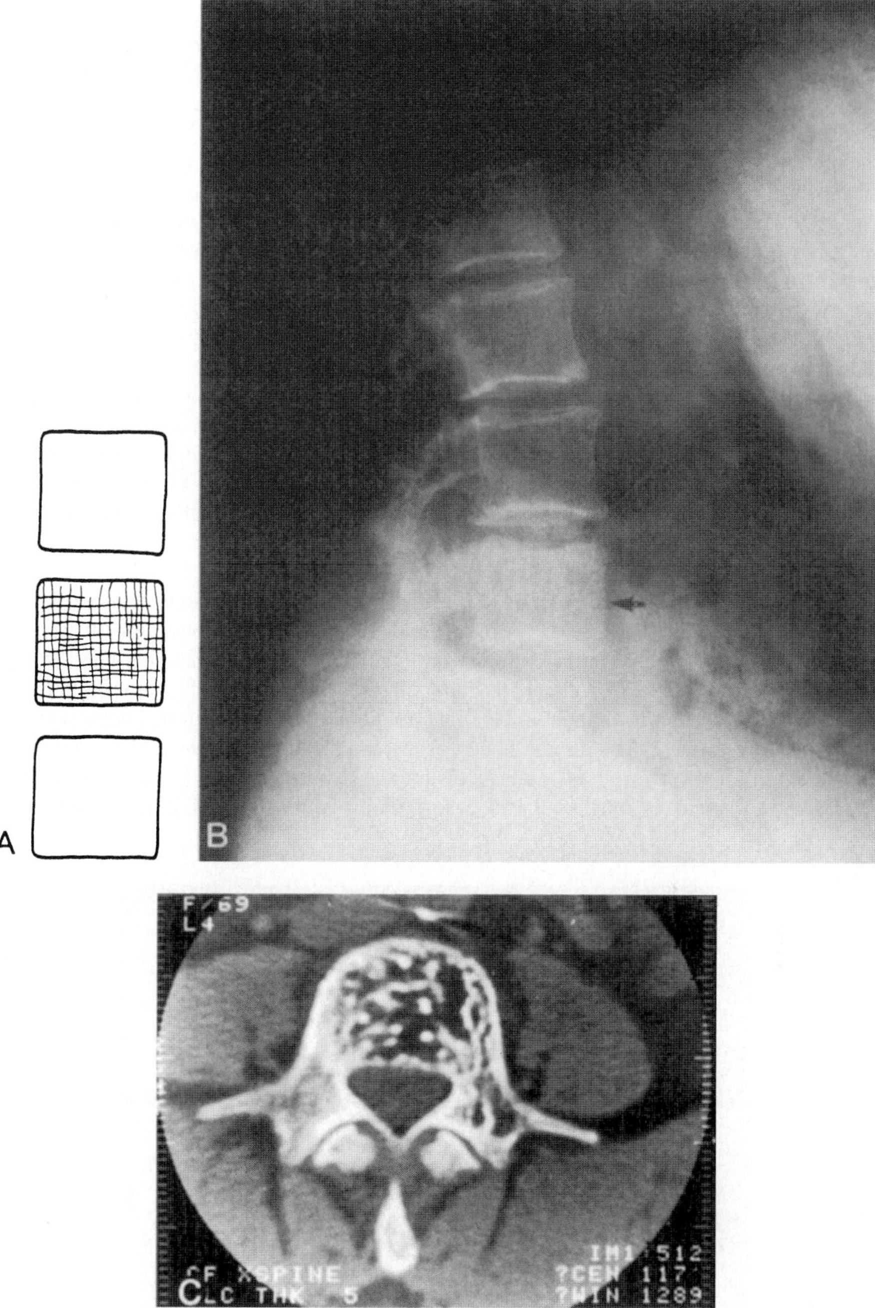

FIGURE 3-21 ● **A:** Diagram to show the characteristic x-ray appearance of the so-called hemangioma of the vertebral body. The vertical and horizontal trabeculae are accentuated giving a corduroy cloth or honey-combed appearance. **B:** Hemangioma on plain x-ray (L4) *(arrow).* **C:** Computed tomography (CT) of hemangioma. (From Macnab I. *Backache.* Baltimore: Williams & Wilkins; 1977:31 with permission.)

Giant Cell Tumor

Although giant cell tumor is a relatively common benign tumor of long bones (most common on either side of the knee joint), it is relatively rare in the spine. When it does occur in the spine, it is most common in the sacrum and more prevalent in the female patient, tending to occur in an individual a little older than one with osteoid osteoma or osteoblastoma.

The clinical presentation is no different from other benign lesions discussed and includes pain with occasional neurologic compromise.

Although the lesion is not commonly malignant, it is certainly more malevolent than benign. From the moment the lytic, expansile lesion with little cortical reaction is seen on MRI (Fig. 3-22), the chase is on—with laboratory tests and pathology examination—to separate it from malignant lesions. All laboratory test results will be normal, and pathologic examination will reveal multiple giant cells. These cells can be confused with aneurysmal bone cysts and brown tumor of hyperparathyroidism.

Treatment requires aggressive total excision of the tumor. Unfortunately, some of the lesions in the sacrum cannot be totally excised because of size and location. Radiotherapy used for these patients has the possibility of increasing the chances of malignant transformation. Of all the benign tumors of the spine, giant cell tumor is the most difficult to treat, and if it is not treated aggressively (12), it will quickly change its behavior to a more aggressive and, eventually, malignant lesion.

Eosinophilic Granuloma

This condition is a proliferative disorder of histiocytes. Vertebral involvement occurs early as a lytic lesion and subsequently as a variable degree of compression of a vertebral body, without any evidence of an adjacent soft tissue mass. In the extreme form, the vertebra is flattened to a thin disc, the so-called vertebra plana (Fig. 3-23). This spontaneous collapse of the vertebral body in children was first described by Calve (3). It was thought to be a manifestation of osteochondritis juvenilis and is still referred to as Calve disease. The disease is part of the complex of histiocytosis X disorders, which includes the more sinister forms of multiple histiocytic deposits in Hand-Schüller-Christian and Letterer-Siwe diseases. As long as the disease remains monostotic, it is the benign form of

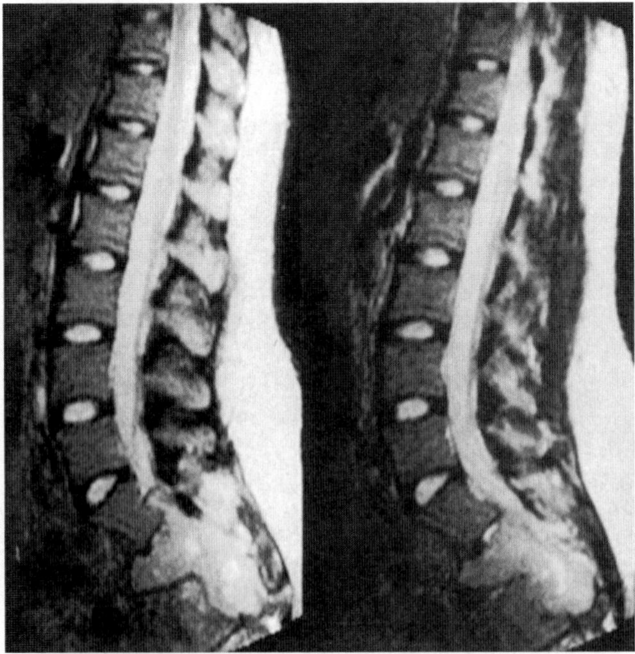

FIGURE 3-22 ● A giant cell tumor is replacing most of the sacrum on magnetic resonance imaging (MRI) (a T2-weighted sagittal: two contiguous sagittal slices).

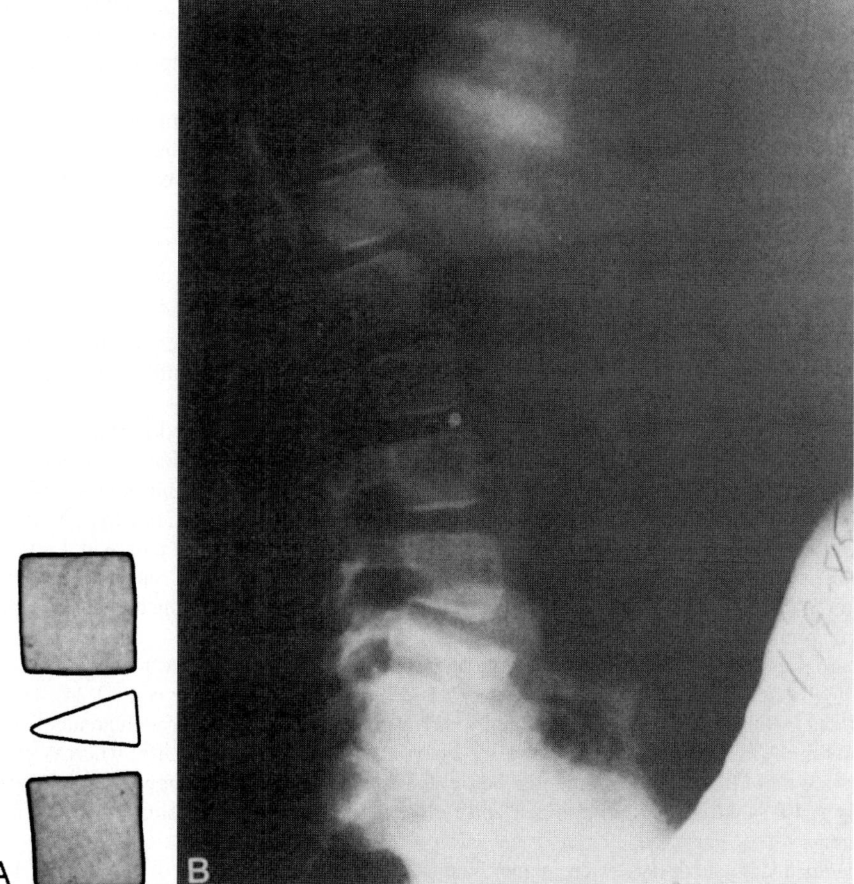

FIGURE 3-23 • **A:** Wedging of the vertebral body associated with Calve disease. (From Macnab I. *Backache*. Baltimore: Williams & Wilkins; 1977 with permission.) **B:** Eosinophilic granuloma, vertebra plana, L5.

eosinophilic granuloma. If a biopsy is performed, the eosinophils may be mistaken for neutrophils, and the diagnosis of osteomyelitis is made; likewise, the phagocytic histiocytes may be erroneously confused with Hodgkin disease.

The prognosis for the solitary lesion is excellent, and no treatment is necessary. A word of caution: Any secondary deposit may cause wedging of a vertebral body, and this possibility must be considered carefully before making the diagnosis of Calve disease.

MALIGNANT TUMORS

Malignant lesions, primary or secondary, are largely afflictions of persons older than 40 years; the incidence of malignant lesions increases with age. The tumors almost invariably involve the body, if primary, and the junction of the body and posterior elements, if secondary.

Backache is the presenting symptom, although neurologic manifestations may arise not only from the expansile lesion but also from vertebral collapse and direct extradural extension. Early in the natural history of the disease, the lesion may not be demonstrated on radiograph. It must be remembered that 30% of the cortex of a bone must be destroyed before a lesion is radiologically evident. When routine radiographs fail to demonstrate any abnormality, a bone scan can be of value in defining the presence of the lesion and the extent of spinal involvement. CT and MR imaging are more sensitive in detecting these lesions before plain radiographic changes occur.

The concept of "disease extent" is critical in the treatment of spinal malignancies. Solitary metastatic lesions have a better prognosis for survival and warrant an active search for the primary lesion, with aggressive surgical or radiotherapeutic measures being applied to the secondary lesions.

The laboratory findings, such as alterations in the blood levels of calcium, phosphorus, alkaline and acid phosphatases, and globulins, may suggest malignant disease and can, on occasion, identify entities such as myeloma. Final confirmation of the nature of the lesion may require percutaneous or open biopsy.

Primary Malignant Tumors

Although primary malignant lesions are rare, the following may be seen.

Chordoma. This is a slowly developing, locally invasive and destructive tumor originating from remnants of notochordal tissue, with a distinct predilection for the midline position at either end of the spinal column.

This lesion is uncommon before the age of 30 years and is found more often in men. It is interesting that, although the tumor is locally aggressive with a 10% incidence of metastases, the symptoms are frequently of long duration; the average length of back pain before diagnosis is commonly more than 1 year. Pain in the lower back, sacrum, and coccyx are early and persistent symptoms. Characteristically, as with all tumors of the spinal column, the pain is not relieved by recumbency. As the tumor encroaches on the sacral foramina, neuropathies and bowel and bladder symptoms appear. Neurologic involvement is usually later in the natural history of the tumor. A rectal examination is very helpful in diagnosing this tumor.

Radiographs reveal a large lytic lesion of the sacrum, with a large soft tissue mass almost indistinguishable from the radiographic appearance of a giant cell tumor (Fig. 3-24). However, chordoma is slightly more common in men, whereas giant cell tumors occur with greater frequency in women. A chordoma is not seen until well beyond the third decade of life, whereas giant cell tumors are more frequently encountered before the age of 30 years. A giant cell tumor progresses usually more rapidly than a chordoma, and unlike a chordoma may be situated away from the midline.

Therapeutically, both lesions present problems. Total excision is the goal of any surgery, because the rate of recurrence is very high.

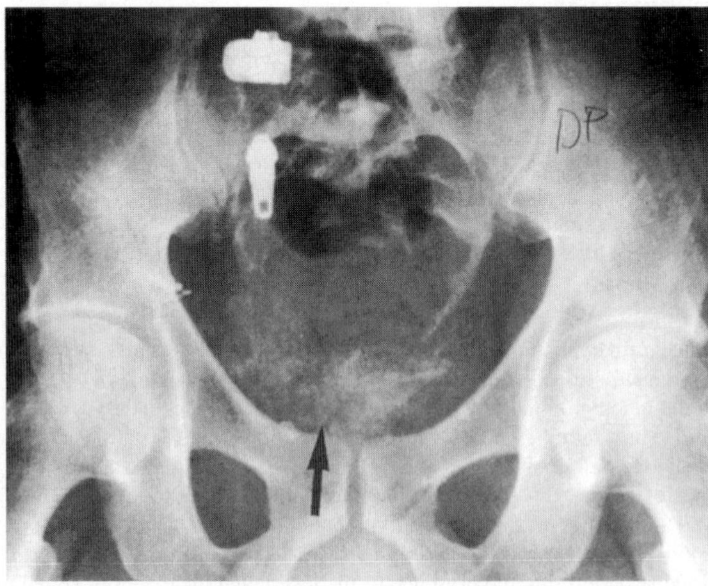

FIGURE 3-24 ● A chordoma on plain radiograph completely replaces the lower half of the sacrum *(arrow).*

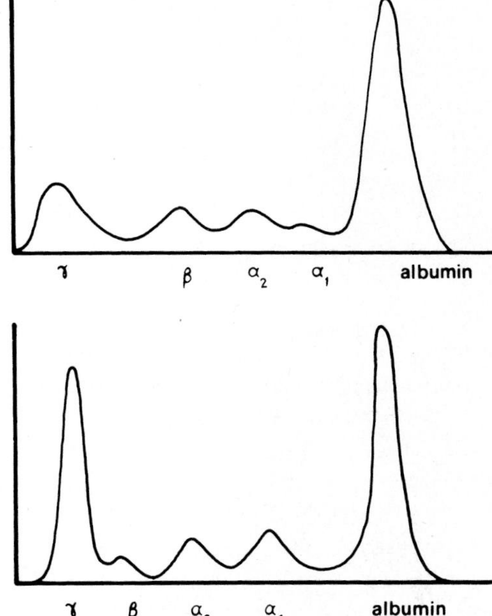

FIGURE 3-25 • **Top:** A normal serum protein electrophoresis (SPEP). **Bottom:** SPEP in multiple myeloma showing a spike in the gamma region.

Sacral tumors in the upper sacral segments can be removed by a combined abdominal and sacral approach. This excision will leave satisfactory anal and bladder sphincter function. Those tumors in the lower sacral segments can be removed posteriorly.

Myeloma. This is the most common primary malignant tumor of the spine. It is a malignant tumor of plasma cells that produce immunoglobulins and antibodies. The disseminated form of myeloma is uncommon before the age of 50 years and is more often seen in men. Clinically, backache, weakness, weight loss, and other constitutional symptoms occur in nearly every patient with the generalized disease. The onset of pain may be sudden and is usually produced by the occurrence of a pathologic fracture.

The ESR is consistently elevated and is usually greater than 50 mm/hour. Almost all of these patients are very anemic. Laboratory investigations may also reveal nonspecific, minor hypercalcemia; hyperuricemia; and an elevation in the alkaline phosphatase level. Characteristically, the disease is associated with abnormal protein levels, which are best demonstrated by serum protein electrophoresis (Fig. 3-25). Bence Jones proteinuria may be demonstrated in approximately 50% of the cases. Generally, when the globulins are normal, the albumin is normal. The albumin decreases when the globulins are elevated, which reflects damage to the renal tubules.

On radiographs, the solitary lesions are purely lytic (Fig. 3-26) and do not show any attempt at regeneration of bone, a fact that renders bone scans negative in a high percentage of cases. The disseminated form frequently shows nothing more than a diffuse osteopenia with or without vertebral body crush. Bone marrow and lesion biopsy are the basis of investigation and will reveal many plasma cells.

Treatment of solitary plasmacytoma lesions is predicated on preservation of spinal stability and cord function. In the absence of gross spinal instability, management with radiotherapy and chemotherapy is probably the best mode of treatment. Spinal instability may require excision of the lesion and bypass bone grafting.

Cord impairment makes decompression mandatory. Depending on the number of segments affected and the type of encroachment on the cord, decompression may have to be performed either anteriorly or posteriorly. Because the neurologic encroachment is coming from an anterior direction, the anterior approach to decompression, if feasible, is the preferred approach. This may seem to be excessive surgery for a malignant lesion, but it should be remembered that solitary lesions have a 5-year survival rate of approximately 60%.

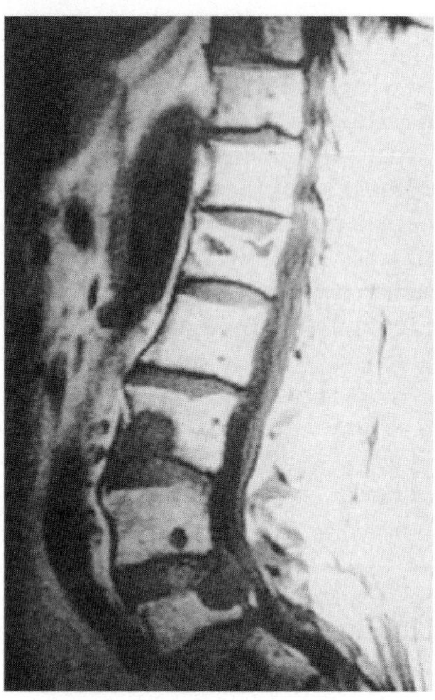

FIGURE 3-26 ● Magnetic resonance imaging (MRI) of multiple sites of myeloma involvement of the lumbar spine (T1).

Other malignant tumors include chondrosarcoma, osteosarcoma, Ewing sarcoma, fibrosarcoma, and lymphoma. They are not unlike any other malignant tumor, and patients present with pain and sometimes neurologic involvement. Treatment depends on cell type and location; most patients with malignant tumors have a poor prognosis.

Metastatic tumors. The spine is the most common site of metastatic spread in the skeleton, and the lumbar vertebrae are the most frequently involved (15). The radiographs of the spine may be normal inasmuch as 30% cortical mass of a bone must be destroyed before a lesion is radiologically apparent. In autopsy specimens, only 15% of grossly affected vertebrae demonstrate recognizable lesions when the excised specimen is radiographed.

Most lesions in the vertebrae are osteolytic. Markedly osteolytic metastases are seen with hypernephroma and thyroid and large bowel carcinoma. Breast, prostate, and lung tumors may produce osteoblastic (increased bone density) metastases. Remember, both renal cell carcinoma and multiple myeloma might be silent when a bone scan is performed, which necessitates a skeletal survey.

Back pain due to spinal metastases may be the presenting finding in approximately 25% of patients suffering from malignant lesions. Any patient older than 50 years who presents with a history of low back pain of sudden onset without provocative trauma, unrelieved by bed rest, and associated with sudden cramps of pain and a significantly elevated ESR should be suspected of suffering from a secondary deposit in the spine unless proved otherwise. The concern is even greater if the patient has a previous history of a malignant lesion.

The radiographs may be normal, or the changes may indeed be minimal. A careful examination of the anteroposterior view of the spine may show the absence of one pedicle, the "winking owl sign" (Fig. 3-27).

When destructive lesions of the vertebral bodies are demonstrated, it is important to distinguish between neoplasms and infections. As a general rule, it may be said that the disc space is involved when infections occur and spared when neoplasms occur (Fig. 3-12). Occasionally, despite a clinical picture that is highly suggestive of secondary deposits in the spine, the only abnormality at radiographic examination is a diffuse osteoporosis of the vertebral column with or without a minor vertebral body crush. In such a patient, a disciplined use of laboratory findings followed, when indicated, by a bone scan and trephine biopsy is necessary to establish the diagnosis and define treatment.

In those patients in whom radiographs show a destructive vertebral lesion irrefutably due to a secondary malignant deposit and in whom there is no evidence of the site of the primary lesion, it is

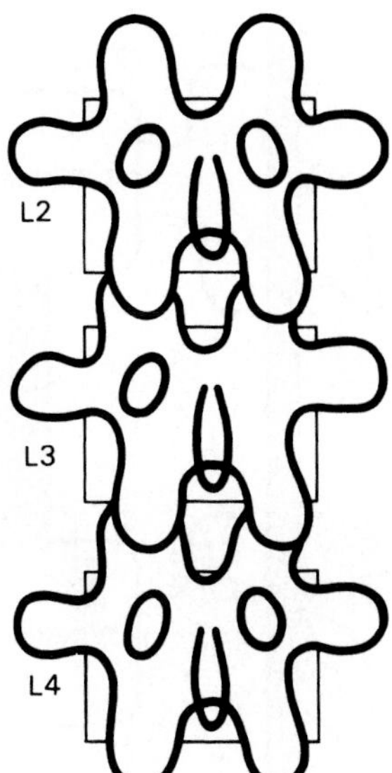

FIGURE 3-27 • Absence of one pedicle (the third lumbar vertebra depicted in this diagram) is often the first and only sign of a secondary deposit in the lumbar spine. The x-ray appearance is sometimes referred to as the "winking owl sign." (From Macnab I. *Backache.* Baltimore: Williams & Wilkins; 1977:36 with permission.)

routine to perform a biopsy. But remember that the cell morphology in the secondary deposit is frequently so altered as to make it almost impossible to diagnose more specifically than "adenocarcinoma" or "epithelial tumor." However, the surgeon has to accept the fact that on occasion a specific diagnosis can be made, such as an unsuspected myeloma or a lymphoma. Under such circumstances, more specific modes of therapy can be instituted, depending on whether the lesion is hormone dependent or chemically controllable. The disease in such patients may run a slow course, and in certain instances, the surgeon might be justified in carrying out a biologic stabilization with a bone graft.

On the other hand, when the prognosis is extremely grave in a patient whose general health is deteriorating, the debilitating pain can be humanely controlled by "grouting" the spine with methyl methacrylate (bone cement). The pain relief obtained by such means can, on occasion, be very gratifying, and the procedure, therefore, is justifiable despite the unremitting, relentless, and often rapid progress of the lesion.

More than one quarter of patients with spinal metastases present with neurologic dysfunction. For tumors that frequently run a long clinical course, this is a disastrous complication. The prognosis is related to the following factors: (a) The level of neurologic dysfunction: More than 80% of tumors producing neurologic defects occur at the thoracic cord level. The more proximal the level of cord involvement, the poorer the prognosis. (b) Duration of neurologic dysfunction: As a rule, the longer the signs are present, the worse the prognosis. (c) The onset of neurologic signs: The more rapid the onset, the less favorable the prognosis. (d) Sphincter involvement: Sphincter involvement is indicative of an extremely poor prognosis.

It can be generally said that two thirds of patients who undergo operation for partial neurologic defects can maintain their preoperative status. One third of those who are unable to walk before the operation can once again, for a period of time, get up and around. This improved prognosis has come about by the use of the anterior approach to remove the affected vertebrae (vertebrectomy). (Fig. 3-28). The less reliable laminectomy, or posterior decompression, for masses that encroach on neurologic tissue anteriorly, has largely been abandoned.

The timing of the decompression is of importance, and it appears that if a decompression is indicated, it must be carried out as an emergency procedure if any measure of recovery is to be expected. The surgical decompression must be performed with the meticulous technique used in the decompression of acute traumatic lesions. Careless handling of the cord can convert a partial lesion into a complete lesion.

The management of metastatic spine lesions ranges from the simple to the complex. Experience, personal philosophy, and the patient are, at times, the only guides to this type of lesion, the most difficult of orthopedic problems.

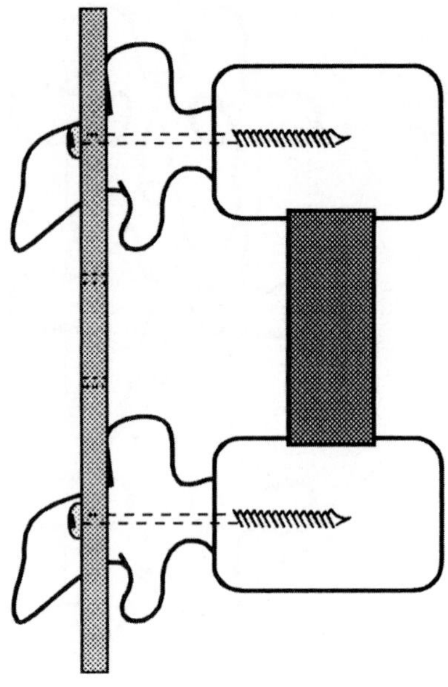

FIGURE 3-28 ● The vertebra has been removed, and a bone graft is substituted and held into place by pedicle screws and plates.

METABOLIC BONE DISEASE: OSTEOPOROSIS

There are many metabolic bone diseases, but in the adult, the most common by far is osteoporosis (9,10). The dynamic model of bone mass is founded on a balance between bone deposition and bone resorption. In osteoporosis, bone resorption is more extensive than bone deposition. The major impact of decreased bone mass is on thin cancellous bone (increased porosity of trabeculae) more than cortical bone (decreased cortical thickness), which weakens skeletal structures to the point where fractures occur with minimal trauma. The susceptible areas are the femoral neck, radius, ribs, and axial skeleton. Osteoporosis affects the axial skeleton through the occurrences of microfractures or gross fractures, which cause back pain (5).

Osteoporosis may be considered as primary or secondary (Table 3-3). Primary osteoporosis is classified into postmenopausal (Type I), senile (Type II), and idiopathic (juvenile or adult).

POSTMENOPAUSAL OSTEOPOROSIS

This is obviously a condition affecting women after menopause (50+ years). It affects 15 to 20 million Americans, resulting in 1.5 million fractures per year.

Although all women, and a few men, are susceptible to osteoporosis, there are very definite risk factors that increase the severity and consequences of osteoporosis (Table 3-4). The effect is primarily on trabecular bone, and the resulting fractures are predominantly to the vertebrae and distal radius.

SENILE OSTEOPOROSIS

Senile osteoporosis decreases both trabecular and cortical bone mass. It affects both sexes who are 70 years of age or older, but the incidence is higher in women compared with men (2:1). Add the effects of senile osteoporosis to postmenopausal osteoporosis, and older women are very vulnerable to fractures.

IDIOPATHIC OSTEOPOROSIS

Idiopathic juvenile osteoporosis is a rare condition affecting children between the ages of 8 and 12. It runs a 2- or 3-year course and then regresses spontaneously. Idiopathic osteoporosis of adults is more common in men. It usually becomes clinically evident at 40 years of age, and the symptoms may persist for 5 to 10 years. The causes of secondary osteoporosis are legion (Table 3-3).

TABLE 3-3

A General Classification of Osteoporosis

Regional	Disuse (immobilization) Post-traumatic osteodystrophy Migratory Inflammatory
General	
Congenital	Osteogenesis imperfecta Homocystinuria
Acquired Primary	Postmenopausal (Type I) Senile (Type II) Idiopathic (adult or juvenile)
Acquired	
Secondary	Nutritional Poor Ca^{2+} intake Poor Ca^{2+} absorption Endocrine Hyperthyroidism (thyrotoxicosis) Hyperadrenocorticism (endogenous or exogenous) Acromegaly Hypogonadism Prolonged use of steroids Neoplastic Multiple myeloma and leukemia Bone metastases Hormone-producing tumors Myeloproliferative Sickle cell anemia Thalassemia
Drug induced	Heparin Anticonvulsants
Compound	Associated with hyperparathyroidism and some cases of osteomalacia

TABLE 3-4

Factors Increasing Risks of Osteoporosis

Females > Males (4:1)
Caucasians and Asians
Small body size
Positive family history
Surgically initiated estrogen deficiency (oophorectomy)
Lifestyle factors: Smoking
Alcohol consumption
Coffee (excessive)
Decreased physical exercise
Poor nutrition

Cause

In postmenopausal and senile osteoporosis, although both formation and resorption of bone are diminished, the rate of resorption exceeds the rate of formation. Many theories have been expounded to explain this curious phenomenon. It has been postulated that estrogen deficiency renders one more susceptible to the action of parathyroid hormone. Predictably, it has been suggested that a long-standing calcium deficiency in the diet leads to secondary hyperparathyroidism and bone resorption. Finally, lack of exercise in the older patient is said to be a contributing cause.

Clinical

The presenting symptom of vertebral osteoporosis is backache. The pain is spondylogenic in nature, being aggravated by general and specific activities and relieved to some extent, but not completely, by recumbency.

The pain has been ascribed to trabecular buckling or fractures. This is an untenable hypothesis in view of the fact that trephine biopsies of the vertebral bodies can be performed painlessly. When considering the cause of pain, it must be remembered that, although the bone mass has been markedly diminished, the size of the vertebral body remains the same. If the quantity of bone has been decreased, the other contents of the vertebral body must increase: the marrow, the fat, and the blood lakes. The fat content of an osteoporotic vertebral body does not increase primarily. Therefore, it must be presumed that the volume of the blood lakes must be greater. This implies venous stasis. The intraosseus venous pressure of a normal vertebra is approximately 28 mm Hg. The intraosseous venous pressure of an osteoporotic vertebral body is approximately 40 mm Hg. It is known that intraosseous venous stasis is seen in juxta-articular bone in osteoarthritis and that this is reversed after osteotomy. The decrease in venous pressure after osteotomy and forage of the hip joint for osteoarthritis probably accounts for the relief of pain experienced in the immediate postoperative period. It is probable that venous stasis in the vertebral bodies plays a significant role in the production of the dull, nagging, constant, boring pain about which these patients so commonly complain.

Although trabecular fractures do not play a role in the reproduction of symptoms, crush fractures of a vertebral body are common and are associated with the sudden onset of severe pain.

Fractures of the vertebral column are usually first noted in the thoracic region. Involvement of several upper thoracic vertebral bodies over a course of time may produce an increasing kyphosis, sometimes referred to as a "dowager's hump." Fractures in the upper thoracic spine may occur without a significant increase in discomfort, because of the support afforded by the rib cage; however, when crush fractures involve the lower thoracic or upper lumbar vertebrae (the usual location), severe pain may result.

Characteristically, the pain has a wide referral over the back and is not localized to the fracture level. This is probably due to widespread muscle spasm.

At physical examination, it is usual to locate the acutely fractured vertebrae with local pressure or percussion on the spinous process. Neurologic changes (radicular or myelopathic) are not present, and if so should alert you to some other cause, such as osteoporosis secondary to multiple myeloma.

The patient, then, will present with the history of a grumbling debilitating back pain punctuated on occasion with one or more episodes of severe incapacitating pain. These episodes of severe pain are usually initiated by some minor mechanical event, such as a slip or lifting. When the history is prolonged, the patients may also relate progressive loss of height and rounding of the upper thoracic spine. At examination, the thoracic kyphosis is noted, with a compensatory increase in the lumbar lordosis. If, over a period of time, the patient has sustained several vertebral crush fractures, the rib cage may come to rest on the iliac crest.

Radiograph

Radiographs of the spine show general loss of trabecular bone density and on closer inspection reveal lack of the horizontally disposed trabeculae. There may be ballooning of the discs into the vertebrae, which results in a fishtail appearance of the vertebral bodies. Compression fractures and endplate fractures are common (Fig. 3-1).

Secondary osteoporosis may produce an identical radiologic appearance, and it is important to exclude the possibility of systemic disease before making the diagnosis of primary osteoporosis.

TABLE 3-5

Hematologic and Biochemical Changes in Common Types of Osteoporosis

Change Factors	Osteoporosis	Osteomalacia	Hyperparathyroidism	Multiple Myeloma	Advanced Metastatic Disease
Hemogram				<10 g%	↓
ESR	No			↑↑↑	↑
BUN/CR	Abnormal			N↑	N↑
Calcium	Values	↓	↑	N↑	↑
Phosphorus		↓	N↓	↑	↓
Alkaline phosphatases	↑	↑	↑	↑	
Acid phosphatases					↑ (prostate)
Uric acid			N↑	↑	↑
Protein electrophoresis				M spike	globulin
Immunoelectrophoresis				M spike	N/ABN

ESR, erythrocyte sedimentation rate; BUN/CR, blood urea nitrogen/creatinine; N, normal; ABN, abnormal.

Laboratory

Idiopathic osteoporosis does not produce any changes in the blood chemistry. Osteomalacia and hyperparathyroidism specifically affect calcium and phosphorous metabolism. Bone activity is reflected by the elevated alkaline phosphatase level in both of these conditions. Multiple myeloma, which may be seen with back pain and a radiograph showing diffuse osteoporosis of the spine, is associated with significant changes in blood chemistry. There are alterations in the albumin and globulin ratios, and abnormal globulins can be detected. The ESR is raised, and frequently there is a significant anemia. The changes in blood chemistry of these various conditions are summarized in Table 3-5.

TABLE 3-6

Methods of Quantifying Osteoporosis

Method	Basis	Drawback
Trabecular index	Count number of trabeculae in volume of bone (usually done in femoral neck)	Difficult to standardize
Cortical thickness	Measure cortical thickness relative to overall width of bone (usually done on metacarpal shaft)	Only measures endosteal bone resorption in cortex; difficult to standardize
Dual energy x-ray absorptiometry (DEXA)	Quantitative radiographic measurement of bone mass	Measures cancellous bone of spine and femur
Quantitative computed tomography	Using standard scanner, comparison of density of an area of bone (vertebral trabeculae) with a "phantom" of vials containing varying analogue	Expensive and time restraints; site specific, that is, if measuring spine, it will not give reliable information about extent of bone loss in femoral neck
Neutron activation analysis	Only available in a few research centers	Not familiar

Measurement

Many attempts have been made to use radiographs to measure the extent of osteoporosis (Table 3-6). All such attempts have limitations and need to be applied and interpreted by someone familiar with the method. Because osteoporosis is such a slow dynamic event, it is also useful to repeat the test of choice over lengthy intervals to measure the progress of the disease and/or response to various treatment modalities.

The most widely used assessment method today is the dual energy x-ray absorptiometry (DEXA) scan. Using radiographic penetration, bone density in the lateral lumbar spine and proximal femur can be quickly assessed (10 to 20 minutes) with minimal radiation (less than 0.1 mrem) (Fig. 3-29). Reproducibility is sufficiently accurate to allow for serial studies in estimating calcium

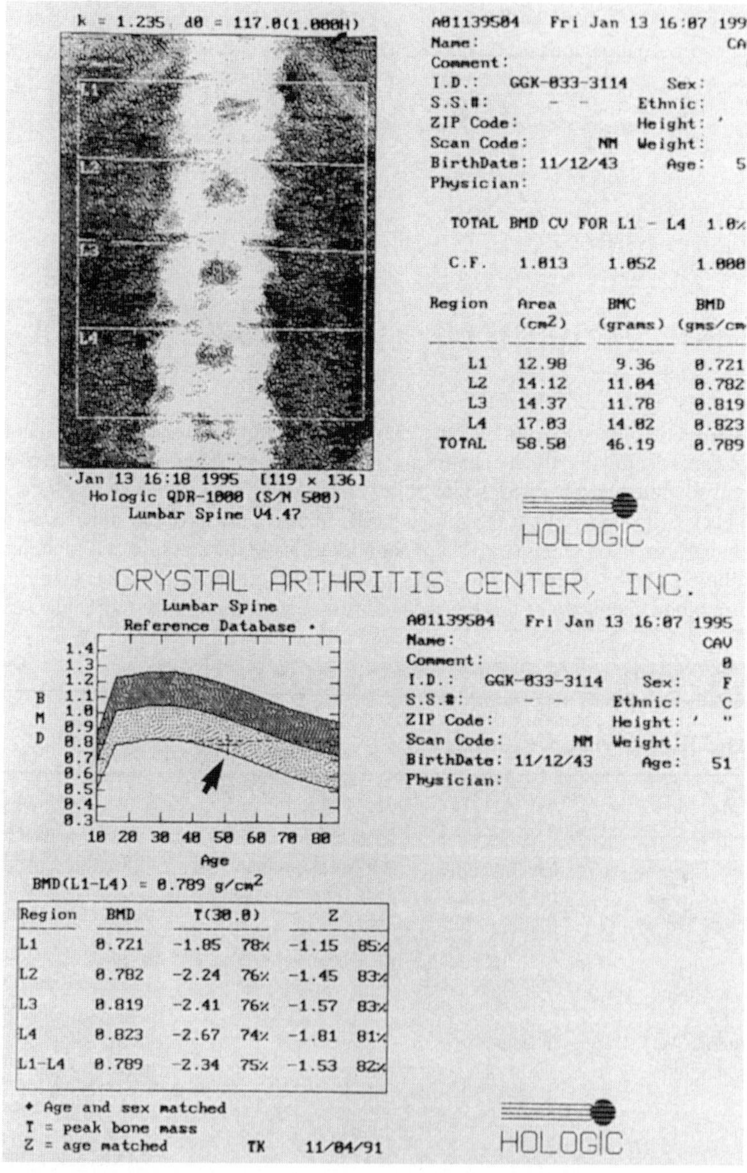

FIGURE 3-29 ● A dual energy x-ray absorptiometry scan of the lumbar spine. **Top:** Figure and table depict the bone mineral density (BMD), which is plotted (below) as an average (cross hairs [*arrow*]) compared with normal (heavy stippled area).

balance. The United Nations World Health Organization has published DEXA scan criteria for a diagnosis of osteopenia (1 to 2.4 standard deviations below the mean) and osteoporosis (≥2.5 standard deviations).

Treatment

The treatment of postmenopausal or senile osteoporosis is more encouraging than in previous years. There are now several medications available that have been shown to build bone in well-controlled clinical trials (2,10).

The risks of many therapeutic measures that are frequently advocated outweigh any possible advantage. Estrogens have been given for the treatment of this condition; they are associated with the nuisance of withdrawal bleeding and the increased risk of endometrial or breast malignancy. Estrogen therapy does not reverse the calcium imbalance. Androgens and anabolic steroids are more likely to increase muscle bulk than bone bulk. The administration of fluorides is sometimes associated with some subjective improvement and an apparent, albeit slight, increase in bone density on radiograph. This may be an artifact occasioned by the fact that fluoride salts are more radiopaque. The side effects of fluorides (gastrointestinal upset, ulceration, and joint stiffness) have limited their usefulness.

Treatment can be divided into two phases.

Prevention. Any disease is best prevented. The treatment of osteoporosis should be directed at young women who are at risk and be designed to eliminate as many risk factors as possible (Table 3-4). The basis of prevention is threefold: hormonal substitute when osteoporosis risk is high (e.g., oophorectomy at a young age and menopause), adequate calcium intake (minimum 1,000 mg/day), and regular exercise. Other lifestyle changes such as elimination of excessive intake of alcohol and coffee should also be encouraged.

SUMMARY

This chapter has presented much information on trauma, tumors, infection, and osteoporosis. Obviously, the information is mainly of summary value, but it also serves as a reminder that when a patient presents with back pain, there are literally hundreds of diagnoses to consider.

REFERENCES

1. Batson OV. The function of the vertebral veins and their role in the spread of metastases. *Ann Surg.* 1940;112:138–142.
2. Bouxsein ML, Kaufman J, Tosi L, et al. Recommendations for optimal care of the fragility fracture patient to reduce the risk of future fracture. *J Am Acad Orthop Surg.* 2004;12:385–395.
3. Calve JA. Localized affection of spine suggesting osteochondritis of vertebral body, with clinical aspects of Pott's disease. *J Bone Joint Surg.* 1925;7:41–46.
4. Carmona R. *Bone health and osteoporosis: A report of the Surgeon General. United States Department of Health and Human Services.* U.S. Government Printing Office, Washington DC; 2004.
5. Cohen LD. Fractures in the osteoporotic spine. *Orthop Clin North Am.* 1990;21:143–150.
6. Coumans JV, Reinhardt MK, Lieberman IH. Kyphoplasty for vertebral compression fractures: 1-year clinical outcomes from a prospective study. *J Neurosurg.* 2003;99(1 suppl):44–50.
7. Garfin SR, Yuan HA, Reiley MA. New technologies in spine: kyphoplasty and vertebroplasty for the treatment of painful osteoporotic compression fractures. *Spine.* 2001;26:1511–1515.
8. Huvos AG. *Bone Tumors: Diagnosis, Treatment and Prognosis.* Toronto: WB Saunders; 1979.
9. Lane JM (ed). Symposium of metabolic bone disease. *Orthop Clin North Am.* 1985;15:596–790.
10. Lane JM, Garfin SR, Sherman PJ, Poynton AR. Medical management of osteoporosis. *Instr Course Lect.* 2003;52:785–789.
11. Lieberman IH, Dudeney S, Reinhardt MK, Bell G. Initial outcome and efficacy of "kyphoplasty" in the treatment of painful osteoporotic vertebral compression fractures. *Spine.* 2001;26:1631–1638.
12. Marcove RC, Weiss LD, Vaghaiwalls MD, et al. Cryosurgery in the treatment of giant cell tumors of the bone. *Cancer (Philadelphia).* 1978;41:957–969.
13. Modic MT, Feiglin DH, Piraino DW, et al. Vertebral osteomyelitis: assessment using MR. *Radiology.* 1985;157:157–166.
14. Rao R, Singrakhia M. Painful osteoporotic vertebral fracture: pathogenesis, evaluation, and roles of vertebroplasty and kyphoplasty in its management *Bone Joint Surg Am.* 2003;85:2010–2022.
15. Wong DA, Fornasier VL, Macnab I. Spinal metastases: the obvious, the occult and the impostors. *Spine* 1990;15:1–4.

CHAPTER 4

Spondylogenic Backache: Soft Tissue Lesions and Pain Mechanisms

"Knowledge of structure of the human body is the foundation on which all rational medicine and surgery is built."

—Mondini de Luzzi

By far, the most important soft tissue syndromes to be described in this chapter are lesions of the disc: disc degeneration with or without disc rupture, and the secondary phenomenon of root encroachment. But no discussion of soft tissue lesions would be complete without including "fibrositis" and "myofascial pain syndromes." When you read Chapter 10, you will note that these syndromes are included in the psychosomatic classification of nonorganic pain and have been given the descriptive term of "the orthopaedic ulcer."

The major factor that has clouded and confused the diagnosis of soft tissue lesions of the back is the phenomenon of referred pain (23). When a deep structure is irritated by trauma, disease, or the experimental injection of an irritating solution, the resultant pain may be experienced locally, referred distally, or experienced both locally and radiating to a distance. The classic example is the patient experiencing myocardial ischemic pain who may report discomfort, numbness, heaviness, and/or a sensation of swelling in the arm along with referred pain to other sites, such as the neck and jaw or the shoulder. It is important to recognize that tenderness may also be referred to a distance. The injection of hypertonic saline into the lumbosacral supraspinous ligament may give rise to pain radiating down the leg as far down as the calf, and the pain may also be associated with tender points commonly situated over the sacroiliac joint and the upper outer quadrant of the buttock (Fig. 4-1).

The complaint of pain and the demonstration of local tenderness may obscure the fact that the offending pathologic lesions are centrally placed and may lead the clinician to believe erroneously that the disease process underlies the site of the patient's complaints. This erroneous belief may apparently be confirmed by the temporary relief of pain on injection of local anesthetic into the site of the referred pain. These points must be borne in mind when the clinician considers soft tissue lesions giving rise to low back pain.

THE NEUROPHYSIOLOGY OF PAIN AND REFERRED PAIN

Pain is a complex neurophysiologic phenomenon, initiated peripherally, appreciated centrally, and in between modified by a complex relationship of fiber tracts (18). Chronic pain carries with it the burden of past experiences and emotional and socioeconomic reactions (18). Is it any wonder that scientists have not solved the puzzle of pain? Add to that the fact that patients cannot describe pain, and we have a foundation of quicksand on which to construct an understanding and treatment of one of the most common presenting complaints in medicine: low back pain.

Let us try to follow pain from its origin to a patient's response to the painful stimulus.

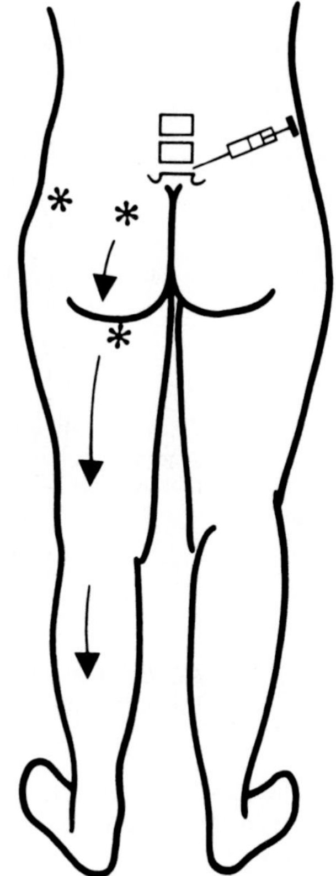

FIGURE 4-1 • The injection of hypertonic saline into the supraspinous ligament between L5 and S1 will give rise to local pain and pain referred down the back of the leg in sciatic distribution. In addition to this, there will be areas of tenderness produced in the lower limb most commonly at the sites noted by the asterisks. (From Macnab I. *Backache.* Baltimore: Williams & Wilkins; 1977:81 with permission.)

PERIPHERAL MODULATION

Step 1

Nerve endings of many different types (encapsulated or free nerve endings) detect the painful stimulus. These nerve endings that detect pain are known as nociceptors.

Step 2

The impulse message of pain travels through afferent sensory nerves in large (fast conduction myelinated A fibers) and smaller and slower conduction nonmyelinated C fibers.

Step 3

The dorsal ganglion (Fig. 4-2) contains the cell bodies for the conduction axons in Step 2. Here, a synapse occurs, and the messages continue on to the dorsal horn of the spinal cord. There is some consideration that a threshold of stimulus has to be reached before the impulse message of pain makes it through the synapse in the dorsal root-ganglion. This represents the first of the various gates that painful impulses have to traverse (23).

Step 4: The Dorsal Horn—The Gate

From the dorsal root-ganglion, impulses travel to the dorsal horn substantia gelatinosa (Fig. 4-3). This is where Wall and Melzack (23) have erected their primary gate construct. They have postulated the presence of a sorting-out center in the dorsal horns of the spinal cord. These sorting-out centers act to increase or decrease the flow of nerve impulses from the peripheral fibers to the central nervous system (CNS). How the gate behaves is determined by a complex interaction of distal afferent stimulation and descending influences from the brain. There is a critical level of pain information that arrives in the dorsal horn and that will stimulate and open the gate and allow for higher transmission (Fig. 4-3).

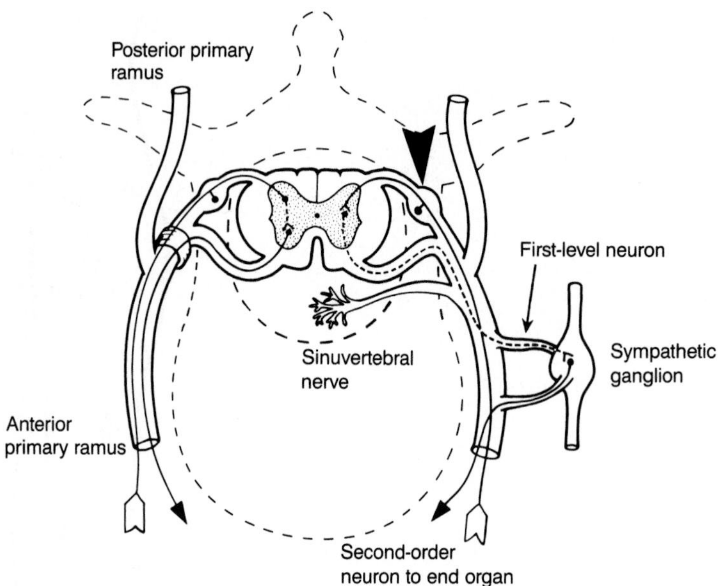

FIGURE 4-2 ● The proximal origins of the peripheral nerve fiber tracts. The dorsal root-ganglion is designated by the *arrowhead* on the right.

The dorsal (sensory) afferent fibers travel in the dorsal root entry zone for one or two segments before entering the dorsal horn (Fig. 4-3). The dorsal horn is made up of six lamina. Which lamina a sensory fiber synapses in is determined by the fiber size:

- C fibers terminate in laminae 1 and subsequently in lamina 2.
- A δ fibers terminate in laminae 2 and 5.

Like computers, these laminae simulate the information delivered, pass it back and forth, and receive descending modulation impulses. It is after this computerized analysis of the information that the pain impulses are ready for collection and discharge up the spinal cord pathways. This section of the dorsal horn is the gate center for pain modulation.

It is thought that activity in the nonmyelinated C fibers tends to inhibit transmission and thus closes the gate; conversely, small myelinated A δ-fiber activity facilitates transmission and opens the gate.

From a clinical point of view, trigger zones in the skin and muscle are postulated to keep the gate open. Anxieties, depression, life situation pressures, and past memories of pain can all serve to keep the gate open and increase the appreciation of pain. Local anesthetic/steroid trigger injections are used to negate this phenomenon. Likewise, transcutaneous electrical nerve stimulation

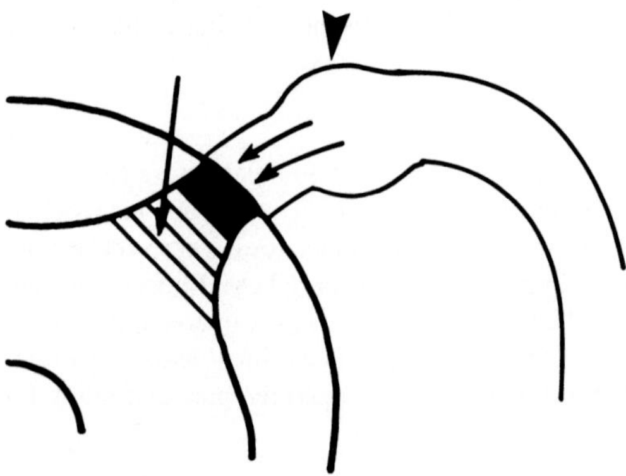

FIGURE 4-3 ● The gate control theory of pain: sensory fibers (*double arrows* and dorsal root-ganglion designated by *arrowhead*) arrive in lamina of dorsal horn. Higher centers *(single arrow)* influence whether or not "gate" opens for transmission of pain impulses to higher centers.

units are used to stimulate the C fibers and close the gate to transmission of pain impulse to higher centers. The most common "gate closers" are obviously analgesics.

Step 5: The Spinal Cord Tracts (Transmission Pathways)

Now, things really get complicated. What is known for sure is that, from the dorsal horn, pain fibers cross to the opposite side to ascend in the spinothalamic tract (Fig. 4-4).

Within the human spinal cord, there are approximately five ascending pathways for the pain impulses:

1. Spinothalamic tract
2. Spinoreticular tract
3. Spinomesencephalic tract
4. Spinocervical tract
5. Second-order dorsal column tract

These tracts are not independent pathways to higher centers but, instead, have many cross-connections. In fact, the spinoreticular and spinomesencephalic tracts are considered one and the same by some neurobiologists (8). They are probably "brainstem" tracts, carrying an altering message to the reticular formation that pain is something with which the body is going to have to contend. These tracts end in the brainstem reticular zones of the medulla and pons.

The last two listed tracts are more theoretical than real and are simply mentioned for completeness.

By far, the most important afferent pain pathway is the lateral spinothalamic tract, which is located in the anterolateral column of the cord and carries crossed pain fibers from the contralateral side of the body. After the afferent fibers leave the dorsal horn gray matter zone, they cross the midline to enter the spinothalamic tract. More caudal fibers are displaced laterally as more cephalad fibers enter the tract from the opposite side (Fig. 4-5).

Pathways for temperature sense travel in close association with the lateral spinothalamic tract. It is the lateral spinothalamic tract that is transected during percutaneous cordotomy for the control of pain.

Step 6: The Higher Centers

Higher centers for receipt of pain fibers. As higher levels in the CNS are observed, the discrete sensory tract blends into many other CNS pathways. To say exactly where every pain pathway goes at this higher level is impossible. Only the most basic concepts are mentioned here:

1. Fibers from the spinothalamic tract go to the thalamus, from whence they are distributed to many higher centers.
2. Other afferent sensory tracts end in the brainstem reticular formation.
3. Fibers from the thalamus going on to higher cortical centers travel through the internal capsule.
4. Many of these fibers will end up in the postcentral gyrus of the cortex, which is considered to be the predominant sensory area of the cerebral cortex.

Summary of concepts presented. When trying to understand the nervous system pathways for pain, one is struck by the multidimensional character of pain:

1. There are multiple nociceptors activating multiple neural systems.

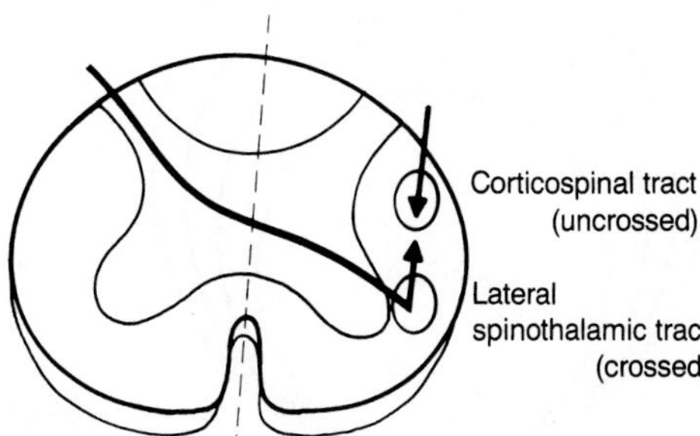

FIGURE 4-4 • Pain fibers cross (in the same segment or one or two cord segments higher) to enter the lateral spinothalamic tract on the opposite side.

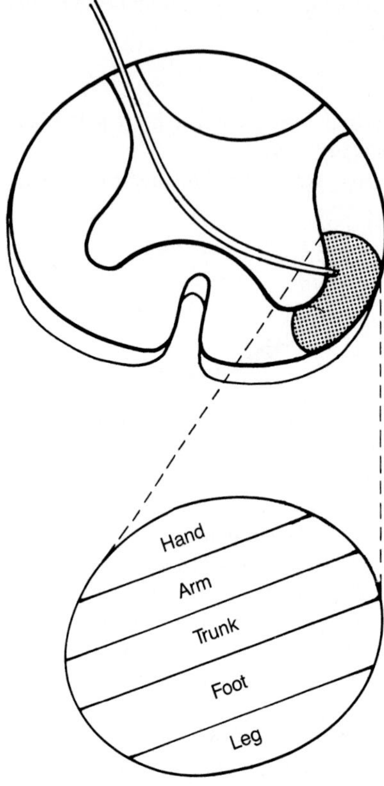

FIGURE 4-5 ● The lamination of fibers in the lateral spinothalamic tract (lower) is such that the later entering (upper extremity) fibers displace the earlier entering (lower extremity) fibers to the periphery.

2. There are multiple ascending tracts.
3. There are multiple CNS receptors.

Step 7: The Psychological Aspects of Pain

The greatest gray area in trying to understand pain lies in the obvious psychological modulation of pain that occurs in every human being. As clinicians, we are aware of patients in whom the slightest amount of pain seems to cause significant disability, and we are also aware of patients in whom a significant amount of pain is accompanied by little alteration in acts of daily living. The reason for this discrepancy and range of pain response lies in understanding the psychological aspects of pain, which are best depicted in Figure 4-6 (14).

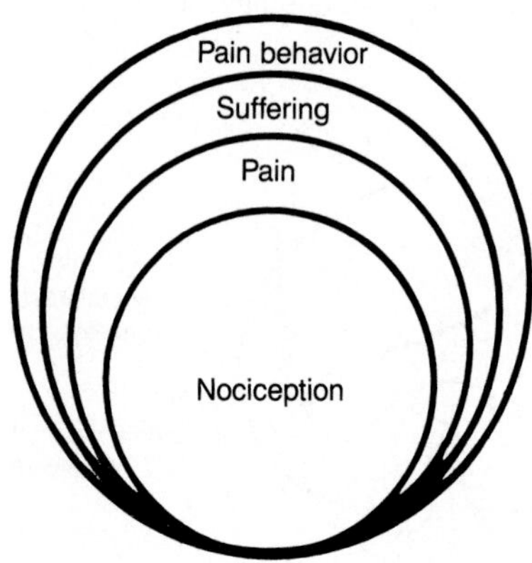

FIGURE 4-6 ● The staging of pain originating with the painful stimulus (received by the nociceptors).

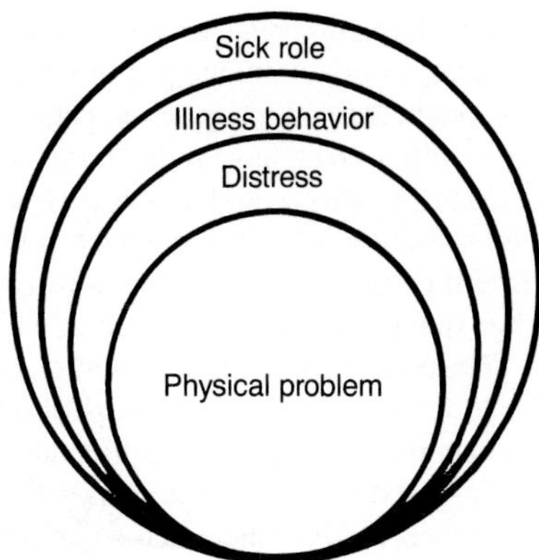

FIGURE 4-7 • Waddell has modified the conceptual model of pain to a more clinically useful model of illness: "an operational model for clinical practice." (From Waddell G. A new clinical model for the treatment of low back pain. *Spine.* 1987;12:632–644 with permission.)

The nociception circle is the actual injury. The pain response is the result of the injury. Without any psychological modification, a patient would suffer with the pain.

The difficult part of this diagram is the pain behavior circle. This is what is manifested by the patient and what doctors and relatives observe in a patient experiencing pain. Pain behavior is wrapped up into the theories of primary and secondary pain and may include moaning, grimacing, limping, excessive talking, excessive silence, refusing to work, seeking health care, and taking medications. The clinician can only conclude that pain is always accompanied by a display of emotions. These emotions are in the form of anxiety, fear, depression, anger, aggression, and so forth, and manifest themselves as pain behavior. Waddell et al. (22) have enhanced this concept with their Glasgow illness model (Fig. 4-7), which is more applicable to the back pain sufferer—plied and enticed by such societal phenomena as accidents, lawyers, courts, and financial awards.

The emotional intensity and pain behavior of the patient are significantly related to genetic makeup, cultural background, and interpretation of past events. It is an extremely complex cognitive process beyond the scope of this book.

From the six previous steps and multiple "hoop jumps," let us try to construct a theory of referred pain!

REFERRED PAIN

From the original work of Kellgren (12) to the more recent work of Mooney and Robertson (17), the concept of referred pain has enjoyed wide support among spine surgeons. Whether this support is correct remains to be seen in light of new work that must be done in this field. The most confusing position has been stated by Bogduk and Twomey (3), which states that if pain traveling down the leg is not associated with neurologic symptoms or signs, it is not true radicular pain. This is obviously incorrect, because many patients with sciatica, especially those in the younger age group, present exclusively with leg pain and marked reduction of straight leg raising (SLR), with little in the way of neurologic symptoms or signs. On investigation, they are found to have a disc herniation; when the disc herniation is treated, these symptoms abate. To conclude that these patients had referred sclerotomal or myotomal pain rather than true radicular pain is obviously an error.

At the other end of the spectrum, there are those in the field who state that any pain that does not go below the knee is referred pain and that any pain that travels below the knee is radicular pain. This also is incorrect because there are many young patients who present with a disc herniation manifested only by high iliac crest or buttock discomfort. On investigation, they are found to have a disc rupture; when the disc rupture is treated, their pain disappears.

Finally, there are patients who have radiating pain down the leg, full SLR, and no neurologic changes and who are also thought to have referred extremity pain. Some of these patients are in the older age group and, on computed tomography (CT) scanning and magnetic resonance imaging (MRI), are found to have various degrees of encroachment in the lateral zone. When these encroachment phenomena are relieved microsurgically, the pain disappears and, obviously, they have had radicular rather than referred discomfort.

For all of these reasons, it is time to repeat the work of Kellgren (12) and Mooney and Robertson (17), knowing exactly the pathology that lies at each segment as documented on CT scan and MRI. It is predicted that many of the patients who have previously been tagged with the label "referred pain" will, in fact, have radicular pain due to the direct involvement of a nerve root.

Many experts would accept patients as having referred pain when they present with a very diffuse sensation in their legs, which is bilateral in nature and not associated either with any radicular pattern or any root tension irritation or compression findings. Provided that those patients do not have spinal stenosis on CT scan or MRI, they probably have referred pain.

The concept of referred pain is one of two types of discomfort. Either it is a deep discomfort felt in a sclerotomal or myotomal distribution or it may be superficial in nature and felt within the skin dermatomes. The fact that gallbladder pain can be felt in the shoulder obviously supports the fact that referred pain is a phenomenon that does occur.

In theory, somewhere in the nervous system is a convergence and summation of nerve impulses from the primary painful area. This is probably lamina 5 in the dorsal horn. The stimulation of this lamina opens a gate and allows central dispatch of the pain message and distal referral of other sensations that indicate referred pain. The essential feature of the relationship between the site of the pain and the distal referral is the common segmental origin of the sensory innervation for both the origin and the distal referral site. Some of that commonality may occur in the complicated ascending pathways in the spinal cord. You can increase the painful sensation by touching the sites of referred pain. These areas are known as trigger zones, and, through various methods of stimulation and anesthetization, referred pain can be altered.

In summary, the concepts of referred pain are likely to be alerted with today's sophisticated investigations in the form of CT scanning and MRI. With these tools in hand, it is time to go back and repeat the outstanding work of Kellgren (12) and Mooney and Robertson (17) in an attempt to further understand the concept of referred pain.

MYOFASCIAL SPRAINS OR STRAINS

Partial tears of the attachment of muscles may occur, giving rise to local tenderness and pain of short duration. There is always a history of specific injury. The pain and tenderness are always away from the midline. This is a young person's injury occurring in strong muscles that are guarding a healthy spine. A similar injury sustained by an older man, with weaker muscles and degenerated disc, is much more likely to result in a posterior joint strain.

The lesions heal quickly with the passage of time despite, rather than because of treatment. Injections of local anesthetic (with or without the addition of local steroids) into the areas of maximal tenderness certainly afford temporary relief of varying duration, but it is doubtful whether they speed the resolution of the underlying pathology.

The symptoms may persist for approximately 3 weeks, during which time the patient is well advised to avoid provocative activity. If symptoms persist beyond this period of time, the problem should be carefully reassessed lest some more significant underlying lesion has been overlooked.

FIBROSITIS (FIBROMYALGIA) AND MYOFASCIAL PAIN SYNDROMES

The name "fibrositis" was first introduced by Sir William Gowers (7) in 1904, when he coined the word to denote nonspecific inflammatory changes in fibrous tissue that he felt were responsible for the clinical syndrome of "lumbago." Fibrositis is now the most common cause of chronic, widespread, nonarticular, musculoskeletal pain in general practice. To date, the underlying pathologic lesion has never been demonstrated histologically and probably does not exist. The so-called fibrositic nodules, or tender points, which are palpable over the iliac crest, are usually localized nodules of fat. These "trigger points" are considered to be one of the hallmarks of fibrositis. Never mind that the examiner forgot to test the skin overlying these trigger points for tenderness or that the point locations have not been submitted to rigid scientific testing to determine validity.

The tender points are situated in an area that is a common site of referred tenderness derived from an underlying spinal lesion and they, along with the overlying skin, may be tender on pressure. The demonstration of a tender nodule associated with back pain and the occasional relief of symptoms by the injection of local anesthetic has lent weight to this clinical concept. Surgical exploration of the nodules has revealed their questionable anatomic nature.

The concept of fibrositis becoming the most common cause of back pain in general practice for nearly half of a century is a classic example of how the phenomenon of referred pain and tenderness have clouded the recognition of the pathologic basis of low back pain derived from soft tissue disorders. There is no reason why the term should not be retained to describe the clinical syndrome: "low back pain of undetermined origin associated with tender points." However, it must be remembered that the term does not denote a specific pathologic process. Rather, it describes a perfectionist or anxiety-laden personality, with diffuse chronic pain, in whom the bones, joints, bursae, and nerves are normal. These patients complain of musculoskeletal pain; nothing can be found on physical examination or investigation (except the tender points), so these patients are lumped into the nebulous category of fibrositis. If their syndrome is localized to one area of the body, such as the low back, there is a tendency to label the entity "myofascial pain syndrome" rather than fibrositis. This hair splitting does little to help us understand the problem.

Much of what we are describing throughout this text conforms to the traditional medical model of disease:

1. A rational collection of symptoms and signs
2. A probable diagnosis
3. Verification of the diagnosis through investigation
4. Resolution through scientifically proven treatment regimens

Fibrositis does not fit this model. Although it is a recognizable collection of symptoms (with few signs) (Table 4-1), it fails the remaining tests of the traditional medical model. By the time the diagnosis is made, you have a despondent patient and a frustrated primary care physician.

There is little question that the syndrome can be modified by psychosocial and economic factors (20).

Treatment of fibromyalgia patients is less than gratifying because the syndrome cannot be cured. Those clinicians with the patience of Job can do a great deal to ameliorate symptoms and lead patients to a better quality of life.

Effective methods of treatment have included some or all of the following:

1. Reassure the patient of the benign nature of the problem.
2. Do not reinforce through excessive investigation or treatment that the problem is serious.
3. Provide extensive education to the patient: make the patient the center of the solution and encourage him or her to take control of the symptoms through:
   a. Behavioral modification.
   b. Loss of weight.
   c. Improved physical fitness.
   d. Abstinence from smoking and excessive alcohol intake.
4. Judiciously use drugs such as mild analgesia/anti-inflammatories and antidepressants.
5. Limit the repetitive use of trigger point injections.
6. Control unlimited use of manipulation, modalities, biofeedback, and so forth, until the patient has a clear understanding of the nature of fibrositis and the noncurative nature of these interventions.
7. Discourage politicians and bureaucrats from liberalizing compensation and Social Security regulations that encourage this syndrome through financial reward.

TABLE 4-1

Clinical Characteristics of Fibrositis

Clinical Characteristics of Fibrositis
Pain: chronic, changing, widespread, deep
Associated stiffness, weakness (nonmeasurable)
Trigger points: numerous, throughout body
Aggravation: by internal (e.g., fatigue) and external (e.g., cold) stimuli
Sleep: nonrestorative sleep pattern

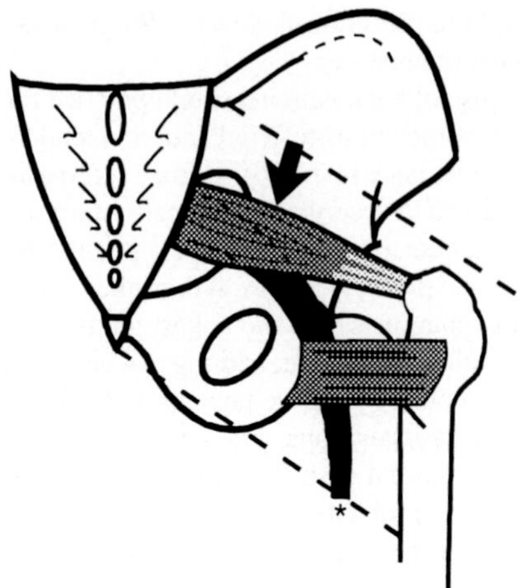

FIGURE 4-8 ● The piriformis muscle *(arrow)* exiting the sciatic notch, with the sciatic nerve (*) in close proximity. Spasm of the piriformis muscle may irritate the nerve.

All too often, the doctor-patient relationship follows two extremes concerning fibrositis: (a) "The condition doesn't exist; all of the patients are crazy and I will not care for them" and (b) "The patients are sick and require extensive investigation and treatment," which some clinicians would describe as overservicing. The best road to follow with these patients is the middle road, helping the patient to understand the psychosomatic nature, placing them in a vigorous self-supervised exercise program and, on occasion, providing low doses of amitriptyline (Elavil) to help with the sleep disorder.

PIRIFORMIS SYNDROME

The piriformis muscle has taken on a high profile as a cause of sciatica. A number of patients with pain down their leg in a sciatic distribution will arrive in the clinician's office with the latest newspaper clip describing how the piriformis muscle (Fig. 4-8) has trapped the sciatic nerve deep in the buttock. This entrapment, theoretically, causes pain radiating down the leg in a sciatic distribution and up into the back. The presentation is identical to lumbosacral root encroachment problems, such as disc herniations and lateral zone encroachment. A variant of this syndrome is the carrying of a fat wallet in one's hip pocket, which in turn puts pressure on the piriformis muscle and irritates the sciatic nerve.

Proponents of this syndrome as a cause of sciatic pain say they can diagnose and treat the condition by stretching the hip into internal rotation (Fig. 4-9). Modalities such as ultrasound and massage to the piriformis area of the buttock have been proposed to reduce muscle spasm and inflammation.

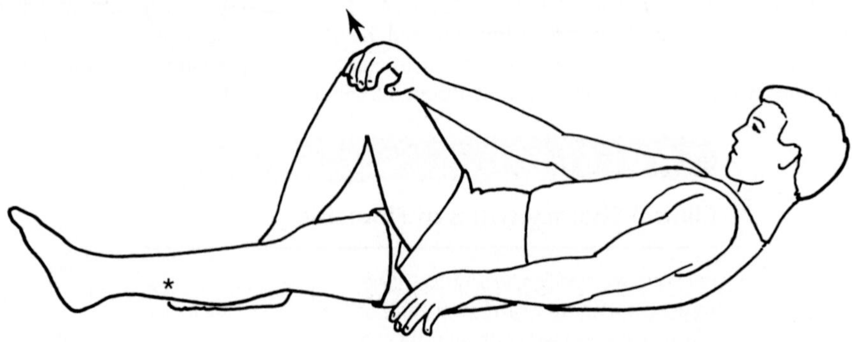

FIGURE 4-9 ● The stretching exercise to relieve piriformis muscle spasm. In the supine position, with the hip and knee flexed and the foot crossed, (*) the hip is adducted *(arrow)*.

The problem with this diagnosis and treatment is the lack of scientific testing of the parameters. Until appropriate studies on the clinical presentation and effective treatment are provided, it is best to see this diagnosis as a low-level possibility in a patient who probably has sciatica due to a disc rupture or subarticular root encroachment.

KISSING SPINES: SPRUNG BACK

Approximation of the spinous processes ("kissing spines"), and the development of a bursa between them, have been indicated as a cause of low back pain. "Sprung back" is a term used to describe rupture of the supraspinous ligament after a sudden flexion strain applied to the spine with the pelvis fixed, as in falling on the buttocks with the legs out straight. It is doubtful whether either of these entities are, in and of themselves, a cause of low back strain (Fig. 4-10).

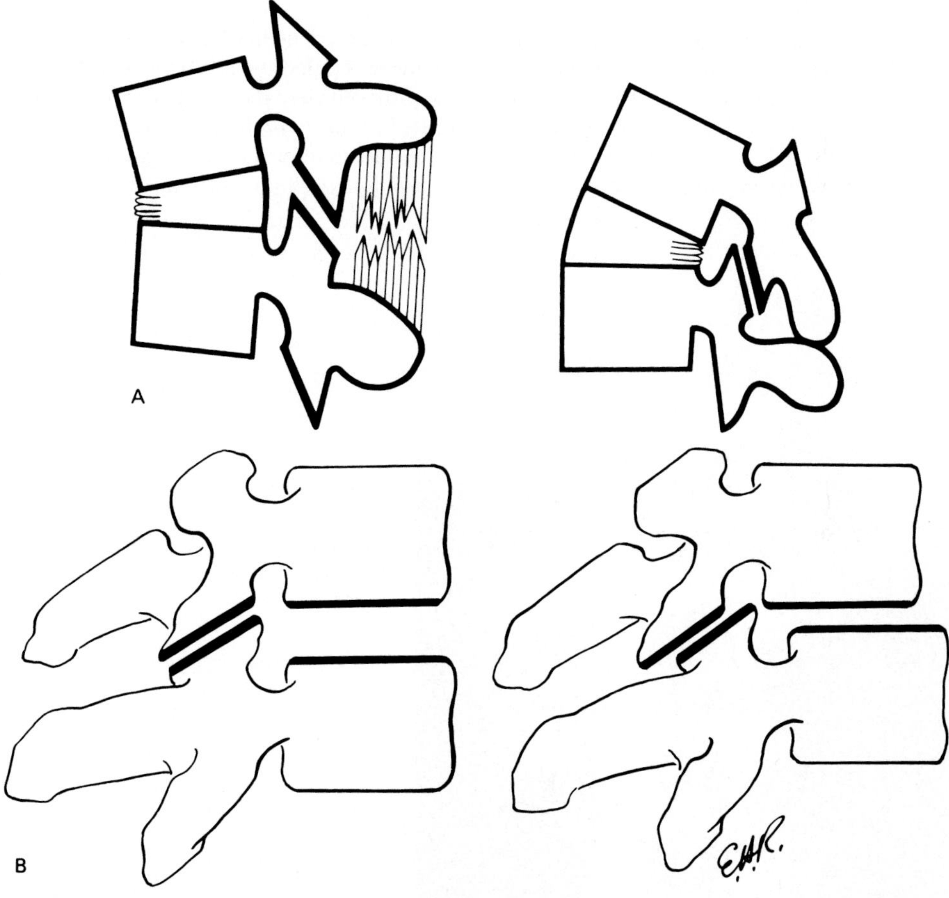

FIGURE 4-10 ● **A:** The radiologic demonstration of apposition of the spinous processes has been referred to as "kissing spines." This anatomic disposition of the spinous processes cannot occur in the absence of an unstable disc segment. In the balance of probabilities, it is the associated disc degeneration rather than the bony apposition of the spinous processes that is the cause of the patient's symptoms. (From Macnab I. *Backache.* Baltimore: Williams & Wilkins; 1977:83 with permission.) **B:** As the intervertebral discs lose height and the vertebral bodies approach one another, the posterior joints must override and assume the position normally held in hyperextension. It is to be noted that owing to the inclination of the posterior joints, as the upper vertebral body approaches the vertebral body beneath it, it is displaced backward producing a retrospondylolisthesis. This posterior displacement of the vertebral body, indicative of posterior joint subluxation, is readily recognizable on routine x-ray examination of the lumbar spine. (From Macnab I. *Backache.* Baltimore: Williams & Wilkins; 1977:88 with permission.)

SACRALIZATION OF A LUMBAR VERTEBRA (BERTOLOTTI SYNDROME)

Bertolotti (1), in 1917, described attachment between the transverse process of L5 with the sacrum and associated this attachment with low back pain (Fig. 4-11). Whether or not the radiographic change that Bertolotti noted is associated with an increased incidence of back pain has been hotly debated since 1917. Although it is possible that some unilateral assimilation between the transverse process of L5 and the sacrum can result in mobile articulations that can develop degenerative changes (Fig. 4-12), it is rare that these changes are symptomatic (4) and even rarer that they should be corrected surgically.

DISC DEGENERATION

To understand the pathogenesis of symptoms derived from degenerative disc disease, it is necessary to have a clear concept of the mechanical changes that may arise from breakdown of an intervertebral disc (26).

The functional components of the intervertebral disc are described in Chapter 1, where it is indicated that the combination of the annulus (fibrous), nucleus pulposus (gelatinous), and hyaline cartilage plate makes for a very efficient coupling unit, provided all of the structures remain intact.

The natural aging process, with or without repeated minor episodes of trauma (the heavy worker), results in loss of the nuclear jelly (because of failure to reproduce the degradated proteoglycans) and weakening of annular support (because of failure of the collagen linking) (11). This

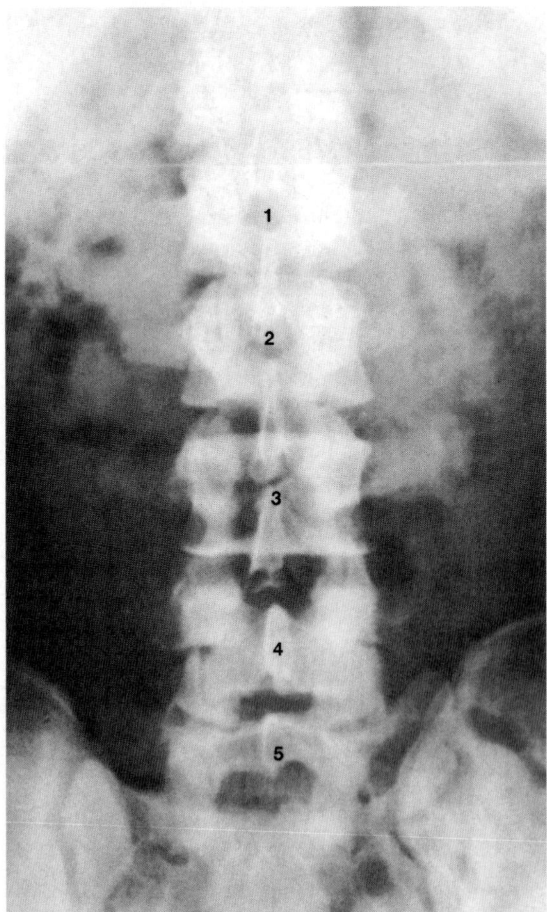

FIGURE 4-11 ● Bertolotti syndrome. Some surgeons would describe these segments as partial sacralization of L5; others would be tempted to number the segments differently (see Chapter 1 for a discussion of congenital lumbosacral anomalies).

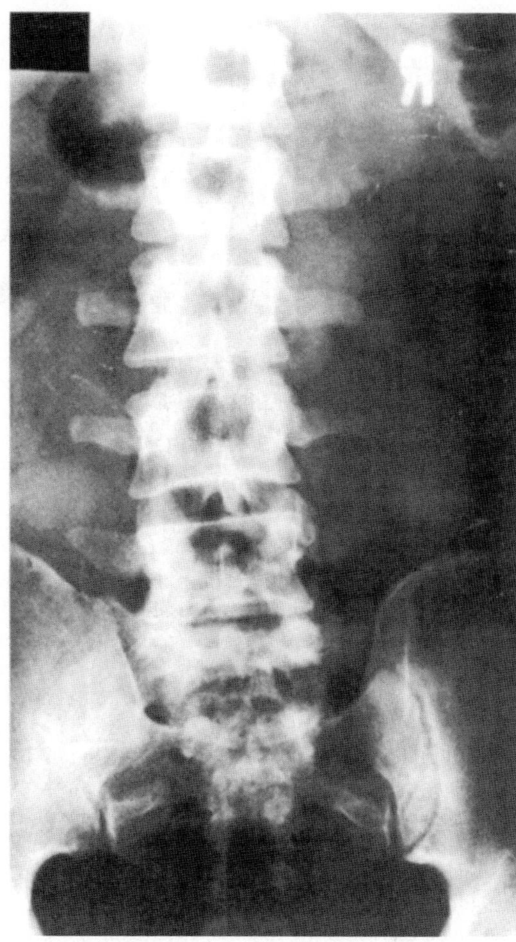

FIGURE 4-12 • Bertolotti syndrome with apparent degenerative changes in articulation.

stage has been labeled by Kirkaldy-Willis et al. (13) as the phase of dysfunction. With advancement of these degenerative changes, any one of the components of the disc loses its biomechanical integrity due to changes such as inspissation of the nucleus pulposus, a tear in the annulus, or a rupture of the hyaline cartilage plate. At this point, a cascading series of events occurs:

1. Fibroblasts fail to reproduce new collagen to replace degradated collagen in the annulus.
2. Chondrocytes fail to reproduce new proteoglycan to replace degradated proteoglycan in the nucleus.
3. Nutritional flow of glucose, O_2, and sulfates to the disc is decreased.
4. These factors (in number 3) change disc metabolism negatively and likely decrease the pH within the disc.
5. The decrease in pH gives the upper hand to degrading enzymes (proteases), which further increases disc degeneration.

SWELLING PRESSURE

Normally, the nucleus pulposus can take on water (swell) or release water (shrink), which allows for the balancing of mechanical loads (Fig. 4-13). With the cascading degenerative changes, the ability to move water in and out of the nucleus is impaired, and swelling pressures can no longer absorb the mechanical load. The balancing act (cushioning) of the disc is upset.

Disc stability or the smooth roller action is lost, and the movement between adjacent vertebral segments becomes uneven, excessive, and irregular. This is the stage of segmental instability, a

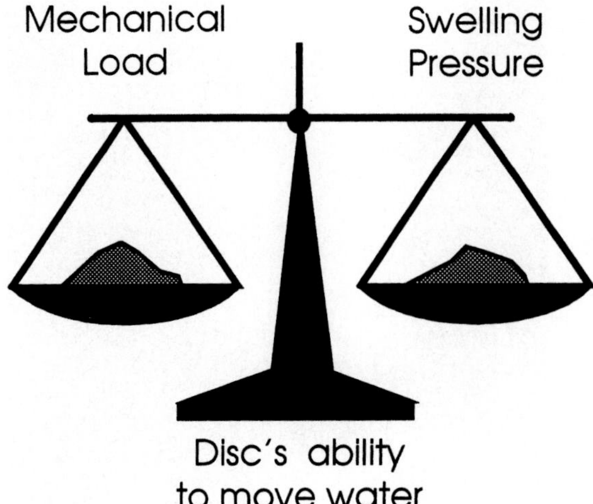

FIGURE 4-13 ● A balancing act exists between mechanical load and swelling pressure; that is, when mechanical pressures increase, the disc gives up water to absorb the load; the reverse occurs when loads decrease (e.g., at night when sleeping).

term first proposed by Harris and Macnab (9), and subsequently relabeled the dysfunctional stage by Kirkaldy-Willis et al. (13). Excessive degrees of flexion and extension are permitted, and a certain amount of backward and forward gliding movements occur as well.

Normally, on flexion of the spine, the discal borders of the vertebral bodies become parallel above the level of L5. This is the maximal movement permitted. In the stage of segmental instability, excessive degrees of extension and flexion are permitted, and a certain amount of backward and forward gliding movement occurs as well (Fig. 4-14).

This abnormal type of movement can be shown by radiographs taken with the patients holding their spines in full extension and flexion. One problem posed by motion studies is the fact that, when a patient is in pain, the associated muscle guarding does not permit adequate flexion and extension radiographs to be taken. However, there are two radiologic changes that are indicative of instability, vacuum sign, (Knuttson's phenomenon of gas in the disc) (Fig. 4-15) and the "traction spur" also known as the Macnab spur (Fig. 4-16).

The traction spur differs anatomically and radiologically from other spondylophytes in that it projects horizontally and develops approximately 1 to 2 mm above the vertebral body edge (15). It owes its development to the manner of attachment of the annulus fibers. In Chapter 1, the mode of

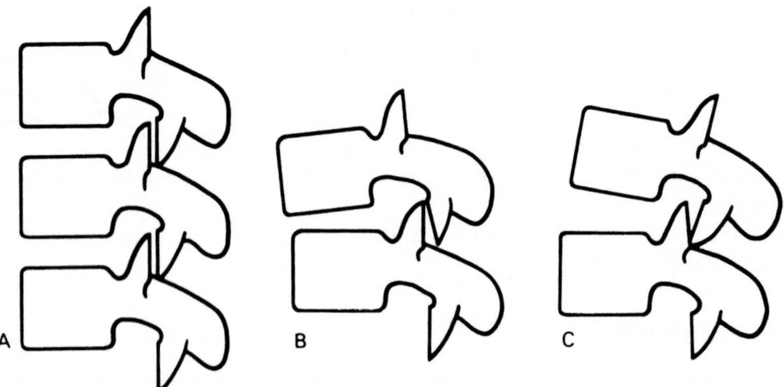

FIGURE 4-14 ● **A:** In the early stages of degenerative disc disease, excessive degrees of flexion and extension are permitted at the involved segment. This abnormal mobility is associated with rocking of the posterior joints (**B** and **C**). (From Macnab I. *Backache.* Baltimore: Williams & Wilkins; 1977:85 with permission.)

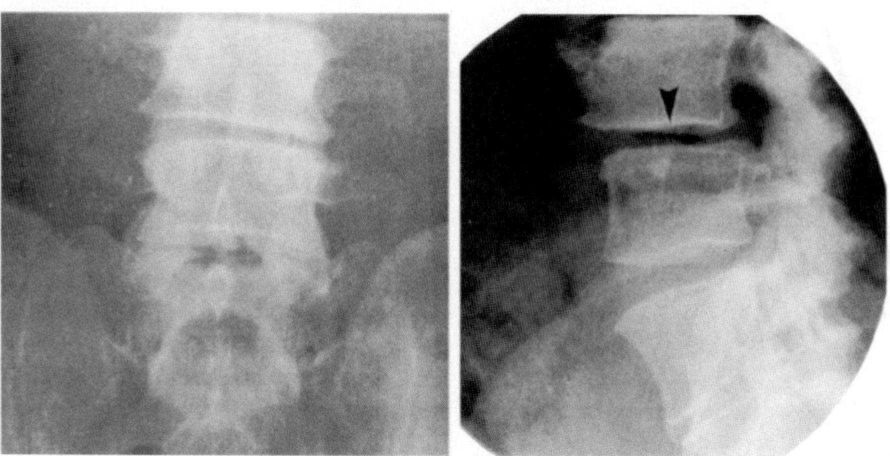

FIGURE 4-15 • Knuttson's phenomenon at a degenerative spondylolisthesis level.

attachment of the outermost fibers to the undersurface of the epiphysial ring is described. With abnormal movements, an excessive strain is applied to these outermost fibers, and it is here that the traction spur develops. It is the small traction spur that is clinically significant in that it is probably indicative of present instability. The large traction spur indicates that this segment has been unstable at some time in the past, but it may be stable now because of fibrotic changes occurring within the disc.

Segmental instability, by itself, is probably not painful, but the spine is vulnerable to trauma. A forced and unguarded movement may be concentrated on the wobbly segment and produce a posterior joint strain or subluxation. Repeated injuries produce secondary degenerative changes in the capsule and cartilaginous surfaces of the facet joints.

The next stage of disc degeneration is segmental hyperextension. Extension of the lumbar spine is limited by the anterior fibers of the annulus. When degenerative changes cause these fibers to lose their elasticity, the involved segment or segments may hyperextend (Fig. 4-17).

A similar change may be seen in the next stage of disc degeneration, disc narrowing. As the intervertebral discs lose height, the posterior joints must override and subluxate, and vertebral body shifts occur (Fig. 4-18). In both segmental hyperextension and disc narrowing, the related posterior

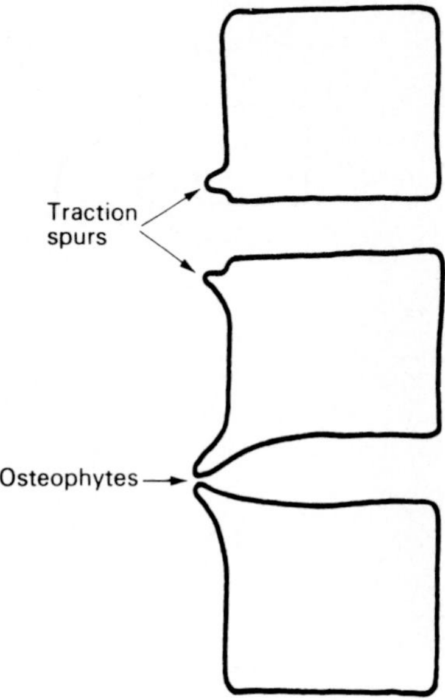

FIGURE 4-16 • The traction spur projects horizontally from the vertebral body about 1 mm away from the discal border. (From Macnab I. *Backache*. Baltimore: Williams & Wilkins; 1977:86 with permission.)

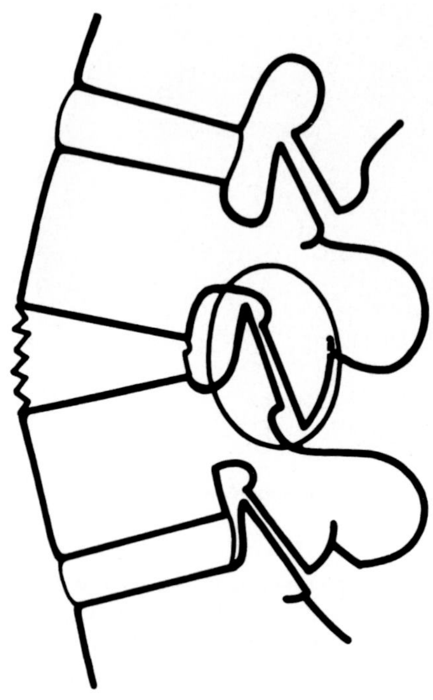

FIGURE 4-17 ● When the anterior fibers of the annulus lose their elasticity, the involved segment falls into hyperextension permitting subluxation of the related posterior joint. (From Macnab I. *Backache.* Baltimore: Williams & Wilkins; 1977:87 with permission.)

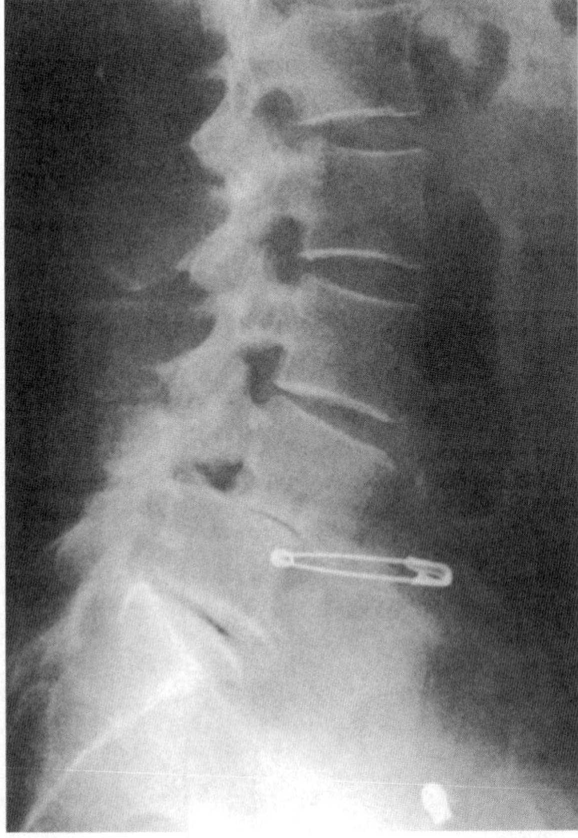

FIGURE 4-18 ● At the level of the safety pin, there is a forward "slip" of L4 on L5 due to degenerative changes in the facet joints. (The safety pin was a radiologic marker—not a form of fixation for the slip!)

joints in normal posture are held in hyperextension, and this postural defect is exaggerated if the patient has weak abdominal muscles and/or tight tensors and is overweight.

When the posterior joints are held at the extreme of their limit of extension, there is no safety factor of movement, and the extension strains of everyday living may push the joints past their physiologically permitted limits and thereby produce pain. Eventually, the posterior joint may subluxate.

Repeated damage to the posterior joints, especially when associated with subluxation, will lead to degenerative changes. This is true osteoarthritis of the spine. Gross lipping to the vertebral bodies, often erroneously referred to as osteoarthritis of the spine, is merely a manifestation of disc degeneration (Fig. 4-19). Gross lipping may be present without associated degenerative changes in the posterior joints.

So much for the morbid anatomic changes associated with disc degeneration. What is the relationship of these changes to the pain experienced? In attempting to answer this, some clinical observations must be noted.

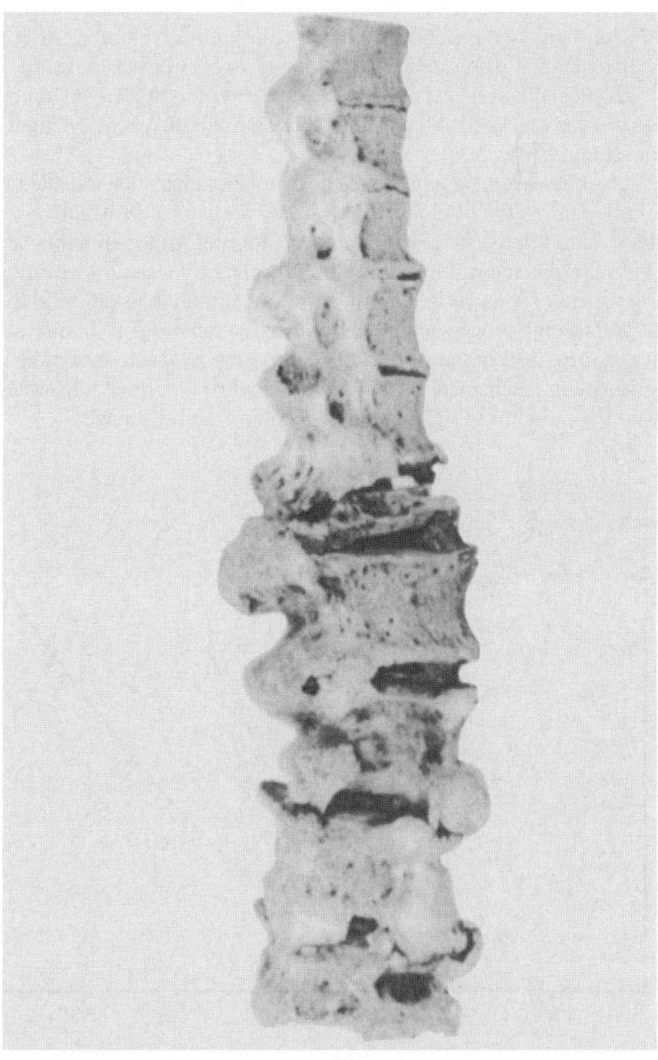

FIGURE 4-19 • Photograph of an excised lumbar spine showing the various bony outgrowths that are associated with disc degeneration. These bony outgrowths are correctly referred to as "spondylophytes." (From Macnab I. *Backache.* Baltimore: Williams & Wilkins; 1977:89 with permission.)

Scoliosis (exclusive of secondary disc degeneration) rarely gives rise to significant back pain, even if left untreated, yet the lesion is associated with very gross posterior joint subluxation at many levels (except in mild idiopathic lumbar scoliosis).

On the premise that the majority of backaches have their first occurrence before the age of 40 years, the radiographs of three hundred 40-year-old laborers, who had been engaged in heavy work all their lives, were reviewed by Dr. Macnab. Of these, 150 had no history of low back pain, and 150 were under treatment for backache at the time of the review. A careful statistical analysis of the radiographs showed no difference in the incidence of anatomic variant and degenerative changes in the two groups studied. Indeed, some of the patients who had been employed in strenuous occupations all their lives without a twinge of back pain showed very marked degenerative changes on radiograph.

If every radiologic sign of disc degeneration is given a numerical rating, and these numbers are added together to give an arbitrary "degenerative index," it can be shown that, although radiologic evidence of degenerative disc disease shows a linear increase with advancing years, the incidence of backache has a peak at 45 years and thereafter tends to decline (Fig. 4-20).

A patient may be seen with severe low back pain, and radiographs taken may show evidence of disc degeneration with segmental instability and posterior joint subluxation. After a period of conservative therapy, the patient's pain subsides, and then he or she returns to heavy work. Follow-up radiographs show identical changes, even though the patient is completely symptom free. This observation serves as more evidence to show that the clinician should assess and treat patients' symptoms and not their radiographs.

On the other hand, it has been the experience of many clinicians that a patient previously incapacitated by low back pain, with radiologic evidence of mechanical insufficiency of the spine due to disc degeneration, can, after a successful spinal fusion, return to strenuous activities without pain. In such an instance, mechanical instability was surely the cause of the original disability.

With our present stage of knowledge, only the following may be stated: (a) disc degeneration does occur as part of the aging process and often remains asymptomatic; (b) disc degeneration may be associated with changes within the disc itself that may be productive of pain; and (c) disc degeneration may give rise to mechanical instability that renders the spine vulnerable to trauma, as a result of which pain may arise from ligamentous or posterior joint damage.

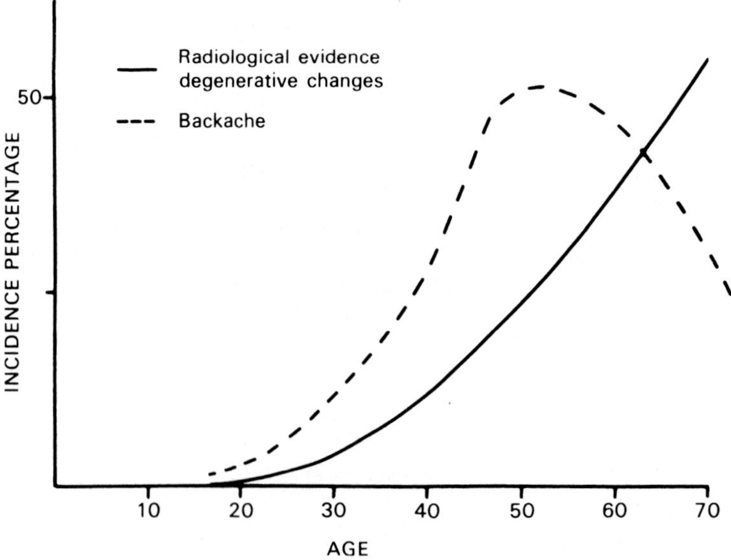

FIGURE 4-20 ● Note from this graph that although the incidence of radiologically demonstrable degenerative changes in the lumbar spine increases with age, the maximal incidence of backache has a peak at 45 and thereafter tends to decline. (From Macnab I. *Backache.* Baltimore: Williams & Wilkins; 1977:90 with permission.)

The pain experienced may remain localized to the back, or there may be both local pain and referred pain, or referred pain only. The experimental injection of hypertonic saline into the supraspinous ligament between D12 and L1 may give rise to pain referred to the low back and both buttocks and as low as the greater trochanter. A similar injection into the supraspinous ligament between L5 and S1 may give rise to buttock pain and pain referred down the leg. The pain referred down the leg in a sciatic distribution rarely goes below the knee, although on occasion it may extend to the ankle. Patients suffering from degenerative changes at the lumbodorsal or lumbosacral junction may present with pain referred in a similar manner.

Posterior joint damage produced by degenerative changes of the L4-5 disc may also produce pain referred to the groin. It is important to emphasize the fact that pain down the leg associated with degenerative disc disease may indeed be referred pain, and the patient's complaint of "sciatica" does not necessarily mean that a nerve root is being compromised.

Degenerative disc disease may lead to nerve root compression under the following circumstances: disc ruptures, bony root entrapment, ligamentous root entrapment, and adhesive radiculitis.

Why Does Disc Degeneration Cause Pain?

The pain of spinal origin can be divided into two groups:

1. Pain originating from the bony column: specifically, its three-joint complex of disc and facet joints.
2. Pain arising as a consequence of direct involvement of the spinal nerve root (which is discussed in the next section of this chapter). Other low back pains, such as those referred from the prevertebral visceral spaces, are not discussed in this chapter.

There continues to be controversy as to whether free nerve endings have a functional presence in spinal structures such as the annulus. Everyone would agree that the deeper annular-nuclear portion of the disc is not innervated. It is well established that the posterior longitudinal ligament is richly supplied with nociceptor fibers from the sinuvertebral nerve. More recently, Yoshizawa et al. (26) and Malinsky (16) have solved the controversy by very definitely demonstrating various types of encapsulated and unencapsulated pain receptors in the outer aspect of all of the annulus. The sources of these fibers have been further documented by Malinsky (16) and include the sinuvertebral nerve, the ventral rami, and the sympathetic gray rami communicantes (Fig. 4-2).

Because it has been extremely difficult to demonstrate nerve fibers in the outer annulus, it is likely that the annulus is reinnervated as the body grows older and as the process of disc degeneration occurs. It is well known that a disc is avascular during most of its adult life, but the disc does become vascularized as it degenerates. Perhaps a similar reaction occurs with nerve supply to the annulus.

Free nerve endings are also present in (a) the fibrous capsule of the facet joint, (b) the sacroiliac joints, (c) the anterior aspect of the dura, (d) the periosteum, (e) the vertebral bodies, and (f) the blood vessel walls. Theoretically, the presence of these nociceptors implies that a stimulus to these areas will be transmitted as a pain impulse. Although this appears to be a simple conclusion, it is not supported by any surgeon who has operated on the spine under local anesthesia and who has palpated the annulus without reproducing pain. In addition, discography can be done in a normal disc, with tremendous pressures placed on the disc, and yet no appreciation of pain on the part of the patient. Thus, the simple presence of these nociceptors does not explain how pain arises in a spinal segment. Further work has to be done with regard to (a) chemical changes that occur with disc degeneration and (b) the influence of abnormal movement.

DISC RUPTURES

There are several sources of nerve root compromise, of which a ruptured intervertebral disc is but one example.

The term "herniated disc" tends to be used so loosely now as to lose much of its clinical significance and, indeed, there has been confusion in terminology (Table 4-2). Sometimes, the operative note will state with disarming simplicity, "a disc was found." To avoid confusion, therefore, it is perhaps advisable to define the pathologic state implied by the term "disc rupture." The height of absurdity was the introduction of the term "concealed disc" (5) to describe a herniated disc that could not be demonstrated at operation.

The exact mechanism of a disc rupture has not been demonstrated, but it is a common misconception that a disc rupture consists of an extrusion of nuclear material through an annular defect

TABLE 4-2

Synonyms for Herniated Disc

Herniated disc	Protruding disc
Prolapsed disc	Bulging disc
Sequestrated disc	Ruptured disc
Soft disc	Extruded disc
Slipped disc	"Disc"

much like toothpaste exuding through a hole in the side of a toothpaste tube. Operative experience belies this impression. It is unusual at surgery to find a disc herniation consisting solely of extravasated nuclear material exuding through a defect in the annulus. The protrusion, extrusion, or sequestration always consists of a varying amount of nucleus, annulus, and cartilage plate.

In an attempt to avoid the confusion of terminology, it is suggested that the following classification be considered. Disc ruptures can be defined as a focal distortion of the normal anatomic configuration of the annulus. Two major pathologic states are to be distinguished: contained disc protrusions and noncontained disc herniations (Table 4-3) (Fig. 4-21). Throughout this discussion you will note we move back and forth between the terminology "ligamentous" (e.g., transligamentous) and "annular" (e.g., subannular). In fact, at L4-5 and L5-S1, the posterior longitudinal ligament is very narrow, and the structures that contain nuclear material are the annular fibers.

CONTAINED DISC PROTRUSIONS

Normally, the annulus fibrosus forms a smooth, continuous ring confining the nucleus pulposus. A protrusion is a localized or focal disc bulge with the annular fibers still continuous and maintaining their Sharpey's fiber attachments to the vertebral body (Fig. 4-22).

This "focal" alteration of disc architecture is to be distinguished from disc collapse (degeneration), with the annulus circumferentially bulging beyond the peripheral rim of the vertebral bodies (Fig. 4-23). The appearance is as though the disc has been made of putty and the vertebral bodies have been compressed together: the middle-aged spread of a middle-aged disc. The annular fibers remain intact, and, at surgery, when a square window is cut in the former (focal protrusion), the nucleus will spontaneously extrude, whereas in nonfocal, diffuse annular bulging, an annular window will not be followed by spontaneous expulsion of disc material.

Subligamentous (Subannular) Extrusion

The displaced nuclear material is still confined by a few of the outermost fibers of the annulus and, if not appreciated beforehand, these fragments can be missed at surgery. The disc herniation has traveled up behind the vertebral body or down behind the vertebral body below (Fig. 4-24). The most common migratory pattern for a disc extrusion is caudally to lie behind the vertebral body below. Disc herniations that rupture in a cephalad direction are more often sequestered than extruded fragments.

TABLE 4-3

Types of Disc Herniations

Contained
1. Protrusions
2. Subligamentous (subannular) extrusion

Noncontained

3. Transligamentous extrusion
4. Sequestered

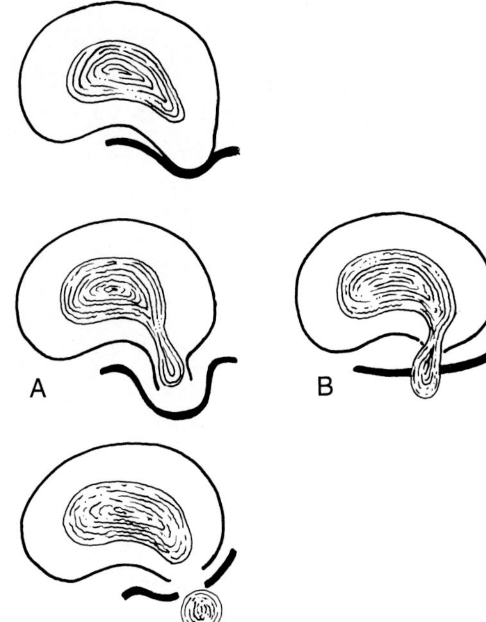

FIGURE 4-21 • There are two basic types of disc herniations, contained and noncontained. **Top row:** Protrusion (contained). **Middle row: (A)** Extrusion: subannular (contained); **(B)** Extrusion: transannular (noncontained). **Bottom row:** Sequestered (noncontained).

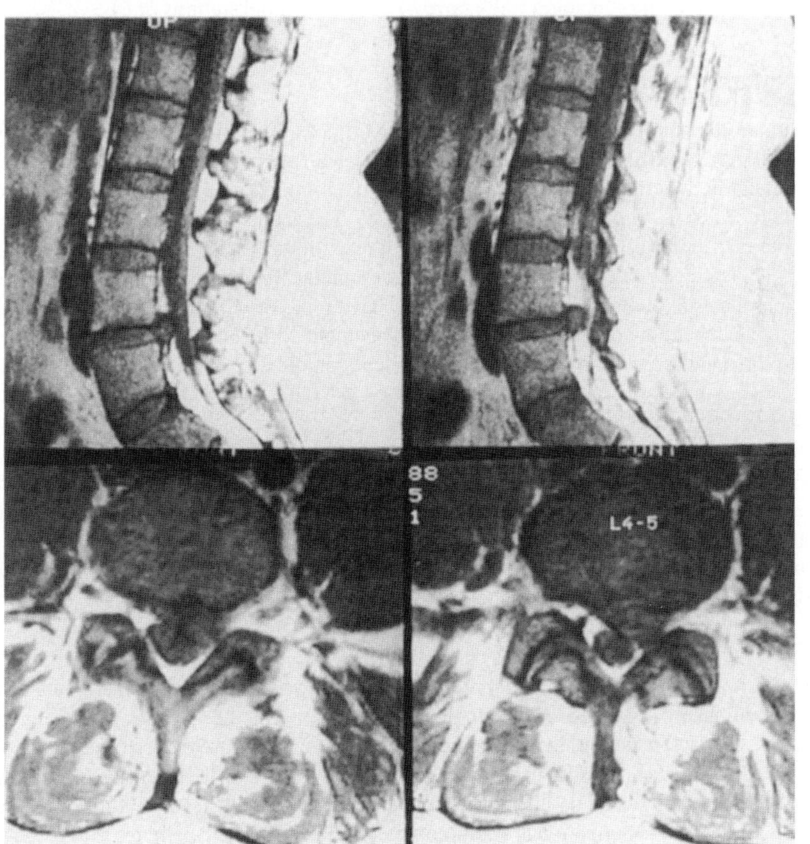

FIGURE 4-22 • Magnetic resonance imaging (MRI) of a disc protrusion. These views are all from a T1 protocol, with two adjacent sagittal slices **(top)** and two adjacent axial slices **(bottom)** showing an apparent contained disc herniation in the first story of the 4th anatomic segment. Note the "focal" prominence of the disc herniation.

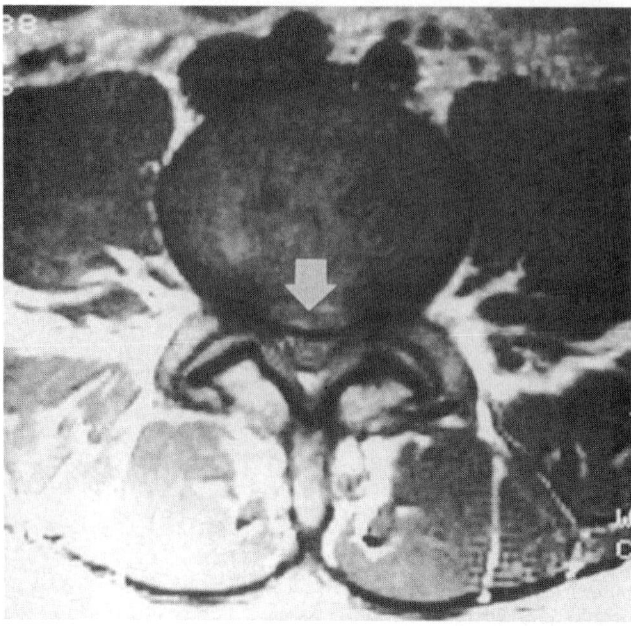

FIGURE 4-23 ● A diffuse annular bulge on T1 axial magnetic resonance imaging (MRI) *(arrow)* adds to a spinal stenosis of L4-5.

NONCONTAINED DISC HERNIATIONS

Disruptions of the annular fibers, whether in their body or at the attachment to the vertebral body margin, will permit extrusion, or sequestration, of nuclear material. In an adult practice, the most common material to herniate is the nuclear material, but as mentioned earlier, annulus and endplate may be included in the ruptured fragment (Fig. 4-25). The inclusion of endplate usually occurs in younger patients and is typical of a juvenile type of disc rupture. After detachment of a segment of the cartilage plate and/or disruption of the posterior annular fibers, a portion of the annulus, along with nuclear material, may be displace posteriorly. Two types of noncontained disc herniations can be recognized, depending on the extent of the displacement of the nuclear material and where it lies relative to the annular/posterior longitudinal ligament complex.

Transligametnous (Transannular) Extrusion

In this lesion, the displaced nuclear material has burst through the posterior fibers of the annulus and the posterior longitudinal ligament to lie in the spinal canal (Fig. 4-26). However, there is still a connection between this extruded discal material and the disc space cavity. If the extrusion remains in its abnormal position long enough, a very thin membrane may form over it, in the body's attempt to separate the discal material from the neurologic structures. This flimsy membrane is not to be confused with annular fibers or posterior longitudinal ligament.

Sequestered Intervertebral Disc

Nuclear material has not only ruptured through the annular/posterior longitudinal ligamentous complex, it has completely separated itself from the nuclear cavity, and the discal fragment lies free in the spinal canal. Characteristically, these disc herniations are either extremely large or have migrated away from the disc space. Discal material can travel posteriorly to lie posterior to the nerve root. Sequestered disc herniations can also travel caudally to lie behind the vertebral body below (Fig. 4-27). A sequestered disc herniation is a common description in surgical pathology; in fact, it does not occur as commonly as disc extrusions. On occasion, the freed portion of the disc may erode or burst through the dura. This is more likely to happen in a patient who has had a previous surgery for a disc herniation and who suffers a sudden rerupture of the same disc on the same side. Because of the scarring of the dura around the root to the disc space, a transdural discal herniation may occur.

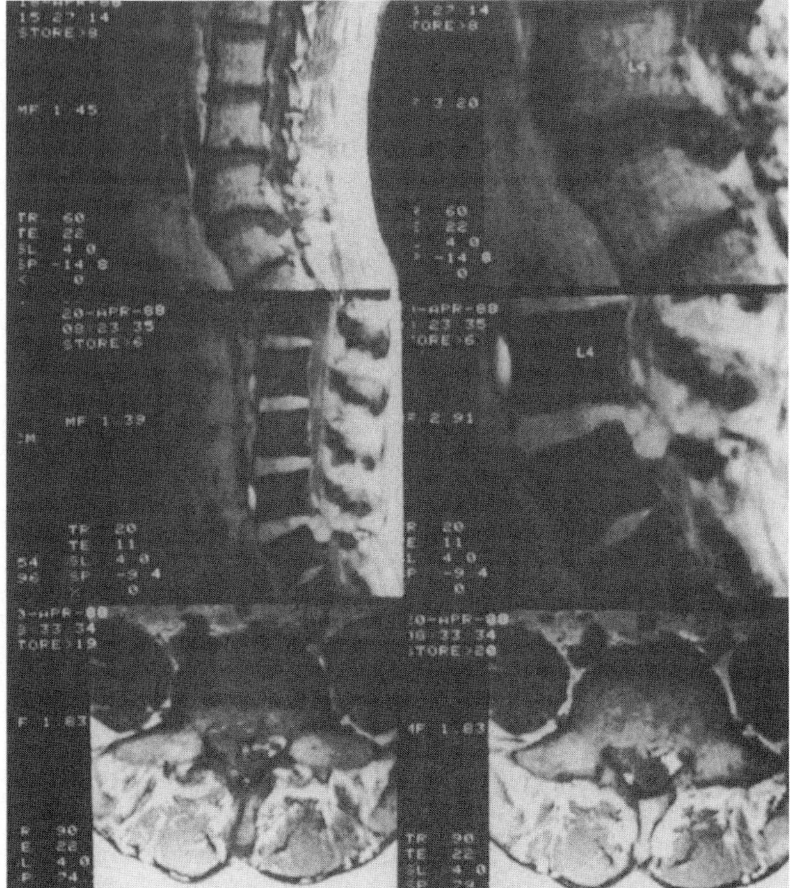

FIGURE 4-24 • Magnetic resonance imaging (MRI) showing a subligamentous disc extrusion from L4-5 to lie in the third story of L5.

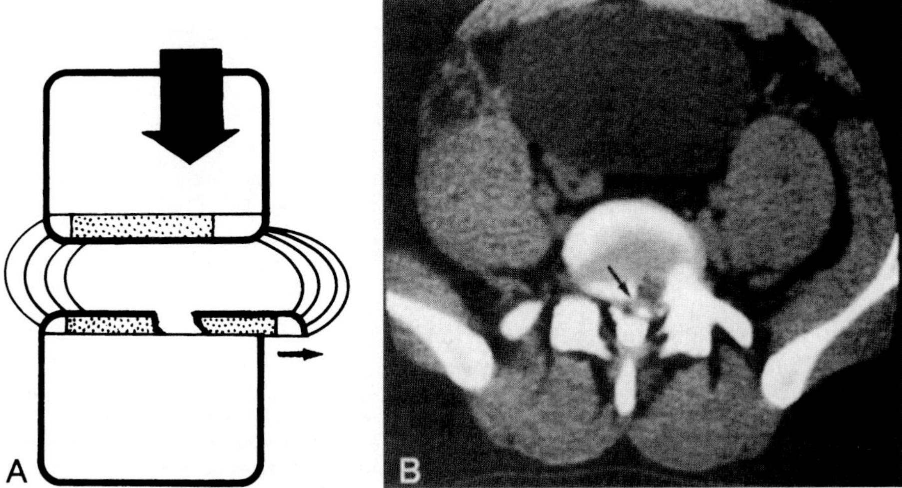

FIGURE 4-25 • **A:** Disc rupture with piece of endplate included *(arrow)*. **B:** CT showing fragment of endplate (L5-S1, left).

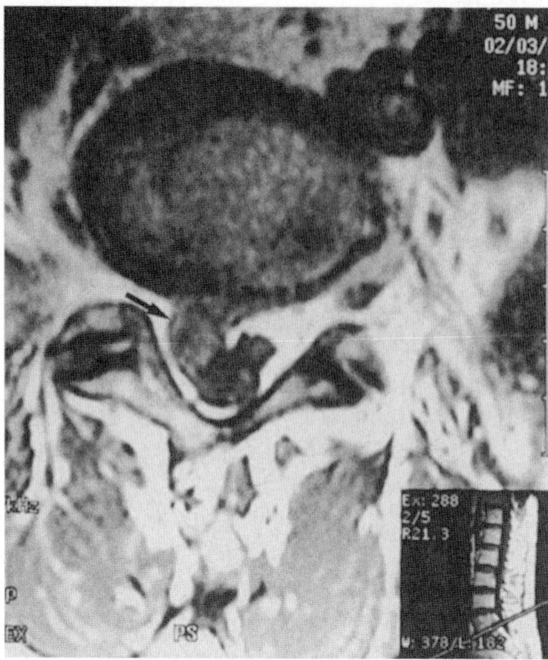

FIGURE 4-26 ● A transannular (or pedunculated) disc rupture *(arrow)* on T1 axial at L5-S1.

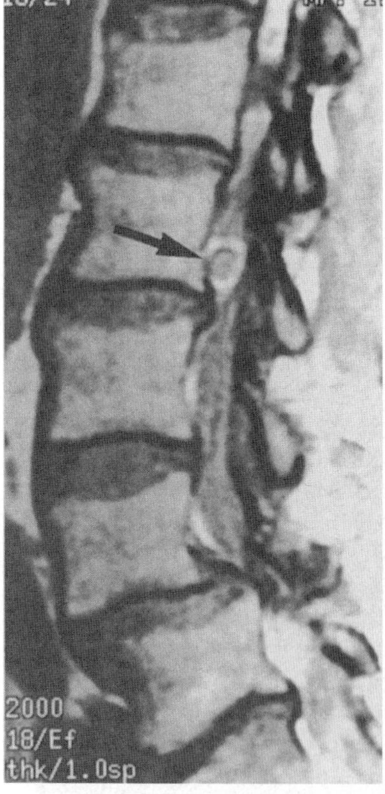

FIGURE 4-27 ● A sequestered disc lying behind the vertebral body of L2 *(arrow).* Did you see anything else on the T1 sagittal MRI? (Do not tell us you missed the degenerative spondylolisthesis at L4-5.)

Intradiscal Rupture (Internal Disc Disruption)

This is largely a theoretical concept. It is believed that on occasion the innermost fibers of the annulus will rupture, with degeneration of nuclear material producing an autoimmune reaction within the disc space. This distention within the nuclear space may produce pain. Unfortunately, this condition is revealed by discography and, when found, can lead to surgery.

PATHOGENESIS OF SYMPTOMS RESULTING FROM DISC RUPTURES

There is no clear, single explanation as to why a disc rupture causes sciatica. Some disc ruptures remain asymptomatic. Myelogram, CT, and MRI performed on asymptomatic patients have shown varying incidence of disc herniations (2,10,25).

In trying to understand the back and leg complaints of a patient with a herniated nucleus pulposus (HNP), a few things are clear. The patient's major complaint is pain. Yet, physical pressure on a peripheral nerve does not produce pain; it produces paresthesia. In examining this problem further, at the conclusion of routine laminectomy for HNP, Macnab instituted placement of a Fogarty catheter underneath the emerging nerve root of a segment above. When the patients had regained consciousness, and before they had been given any analgesics, the catheters were distended. It was found that although distention of the catheter underneath an involved, angry, red, inflamed nerve root reproduced the sciatic pain, distention of the catheter underneath the normal nerve root produced paresthesia only.

It is likely that no one neuromechanical theory can explain the mechanism of symptom production in an HNP (6). In the routine consideration of simple sciatica, there are many clinical observations that are not easy to explain:

1. The description of sciatica from patient to patient is so variable that there are obviously many factors involved in the production of symptoms.
2. In the early phases of a disc herniation (a few hours to a few days), a patient may report only back pain immediately after the "snap" sensation heralding the disc rupture. During this time, leg pain is absent as a symptom; root tension (SLR reduction) is present as a sign; and the results of the CT or MRI, if done, will be positive.
3. Some patients in the early phases of sciatica will report only paresthesia, which gives rise to an irritating, diffuse, ill-localized numbness in the lower leg and foot.
4. Patients with an HNP have more pain and more SLR reduction than those patients with lateral zone stenosis, yet the latter group of patients have more root encroachment. Rupture a piece of disc into a root that is already squashed in a narrowed subarticular gutter, and you have a patient with incredible leg pain, reasonable SLR ability, and neurologic symptoms and signs (Fig. 4-28).
5. Young patients with an HNP have a lower incidence of neurologic findings than the average 40-year-old patient with an HNP.

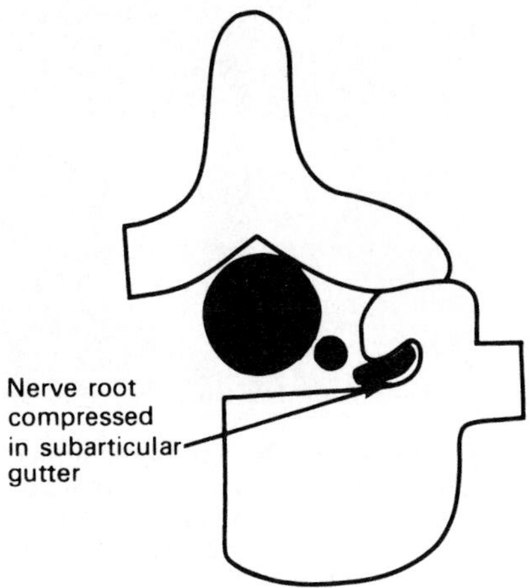

FIGURE 4-28 ● The nerve root as it courses through the subarticular gutter may be compressed between a hypertrophied arthritic posterior joint and the dorsum of the vertebral body. (From Macnab I. *Backache.* Baltimore: Williams & Wilkins; 1977:100 with permission.)

6. The average 40-year-old patient with an HNP is more likely to have neurologic changes than the older patient with lateral zone stenosis whose nerve root is usually severely compromised in the subarticular zone.
7. A patient with a foraminal disc herniation has the most severe pain of all; this phenomenon raises the question as to the mechanism of pain production when a disc herniation lies on the dorsal root-ganglion (24).
8. It has been documented that patients undergoing myelography, CT, or MRI, after bed rest has relieved sciatica, may still have positive study results. This phenomenon had been reported up to 15 months after sciatica has disappeared (6).
9. In some patients undergoing successful chemonucleolysis, the CT scan defect has persisted despite relief of symptoms and recovery from nerve root tension and compression (17) (Fig. 4-29).
10. Infrequently, a patient presents with the sudden onset of severe leg pain, which is quickly followed by a profound neurologic lesion (e.g., drop foot), followed by an equally dramatic disappearance of pain and root tension in a few hours to a few days. Prolonged observation of these patients often reveals a significant degree of neurologic recovery.
11. Pain is an unpleasant emotional state. So much depends on past experiences of the patient and his or her emotional state and needs at the time of discomfort.
12. If a patient with diabetes is unfortunate enough to also develop an HNP, the degree of pain experienced is often so much more than usual. Are the diabetic patient's nerves extra sensitive to compression factors?

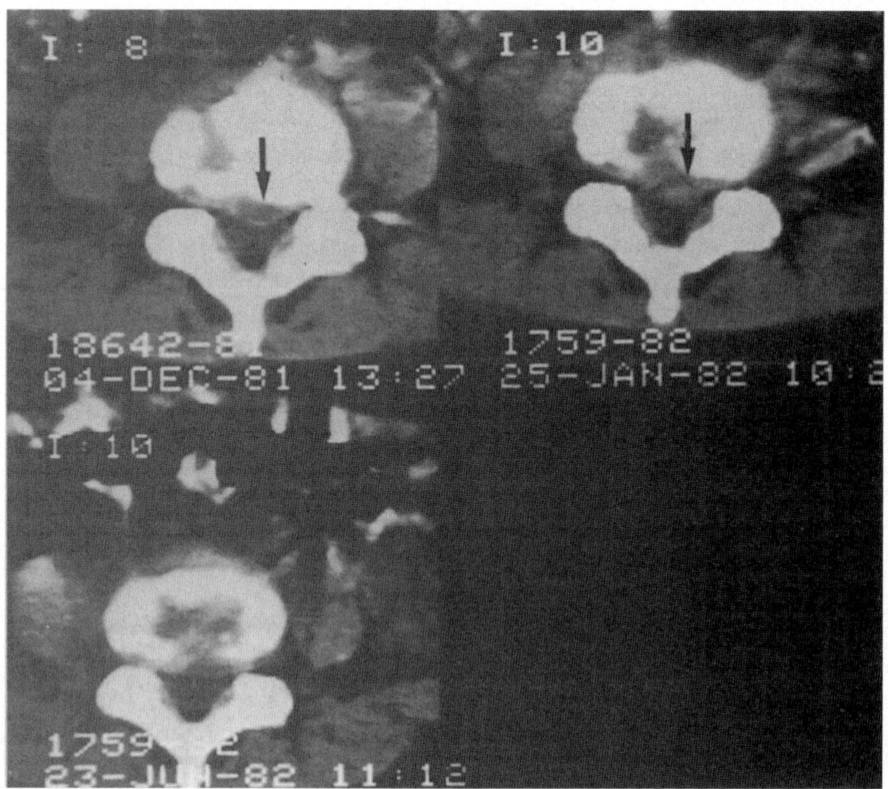

FIGURE 4-29 ● Computed tomography (CT) before and after chemonucleolysis. **Top left:** Before chymopapain. Herniated nucleus pulposus (HNP), L4-5, left *(arrow).* **Top right:** 1 month after chemonucleolysis. Leg pain has been relieved but the CT scan defect is still evident *(arrow).* **Bottom left:** 6 months after chemonucleolysis. No further treatment, no further symptoms; the defect has gone.

ANATOMIC LOCATION OF THE PRESSURE ON THE ROOT-GANGLION

The potential anatomic locations for pressure of an HNP are as follows:

1. Cauda equina
2. Single root
   a. Motor
   b. Sensory
3. Sympathetic fibers
4. Dorsal root-ganglion (24)

Two things are apparent. First, patients who have a foraminal disc herniation with implied direct pressure on the dorsal root-ganglion tend to have more severe pain than do patients with any other type of disc herniation. Second, many patients describe a change in temperature with their sciatic discomfort, which implicates some upset in vascular tone that is almost certainly due to stimulation of the sympathetic nervous system. (Some experts might argue that the sympathetic chain ends at L1–L2, and there are no sympathetic fibers in the lower lumbar roots. The frequent occurrence of "coldness" as a symptom in disc ruptures signifies that some sympathetic fibers in the area are being irritated.)

DORSAL ROOT-GANGLION

There is a very large potential role for an irritated dorsal root-ganglion to modulate pain in low back disorders. The effect may arise through direct irritation from an HNP or indirect stimulation through some unknown mechanism. Weinstein (24) has called the dorsal root-ganglion the "brain" of the motion segment.

The net effect of ganglion irritation is the release of neuroactive peptide (e.g., substance P) (21) that has long been identified as a resident compound of the dorsal ganglion. Only recently has an increase in retrievable substance P been documented on vibratory stimulation (24). This phenomenon is secondary to stimulation of unmyelinated and thinly myelinated fibers.

ULTIMATE PATHOLOGIC CHANGES

Obviously, the compression of nerve tissue by a disc rupture upsets normal neural function and thus produces symptoms. Nerve function is dependent on the adequate supply of oxygen and other nutrients by way of the intraneural microcirculation. It is most likely that one of the significant events in the pathogenesis of sciatica is the primary upset in vascular supply to a nerve root, with the secondary phenomenon of interference with nerve root nutrition, both of which upset neurophysiologic function.

NERVE ROOTS ARE DIFFERENT FROM PERIPHERAL NERVES IN TWO RESPECTS

1. Nerve roots do not have the protective connective tissue covering of a peripheral nerve; for example, the dura substitutes for epineurium, the cerebrospinal fluid substitutes for perineurium.
2. The microcirculation of a radicular nerve is provided through surface arteries. Radicular nerves come from both a proximal and distal direction, with an anastomotic zone that is vulnerable to a decrease in blood flow. Using the vital microscope and direct observation, Rydevick et al. (21) have shown that compression and tension of a nerve root decreases its blood supply. This results in changes in intraneural blood, an increase in vascular permeability that results in edema, and an upset in axonal transport. If these changes are longstanding, intraneural fibrosis ultimately occurs.

Myelinated fibers are more susceptible to this distortion; these fibers demonstrate wallerian degeneration if enough pressure for enough time has been brought to bear on a nerve root (19).

Neurophysiology

In the end, there is a decreased capacity of the nerve root to transmit impulses. There may also be hyperexcitability and generation of ectopic activity. This results in the numerous symptoms that occur in sciatica, including pain, tingling, pins and needles, and weakness.

Summary

Considering that (a) ruptured nuclear material may compress motor, sensory, and sympathetic fibers, or the dorsal root-ganglion; (b) the effect of an HNP on a nerve root can be compression, tension, or inflammation, separately or together; and (c) with time, the pathologic changes in a nerve root can be inflammation, edema, intraneural fibrosis, demyelination, axonal degeneration and regeneration. It is thus easy to understand that there is no one cause of sciatica and there is not one classic presentation of sciatica. Sciatica due to an HNP has many faces.

OTHER MODES OF NERVE COMPRESSION—SPINAL STENOSIS

A ruptured intervertebral disc is not the only cause of nerve root irritation in association with disc degeneration in the lumbar spine.

Spinal stenosis is defined as a narrowing of the spinal canal that may produce a bony-soft tissue constriction of the cauda equina and the emerging nerve roots. This bony-soft tissue encroachment may in turn produce symptoms. The bony-soft tissue constraint can be considered anatomically as being lateral in the canal (giving rise to compression of the emerging nerve roots), midline (giving rise to compression of the cauda equina), or both simultaneously. These constraints may be congenital (developmental) or acquired in origin. Most cases are probably a combination of the two etiologies. This condition is described in great detail in Chapter 12.

Bony compression of the emerging nerve roots may arise as a result of subarticular entrapment, pedicular kinking, or foraminal impingement due to posterior facet joint subluxation.

Subarticular Entrapment

The nerve roots course downward and outward, passing underneath the medial border of the superior articular facets before they swing around the pedicle to emerge through the foramen. Hypertrophy of the superior articular facet may compress the nerve root between the facet and the dorsal aspect of the vertebral body (Fig. 4-30).

Pedicular Kinking

When advanced intervertebral disc degeneration is associated with marked asymmetric narrowing of the disc, the tilting of the vertebral body may on occasion kink the emerging nerve root (Fig. 4-31).

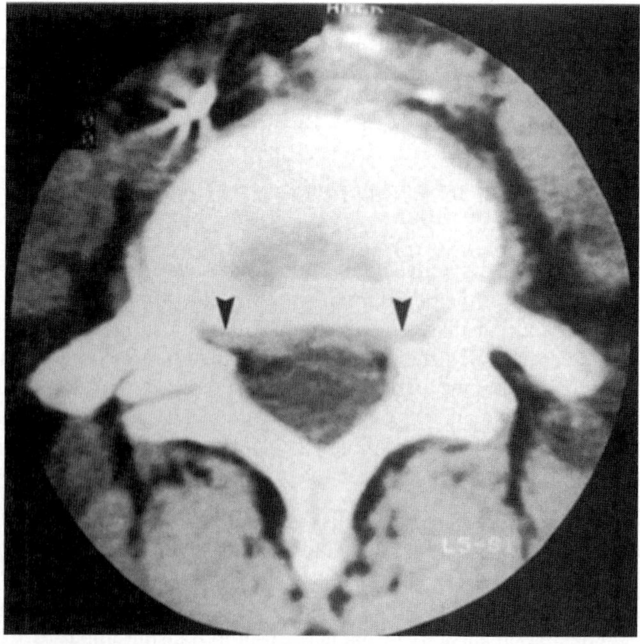

FIGURE 4-30 ● A computed tomography (CT) scan showing bilateral subarticular stenosis at L5-S1 *(arrows).*

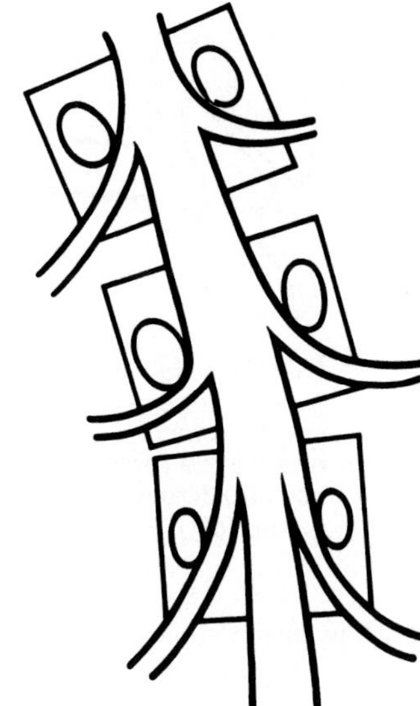

FIGURE 4-31 • With asymmetrical collapse of the disc and tilting of the vertebral body, the nerve root may be kinked by the pedicle, giving rise to severe compression. (From Macnab I. *Backache.* Baltimore: Williams & Wilkins; 1977:100 with permission.)

Commonly, however, the nerve root is seen to be compressed in a gutter formed by a diffuse lateral bulge of the disc and the pedicle above (Fig. 4-32).

Foraminal Encroachment

As the root emerges through the foramen, it lies in close relation to the tip of the superior facet of the vertebra below. As the intervertebral disc narrows, the posterior joint overrides, and the root may, on occasion, be compressed by the superior articular facet (Fig. 4-33).

Midline Compression

Midline compression may be a sequel of disc degeneration when, after narrowing of the intervertebral disc, the spinal canal is constricted by the presence of a diffuse annular bulge, anterior buckling

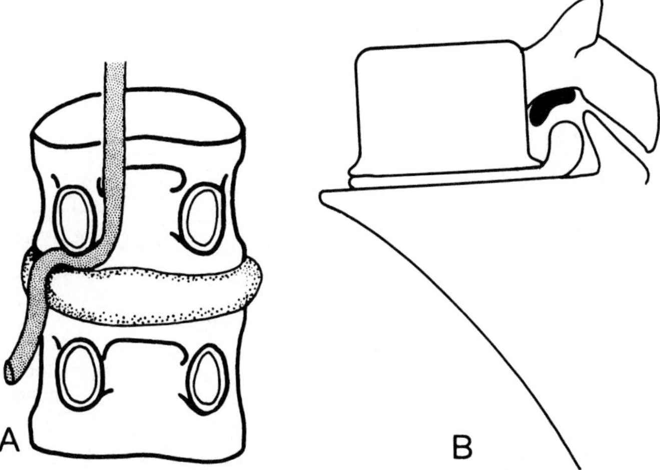

FIGURE 4-32 • **A:** In patients suffering from pedicular kinking of the nerve root, it is very common to find at operation that the nerve root is trapped in a gutter formed between a diffuse lateral bulge of the disc and the pedicle above. From Macnab I. *Backache.* Baltimore: Williams & Wilkins; 1977:101 with permission.) **B:** Sagittal schematic of Figure 4-22A, depicting disc space narrowing, lateral and superior bulging of disc to compress the nerve root in the lateral zone.

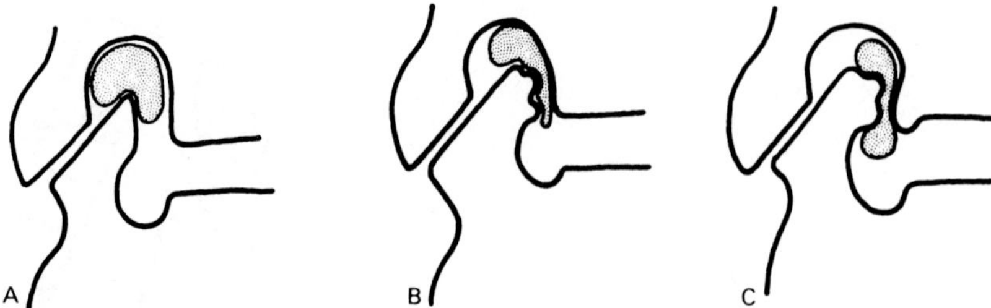

FIGURE 4-33 ● The nerve root may be trapped in the foramen. It may be compressed between the tip of a subluxated facet and the pedicle above **(A);** it may be compressed by osteophytic outgrowths on the superior articular facet **(B);** or it may be compressed between the facet and the dorsal aspect on the vertebral body **(C).** (From Macnab I. *Backache.* Baltimore: Williams & Wilkins; 1977:101 with permission.)

of the ligamentum flavum, and shingling of the laminae posteriorly. This constraint may be further aggravated by overgrowth of the arthritic posterior joints that may, indeed, also encroach on the midline (Fig. 4-34).

Forward displacement of the laminae seen in degenerative spondylolisthesis and the thickening of the lamina seen in certain pathologic states, such as fluoridosis and occasionally Paget disease, may produce a posterior encroachment of the spinal canal. Any technique of spinal fusion that involves decortication of the laminae, with or without the addition of a bone graft, may produce a diffuse hypertrophy of the posterior elements, which leads to constriction of the spinal canal. Postfusion spinal stenosis is, of course, more likely to occur if, before surgery, the patient was suffering either from a congenital narrowing of the spinal canal or a narrowing produced by degenerative change of the type previously described. This is most commonly seen at the L4-5 level.

Various combinations and permutations of laminar and apophyseal compression are seen. For example, the fifth lumbar nerve root may be compressed as it courses under the superior articular facet of L5 (Fig. 4-30). Although laminar compression may occur by itself at times, it is frequently associated with lateral recess or apophyseal root entrapment that may arise at the same segment, or the laminar and apophyseal compressions may be at different segments (Fig. 4-35).

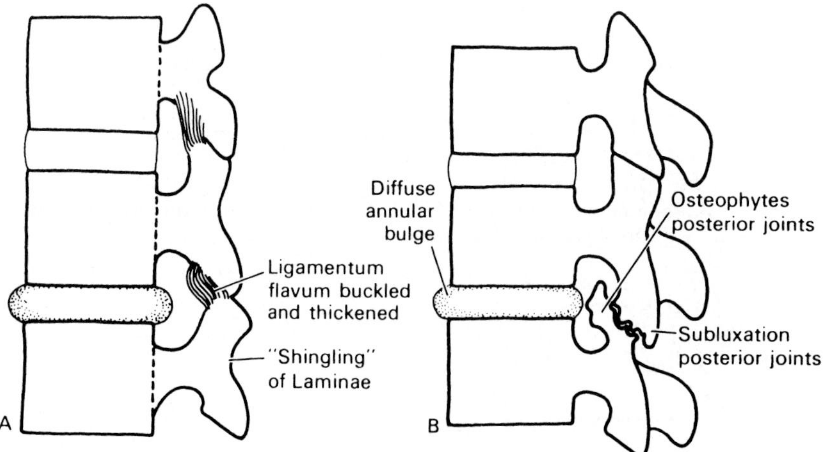

FIGURE 4-34 ● In degenerative spinal stenosis, the spinal canal is narrowed by shingling of the laminae and by bucking of the ligamentum flavum. The arthritic posterior joints may hypertrophy and also encroach on the midline, giving rise to further compression of the cauda equina. The emerging nerve roots are commonly compressed as they course through the narrow subarticular gutter. (From Macnab I. *Backache.* Baltimore: Williams & Wilkins; 1977:102 with permission.)

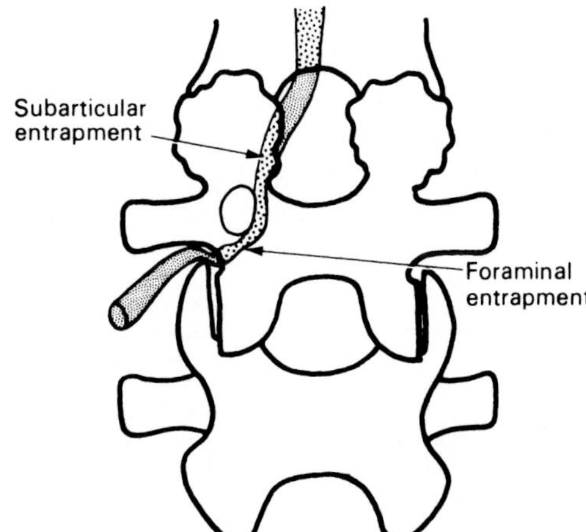

FIGURE 4-35 • In apophysial stenosis an emerging nerve root may be compressed at two sites. For example, as in this diagram, it may be compressed as it passes through the subarticular gutter, and it may also be trapped in the foramen by the tip of the superior articular facet. (From Macnab I. *Backache.* Baltimore: Williams & Wilkins; 1977:102 with permission.)

ROLE OF HNP IN BONY ENCROACHMENT

The compression produced in the subarticular gutter or recess by hypertrophy of the facet joints may be aggravated by a localized protrusion of the annulus, and a diffuse annular bulge may critically occlude a segment with a congenital narrowing of the spinal canal. However, although these spatial disc changes augment the degree of compression present, it is important to emphasize the fact that they are not the sole source of compression, and discectomy alone will not relieve the symptoms entirely.

Bony root entrapment, then, results from narrowing of the spinal canal. This narrowing may be apophyseal and may compress the nerve roots at their point of emergence at one or more segments. The compression may be in the midline and produced by the lamina, or the root compression may be the result of a combination of both of these mechanisms at the same level or at different segments. It is important to emphasize that the most common cause of symptoms in spinal stenosis is compression of a nerve root by osteophytic overgrowth of facets and ligamentum flavum infolding and hypertrophy.

The resulting radicular pain mimics the radicular pain due to a disc rupture. However, the sciatic pain due to a bony root entrapment frequently presents a claudicant character. In contradistinction to the intermittent claudication of vascular insufficiency, the symptoms do not abate on standing still. The patient will report that, if the pain strikes while walking down the road, he or she will lean forward and rest his or her hands on the knees to keep the spine in flexion to relieve the symptoms. The claudicant nature of the sciatic pain produced by apophyseal compression of a nerve root differentiates it from sciatica due to a disc rupture.

There are, in addition, several other features that differentiate bony root entrapment and compression from disc herniation. The first important difference is the age incidence. Root entrapment by bone is more common in patients older than 50 years, whereas disc ruptures are more common in patients younger than 50 years. Patients with bony root entrapment will usually have a history of longstanding backache, with the recent gradual onset of sciatica. On examination of a patient with a neurogenic claudication, despite severe sciatic pain, one of the remarkable findings is that SLR is rarely significantly restricted. The bowstring sign and the crossed SLR are negative. Neurologic changes are minimal but, when present, often incriminate more than one root. A true disc rupture, with extrusion of nuclear material, very rarely occurs at more than one segment simultaneously. This fact is not sufficiently recognized.

CONCLUSION

It is obvious that the pathogenesis of sciatica is multifactorial and not easily explained. The nature of the pressure of the discal fragment of the nerve root-ganglion complex, the location of the root-ganglion complex, and the resulting pathology determine the multifaceted nature of sciatica discomfort. Less important, but also bearing on the patient's symptom complex, is the age of the patient and, thus, the age of the nerve root and the presence of other diseases that might decrease the resistance of the nerve root to these compressive changes.

REFERENCES

1. Bertolotti M. Contributo alla conoscenza dei vizi differencazione regionle del rachid con speciale riguardo all'assimilazione sacrale edlla v lombare. *La Radiologia Medica.* 1917;4:113–144.
2. Bogduk N, Twomey LT. *Clinical Anatomy of the Lumbar Spine.* Melbourne, Edinburgh, London and New York: Churchill Livingstone; 1987.
3. Boden SD, Davis DO, Dina T, Patronas HJ, Wiesel SW. Abnormal magnetic resonance scans of the lumbar spine in asymptomatic subjects. *J Bone Joint Surg Am.* 1990;72:403–408.
4. Castellvi AE, Goldstein LA, Chan DPK. Lumbosacral transitional vertebrae and their relationship with lumbar extradural defects. *Spine.* 1984;9:493–495.
5. Dandy WE. Concealed ruptured intervertebral disks. *JAMA.* 1941;117:821–826.
6. Falconer MA, McGeorge M, Begg CA. Observations on the cause and mechanism of symptom production in sciatica and low back pain. *J Neurol Neurosurg Psychiatry.* 1948;11:13.
7. Gowers WR. Lumbago. Its lessons and analogues. *Br Med J.* 1904;1:117–121.
8. Guyton AC. *Textbook of Medical Physiology.* Philadelphia: WB Saunders; 1986.
9. Harris RI, Macnab I. Structural changes in the lumbar intervertebral discs. *J Bone Joint Surg Br.* 1954;36:304–322.
10. Hitselberger WE, Witten RM. Abnormal myelograms in asymptomatic patients. *J Neurosurg.* 1968;28:204–210.
11. Holm S. Pathophysiology of disc degeneration. *Acta Orthop Scand.* 1993;64(suppl 251):13–15.
12. Kellgren JH. On the distribution of pain arising from deep somatic structures with charts of segmental pain areas. *Clin Sci Mol Med.* 1939;4:35–46.
13. Kirkaldy-Willis WH, Wedge JH, Yong-Hing K, Reilly J. Pathology and pathogenesis of lumbar spondylosis and stenosis. *Spine.* 1978;3:319–328.
14. Loeser JD. Concepts of pain. In: Stanton-Hicks M, Boas RA, eds. *Chronic Low Back Pain.* New York: Raven Press; 1982.
15. Macnab I. The traction spur: an indication of segmental instability. *J Bone Joint Surg Am.* 1971;53:663–670.
16. Malinsky J. The ontogenetic development of nerve terminations in the intervertebral disc of man. *Acta Anat.* 1959;38:96–113.
17. Mooney V, Robertson J. The facet syndrome. *Clin Orthop.* 1976;115:149–156.
18. Noordenbos W. Prologue. In: Wall PD, Melzack R, eds. *Textbook of Pain.* Edinburgh, Scotland: Churchill Livingstone; 1984.
19. Parke WW, Gammell K, Rothman RH. Arterial vascularization of the cauda equina. *J Bone Joint Surg Am.* 1981;63:53–62.
20. Reilly PA, Travers R, Littlejohn GO. Epidemiology of soft-tissue rheumatism: the influence of the law. *J Rheumatol.* 1991;18:1448–1449.
21. Rydevick B, Brown M, Lundborg G. Pathoanatomy and pathophysiology of nerve root compression. *Spine.* 1984;9:7–15.
22. Waddell G, Morris EW, DiPaola MP, et al. A concept of illness tested as an improved basis for surgical decisions in low-back disorders. *Spine.* 1986;11:712–719.
23. Wall PD, Melzack R. *Textbook of Pain.* Edinburgh, Scotland: Churchill Livingstone; 1984.
24. Weinstein J. Mechanisms of spinal pain: the dorsal root ganglion and its role as a mediator of low-back pain. *Spine.* 1986;11:999–1001.
25. Wiesel SW, Tsourmas N, Feffer HL, et al. A study of computer-assisted tomography: i. The incidence of positive CAT scans in an asymptomatic group of patients. *Spine.* 1984;9:549–551.
26. Yoshizawa H, O'Brien JP, Smith WT, et al. The neuropathology of intervertebral disc removed for low back pain. *J Pathol.* 1980;132:95–104.

CHAPTER 5

Epidemiology and Natural History of Spondylogenic Backache

"It's not so much the pain the man has, it is more the man who has the pain."

—Ian Macnab (1950s)

Although backache (with or without sciatica) is a benign, often self-limiting condition, it drains up to $90 billion per year (18) from the American government's health care budget. This has increased approximately $30 billion since the mid-1980s (7). The cost of both time lost from work (with loss of productivity) and medical care, as well as the cost of litigation and disability claims, make back pain an industry unto itself. Competing for attention for this "cash flow" are members of all manners of disciplines, each claiming to have the "answer."

FACTS AND FACTORS

Epidemiologic studies generate two sets of statistics:

1. Facts: The incidence (new cases per period of time) and the prevalence (all cases) as a measure of the natural history of the disease
2. Factors: Environmental (especially industrial) and individual factors that affect the incidence of low back pain and can be altered to decrease morbidity

FACTS

Low back pain is a high-profile symptom in industrialized societies. A study in England (8) revealed that 2% of the population annually sought medical care for back pain. Frymoyer et al. (9) have shown that during a lifetime, 70% of men will have an episode of low back pain.

Further facts that reveal the extent of low back pain as a problem for society are as follows:

1. In the United States, 2.5 million workers are injured per year (14).
2. Each year, 2% of all employees have a back injury (14).
3. Each year, 28.6 days per 100 workers are lost (14) (this amounts to 17 million work days per year in the United States).
4. At any one time, there are 1.2 million low-back-disabled adults in the United States (14).
5. In the United Kingdom, 1 in 25 men changes his job each year because of a low back injury (10).

In the industrial commission field, Snook and Jensen (24) have pointed out how difficult it is to calculate the cost of low back pain, because there are so many sources of payment to an injured worker. These include (a) wages that are paid during the waiting period before compensation from workmen's compensation insurance, (b) group and individual health insurance plans, and (c) Social Security benefits. The direct cost of back injuries to the industrial commissions in the United States totals $11 billion per year (24). Back injuries account for 20% of all compensable injuries but incur one third of the cost per year. It is estimated that the average cost per case is $6,000 and that, within the category of low back pain, 25% of the injuries account for 90% of the costs.

Low back pain accounts for a considerable annual volume of surgery in the United States. Approximately 150,000 patients undergo a simple laminectomy for removal of a herniated disc, and another 150,000 per year undergo spine surgery for some other degenerative condition (5). As the number of specialists who call themselves spine surgeons increases, so does the number of operations. To date, no investigator has been able to determine if Americans are better off as a result of the increase in back-spine specialists (23).

FACTORS AFFECTING INCIDENCE OF LUMBAR DISC DISEASE (DISC DEGENERATION AND DISC HERNIATION)

Age

Low back pain is most prevalent between the ages of 35 and 55 years. However, most patients in this age group have had a prior episode of back pain before age 35 years. Most operations for low back degenerative conditions occur between the ages of 35 and 55: younger patients usually undergo operations at the L5-S1 level, whereas surgery for the older patient usually involves the L4–5 level (13).

A herniated nucleus pulposus is more likely to occur between the ages to 30 and 40 years (13,22), at which time the disc is on its way to degeneration through a decrease in its water content. In patients younger than the age of 30 years, the resilience of the disc protects it from herniation; in patients older than the age of 40 years, a disc has developed some degree of inherent stability through fibrous changes that occur with the loss of turgor (14). However, there are so many exceptions to these age rules that they serve as little more than general guidelines.

Sex

In the general population, the incidence of low back pain appears to be equally distributed between men and women. It is well known that workers exposed to heavy work, especially twisting and lifting, have a higher incidence of back pain. A female worker is more exposed to injury through these forces, but because there are so many more men in the heavy work force, the incidence of back injury in the working population is heavily weighted toward men (13).

Body Build (Anthropometry)

There does not appear to be any strong correlation between height, weight, body build, and the occurrence of low back pain (6).

Posture

Postural deformities such as scoliosis, kyphosis, hypo- and hyperlordosis, and leg length discrepancy do not predispose to low back pain.

Spine Mobility and Strength

After injury there is a decrease in low back strength and mobility (22). There is some question as to whether this strength decrease is primarily responsible for the injury or secondary to the injury. Numerous studies are being undertaken now to determine if there is any predictive value in measuring the mobility and strength of a worker engaged in heavy-duty activity before injury. Studies have shown that the risk of back injury is increased if strength requirements on the job are greater than the isometric strength requirements measured in job simulation (16). On the other hand, Bergquist-Ullmann and Larsson (2) have shown that there is no difference in the rates of recovery from acute low back pain when fit individuals are compared with unfit individuals.

Smoking

One fact is certain: If you smoke, your chances of developing low back pain are greatly increased (6,9). Nothing has yet been proved about the causative factors related to this increased incidence, but theories abound:

- Smoking induces osteoporosis.
- Smoking induces coughing, which may cause microfractures in thinned trabeculae as well as increased intradiscal pressure.

- Smoking impairs blood flow, which is already very limited to a disc; this impairment in turn interferes with disc nutrition.
- Smoking decreases the O_2 carried by hemoglobin, which may interfere with cell survival within a disc.

Occupational Low Back Pain

Approximately one third of back injuries occur at work and are the result of lifting and twisting accidents (4). Another third of low back injuries also occur at work but are the result of slips and falls. The final third of low back injuries are not related to any particular work incident but, instead, occur spontaneously outside the work environment.

There is no uniform agreement on the type of job that is most likely to precipitate a low back injury (19,20). The injury rates and severity rates appear to be increased when heavy objects have to be lifted, especially from the floor level and especially when a twisting component is involved (11). Bulky objects and objects requiring frequent lifting also increase the incidence of low back complaints (15).

Individuals who have to drive as an occupation have a higher incidence of low back complaints (12). Some of this is likely related to the vibratory forces that are part of the job. Wilder et al. (30) have pointed out that the vibratory frequencies found in certain truck seats are a particular problem for truckers. Anyone who spends more than 50% of their time sitting at their job also has a threefold increase in the incidence of a disc herniation (12).

The cost to industry for low back problems is staggering, exceeding that spent on all other industrial injuries combined (25). Adding to the incalculable cost is the fact that injury usually strikes in the peak productive years of ages 35 to 55 (1,26).

Snook and Jensen (24) made the following observation on cost:

- One third of the cost per industrial claim goes to medical care, and two thirds goes to disability payments.
- Ninety percent of the compensation costs are consumed by 25% of the injury claimants.

Further evidence of the serious impact of low back pain in industry is the fact that workers with back complaints who are absent from work for longer than 6 months have only a 50% chance of returning to productive employment (21). Extending the work absence to 2 years virtually wipes out any chance that those workers will return to gainful employment. When exhorting an individual to work harder at physical therapy, remember that a return to work is inhibited more by whether or not the worker likes his or her boss and/or job than by his or her physical capacities (3).

Emotional State

Although much is said and written about low back pain, stress, and mental health, there is no body of scientific study suggesting that those individuals with emotional illness have an increased incidence of low back pain and sciatica (3). It is more likely that low back pain and emotional illness can coexist independently for a short time, but eventually (and occasionally, immediately) emotional lability will increase the degree of disability, sometimes beyond the bounds of the clinician's reason. Most studies (1,3,9) tend to show that the chronically back-injured worker is of poor intellectual capacity, with less ability to establish emotional contact and less in the way of a philosophical attitude toward injury. Whether this mental status precedes or results from the low back injury is open to question. Everyone would agree that worker dissatisfaction is high on the list of factors that make a worker vulnerable to a low back disability.

Radiographic Factors

Back pain is more frequent in persons with multilevel degenerative disc disease (28). Individuals with a spondylolysis or spondylolisthesis also have an increased incidence of back pain, especially when asked to do heavy work (29).

Most studies suggest that congenital lumbosacral anomalies do not increase the incidence of low back pain (27). The incidence of these anomalies across the general population appears to be approximately 5%; yet when one looks at studies on low back pain sufferers, the incidence of congenital lumbosacral anomalies on radiologic examination approaches 10%. This doubling of the incidence of congenital lumbosacral anomalies compared with the incidence of low back pain in the general population requires further study before anyone can dismiss these radiologic changes as being insignificant.

THE NATURAL HISTORY OF SPONDYLOGENIC LOW BACK PAIN

Waddell (29) has rightly pointed out that, because so many people suffer from low back pain at one time or another in their life, perhaps we should see this as normal and designate those who do not suffer from back pain as being abnormal! If spondylogenic back pain is so common, why aren't the hospital wards and doctors' offices full of the afflicted? Why should a disease, second only to the common cold in disabling those younger than age 45 years, consume up to $90 billion per year in America? Waddell has again hit the nail on the head in stating that in those countries where there are no caregivers for low back pain (e.g., Africa), there is no back disability!

The most important statement we can make in this book is as follows: *Spondylogenic low back pain is a self-limiting symptom (not a disease) that should require low cost for care.*

Ninety percent of patients with low back pain improve after 2 months (2). Those patients who recover face a 60% recurrence rate during the following 2 years.

Kirkaldy-Willis et al. (17) has provided us with the framework for understanding the natural history of spondylogenic low back pain (Fig. 5-1). They divided the spectrum of degenerative disc/facet joint disease into three phases.

PHASE I: DYSFUNCTION

Minor pathology causes limited abnormal function in the disc and/or facet joints, which leads to pain.

PHASE II: INSTABILITY

This is the intermediate phase in which continuing microtrauma leads to further degeneration in the disc and facet joints, producing laxity of the annulus and facet joint capsules. The resulting instability leads to more prolonged episodes of back pain.

PHASE III: STABILIZATION

This is the final stage that not all patients reach. Fibrosis of the nuclear-annular complex and the facet joint capsule, along with osteophyte formation, represents the body's attempt to stabilize the motion segment. Narrowing of the disc and settling of the facet joints probably adds further mechanical stability to the segment. Many patients, as they age, will volunteer that they are not as flexible as they used to be. It is fortunate for them, because this protects them from symptoms!

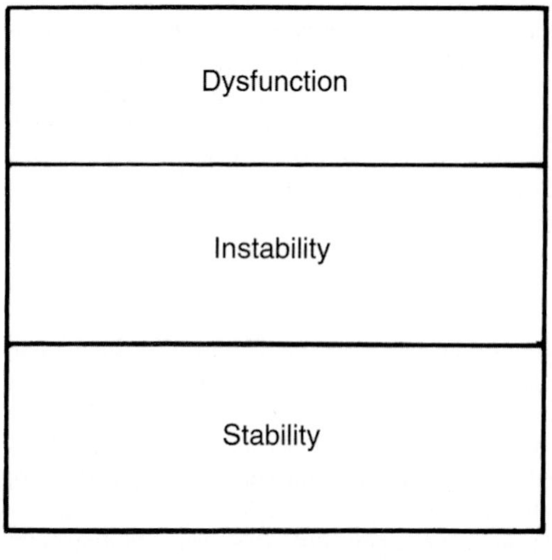

Dysfunction
Instability
Stability

FIGURE 5-1 ● The three phases of disc degeneration as depicted by Kirkaldy-Willis.

SUMMARY

Low back pain is an epidemic, and more and more studies are bringing this fact to our attention. There is a greater understanding of low back pain and of the facts and factors that result in the significant cost to society of treating this condition. Fortunately, the majority of sufferers have a propensity for spontaneous resolution of symptoms. Unfortunately, a subset of patients become long-term, disabled individuals and extract a significant number (billions) of dollars from the medical care system. These factors are now coming under more scrutiny from the medical community and those paying for patient care. Change in the way we handle low back pain from degenerative conditions of the spine is upon us.

REFERENCES

1. Anderson GBJ. Epidemiologic aspects on low-back pain in industry. *Spine.* 1981;6:53–60.
2. Bergquist-Ullmann M, Larsson U. Acute low back pain in industry. *Acta Orthop Scand Suppl.* 1977; 170:1–117.
3. Bigos SJ, Battie MC, Spengler DM, et al. A prospective study of work perceptions and psychological factors affecting the report of back injury. *Spine.* 1991;16:1–6.
4. Brown JR. Factors contributing to the development of low back pain in industrial workers. *J Am Ind Hyg Assoc.* 1975;36:26–31.
5. *Commission on Professional Hospital Activity of Ann Arbor, Michigan: Hospital Records Study.* Ambler, PA: IMS America Ltd; 1978.
6. Deyo RA, Bass JE. Lifestyles and low back pain: the influence of smoking, exercise, and obesity. *Clin Res.* 1987;35:577A.
7. Deyo RA, Tsui-Wu YJ. Descriptive epidemiology of low back pain and its related medical care in the United States. *Spine.* 1987;12:264–268.
8. Dillane JB, Fry J, Katon G. Acute back syndrome—A study from general practice. *Br Med J.* 1966;2:82–84.
9. Frymoyer JW, Pope MH, Clements JH, et al. Risk factors in low back pain. *J Bone Joint Surg Am.* 1983;65:213–218.
10. Harris AI. *Handicapped and Impaired in Great Britain, Part I.* London, England: Social Survey Division, Office of Population Census and Surveys. Her Majesty's Stationary Office; 1971.
11. Kelsey JL. An epidemiological study of the relationship between occupations and acute herniated lumbar intervertebral discs. *Int J Epidemiol.* 1975;4:197–205.
12. Kelsey JL. An epidemiological study of acute herniated lumbar intervertebral disc. *Rheumatol Rehabil.* 1975;14:144–159.
13. Kelsey JL, Ostfeld AM. Demographic characteristics of persons with acute herniated lumbar intervertebral disc. *J Chronic Dis.* 1975;28:37–50.
14. Kelsey JL, White AA. Epidemiology and impact of low back pain. *Spine.* 1980;5:133–142.
15. Kelsey J, White A, Pastides H, Brobee G. The impact of musculoskeletal disorders on the population of the United States. *J Bone Joint Surg.* 1979;61:959–964.
16. Keyserling WM, Herrin GD, Chaffin DB. Isometric strength testing as a means of controlling medical incidents on strenuous jobs. *J Occup Med.* 1980;22:332–336.
17. Kirkaldy-Willis WH, Wedge JH, Yong-Hing K, Reilly J. Pathology and pathogenesis of lumbar spondylosis and stenosis. *Spine.* 1978;3:319–328.
18. Luo X, Pietrobon R, Sun SX, et al. Estimates and patterns of direct health care expenditures among individuals with back pain in the United States. *Spine.* 2004;29:79–86.
19. Magora A. Investigation and relation between low back pain and occupation. *Scand J Rehabil Med.* 1975;7:146–151.
20. Magora A, Schwartz A. Relation between the low back pain syndrome and x-ray findings. *Scand J Rehabil Med.* 1976;8:115–125.
21. McGill CM. Industrial back problems: a control program. *J Occup Med.* 1968;10:174–178.
22. Miller JA, Schmaalz C, Schultz AB. Lumbar disc degeneration: correlation with age, sex and level in 600 autopsy specimens. *Spine.* 1987;13:173–178.
23. Nachemson AL. The lumbar spine—an orthopedic challenge. *Spine.* 1976;1:59–71.
24. Snook SH, Jensen RC. Cost. In: Pope MH, Frymoyer JW, Anderson G, eds. *Occupational Low Back Pain.* New York: Praeger; 1984:115–121.
25. Spengler DM, Bigos SJ, Martin NA, et al. Back injuries in industry: a retrospective study. Overview and costs analysis. *Spine.* 1986;11:241–245.
26. Svenson HO, Anderson GB. Low back pain in forty- to forty-seven-year-old men, work history and work environment factors. *Spine.* 1983;8:272–276.
27. Tilley P. Is sacralization a significant factor in lumbar pain? *J Am Osteopath Assoc.* 1970;70:238–241.
28. Torgerson BR, Dotter WE. Comparative roentgenographic study of asymptomatic and symptomatic lumbar spines. *J Bone Joint Surg.* 1976;58:850–853.
29. Waddell G. 1987 Volvo Award in Clinical Sciences. A new clinical model for the treatment of low back pain. *Spine.* 1987;12:632–644.
30. Wilder DG, Woodworth BB, Frymoyer JW, et al. Vibration and the human spine. *Spine.* 1982; 7:243–254.

CHAPTER 6

Spondylolysis and Spondylolisthesis

"False facts are highly injurious to progress of science, for they often endure long; but false views, if supported by some evidence do little harm, for everyone takes a salutary pleasure in proving their falseness."

—Charles Darwin

SPONDYLOLYSIS

With the significant increase in sporting effort in high school athletes ("My son is the best linebacker in his high school's history!"), there is an epidemic of spondylolysis. Up until recently, we have considered this condition a routine problem. More recently, with the use of computed tomography (CT) scanning and single photon emission computed tomography (SPECT) scanning, it has been found that the condition is far from routine, and it is difficult to be dogmatic with regard to the criteria for diagnosis and treatment.

ETIOLOGY OF SPONDYLOLYSIS

The classic teaching of causation for spondylolysis has been that an individual is born with a weakness in the pars interarticularis, and at approximately age 6, a fatigue injury occurs that breaks the pars (7). Later, in high school, with the weightlifting and contact stresses of football or the extension stresses of gymnastics or wrestling, the latent fracture is irritated and becomes symptomatic.

Another group of teenagers exists who present with an acute lesion. They have no history of injury, and they suffer a significant hyperextension injury or compressive force to their lumbar spine, which is followed by the immediate and sudden onset of very severe low back pain. Radiographs reveal a fresh fracture, and these patients have a very hot bone scan (Fig. 6-1) (10). These patients are in the minority and represent a special treatment situation.

Finally, remember that 5% of the general population walks around with a spondylolysis that is completely asymptomatic (10). Spondylolysis may be unilateral in up to one third of these patients.

CLINICAL PRESENTATION

A wide spectrum of presentations exists in these young patients, ranging from an acute disabling episode of back pain to mild low back discomfort when the patient engages in certain activities. The back pain may be dominant to one side, but more often is across the lumbosacral junction. Radiating leg pain is rare in spondylolysis, but hamstring tightness on straight leg raising testing is common. Neurologic symptoms and signs are absent.

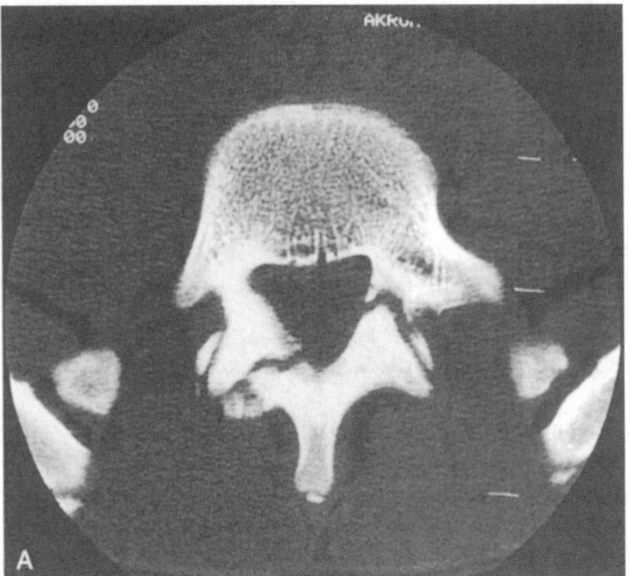

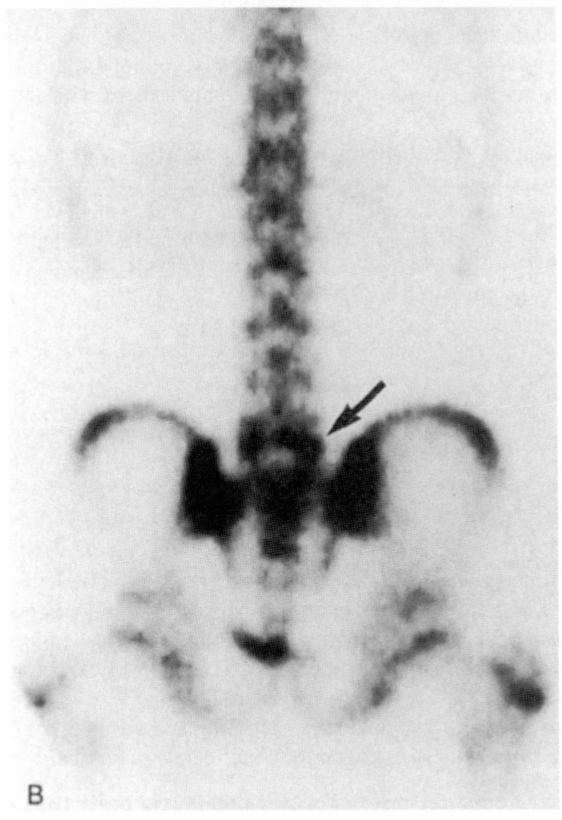

FIGURE 6-1 ● **A:** Axial CT of spondylolysis, L5. **B:** Bone scan in same patient showing bilateral "hot" pars interarticularis *(arrow)*.

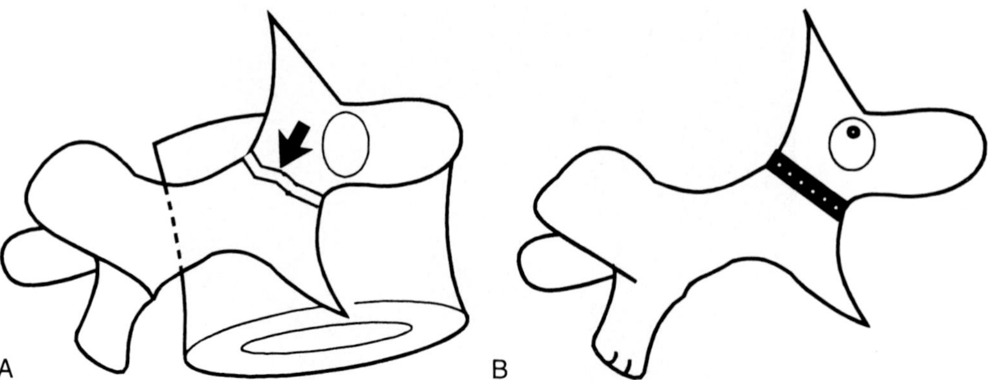

FIGURE 6-2 ● **A:** Schematic of oblique view of spondylolysis *(arrow)*. **B:** Note how lesion looks like a collar on a Scottish terrier.

RADIOGRAPHIC FINDINGS

The radiographic findings have no set pattern. Although most teenagers will have a defect that is seen on oblique radiographs (Fig. 6-2), enough negative oblique radiographs occur (Fig. 6-3) to require additional radiologic investigation in a young patient with unexplained mechanical back pain.

Additional investigative steps include a SPECT scan (Fig. 6-4) and a CT scan (Fig. 6-5). Experience has shown us that there is no pattern to the findings in these three tests (oblique lumbar radiographs, SPECT scan, and CT scan). You can almost pick whichever combination you wish: for example, positive oblique radiographs/negative SPECT and CT; negative oblique radiographs and SPECT/positive CT; positive oblique radiographs, SPECT, CT; and so on. In addition, the CT scan findings are by no means uniform (Fig. 6-6).

LEVEL OF LYSIS

The majority of spondylolytic lesions occur at L5, but a few will be present at higher lumbar levels.

TREATMENT

After many years of programmed treatment (e.g., a hot bone scan means a fresh fracture that must be immobilized), we have reduced our advice to two rules for two different groups of patients:

1. If the patient has low back pain and any one of the three tests is positive, take the patient out of the sport, put them in exercise physical therapy, and brace them. When they become asymptomatic, they join Group 2.
2. If the patient has no symptoms, do not restrict activities and do not brace them (or take them out of a brace), despite the results of radiographs, bone scan, and CT scan.

Unfortunately, many young persons fall between these two groups and require some form of activity restriction, therapeutic exercise, and bracing. The real problem comes when trying to determine the duration of treatment. Remember, "my son is the best linebacker in his high school's history," which is a statement usually associated with an important game in the near future at which all the college scouts will be in attendance! In this pressure situation of having to treat the patient/parent team, do what is best for the patient. If the patient is asymptomatic, let them play regardless of the investigation results. If the patient is symptomatic, restrict activities (regardless of the investigation results).

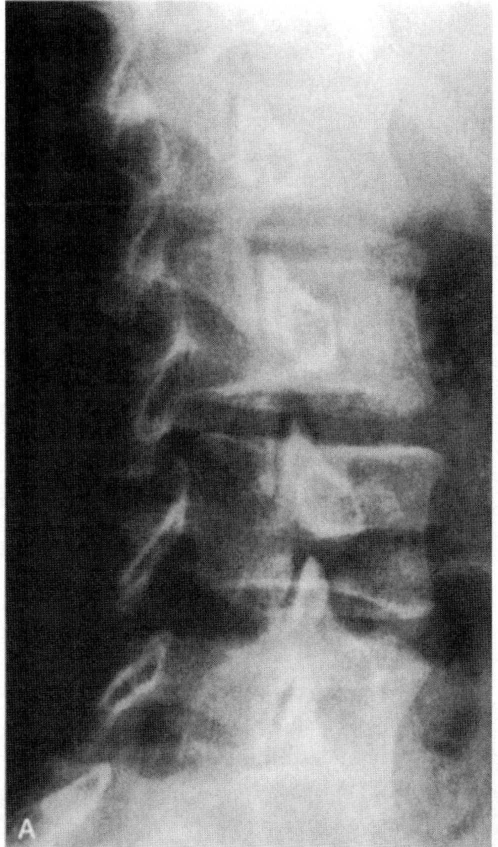

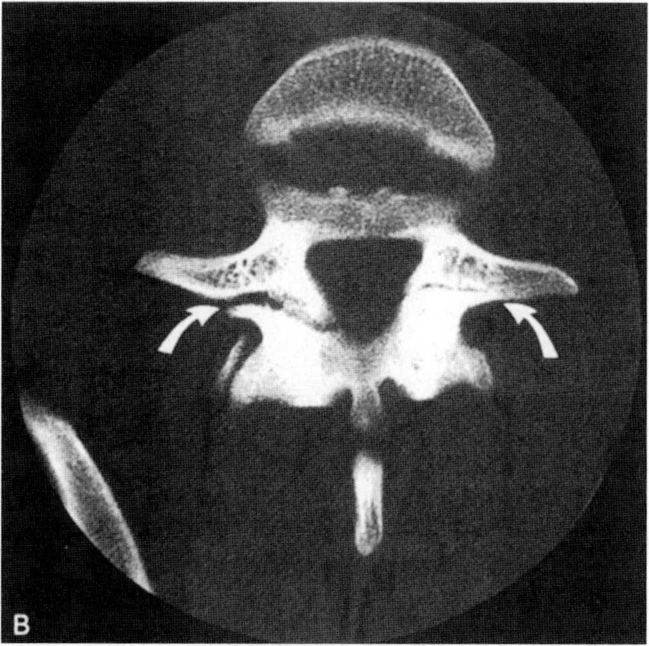

FIGURE 6-3 • **A:** An oblique radiograph of an adolescent who, after a football injury, developed low back pain; there is no apparent fracture. **B:** CT scan done at the same time showing bilateral pars defects *(arrows)*. *(continued)*

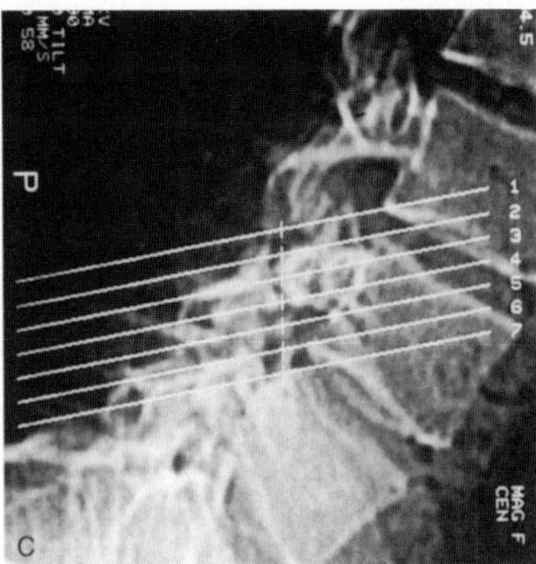

FIGURE 6-3 ● *(Continued)* **C:** The reverse gantry angle technique used to show defect in **B.**

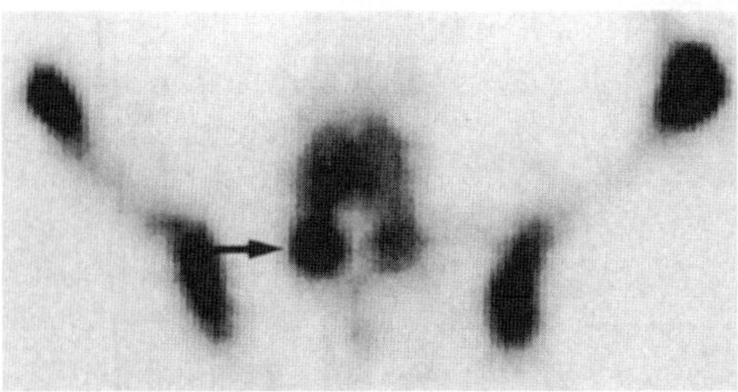

FIGURE 6-4 ● SPECT of spondylolysis *(arrow).*

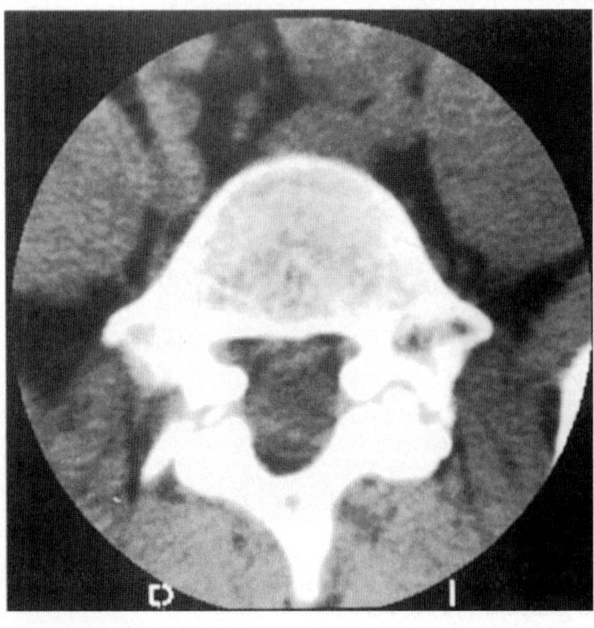

FIGURE 6-5 ● A CT scan of an old lysis (L5 bilateral).

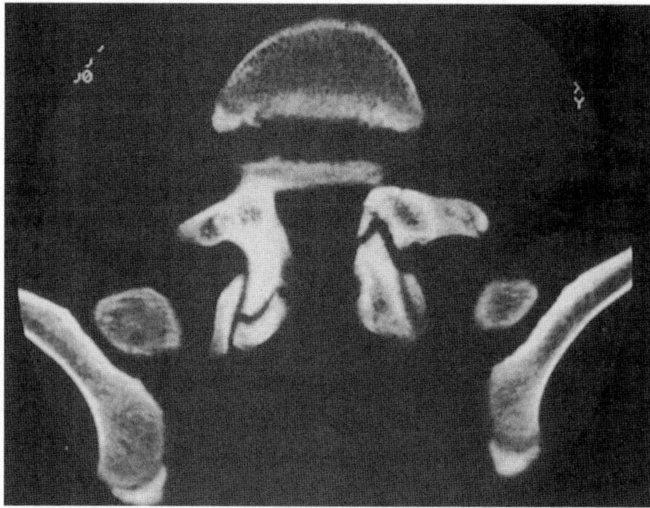

FIGURE 6-6 • Compare this CT of spondylolysis to Figures 6-5 and 6-3; each scan shows a different fracture pattern.

SPECIFIC TREATMENT OF SPONDYLOLYSIS

Conservative Treatment

Patients are treated with modalities and a flexion exercise program. Once symptoms start to improve, a generalized conditioning program and specific equipment-based exercises are instituted to strengthen the low back. During this program, the patient is abstaining from the aggravating activity (sport), which in itself may be the most important treatment step.

On relief of symptoms, the patients gradually return to sports. The most difficult aspect of judging the rate of return to sports is to balance what a stoical teenager who wants to "mix it up" with his or her peers is telling you about ongoing symptoms with what you, the treating physician, observe on examination.

Surgical Treatment

It is rare that a young patient cannot improve with conservative treatment. In these situations, direct surgical repair of the defect can be considered. Figure 6-7 shows the various ways of accomplishing this repair.

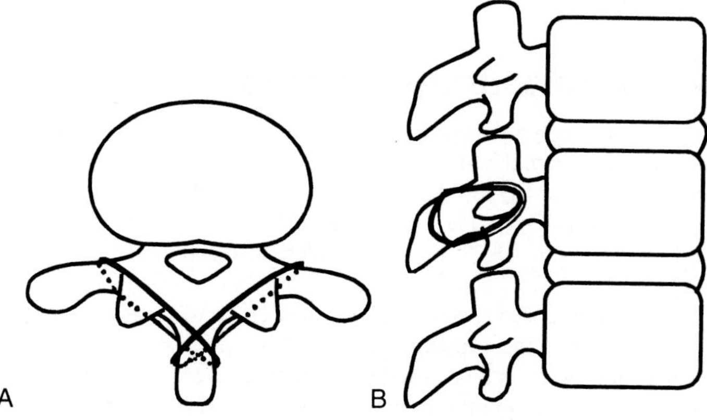

FIGURE 6-7 • **A:** Axial view of repair of spondylolysis with wire around spinous process and transverse processes. **B:** Sagittal view of the same repair.

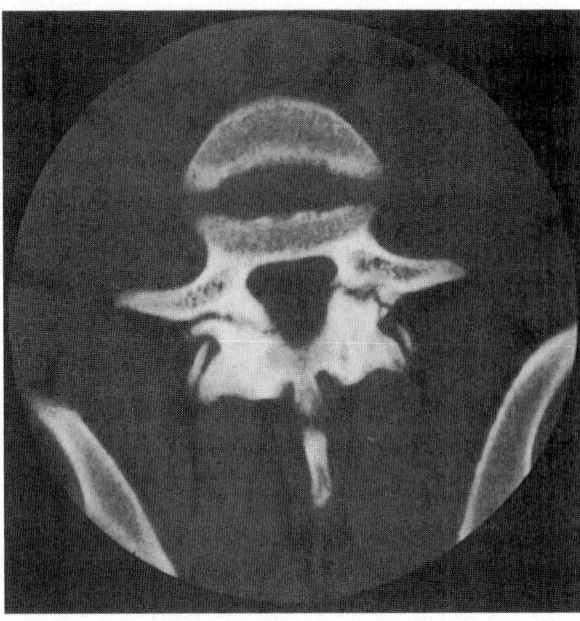

FIGURE 6-8 ● This is the CT scan of the same patient in Figure 6-3, 5 months later; the patient experienced no pain and was playing sports. The pars interarticularis fractures are still obvious.

FOLLOW-UP

On follow-up, plain radiograph, and CT scan, we have seen a minority of these lesions heal despite the patient becoming asymptomatic (Fig. 6-8). We simply follow up these patients every 6 months to a year with a standing lateral lumbar spine radiograph. If they start to develop a slip (spondylolisthesis), we become more aggressive with treatment intervention.

SPONDYLOLISTHESIS

Forward slip of the fifth vertebra is resisted by the bony locking of the posterior facets, the intact neural arch and pedicle, normal bone plasticity preventing stretch of the pedicle, and the intervertebral discs bonding the vertebral bodies together (Fig. 6-9). Breakdown of this normal locking mechanism occurs with articular defects and defects in the neural arch. These pathologic defects produce five recognizable clinical groups of spondylolisthesis (6) (Tables 6-1 and 6-2): dysplastic, isthmic, degenerative, traumatic, and pathologic.

DESCRIPTION OF SPONDYLOLISTHESIS ON RADIOGRAPH

Before describing the various types of spondylolisthesis, it is best to understand the terms used to measure the extent of the vertebral body slip.

The classic measurement of the slip degree has been that of Myerding (4), an obstetrician who described four degrees of slip (Fig. 6-10) (Grade 1 = 25%, Grade 2 = 25% to 50%, Grade 3 = 50% to 75%, and Grade 4 = 75% to 100% slip). A complete dislocation of L5 on S1 (Fig. 6-25) was called a spondyloptosis.

Wiltse and Winter (8) proposed a more sophisticated group of measurements (Fig. 6-11). The reason for this was to separate the tangential movement in the low-grade slips (Grades I and II) from the angular/tangential slips that occurred in the higher levels of slip. In fact, this more complete classification has served to point out that the low-grade slips behave like degenerative disc disease, and the high-grade slips are more like a spinal deformity that requires a whole new set of management principles. This distinction is covered in the following sections.

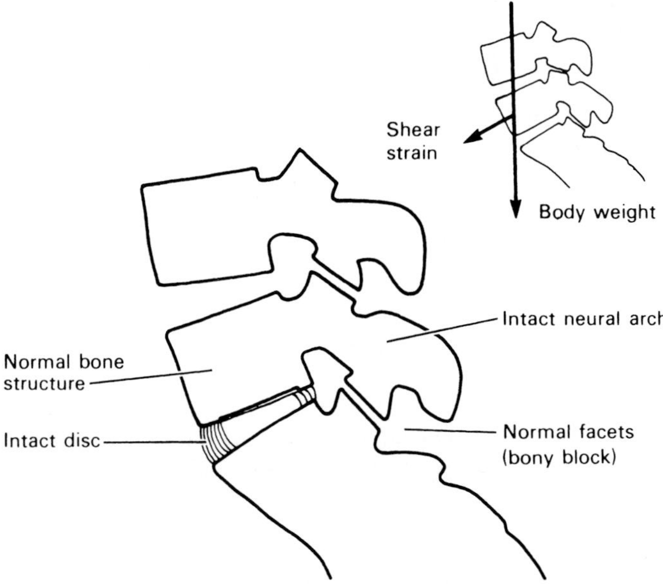

FIGURE 6-9 ● The normal locking mechanisms resisting forward displacement of the fifth lumbar vertebral body. (From Macnab I. *Backache.* Baltimore: Williams & Wilkins; 1977:45 with permission.)

TABLE 6-1

Working Classification of Spondylolisthesis

	Etiology	
Bony Location of Defect	**Congenital**	**Acquired**
Pars	Isthmic (fatigue fracture)	Traumatic fracture
Facet joint	Congenital absence or dysplasia	Degeneration of facet joint
Bone	0	Weak or 'plastic' bone

TABLE 6-2

Commonly Accepted Clinical Classification of Spondylolisthesis

Type	Classification	Description
I	Dysplastic	Congenital abnormalities of upper sacrum or arch at L5
II	Isthmic	Lesion in pars interarticularis Lytic—fatigue fracture Elongated but intact pars Acute fracture
III	Degenerative	Facet joint degeneration
IV	Traumatic	Fractures in areas of arch other than pars
V	Pathologic	Secondary to generalized or localized bone disease

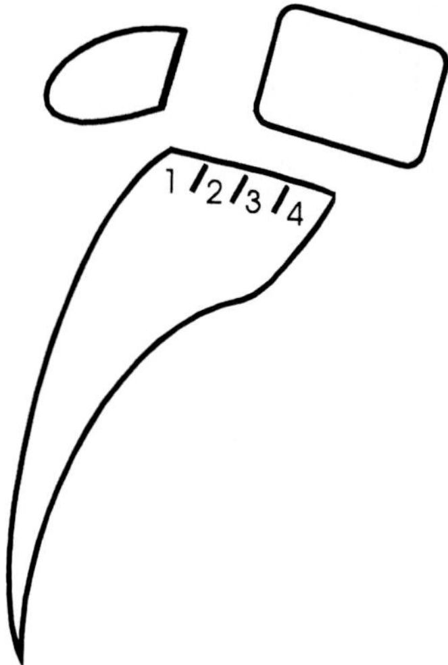

FIGURE 6-10 ● Myerding (4) classification of slip grades, which divides the sacrum into "quarters." This is a drawing of a Grade II slip.

TYPE I CONGENITAL OR DYSPLASTIC SPONDYLOLISTHESIS

Congenital spondylolisthesis with forward displacement of a vertebral body at birth is a clinical curiosity. The spinal defect is usually only one of multiple congenital anomalies, and the clinical problem presented is not the management of the spondylolisthesis but the management of the associated congenital scoliosis.

In a true dysplastic spondylolisthesis, the lesion may be either dysplasia of the upper sacrum, specifically in the facet joints (Fig. 6-12), or an attenuation of the pars interarticularis that gets pulled out and thinned as though it were made of a malleable plastic (Fig. 6-13). As the slip increases, and as the pars interarticularis becomes increasingly stretched, it may eventually break, but this break is secondary to the slip and is not the cause of the slip. This concept represents a slight deviation from the Wiltse-Newman-Macnab classification (6), the reason for which is explained in

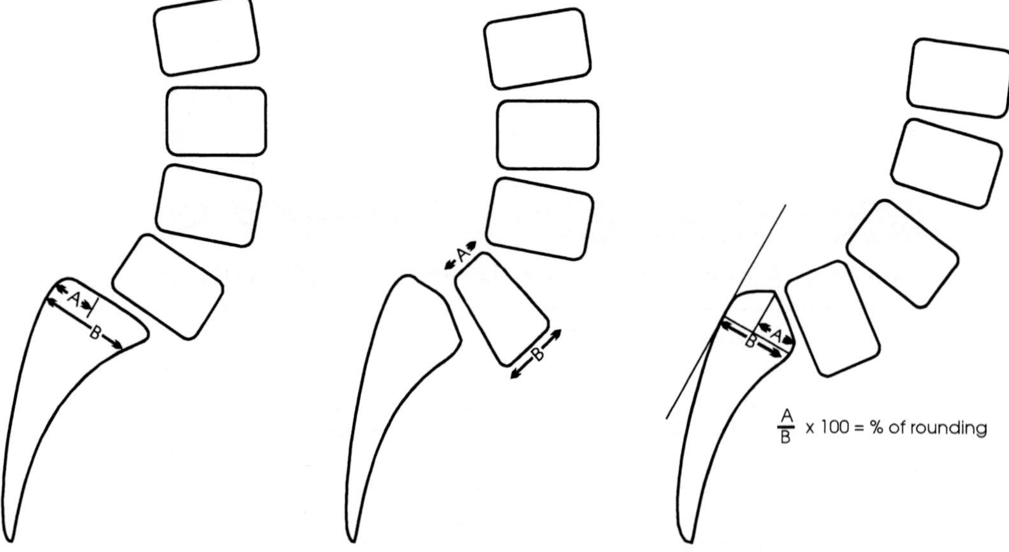

FIGURE 6-11 ● The Wiltse-Winter nomenclature. **Left:** The degree of slip is expressed as the percentage A is of B. **Middle:** Vertebral wedging—again, what percent A is of B. **Right:** Sacral rounding.

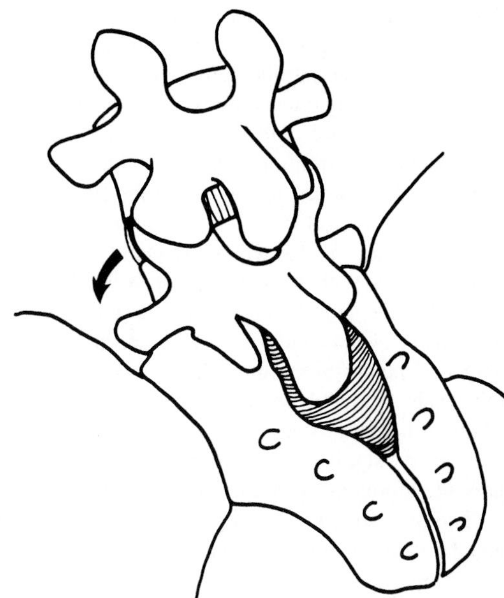

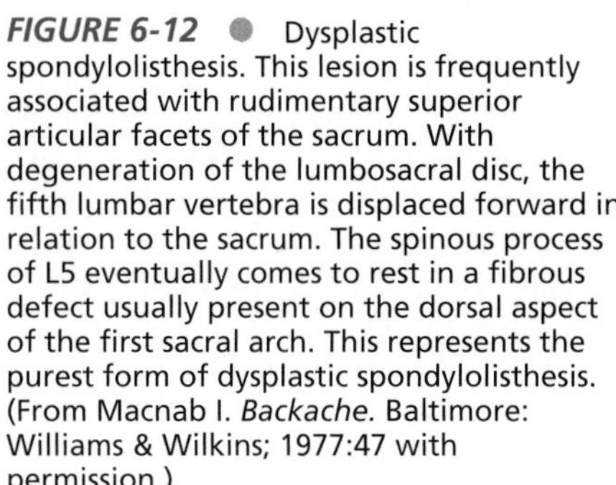

FIGURE 6-12 ● Dysplastic spondylolisthesis. This lesion is frequently associated with rudimentary superior articular facets of the sacrum. With degeneration of the lumbosacral disc, the fifth lumbar vertebra is displaced forward in relation to the sacrum. The spinous process of L5 eventually comes to rest in a fibrous defect usually present on the dorsal aspect of the first sacral arch. This represents the purest form of dysplastic spondylolisthesis. (From Macnab I. *Backache.* Baltimore: Williams & Wilkins; 1977:47 with permission.)

the legend of Figure 6-12. On occasion, there may be a subluxation of the posterior joints between L5 and the sacrum due to a lack of development of the first sacral arch, with absence or dysplasia of the superior articular facets of the sacrum. The only structure preventing forward slip of the fifth lumbar vertebra is the lumbosacral disc. When this breaks down, the fifth lumbar vertebra slips forward, with the inferior facets gliding over the rudimentary superior articular facets. The spinous process of L5 eventually comes to rest in the fibrous defect in the first sacral arch (Fig. 6-12). However, this by itself would not allow a very marked slip. Further slipping must involve attenuation and elongation of the pars interarticularis.

In this form of spondylolisthesis, slipping occurs early in life and is permitted by virtue of detachment of the hyaline cartilage plate. The degree of slip is usually quite marked (2). In severe

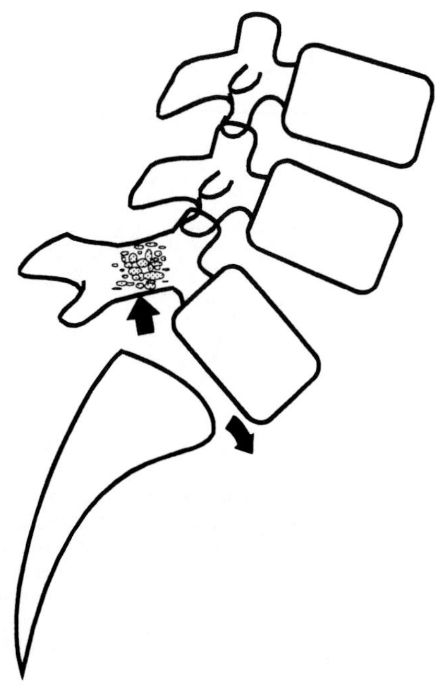

FIGURE 6-13 ● An elongated pars may allow for a spondylolisthesis.

degrees of slip, the basic pathology is frequently overlooked because when severe degrees of slip are noted on radiograph, it has always been assumed that there must be a defect in the pars interarticularis. The fact that the defect may not be shown on the radiograph has been ascribed to difficulties in radiologic techniques. The important clinical feature of the lesion is the fact that often there is lack of a defect in the pars interarticularis. Because there is no defect, the neural arch comes forward with the slipping vertebra, and the cauda equina may be compressed between the laminae of L4 and L5 and the dorsal area of the first sacral body. Lane in 1893 described a young woman who had the misfortune to be the serving maid of a man who suffered from the delusion that life was all cricket (5). He would frequently strike her in the rear with a cricket bat that he always carried around with him. She gradually became paraplegic. Lane, describing his operative findings, stated that the neural arch was intact, and as the arch had slipped forward, it had compressed the dura mater of the cauda equina. According to Lane, the spinous process of L5 lay in the fibrous defect of the dorsal sacrum. This is a beautiful description of the pathology of dysplastic spondylolisthesis. Although examples of cauda equina compression are sometimes seen with this type of spondylolisthesis, the attenuation and elongation of the isthmus that inevitably occur usually prevent any significant distortion of the cauda equina (Fig. 6-14). In fact, the majority of patients present without any evidence of nerve root irritation at all.

The average age of symptom onset may be very young but is most often 14 years in girls and 16 years in boys (±4 years), the final growth spurt age. The onset may be quite sudden and dramatic and is aptly termed a "listhetic crisis." The patient experiences a sudden onset of backache and, on examination, characteristically presents with a rigid lumbar spine that is commonly associated with a spastic or functional scoliosis. The pelvis is rotated anteriorly, giving rise to a flat sacrum; hamstring spasm is frequently seen, which makes the patient walk with bent knees (Fig. 6-15).

The reason for differentiating this group of spondylolisthesis from the others is that the indications for surgery are much more clear-cut than in the next group, isthmic spondylolisthesis. If a dysplastic spondylolisthesis progresses to the stage of producing severe symptoms before the age of 21 years, with or without signs of nerve root irritation, it is unlikely that the patient will make a complete recovery without surgical intervention. Patients presenting with a first- or even second-degree slip will probably continue to slip more if seen in their early teens. Evidence has substantiated the view that fusion performed at this stage will prevent further slip.

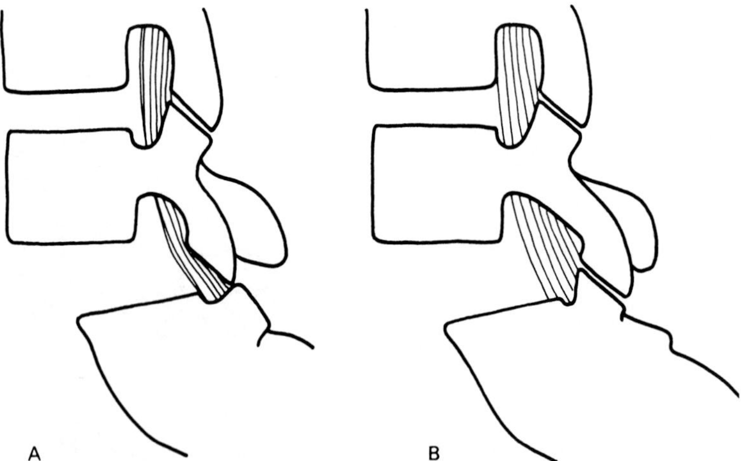

FIGURE 6-14 ● Dysplastic spondylolisthesis. In the presence of a normal pars interarticularis, forward dislocation of the fifth lumbar vertebra in relation to the sacrum is likely to produce compression of the cauda equina **(A).** The elongation of the pars interarticularis associated with the forward displacement of the fifth lumbar vertebra in dysplastic spondylolisthesis maintains the diameter of the spinal canal and obviates compression of the cauda equina **(B).** (From Macnab I. *Backache.* Baltimore: Williams & Wilkins; 1977:48 with permission.)

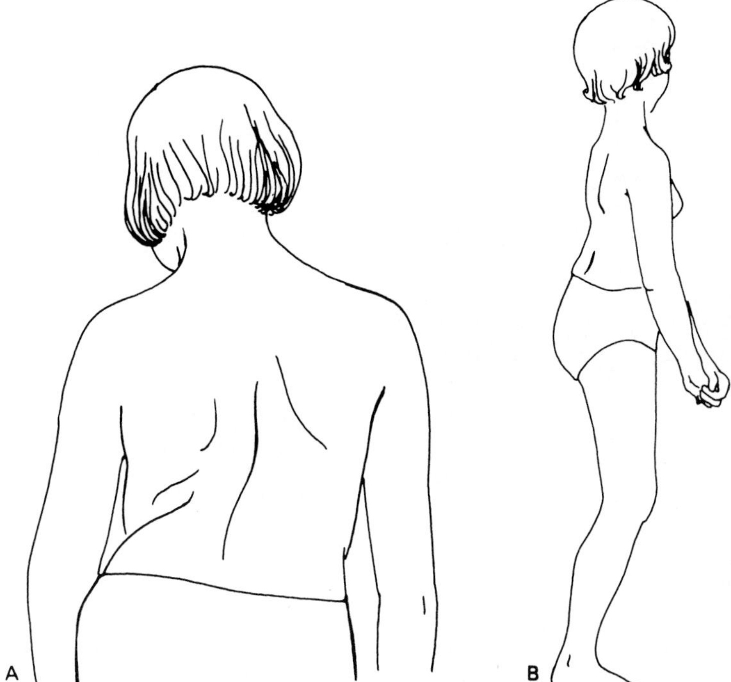

FIGURE 6-15 ● A "listhetic crisis" is frequently associated with a functional scoliosis **(A).** Hamstring spasm is common despite anterior rotation of the pelvis, and the patient frequently stands and walks with bent knees **(B).** (From Macnab I. *Backache.* Baltimore: Williams & Wilkins; 1977:49 with permission.)

The slip angle (lumbosacral kyphosis) contributes significantly to deformity, including the prominence of the buttocks and the sagittal imbalance with forward thrust of the torso. Reducing this slip angle is far more valuable than reducing the translation.

In the surgical management of this condition, the following points must be borne in mind: It is unwise to attempt to reduce the slip translation. Patients who present evidence of root tension or impairment root conduction will require laminectomy and, on occasion, decompression of the involved root or roots. All patients will require stabilization and fusions, and the best method of fusion devised to date is the ala transverse fusion (Fig. 6-16). Numerous methods have been described.

ISTHMIC SPONDYLOLISTHESIS

Lytic: Fatigue Fracture of Pars

In isthmic spondylolisthesis, the basic lesion is a defect in the pars interarticularis of the neural arch (Fig. 6-17). The etiology of this lesion is unknown, but Wiltse et al. (6) and others postulate that it is a fatigue fracture of the pars. This lesion likely occurs in a congenitally weakened pars (9). The neural arch defects occur most commonly between the ages of 5 and 7 years. Forward slipping of the vertebral body occurs most frequently between the ages of 10 and 15 years and rarely increases after age 20 years.

Despite the uncertainty relating to the etiology of the neural arch defect, the radiologic appearance is well known in general. The patient with low back pain presents an irksome problem for the orthopedic surgeon. The diagnosis is usually obscure or cannot be proved. Treatment perforce is empirical, and the results of treatment, in many instances, are unrewarding. Therefore, the demonstration on radiograph of a gross abnormality of this type is generally greeted with a sigh of relief: Here is a recognizable cause of backache; here is an easily understood and treatable lesion.

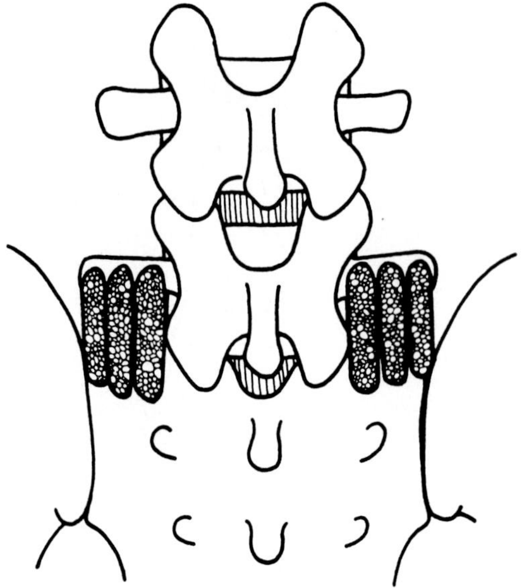

FIGURE 6-16 ● Ala transverse fusion using corticocancellous grafts bridging the gap between the transverse process of L5 and the ala of the sacrum. (From Macnab I. *Backache*. Baltimore: Williams & Wilkins; 1977:50 with permission.)

However, a word of caution must be interjected. Severe degrees of slip may be present in patients who engage in very vigorous activities, and yet they never suffer from backache (3). As with disc degeneration, the degree severity of the radiologic abnormality does not correlate with the severity of the symptoms.

Because there is no doubt that lytic spondylolisthesis can and does occur without producing symptoms, the mere radiologic demonstration of the defect in a patient with back pain does not indicate that the source of the symptoms has necessarily been demonstrated. Other anatomic variants have in the past been thought to be a cause of backache. It is now generally accepted that none of these anatomic variants is, by itself, a cause of low back pain. The question must arise, therefore, as to whether a neural arch defect, with or without a slip of the vertebral body, is yet another example of an anatomic variant incorrectly blamed as a cause of low back pain.

However, it is not unusual that patients with spondylolisthesis may become completely symptom free after a successful spinal fusion. In trying to explain this apparent contradiction, many years ago Dr. Macnab divided patients with back pain into three age groups (younger than 25, 26–40, and older than 40 years), and the incidence of spondylolisthesis was studied in each group (Table 6-3). Older than age 40 years, the incidence was approximately the same as the population as a whole, whereas younger than age 25 years, nearly 19%, a significant number, showed the defect. From these findings, it can be said that if the radiograph of a patient with back pain shows a lytic spondylolisthesis and the patient is younger than 26 years, the defect is probably the cause of the symptoms; between ages 26 and 40 years, the defect is only possibly the cause; and older than age 40 years, it is rarely, if ever, the sole cause of symptoms. In the management of lytic spondylolisthesis associated with neural arch defects, the age of the patient, therefore, is of prime importance.

When considering the pathogenesis of symptoms in this group, the following points must be remembered. The lesion may be asymptomatic. If the syndesmosis firmly bonds the two halves of the neural arch together, there is no mechanical instability and probably no mechanical reason for pain. If, however, the syndesmosis is loose, separation occurs on flexion (Fig. 6-18), and a strain is applied to the fibrous syndesmosis and the supraspinous ligament as well. Repetitive strains of this nature could give rise both to local and referred pain in a sciatic distribution.

Root irritation is not uncommon. With forward slip of the vertebral body, the intervertebral foramen is generally enlarged, and the nerve root may not be encroached on because the neural arch is left behind as the vertebral body slips forward. However, nerve root compression can occur in the following circumstances. On occasion, when the vertebral body slips forward, the neural arch will rotate on the pivot formed by its articulation with the sacrum and may encroach on the foramen (Fig. 6-19). A second form of root encroachment is a small hook frequently found on the proximal edge of the isthmic defect that engages the nerve root (also sometimes called the mushroom cap

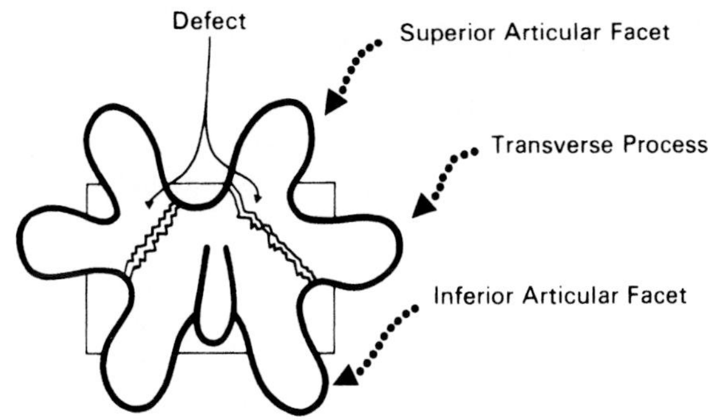

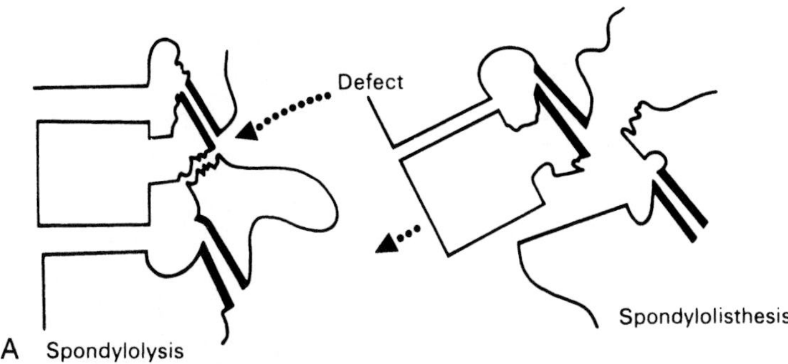

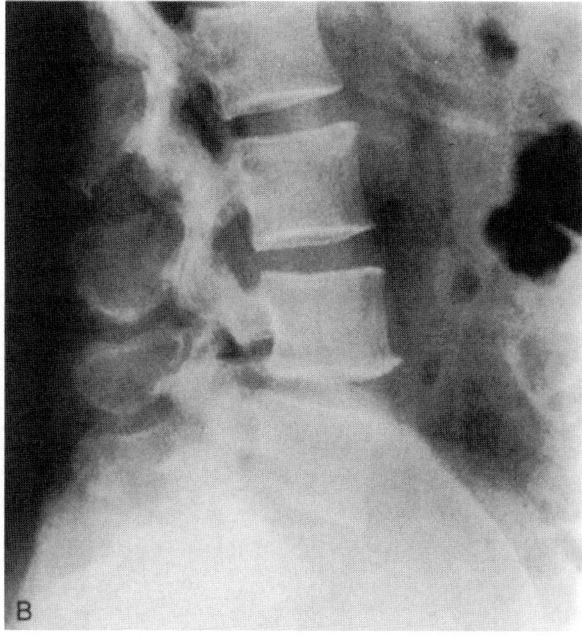

FIGURE 6-17 • **A:** Isthmic spondylolisthesis. The basic lesion is a defect in the neural arch across the pars interarticularis. When degenerative changes occur in the subjacent disc, the vertebral body will displace forward carrying, with it the superimposed spinal column and leaving behind the inferior articular facets, lamina, and spinous process. (From Macnab I. *Backache.* Baltimore: Williams & Wilkins; 1977:51 with permission.) **B:** Lateral radiograph of spondylolisthesis at L4-5.

TABLE 6-3

Incidence of Spondylolisthesis

Age (years)	No. of Patients	Arch Defects	Percentage
Younger than 26	116	22	18.9
26–40	350	26	7.6
Older than 40	530	28	5.2
Total	996	76	7.6

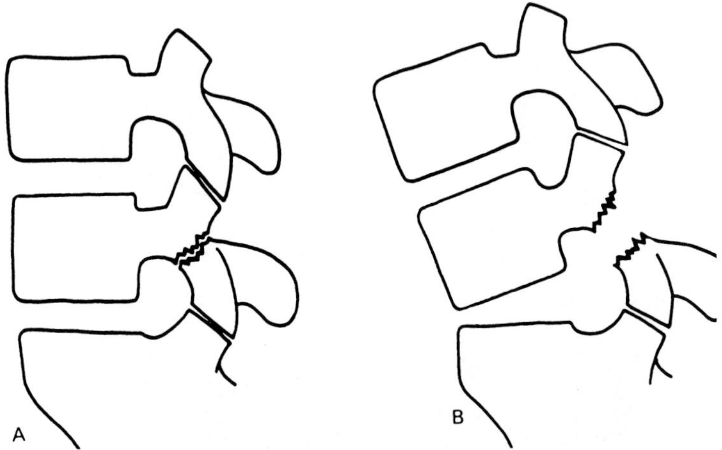

FIGURE 6-18 ● In isthmic spondylolisthesis, although the defect may be closed when the patient holds the spine in extension **(A),** separation may occur to a marked degree on flexion **(B).** (From Macnab I. *Backache.* Baltimore: Williams & Wilkins; 1977:52 with permission.)

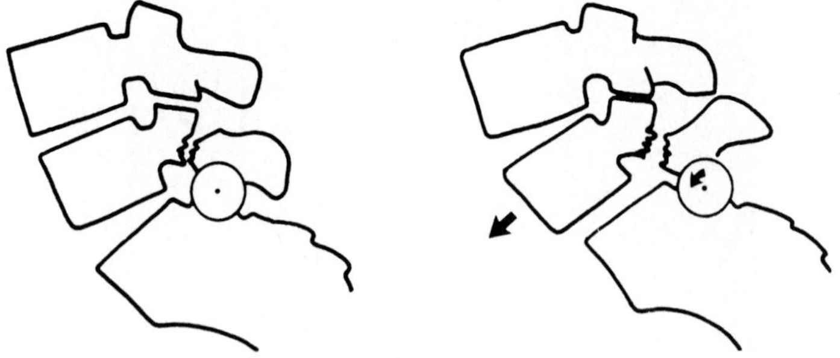

FIGURE 6-19 ● When the vertebral body slips forward, the traction applied to the free neural arch may cause it to rotate on the pivot formed by its articulation with the sacrum. When this occurs the anterior aspect of the neural arch defect may encroach on the foramen and compress the emerging nerve root. (From Macnab I. *Backache.* Baltimore: Williams & Wilkins; 1977:53 with permission.)

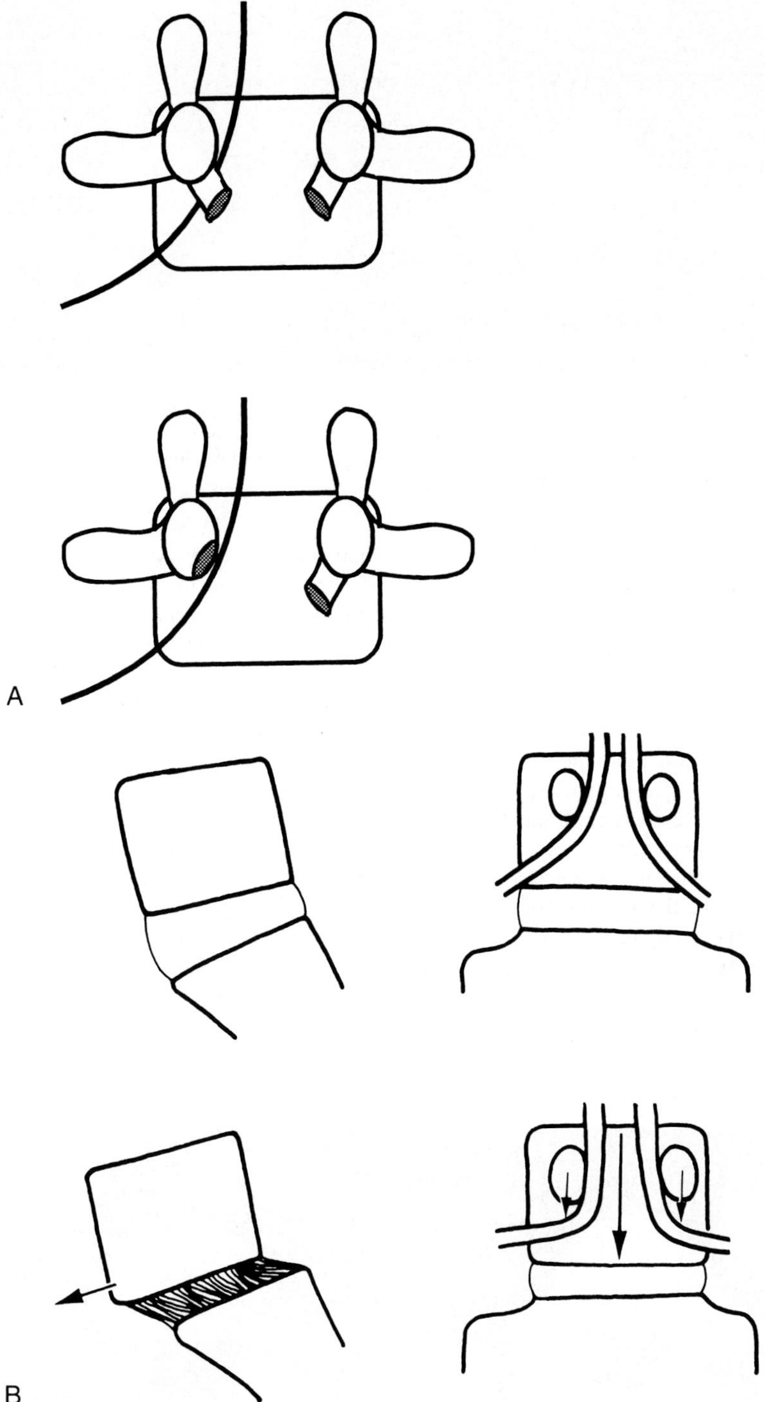

FIGURE 6-20 • **A:** The hook on proximal portion of the defect *(top schematic)* has been excised along with a portion of the pedicle *(shaded)* in the bottom schematic. **B:** Kinking of the nerve roots by the pedicles as the body of L5 slips downward and forward. (From Macnab I. *Backache.* Baltimore: Williams & Wilkins; 1977:54 with permission.)

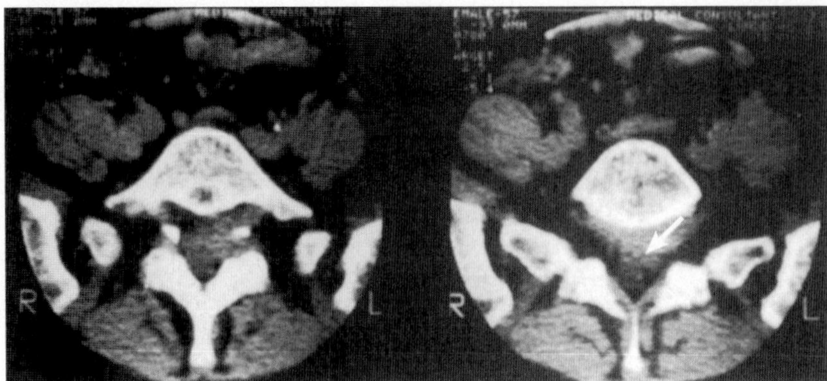

FIGURE 6-21 ● A lytic spondylolisthesis with ossified portion to fibrocartilaginous contents of defect. This small ossicle of bone is often lying on the nerve root to cause compressive symptoms. Did you notice the large herniated nucleus pulposus on the left in the axial slice to the right *(arrow)*?

osteophyte.) (Fig. 6-20). The likelihood of foraminal entrapment of the nerve root is increased if disc space narrowing occurs, which allows the pedicle to guillotine the nerve root (Fig. 6-20). The fibrocartilaginous contents of the pars interarticularis defect may also encroach on the nerve root (Fig. 6-21). The least common cause of root involvement is disc rupture at the slip level (Fig. 6-22) or a different level.

The nerve root, after it has emerged through the intervertebral foramen, is more or less fixed as it courses through the large muscle masses. With spondylolisthesis, the vertebral body glides forward and downward along the inclined plane of the superior surface of the vertebral body below. This downward drop is particularly marked at L5-S1. With this movement of the vertebra, the pedicles descend on the nerve roots and kink them as they emerge through the foramen (Fig. 6-20).

Forward slipping will not occur without some degenerative changes occurring in the underlying disc. This generally takes place as a slow attrition of the disc, but sometimes the disc collapses and bulges out around the periphery of the vertebral body just like squashed putty. The nerve root may get buried in this bulging mass after it has emerged from the foramen.

There is a strong ligamentous band that runs from the undersurface of the transverse process to the side of the vertebral body, the corporotransverse ligament (Fig. 6-23). At L5, the fifth lumbar nerve root runs between the ligament and the ala of the sacrum. With marked forward slip and downward descent of L5, the ligament comes down like a guillotine on the fifth lumbar root and

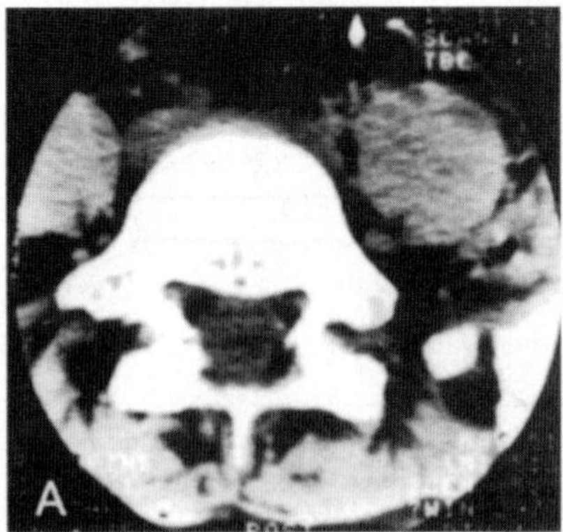

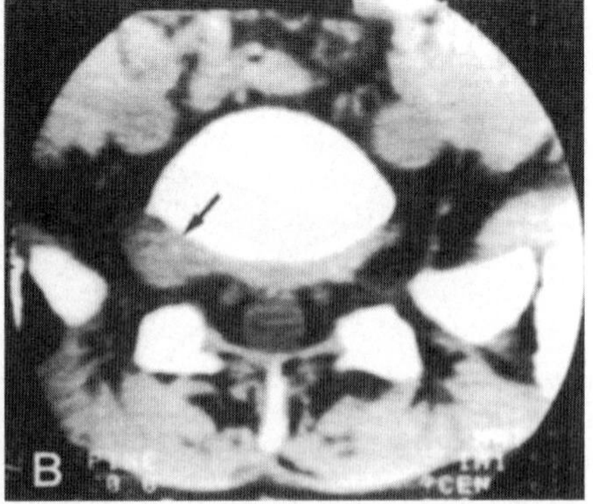

FIGURE 6-22 ● **A:** A CT scan (unfortunately a soft tissue window) showing a lytic spondylolisthesis. **B:** The next slice caudally shows the reason for the severe right leg pain in this patient—a large foraminal herniated nucleus pulposus of the slip level (L5-S1) *(arrow)*.

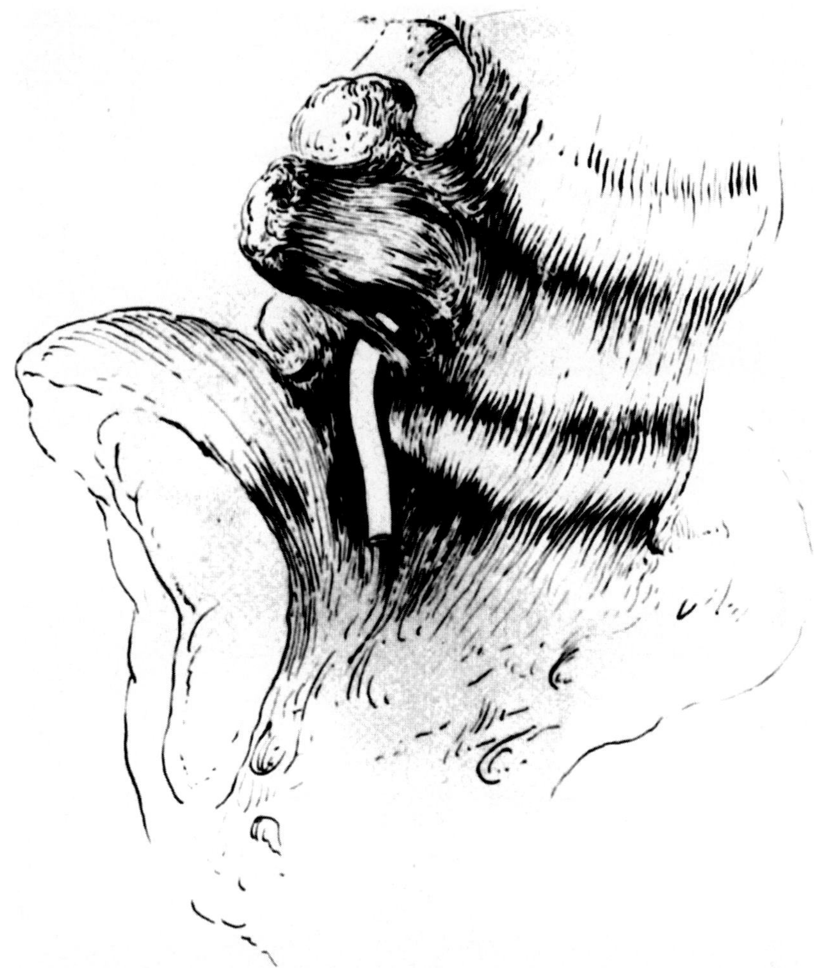

FIGURE 6-23 • The relationship of the fifth lumbar nerve root to the corporotransverse ligament. (From Macnab I. *Backache.* Baltimore: Williams & Wilkins; 1977:55 with permission.)

may entrap it against the ala of the sacrum. Kinking of the nerve root by the pedicle and extraforaminal entrapment of the nerve all encroach on the nerve emerging through the foramen at the site of the slip. With slipping of the fifth lumbar vertebra, it is the fifth lumbar root that is involved. Another possible cause of fifth lumbar root compression in a patient with an L5-S1 slip is, of course, a disc herniation at L4-L5.

Spondylolysis predisposes to premature disc degeneration in the subjacent disc, and spondylolisthesis eventually causes disc degeneration. These degenerative changes may of themselves be painful, giving rise to local or referred pain in sciatic distribution without root irritation.

Therefore, the local causes of pain in spondylolysis, with or without a slip, are instability, foraminal encroachment of the nerve root, extraforaminal entrapment of the nerve root, and disc degeneration.

Older than the age of 30 years, other sources of pain become increasingly common, and these must of course influence treatment. A disc rupture may occur in association with spondylolisthesis. Although the rupture may occur at the disc involved in the slip (Figs. 6-21 and 6-22), much more commonly it is seen at the disc above the slip (Fig. 6-24). When a disc rupture occurs at the segment above the slipping vertebra, one has to accept the fact that the patient's symptoms may be stemming solely from the herniated disc and that the spondylolisthesis may be asymptomatic. In

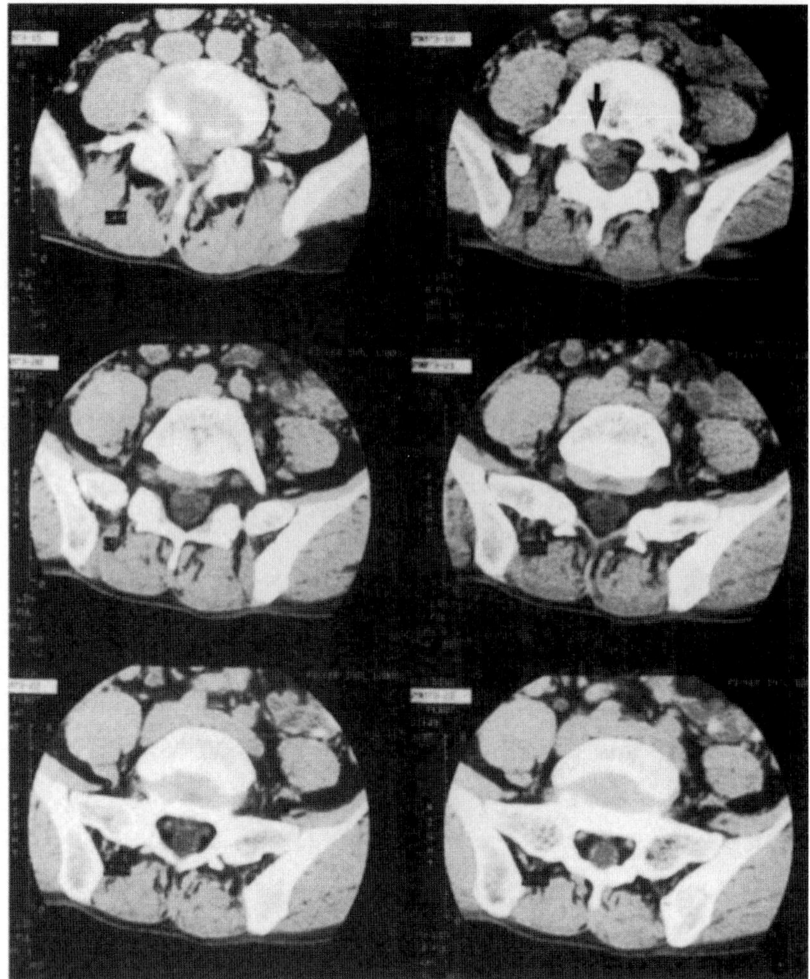

FIGURE 6-24 ● CT scan showing a lytic spondylolisthesis (L5-S1) with large herniated nucleus pulposus, L4-5, right *(arrow).*

some instances, discectomy alone is sufficient to give complete relief of symptoms. This is particularly true in patients who have never experienced any back disability previously.

Symptomatic disc degeneration, as distinct from disc herniation, may occur above the level of the slip. This may produce local pain or referred leg pain.

Unlike dysplastic spondylolisthesis, in which severe slips are associated with pelvic rotation and flattening of the back, in lytic spondylolisthesis, a forward slip of more than 50% is frequently associated with hyperlordosis above the slip and a kyphosis at the slip level. These high-degree slips [Grades 3, 4, and 5 (spondyloptosis)] (Fig. 6-25) are, in essence, kyphotic deformities of the lumbosacral junction causing as much, or more, deformity than backache. Extensive discussion of these deformities can be found in other texts (1,2). When this occurs, the hyperlordosis, by itself, may cause part or all of the symptoms complained of, and the symptoms derived from this source will, of course, persist after a spinal fusion.

With long-standing lumbosacral pathology, the lumbodorsal junction becomes the site of maximal movement, and in patients older than age 35 years, degenerative changes of a marked degree are frequently seen in the discs and posterior joints in this area. Patients with degenerative changes in this region may present with low back pain as the sole symptom. The fact that changes at the lumbodorsal junction play a role in the production of the patient's low back pain can be

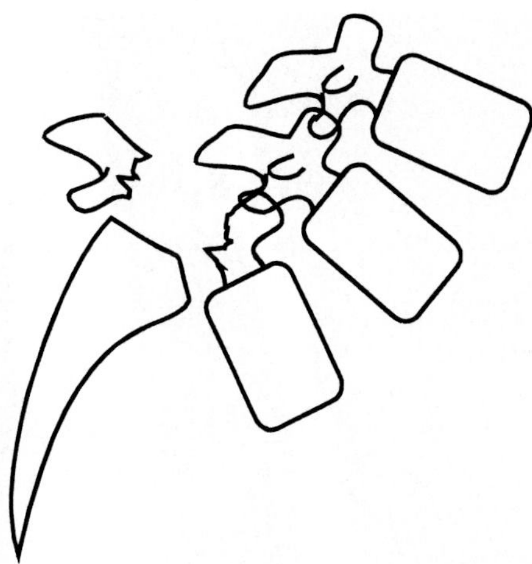

FIGURE 6-25 • Spondyloptosis: the back of the slipped vertebrae (L5) is in front of the sacrum.

demonstrated on clinical examination. With the patient lying on his or her side, with hips and knees flexed to flatten the lumbar curve, the examiner applies firm lateral pressure to the spinous processes of the vertebrae at the lumbodorsal junction. If there is disc instability at this region, and pressure is applied to the spinous processes and maintained for a moment, the patient will experience pain referred down to the lumbosacral region.

It must always be remembered that a spondylolisthesis may be asymptomatic; consequently, the possibility of other sources of back pain must never be forgotten.

If the pain is indeed spinal in origin, it may be due to instability at the defect, root pressure due to disc herniation above or below the slip, foraminal encroachment of the nerve root, or extraforaminal entrapment of the nerve root. The pain, however, may arise elsewhere in the spine, being due to disc degeneration above the slip, hyperlordosis, or thoracolumbar disc degeneration. Finally, the pain may stem from an entirely unrelated cause, such as a metastatic malignancy in the spine.

TREATMENT

Even if the patient's symptoms are indeed due to the spinal lesion, the mere radiologic demonstration of a spondylolysis or spondylolisthesis does not indicate that operative intervention is mandatory. There are, of course, certain unusual instances in which operative intervention is unavoidable, such as evidence of cauda equina compression or evidence of unresolving or increasing impairment of root conduction. Apart from such examples, primary treatment should be conservative. Unlike dysplastic spondylolisthesis, further slipping is unlikely to occur in the older age group, and surgery, therefore, is not indicated to prevent further forward displacement. Continuing disabling pain constitutes the sole indication for surgery in this group of patients.

The type of surgical intervention required demands very careful evaluation of the patient. If the patient presents evidence of root tension or impairment of root conduction, the level of the lesion must be determined by clinical examination and confirmed by CT or magnetic resonance imaging (MRI). In instances of foraminal encroachment of the root, diagnostic root sleeve infiltration is a very useful ancillary measure. The technique of nerve root infiltration is described in Chapter 15. When the patient's complaints are mainly of pain of a sciatic distribution due to foraminal encroachment of the fifth lumbar root, a foraminotomy may be all that is required. If the patient has an acute unilateral radicular syndrome due to a disc herniation, with no back pain, all that is required is disc excision. This will be needed, obviously, at the level of the disc rupture—L4-5 more frequently than L5-S1. The decision to fuse the spine is determined by a history of repeated episodes or continuing back pain of incapacitating severity. If the discs above the level of an L5-S1 slip are normal on T2 weighted MRI (Fig. 6-26), a localized lumbosacral fusion is all that is required. The most reliable method of obtaining a single segment fusion in slips up to 50% is to fuse the transverse process of L5 to the ala of the sacrum (Fig. 6-27).

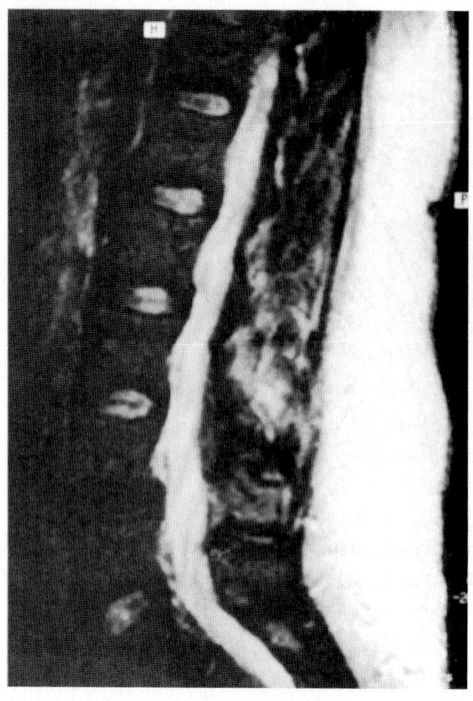

FIGURE 6-26 ● A T2 sagittal MRI with normal discs above and below an L4-5 slip.

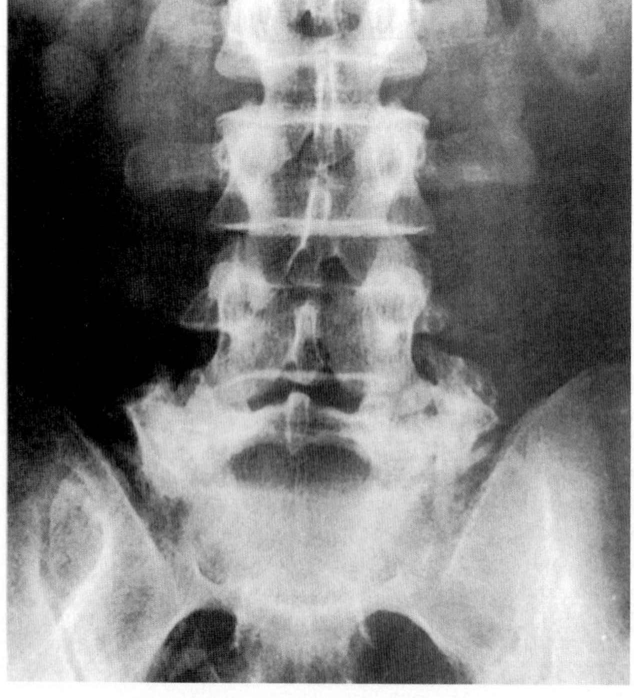

FIGURE 6-27 ● An anteroposterior radiograph of an L5-S1 fusion for spondylolisthesis.

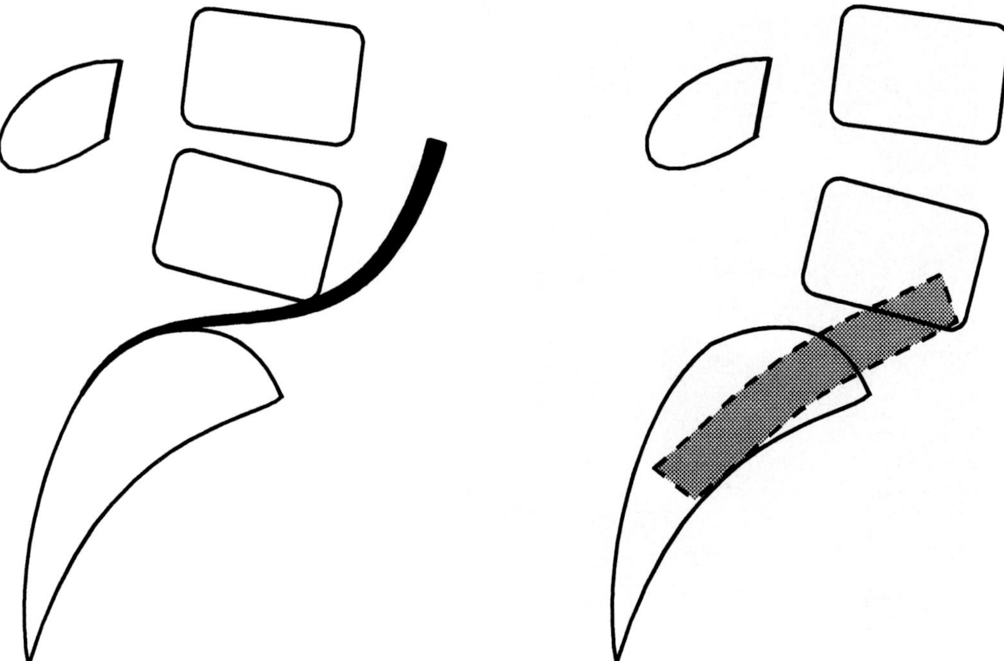

FIGURE 6-28 ● A reduction of the spondylolisthesis through an anterior approach *(left),* followed by a fusion *(right).*

When the forward displacement is more than half of the width of the sacrum, or when T2 MRI reveals degenerative changes at the L4-L5 disc, the accepted method of treatment is a fusion extended up to the transverse process of L4. Some authors skilled in deformity surgery have advocated reduction of the high-grade slips through anterior and posterior combined approaches (Fig. 6-28) (1).

The necessity for a three-segment fusion arises from time to time, for example, a spondylolysis of the last three lumbar segments. A similar problem is presented by an L5-Sl slip with symptomatic degenerative changes at L3-L4 and L4-L5, an L4-L5 slip with disc degenerative changes at the segments above and below the slip, or an L3-L4 lesion with symptomatic degenerative changes in the subjacent discs. Reviews of three-segment fusions for disc degeneration reveal a pseudarthrosis rate of 40%. To avoid this high pseudarthrosis rate, these cases are probably best treated by instrumentation; the various pedicle screw systems are the preferred choice.

TYPE IIB ELONGATED

Isthmic spondylolisthesis with an elongated pars (Type B) represents repeated microfractures of the pars that later heal in the elongated position. It is an acquired lesion with no congenital facet changes, which serves to distinguish it from the orphan mentioned under the discussion of dysplastic spondylolisthesis. This condition rarely causes significant back pain.

TYPE IIC TRAUMATIC

This condition was discussed in the opening section on spondylolysis. A neural arch defect across the pars interarticularis may also occur on rare occasions as a result of trauma, either from a forced hyperextension or from a forced flexion strain. Here again, the problem always arises as to whether the defect resulted from the accident or whether the patient had the defect before the accident. The sites and types of defects are frequently unusual. Healing of the lesion on immobilization is irrefutable evidence of the traumatic origin of the lesion.

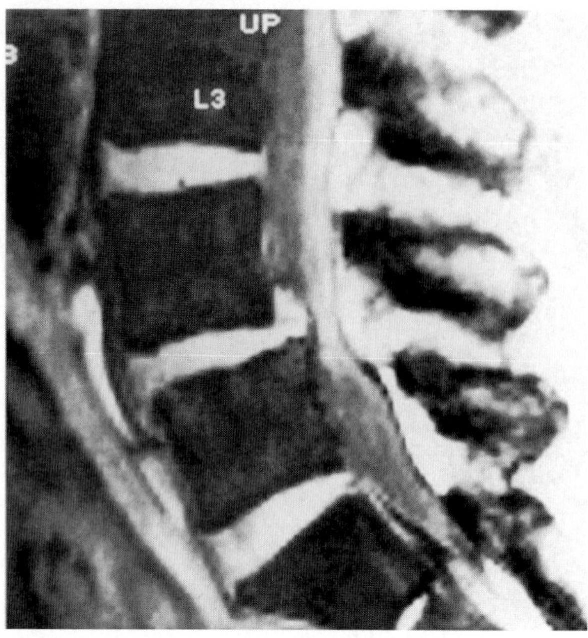

FIGURE 6-29 ● A gradient echo sagittal MRI showing a low-grade slip in degenerative spondylolisthesis with associated encroachment on the common dural sac.

TYPE III DEGENERATIVE SPONDYLOLISTHESIS

In degenerative listhesis, the primary pathology is degeneration of the disc followed by facet degeneration, but the neural arch is intact. The slip is never very great (Fig. 6-29), and most commonly it occurs at the L4-L5 interspace. The L4-L5 segment of the lumbar spine is normally the site of the greatest mobility. In an L4-L5 degenerative spondylolisthesis, it is this excessive mobility (Fig. 6-30), combined with a more sagittal alignment of the facet joints, that results in the lesion. Excessive movement is postulated to cause the breakdown in the posterior joints, which results in the slip. This condition predominantly affects women, with the age of onset of symptoms usually older than 50 years. This form of spondylolisthesis is really a manifestation of disc degeneration that may produce back pain because of the gross segmental instability and associated posterior joint damage. The usual patient presentation is bilateral neurogenic claudication due to root entrapment. This may be produced by a combination of a diffuse annular bulge at the level of the slip, shingling of the laminae, and buckling of the ligamentum flavum (Fig. 6-31). The spinal canal is further narrowed by subluxation of the posterior joints, which are enlarged by osteophytic outgrowths. All of these factors combine to produce entrapment of the nerve roots as they course through the spinal canal or the subarticular gutters. Degenerative spondylolisthesis with narrowing of the spinal canal or lateral zone is the most common form of spinal canal stenosis and is discussed in detail in Chapter 12. In summary, the nature and pathogenesis of the lesion make it obvious that the management of degenerative spondylolisthesis is indeed not unlike the management of degenerative disc disease with or without nerve root irritation.

TYPE IV TRAUMATIC SPONDYLOLISTHESIS

Forward slipping of a vertebral body may occur as the result of a dislocation of the posterior joints, or because of a fracture of a spinous process extending into the lamina at the pars interarticularis. These are really examples of fracture dislocations of the spine and are classified as traumatic spondylolisthesis. A fracture through the pars interarticularis (Type IIC) with forward slip of the vertebral body, a true traumatic spondylolisthesis, is rare. When a patient who has been involved in a severe accident demonstrates a spondylolisthesis on radiograph, it is difficult to say whether or not the patient had a pre-existing spondylolisthesis. Clearly defined fracture edges of the pars of L5 and a sharply pointed anterior margin of the sacrum are both suggestive of an acute lesion. A positive bone scan (SPECT scan) will resolve the legal issues. In contradistinction to spondylolytic and

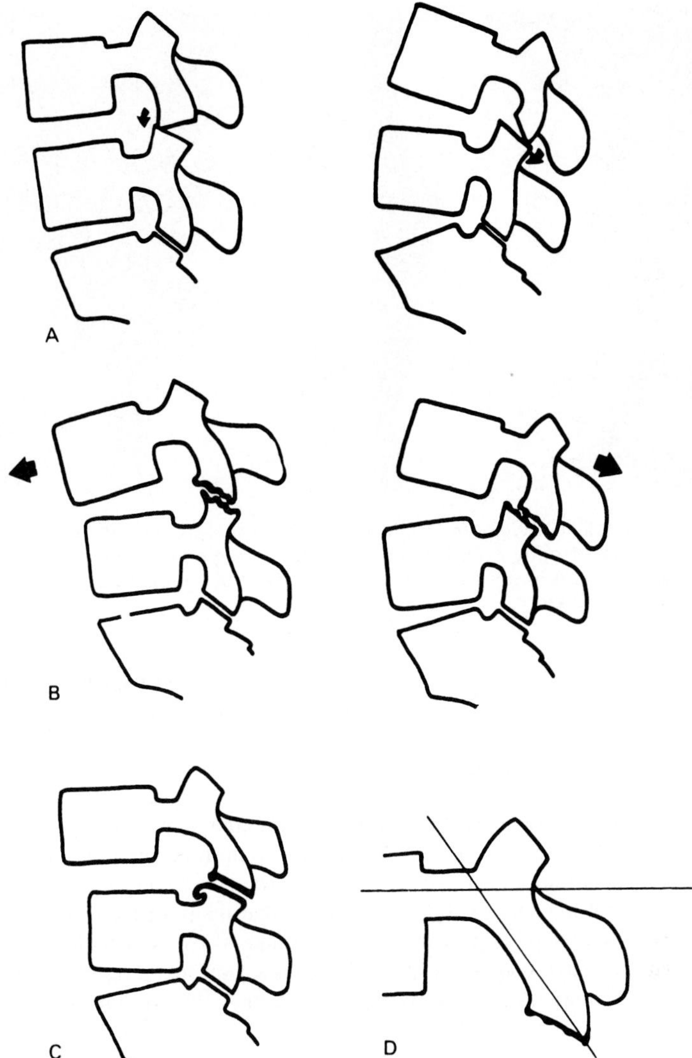

FIGURE 6-30 ● Mechanical insufficiency of an intervertebral disc permits excessive movement on flexion and extension **(A)**. The posterior joints undergo degenerative changes because of this abnormal movement and with increasing breakdown, permit forward and backward gliding of the involved vertebral bodies **(B)**. Subluxation of the arthritic zygapophysial joints permits forward displacement of the vertebral body **(C)**, and the displacement becomes fixed because of an increase in the angle between the pedicle and the inferior processes **(D)**. (From Macnab I. *Backache.* Baltimore: Williams & Wilkins; 1977:61 with permission.)

isthmic spondylolisthesis, an acute traumatic slip can be openly reduced and maintained in the reduced position with the use of instrumentation and fusion.

TYPE V PATHOLOGIC SPONDYLOLISTHESIS

On occasion, generalized bone disease such as osteogenesis imperfecta, osteomalacia, achondroplasia, or a localized bony change such as a secondary deposit or Paget's disease may allow attenuation of the pedicles and thereby permit the vertebral body to slip forward. It is to be noted that, unlike the other types of spondylolisthesis (except Type IIB), forward displacement of the vertebral body in pathologic spondylolisthesis is permitted by elongation of the pedicle (Fig. 6-32).

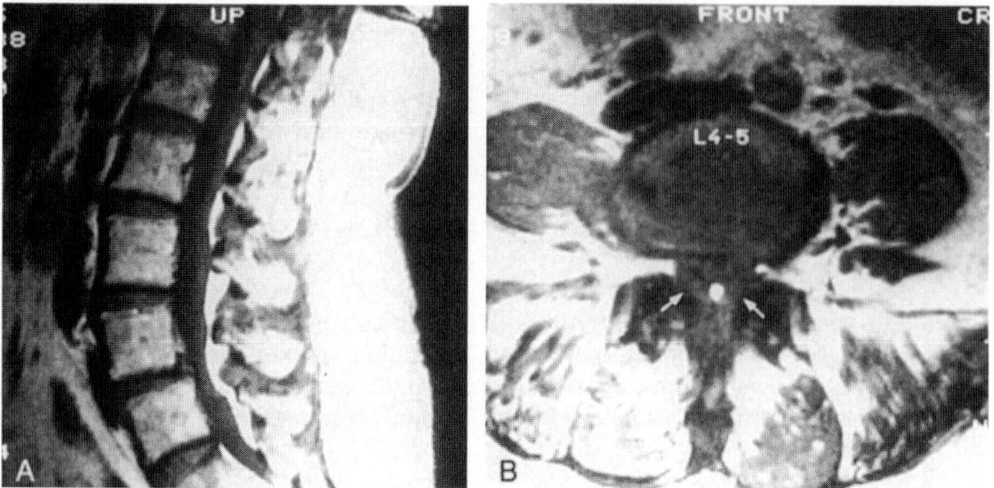

FIGURE 6-31 ● **A:** MRI (T1 weighted sagittal) of spinal canal stenosis at L4-5 due to ligamentum flavum hypertrophy from behind and annular bulging in front. **B:** MRI (T1 weighted axial) of spinal canal stenosis in same patient showing extent of ligamentum flavum encroachment *(arrows)* on common dural sac.

Obviously, the management of the local lesion in this group of cases depends on the management of the cause of the primary disease. This particular problem is rare in clinical practice.

IATROGENIC SPONDYLOLISTHESIS

Spondylolisthesis secondary to aggressive surgical intervention that destabilizes a spinal segment is not included in the Wiltse-Newman-Macnab classification. It occurs most commonly in spinal stenosis decompression without fusion, when too much (or all) of a facet joint is removed, which allows for a later slip at the surgical level. It is likely that many of these patients had a subtle, unrecognized slip at the time of surgery that simply became worse (and obvious) at a later date. A variant of iatrogenic spondylolisthesis is spondylolisthesis acquisita, a vertebral body slip above a lumbar fusion. This is simply a degenerative spondylolisthesis that occurs because a solid fusion

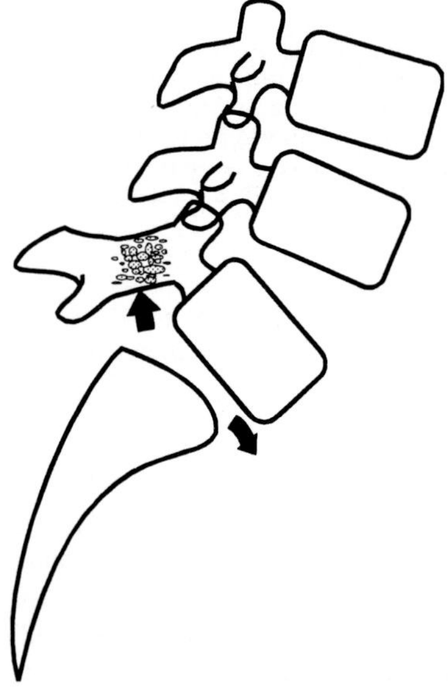

FIGURE 6-32 ● Pathologic spondylolisthesis *(curved arrow)* due to softening and elongation of bone in pars interarticularis *(straight arrow)*.

transfers motion to the segment above. The increase in facet joint and disc forces may result in degeneration and a subsequent spondylolisthesis.

SUMMARY

Although spondylolisthesis presents a dramatic picture on radiograph, it may be asymptomatic and remain asymptomatic for the lifetime of the patient. When the lesion does indeed produce symptoms, the pathogenesis of the symptoms (instability, root compression, and so on) must be established before treatment is instituted.

REFERENCES

1. Bradford DS. Spondylolysis and spondylolisthesis in children and adolescents. In: Bradford DS, Hensinger RN, eds. *Pediatric Spine.* New York: Thieme and Stratton; 1985.
2. Bradford DS, Lonstein JE, Moe JH, et al. *Moe's Textbook of Scoliosis and Other Spinal Deformities.* Philadelphia: WB Saunders; 1987.
3. Eisenstein SMC. Spondylolysis. A skeletal investigation of two population groups. *J Bone Joint Surg Br.* 1973;60:488–494.
4. Myerding H. Spondylolisthesis: surgical treatment and results. *Surg Gynecol Obstet.* 1932;54:371–377.
5. Neuwirth MG. Spondylolysis and spondylolisthesis in children and adults. In: Camins MB, O'Leary PF, eds. *The Lumbar Spine.* New York: Raven Press; 1987:257–273.
6. Wiltse LL, Newman PH, Macnab I. Classification of spondylolisthesis. *Clin Orthop.* 1976;117:23–29.
7. Wiltse LL, Jackson DW. Treatment of spondylolisthesis and spondylolysis in children. *Clin Orthop.* 1976;117:92–98.
8. Wiltse LL, Winter RB. Terminology and measurement of spondylolisthesis. *J Bone Joint Surg Am.* 1983:65: 768–772.
9. Wynne-Davis R, Scott JHS. Inheritance and spondylolisthesis: a radiographic family survey. *J Bone Joint Surg Br.* 1979;61:301–305.
10. Yu C, Garfin SR. Recognizing and managing lumbar spondylolisthesis. *J Musculoskeletal Med.* 1994;11:55–63.

CHAPTER 7

Inflammatory Spondyloarthropathies and Lesions of the Sacroiliac Joints

"Who is this that darkeneth counsel by words without knowledge?"

—Job 38:2

INFLAMMATORY SPONDYLOARTHROPATHIES

Degenerative conditions of the lumbar spine are a common cause of low back pain, and unless a careful history of the patient's pain is taken, it is very easy to neglect the diagnosis of spondyloarthropathies. In closing, ankylosing spondylitis as a cause of back pain is often neglected in the absence of severe flexion deformities.

In addition to ankylosing spondylitis (AS) other spondyloarthropathies include enteropathic arthritis (ulcerative colitis and Crohn's disease), psoriatic arthritis (PA), and reactive arthritis (ReA) [including Reiter's syndrome (RS)]. These conditions are frequently grouped together because they share a common symptom pattern and have a strong familial aggregation and genetic association. They are clearly overlapping entities with a likely common pathogenesis. These conditions are characterized by inflammatory involvement of the sacroiliac (SI) and spinal joints. The condition is frequently associated with peripheral enthesopathies and peripheral arthritis and extra-articular manifestations (ocular, genital, and mucocutaneous).

Less advanced and subtle presentations of these conditions are frequently missed. It is believed that there is a significant underestimation of the prevalence of these diseases. These conditions all have a strong association with the human leukocyte antigen (HLA)-B27 and have an absence of rheumatoid factor (seronegative).

INFLAMMATORY LESIONS OF THE SI JOINT

With a clearer understanding of the clinical syndromes affecting the lumbar spine, SI strains become less of a viable diagnosis on which to base treatment decisions. The flip side of the coin is to have blinders on and see degenerative conditions of the lumbar spine in every patient presenting with low back pain only to miss the very real, and not uncommon, sacroiliitis due to an inflammatory lesion. These so-called seronegative spondyloarthropathies include AS, RS, PA, and enteropathic arthropathy. The most commonly recognized inflammatory lesion of the SI joint is AS.

ANKYLOSING SPONDYLITIS

At one time AS was regarded as the spinal variant of rheumatoid arthritis. It is now known that these two diseases are distinct entities. The name is derived from the Greek roots *ankylos* (bent, or fusion) and *spondylos* (spinal vertebrae).

TABLE 7-1

Natural History of Spondyloarthropathy

The onset is insidious.
There are exacerbations and remissions.
Morning stiffness becomes a dominant symptom.
Spinal movement limitation and deformity are progressive.
If peripheral joints are involved, it happens early.
Iritis is early and recurrent.
A more severe course has an earlier onset.
The course in women is milder than in men.

Adapted from Little H. The natural history of ankylosing spondylitis [Editorial]. *J Rheum.* 1988;15:1179–1180.

Epidemiology

With the standardization of criteria for the diagnosis of spondyloarthropathy (2), better epidemiologic studies have been completed. Initially, spondyloarthropathy was thought to be a disease predominantly affecting men (M:F = 10:1), but more recent studies suggest that women are affected quite commonly, although with a milder form of the disease. AS usually has its insidious onset during the ages of 20 to 35 years and is rare in onset after the age of 40 years.

The progress of the lesion and its major pathologic features are well demonstrated on repeated radiographic examinations. Because the disease does not have a clear clinical presentation, a criteria approach to diagnosis is used (Tables 7-1 and 7-2).

Etiology

The cause of AS is unknown, except that individuals who have inherited the HLA-B27 gene are predisposed to develop the syndrome. The overall incidence of AS in North American Caucasians is 0.1% to 0.2%, whereas the incidence of AS in Caucasians with the HLA-B27 gene is 10% to 20%. There is a 20-times greater incidence of AS among relatives of persons with AS. These relatives have a much higher incidence of HLA-B27 than the normal population. Whether the B27 gene/antigen is the primary cause or whether it acts as a receptor for an infective and/or environmental agent that triggers the disease is unknown.

Pathology

AS affects both synovial and fibrous joints; the pathologic changes take the form of chronic synovitis. The chronic synovitis is followed by cartilage destruction, erosions, sclerosis of underlying bone, and finally, fibrosis and ankylosis of the affected joints. The SI joints are involved most of

TABLE 7-2

Clinical Criteria Suggesting Ankylosing Spondylitis

1. Insidious onset of discomfort
2. Age younger than 40 years
3. Persistence for more than 3 months
4. Association with morning stiffness
5. Improvement with exercise

From *Primer on the Rheumatic Disease,* 9th ed. 1988:145.

TABLE 7-3

Less Common Symptoms in Spondyloarthropathy

Constitutional symptoms, such as fatigue and weight loss
Chest pains from costosternal involvement
Eye symptoms (acute iritis)
Extra-articular bony tenderness (enthesopathy, enthesitis)
Heart and ascending aorta lesions
Apical fibrosis of lung

Adapted from Primer on the Rheumatic Disease, 9th ed. 1988.

the time; the intervertebral discs, symphysis pubis, and manubriosternal joints are frequently involved. Two categories of extra-articular involvement are characteristic:

1. Inflammatory lesions of articular capsule and ligament insertion into bone occur (enthesitis).
2. Extraskeletal lesions may occur in the eye [uveitis (25%–30%), aortic root (1%–4%), and pulmonary tree] (Table 7-3).

Clinical Features

The usual presentation is in a young (adolescent or early adulthood) man who reports the insidious onset of grumbling low back pain. Characteristically, there are remissions and exacerbations over the months. The pain may refer to the buttocks and upper thigh and may even be unilateral, leading readily to confusion with the diagnosis of a ruptured disc. Typical of AS is the absence of neurologic symptoms and the presence of good straight leg raising, which should make the diagnosis of a disc rupture immediately suspect. The next most prevalent complaint is stiffness of the lumbosacral area, especially in the morning, with a hot shower and/or the morning's activity alleviating this complaint. Prolonged periods of inactivity worsen the back pain and stiffness. At times, back pain may awaken the patient at night, and often this pain is at the thoracolumbar junction as well as the low back. Eventually, the pain and stiffness affect the entire spine, causing clinically detectable loss of range of movement. Spread to the peripheral skeleton occurs and most often affects the shoulders and hips. Other symptoms are listed in Table 7-3.

Physical Findings

Early in the disease, there is little to find on clinical examination, which leads to a delay in diagnosis. Probably the two most commonly mistaken diagnoses are to label the patient as having "fibrositis" or to mistake unilateral SI pain for a disc rupture. To the careful examiner, there will be detectable loss of lumbar motion in all three planes: flexion, extension, and lateral flexion. This is in contrast to a patient with a herniated nucleus pulposus, who usually has limited flexion, good backward extension, and limitation of lateral flexion to one side more pronounced than the other (determined by the location of the disc fragment on the nerve root). In AS, there may be pain on direct pressure on the SI joint, and various tests that stress the SI joint may increase the pain.

As the disease progresses, there is loss of lumbar lordosis and a decrease in ability to expand the rib cage. Contrary to other reports, these two changes occur early in the natural history of the disease (3). The loss of chest cage mobility occurs because of involvement of the posterior costovertebral and costotransverse articulations and the anterior costochondral junctions. The normal chest expansion (measured at the level of the fourth rib) is reduced from more than 5 cm to less than 2 cm.

The final stage of advancement in the disease is ankylosis of the spine, and if this occurs in a poorly supervised or poorly motivated patient, severe flexion deformities of the spine may occur (Fig. 7-1).

Extra-articular manifestations include ocular inflammation, psoriasis and psoriasiform nails, keratodermia blennorrhagicum, mucosal ulcers, balanitis aortitis and myocarditis, and apical pulmonary lesions.

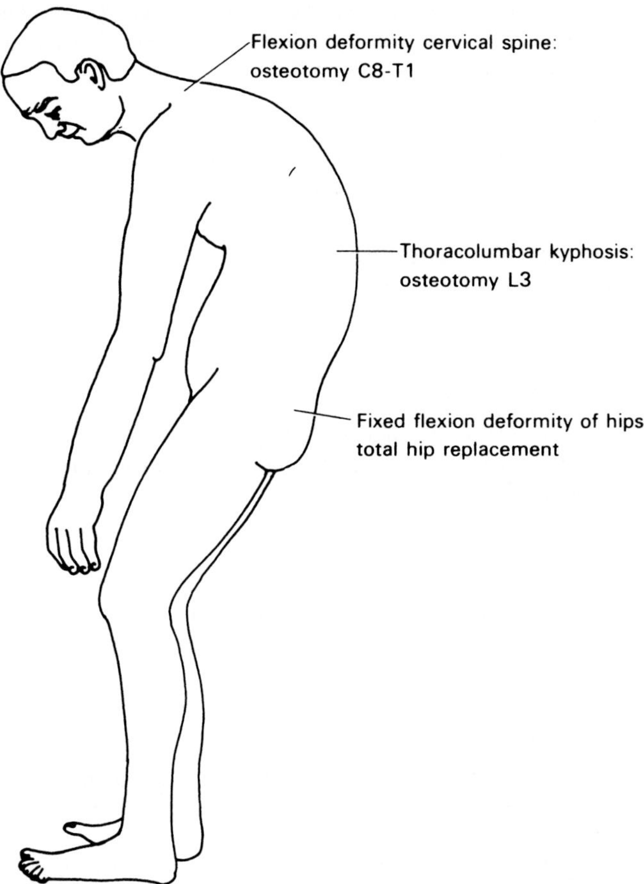

FIGURE 7-1 ● The surgical correction of the fixed flexion deformities associated with ankylosing spondylitis is dependent on the type and site of the maximal deformity. (From Macnab I. *Backache.* Baltimore: Williams & Wilkins; 1977:76 with permission.)

Early in the disease, the enthesopathy may present as tenderness over bony prominences of the ischial tuberosity, greater trochanter, calcaneus, spinous processes, and other bony prominences.

The course of AS is unpredictable. Women tend to have a less severe form of involvement, as do men with later onset. The most severely involved tend to be younger men, but the variability in progression is striking. With proper supervision and an exercise regimen, even the most severely affected can maintain long-term, gainful employment.

Aside from severe extraskeletal involvement of the aorta and pulmonary tree, the most limiting symptoms come from ankylosis of the hips (25%), a spondylodiscitis causing severe back pain, or an atlantoaxial subluxation causing severe neck pain.

The patient with AS is very susceptible to accidents causing fractures of the spine. These fractures are more common in the cervical spine but can occur anywhere in the ankylosed spine. The trauma is usually minor, and the fracture is often missed on initial examination. If a neurologic lesion (paraplegia/quadriplegia) occurs at the time of the spinal fracture, the prognosis for recovery is dismal.

Laboratory Tests for AS

Ninety percent of symptomatic patients have positive blood test results for HLA-B27. The incidence of HLA-B27 in the normal Caucasian population is 6% to 8%. Most patients will have some elevation in the erythrocyte sedimentation rate and C-reactive protein (CRP), although this elevation is rarely dramatic. There is no association with rheumatoid factor and antinuclear antibodies, thus the designation "seronegative spondylarthropathies."

Radiographic Findings

The diagnosis of AS is confirmed by radiograph. The characteristic involvement of the SI joints in the presence of several of the clinical criteria listed in Table 7-2 confirm the diagnosis.

Stages of Radiographic Changes in the SI Joints. (The radiographic involvement is usually symmetric despite lateralization of symptoms.)

Early Stages (Fig. 7-2)

- Blurring of the joint margins
- Erosions and sclerosis of bone

Both of these changes may occur throughout the SI joint but are seen earliest in the lower two thirds (the synovial portion) of the SI joint. The erosions eventually leave the appearance of widening (pseudowidening) of the SI joints.

Late Changes (Fig. 7-2)

- With disease progression, calcification and interosseous bridging of the SI joints occur.

These radiologic changes (early) must be distinguished from osteitis condensans ilii. In this lesion, almost invariably found in multiparous women, there is a wedge-shaped area of sclerosis confined to the iliac side of the joint (Fig. 7-17B).

Development of Syndesmophytes

Initially, there is inflammation of the annulus fibrosus and the corners of the vertebral bodies. With subsequent erosions of the corners of the vertebral bodies, the anterior aspect of the vertebral body appears squared (Fig. 7-3). This is soon followed by ossification of the annulus fibrosus, which bridges the disc space (syndesmophytes) (Fig. 7-4). The ultimate fate is ossification of all ligaments of the spine and the complete fusion of the vertebral column (bamboo spine) (Fig. 7-5).

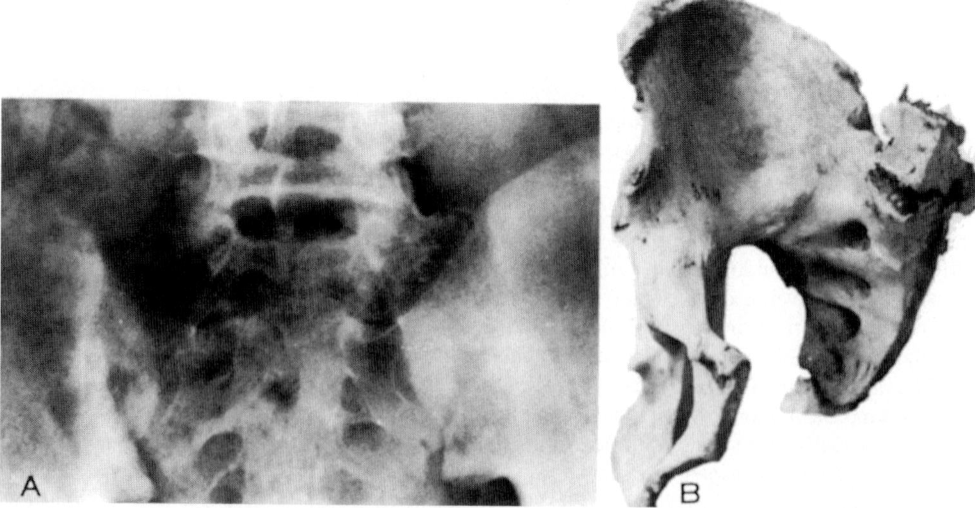

FIGURE 7-2 ● **A:** X-ray demonstrating the irregular definition ("fuzziness") of the sacroiliac joints commonly seen in the early stages of ankylosing spondylitis. **B:** In the later stages of the disease, the sacroiliac joint is completely obliterated by a bony ankylosis as shown in this specimen.

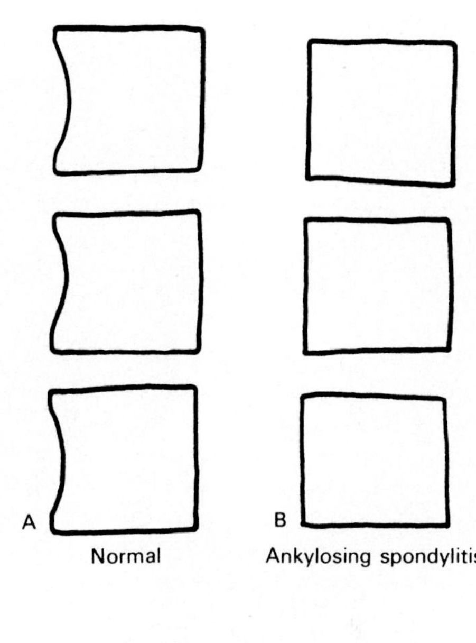

FIGURE 7-3 • **A:** The lateral view of a normal lumbar vertebral body presents a slight concavity anteriorly. **B:** In the early stages of ankylosing spondylitis, this concavity is filled in with the result that the vertebrae appear to be "squared off." (From Macnab I. *Backache.* Baltimore: Williams & Wilkins; 1977:72 with permission.)

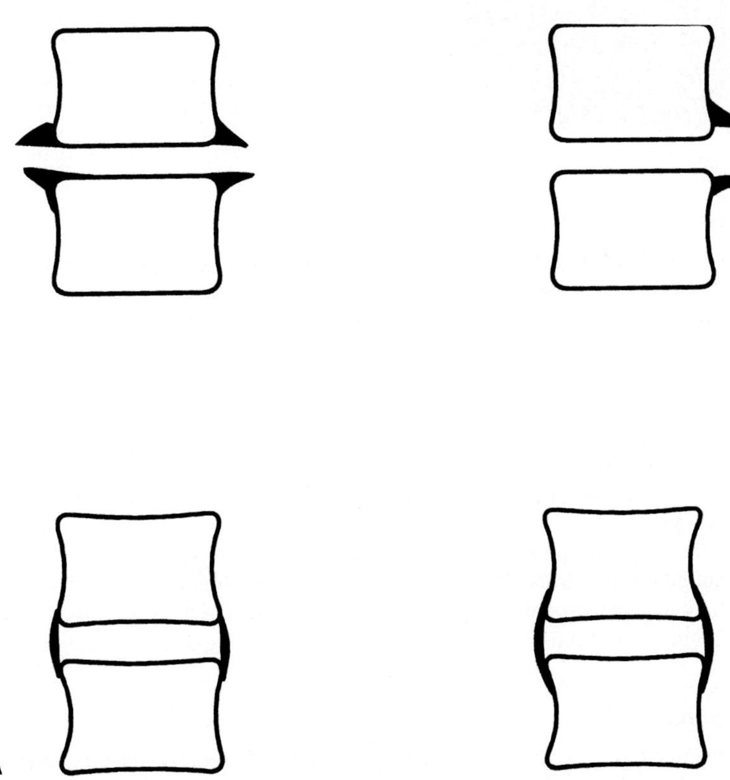

FIGURE 7-4 • **A:** Osteophytes *(top left)* occur in degenerative disc disease; traction spurs *(top right)* are seen in instability; marginal syndesmophytes *(bottom left)* are drawn with other spur-like bony prominences that develop on the edge of vertebral bodies adjacent to disc spaces; non-marginal syndesmophytes *(bottom right)* are characteristic of diffuse idiopathic skeletal hyperostosis. *(continued)*

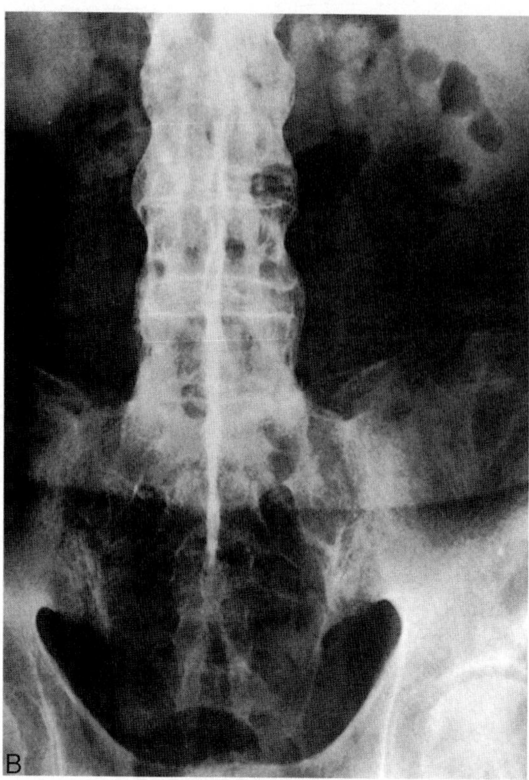

FIGURE 7-4 ● *(Continued)*
B: Radiographs of marginal syndesmophytes in severe AS (causing a bamboo spine).

Other Skeletal Radiographic Changes

Characteristic changes may occur in the manubriosternal joint (Fig. 7-6). Bony erosions and whiskering at sites of osseous-tendon attachments may be seen on radiograph (Fig. 7-7). Figure 7-8 summarizes the clinical and radiographic findings in AS.

Diagnostic Choices Early in the Disease

The clinician who sees many patients with low back pain is usually very sensitive to diagnosing AS. When AS is suspected clinically but not supported by plain radiographic films of the SI joints, what radiographs should be done? It has been suggested that the following radiographic studies are useful: special views of the SI joints, bone scans of the SI joints, and computed tomography (CT) scans of the SI joints.

The yield of useful information with these tests is so low that when balanced against the financial cost of routine use, it is probably not worth doing the tests. Providing other disease entities have been ruled out, the most reasonable choice is to treat the patient as having suspected AS and repeat the plain radiographs in a number of months, rather than chasing down the diagnosis with expensive tests.

Treatment of AS

No specific treatment of a curative nature presently exists. The role of the physician is diagnostic awareness of the disease, amelioration of the symptoms with the carefully controlled use of anti-inflammatory medications, patient education, attention to the possibility of spinal deformities, and management of peripheral joint arthropathies.

It is essential for the patient to understand the natural history of the disease in order that he or she understands the need for reasonable rest and a continuing program of postural education and exercises.

Nonsteroidal anti-inflammatory drugs (NSAIDs) provide the first-line treatment. Generally, salicylates are not very effective for joint pain. Trial and error may be required to identify the most

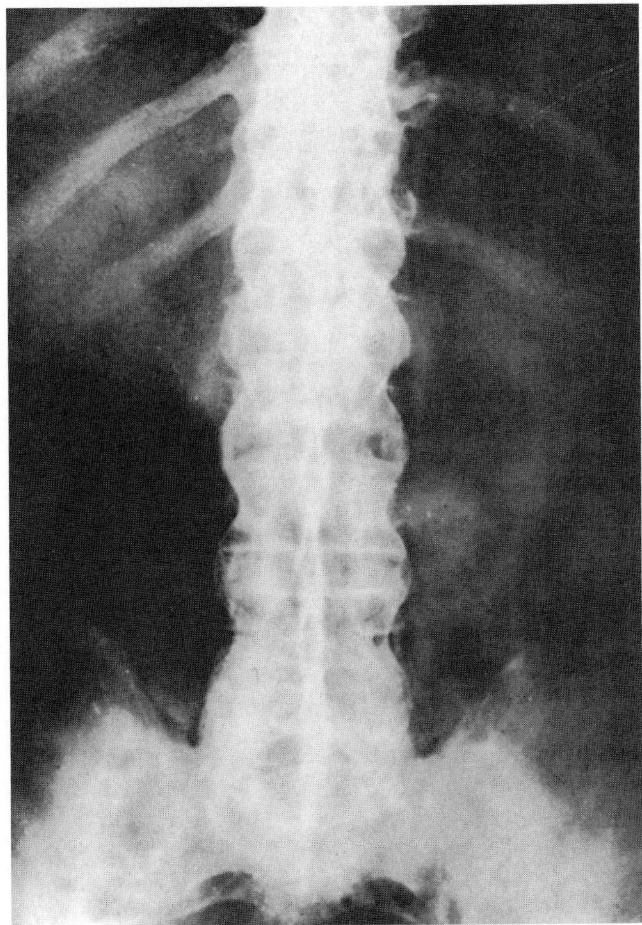

FIGURE 7-5 ● The "bamboo spine." (From Macnab I. *Backache*. Baltimore: Williams & Wilkins; 1977:73 with permission.)

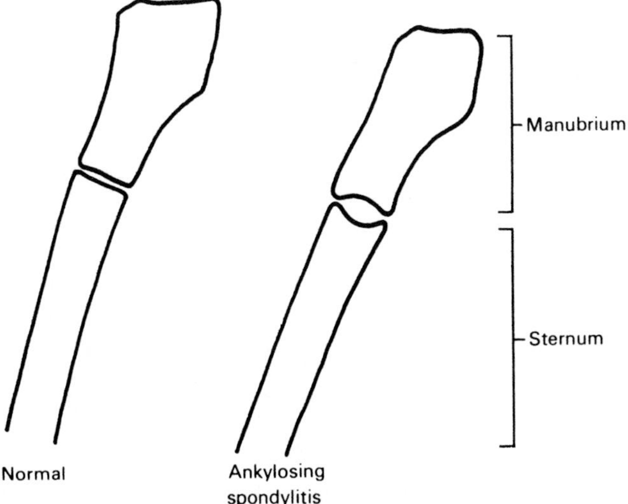

FIGURE 7-6 ● In ankylosing spondylitis, the manubriostructural joint may present a biconcave appearance on x-ray. (From Macnab I. *Backache*. Baltimore: Williams & Wilkins; 1977:74 with permission.)

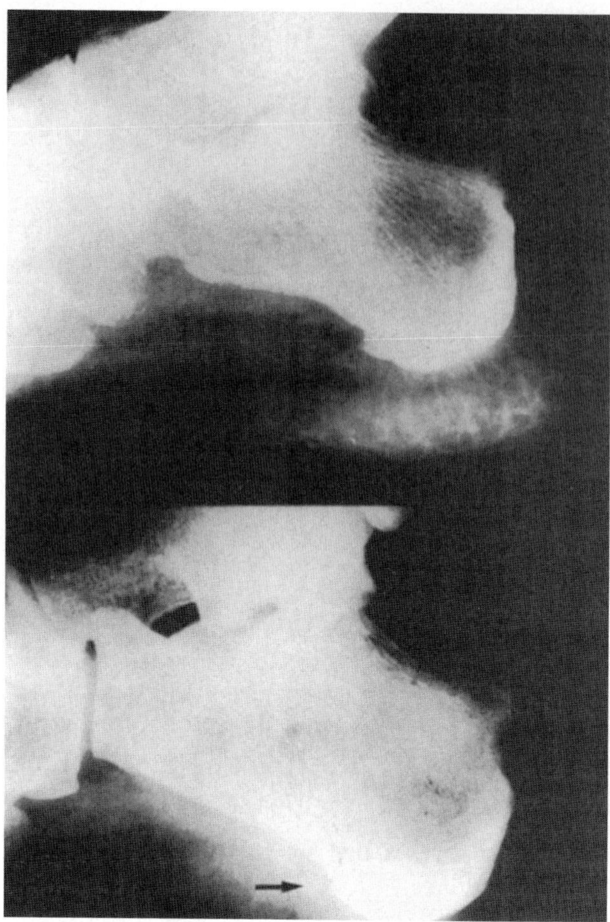

FIGURE 7-7 • Enthesopathy–whiskering along inferior border of os calcis *(arrow)*.

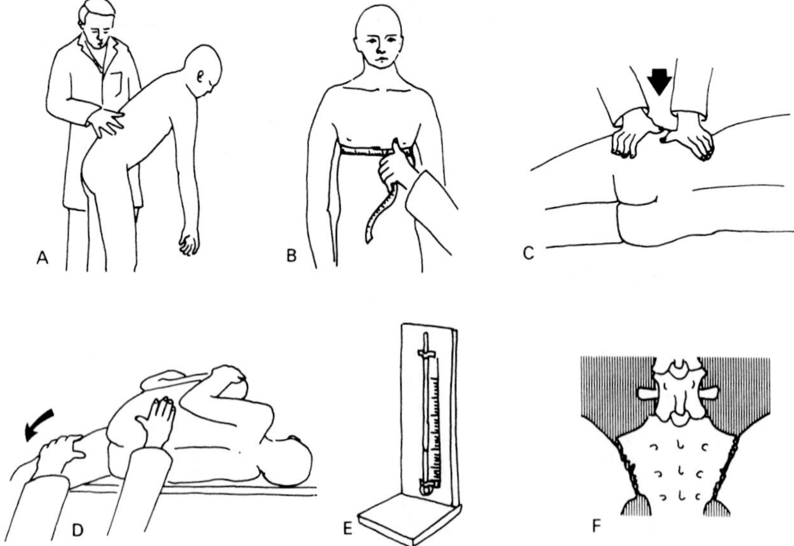

FIGURE 7-8 • Summary of major findings in ankylosing spondylitis. **A:** Rigidity of lumbar spine on forward flexion. **B:** Decrease in chest expansion. **C:** Pain on side-to-side compression of the pelvis. **D:** Pain on Gaenslen's test. **E:** Elevated sedimentation rate. **F:** "Fuzziness" of sacroiliac joints on x-ray. (From Macnab I. *Backache*. Baltimore: Williams & Wilkins; 1977:75 with permission.)

effective anti-inflammatory for any individual. In the author's experience, indomethacin has been the most effective, but it also has more side effects.

Corticosteroids are generally not used for inflammatory spondyloarthropathies.

The exercise program is designed to maintain a straight spine or to attempt to increase lumbar lordosis. Every attempt must be made to maintain the already reduced respiratory excursion.

Occasionally, despite anti-inflammatory medication and excellent continued physical therapy, the spinal deformities progress relentlessly and inexorably to a stage at which the patient can only see a few feet in front of him or her when standing and may have difficulty in sitting and eating. In such instances, surgical correction of the deformities must be considered. Operative correction is undertaken at the site of the maximal deformity, taking into full account the serious surgical hazards of respiratory problems and the danger of producing irreversible neurologic damage (Fig. 7-1).

SPONDYLITIS ASSOCIATED WITH CHRONIC INFLAMMATORY BOWEL DISEASE: ENTEROPATHIC ARTHRITIS

It has been found that spondylitis and a peripheral seronegative arthritis occur in 5% to 20% of patients suffering from Crohn's colitis and chronic ulcerative colitis.

The etiology and pathogenesis of the peripheral arthropathy are unknown. Several distinguishing features have been noted: the gradual onset, involvement of weight-bearing joints, a migratory pattern, and a short-lived course. The spondylitis is clinically and roentgenographically indistinguishable from idiopathic AS. In this regard, it is interesting to note that nearly 80% of the patients with spondylitis associated with inflammatory bowel disease are HLA-B27 positive.

If a patient being treated for Crohn's disease or ulcerative colitis subsequently develops a grumbling backache, the possibility of sacroiliitis with spondylitis must be suspected. One must be aware that spondylitis can occur before the onset of intestinal disease and does so in at least one third of cases. Whereas the severity of the arthropathy correlates with the activity of the bowel disease, the spondylitis appears to progress independently of the primary lesion, and medical and surgical treatment of the bowel disease does not alter progression of the spondylitis.

SPONDYLITIS ASSOCIATED WITH PSORIASIS

Almost identical radiologic changes in the SI joints and lumbar spine may be seen in patients suffering from PA. The age of onset of PA is generally in the second or third decade, with women equally afflicted as men. The etiology and pathogenesis have not been clarified.

The clinician must always be mindful of the fact that the skin lesion of psoriasis does not protect patients from developing simple mechanical backache. Not every patient with psoriasis and back pain is suffering from spondylitis; nevertheless, if the patient has a peripheral arthritis, the possibility of a psoriatic sacroiliitis or spondylitis must be suspected, and appropriate radiographs should be ordered.

Symptom pattern is usually monoarthritis or symmetrical oligo or polyarthritis.

SPONDYLITIS ASSOCIATED WITH RS (REACTIVE ARTHRITIS)

Back pain may be the presenting symptom of RS. It is difficult to define Reiter's disease precisely. Historically, it was considered to be a triad of nonbacterial urethritis, arthritis, and conjunctivitis, but this rigid classification inhibited an understanding of the complexity of the disease. After much debate (6), RS is now defined as an episode of peripheral arthritis of more than 1 month's duration, occurring in association with urethritis and/or cervicitis. Other clinical situations that may coexist are conjunctivitis, mucous membrane lesions, and other cutaneous lesions. The onset is most common between the ages of 20 and 40 years, with men predominantly affected. The known causative organisms include nongonococcal genitourinary (GU) infections (*Chlamydia, Mycoplasma, Ureaplasma*) and enteric infections (*Salmonella, Shigella, Yersinia, Campylobacter jejuni*).

Any one of the clinical manifestations may be the presenting symptom, although urethritis is by far the most common initial feature. The arthritis is marked by acute onset and asymmetrical involvement of a few joints. The large weight-bearing joints, the joints of the midfoot, and the metatarsophalangeal and interphalangeal joints of the toes are the most commonly afflicted.

A high percentage of patients with RS show radiographic evidence of sacroiliitis, but it is only a small percentage that develop a spondylitis. When spondylitis occurs, it is late in the disease evolution and is noted, therefore, as an association rather than a presenting finding.

LESIONS OF THE SI JOINT

The SI joint is an enigma. It is obviously an important set of joints that anchor the pelvis to the sacrum, which in turn act as a supporting "door frame" for the mobile lumbar spine and even more mobile legs. So why shouldn't the resultant concentration of forces cause pain in this joint? Chiropractic, osteopathic, and physical therapy practitioners believe and promote the SI joint "dysfunction" as a source of low back pain (5), whereas physicians are reluctant to accept this proposal. The problem in understanding SI joint sprains, strains, and injuries is the lack of scientific evidence to support the manual therapists' proposal of this joint as a source of pain to be corrected by their particular brand of administrations.

STRUCTURE AND FUNCTION OF THE SI JOINT

The SI joint is a combination of a synarthrodial and diarthrodial joint—a unique joint in the body. The major portion of the joint is a syndesmosis (diarthrodial) joint and is characterized by a very irregular topography, strong fibrous connections within the joint, and strong extra-articular supporting ligaments. The message from study of joint morphology is that this joint moves very little. The inferior portion of the joint is synovial, but it offers up no increased mobility. The joint is said to move two to three degrees in any one direction (4), a phenomenon that decreases with aging changes that stabilize the joint. These aging changes start by age 30 years and obviously decrease movement in the joint, just as patients enter the decades of backache (30 to 60 years of age).

THE SACROILIAC JOINT SYNDROME (SIJS)

The SIJS is said to have a classic presentation (5):

1. There is pain over the SI joint.
2. The SI joint is locally tender to palpation (hard enough pressure can make any SI joint tender!).
3. The pain may be referred to the groin, trochanter, and buttock.
4. The pain is aggravated by provocation tests.
5. There is clinical evidence of increased movement or asymmetry of the SI joint.
6. There is no other apparent cause of the patient's SI joint pain localization (if it is not . . . ., therefore it must be sacroiliac joint syndrome!).

SI SPRAINS

The concept of a "sacroiliac sprain" as a common cause of backache and sciatica was introduced by Goldthwaite (1) in 1905. To this day, little scientific evidence exists to support the fact that SI joint sprain or strain is a symptom-producing condition. A common finding in patients suffering from mechanical backache is pain situated over the SI and tenderness in this region. This does not mean that the SI joint is the source of pain. Rather, this finding is usually a manifestation of the confusing phenomenon of referred pain. Mechanical lesions of the lumbosacral junction associated with disc degeneration frequently give rise to pain referred to the SI region, and such patients will exhibit local tenderness in that region. It is understandably tempting to ascribe these findings to a pathologic lesion in the underlying SI joint. However, the true source of this SI joint pain can be demonstrated by experimental reproduction of the pain by hypertonic saline injection of the supraspinous ligaments at the lumbosacral junction, and by reproduction of the pain by discography of the L4-L5 and L5-S1 discs.

The anatomic configuration of the components of the SI joint makes the joint extremely stable (Fig. 7-9), and this inherent stability is reinforced by the powerful, massive posterior interosseus

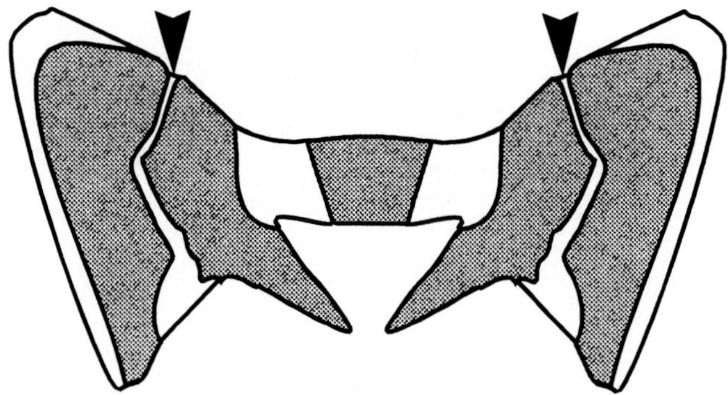

FIGURE 7-9 • The sacroiliac (SI) joints *(arrows)* are very stable joints simply by their construct.

ligaments and by the strong accessory ligaments—the iliolumbar, the sacrotuberous, and the sacrospinous ligaments.

In patients older than the age of 35 years—the backache years—in 30% of the population, the anterior capsule of the SI joint is ossified and, in these patients at least, the SI joints may be exonerated from the blame of backache. In patients younger than the age of 35 years, minimal sliding and rotary movements occur, but considerable force, such as that generated by falls from heights or motor vehicle injuries, is required to push the SI joint beyond its physiologically permitted range, either dislocating or fracturing the joint. This leads to true post-traumatic painful osteoarthritic degeneration of the joint that has an unequivocal clinical presentation.

POST-TRAUMATIC PAINFUL OSTEOARTHRITIC DEGENERATION OF THE SI JOINT: SI JOINT INSTABILITY

Violence severe enough to injure the SI joint will usually be associated with a fracture of the pelvis but, in the unusual circumstances in which the whole brunt of the blow is absorbed by the supporting ligamentous structures of the SI joint, the findings are specific and pathognomonic:

1. There is tenderness over the lower third of the SI joint below the posterior inferior iliac spine.
2. The pubic symphysis is tender on palpation. The pelvis is a closed ring and cannot undergo stretching at one site only. In the absence of a fracture of the pelvic ring, if the SI joint is displaced, the symphysis pubis must also suffer some disruption (Fig. 7-10).

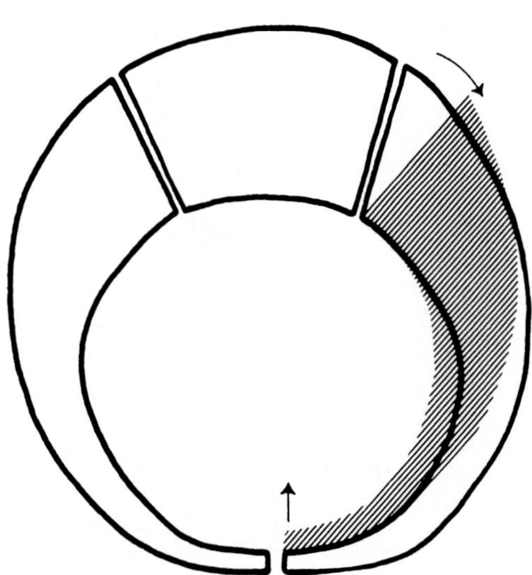

FIGURE 7-10 • Diagram showing that any movement of the sacroiliac joint must be associated with corresponding displacement at the symphysis pubis. (From Macnab I. *Backache.* Baltimore: Williams & Wilkins; 1977:65 with permission.)

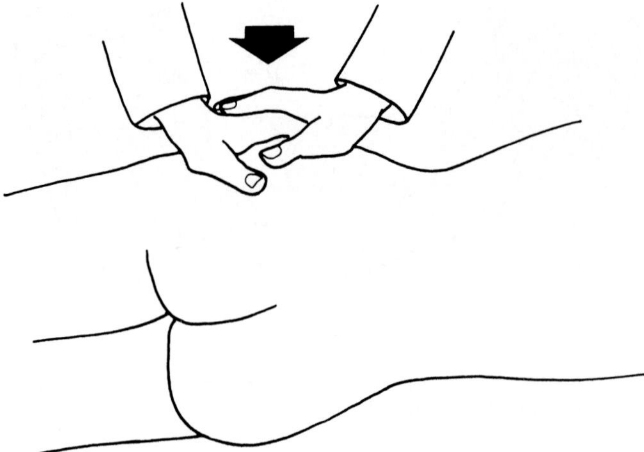

FIGURE 7-11 ● With the patient lying on his/her side, the sacroiliac joint can be stressed by manually applying compression to the pelvis. (From Macnab I. *Backache.* Baltimore: Williams & Wilkins; 1977:66 with permission.)

3. The symptoms experienced clinically may be reproduced by stressing the SI joint with any of the following maneuvers:
   a. Lateral manual compression of the iliac crest (Fig. 7-11).
   b. Resisted abduction of the hip joint. When the gluteus medius contracts to abduct the hip, it pulls the ileum away from the sacrum. With SI joint lesions, abduction against resistance is painful (Fig. 7-12).
   c. Hyperextension of the hip on the affected side against a stabilized pelvis. Although this maneuver, Gaenslen's test (Fig. 7-13), was originally described for eliciting SI joint pain, the test is not specific (3). Hypertension of the hip performed in this manner will also be painful in the presence of pre-existing hip disease (a positive Ely's test), and patients suffering from irritation of the fourth lumbar nerve root may experience anterior thigh pain on this form of hyperextension of the hip (a positive femoral stretch test).

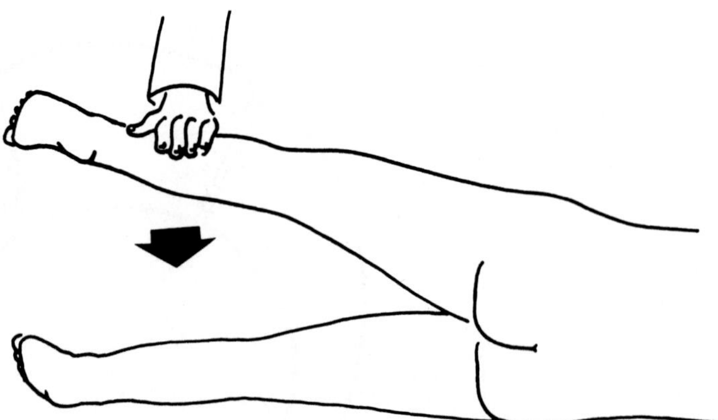

FIGURE 7-12 ● In the absence of hip joint disease, pain experienced over the sacroiliac joint on resisted abduction of the leg is highly suggestive of a sacroiliac joint lesion. (From Macnab I. *Backache.* Baltimore: Williams & Wilkins; 1977:66 with permission.)

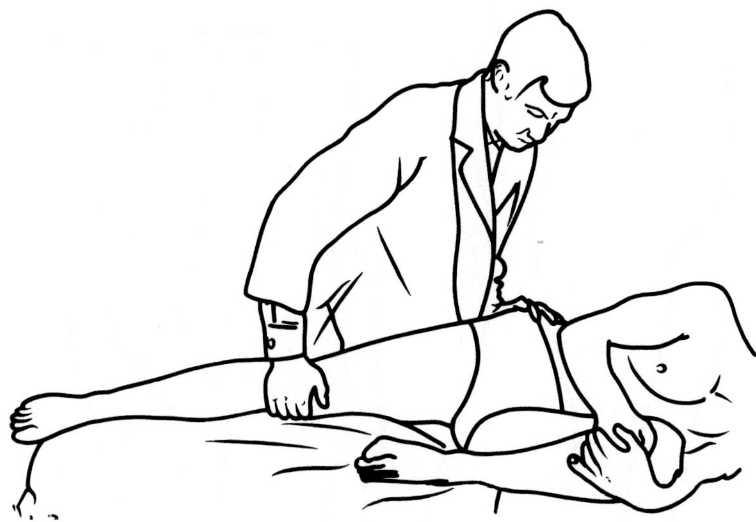

FIGURE 7-13 • Gaenslen's test. (From Macnab I. *Backache.* Baltimore: Williams & Wilkins; 1977:67 with permission.)

   d. Forced external rotation of the affected hip in the supine position (Patrick's test, or faber sign) (Fig. 7-14) causes pain in the SI joint.
4. Patients with painful SI joints may develop gluteal inhibition, with a resulting Trendelenburg lurch when walking (Fig. 7-15).
5. There are often accompanying degenerative changes in the symphysis pubis.

In addition to post-traumatic osteoarthritic degeneration of the SI joint, there is another obvious source of SI joint pain—pregnancy.

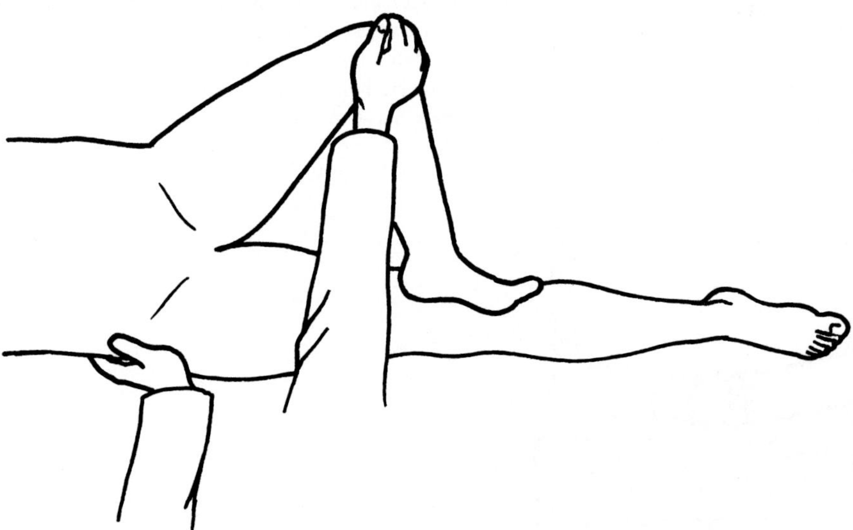

FIGURE 7-14 • Faber test, also known as the Patrick test, is done with the hip on the test side in flexion *(f),* abduction *(ab),* and external rotation *(er),* (thus faber). Downward pressure on the knee while fixing the opposite side of the pelvis will stress the left sacroiliac (SI) joint.

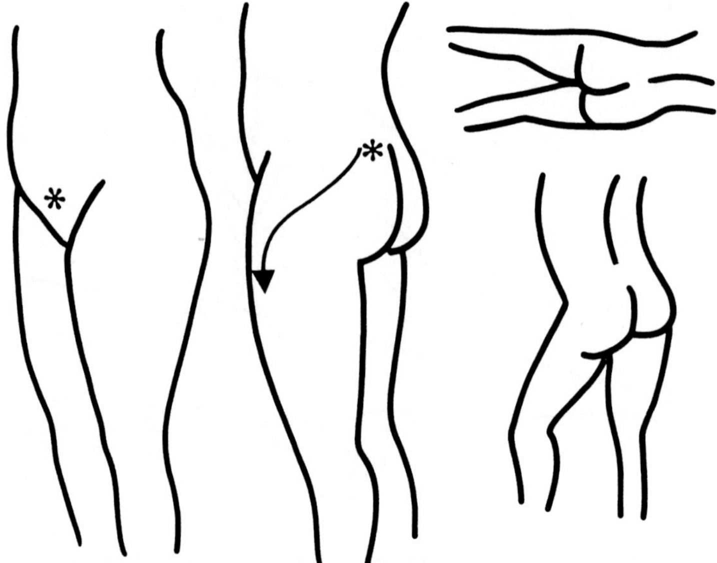

FIGURE 7-15 ● Summary of findings in sacroiliac joint disease. Tenderness can be elicited not only over the sacroiliac joint but over the symphysis pubis as well. The pain usually radiates over the lateral aspect of the great trochanter and down the front of the thigh. The patients exhibit pain on abduction of the hip on the affected side and walk with a Trendelenburg lurch. (From Macnab I. *Backache.* Baltimore: Williams & Wilkins; 1977:67 with permission.)

THE PAINFUL SI JOINT OF PREGNANCY

During the latter months of pregnancy, the supporting ligaments of the SI joints become "relaxed" to allow enlargement of the birth canal. At this time, and during parturition, the joints are indeed susceptible to strain as a result of trivial trauma. Patients complain of pain localized to the involved SI joint, and the pain radiates around the greater trochanter and down the anterolateral aspect of the thigh. Patients exhibit, on examination, the specific physical findings previously described.

The symptoms of true SI sprains generally subside rapidly with bed rest, analgesics, and anti-inflammatory medications. The use of a trochanteric belt can give relief while walking and can obviate the antalgic gait (Fig. 7-16). In a few patients whose symptoms persist, administration of intra-articular steroids may be necessary.

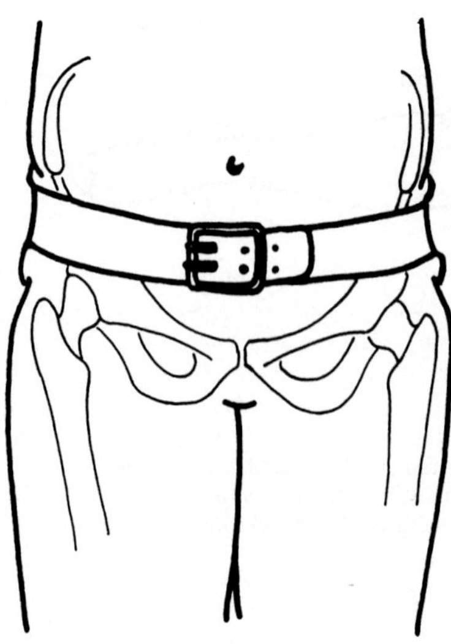

FIGURE 7-16 ● Trochanteric cinch. (From Macnab I. *Backache.* Baltimore: Williams & Wilkins; 1977:68 with permission.)

OSTEITIS CONDENSANS ILII

Osteitis condensans ilii is a condition of mild-to-moderate SI joint pain occurring in postpartum women 30 to 40 years of age. The major problem with this disease is its confusion with AS. The cause is unknown, but its very high prevalence in women suggests some relationship to the laxity of the SI joint late in pregnancy and delivery being the cause.

The symptoms are rarely severe, and the radiographic presentation is classic (Fig. 7-17). The triangular sclerosis is confined to the iliac side of the SI joint, with no evidence of the destruction of the SI joint that occurs in AS.

The course of osteitis condensans ilii is almost always benign. Treatment consists of an explanation to the patient of the benignity of the problem and simple measures such as heat or ice and mild analgesic/anti-inflammatory medicine. With time, the symptoms almost always disappear.

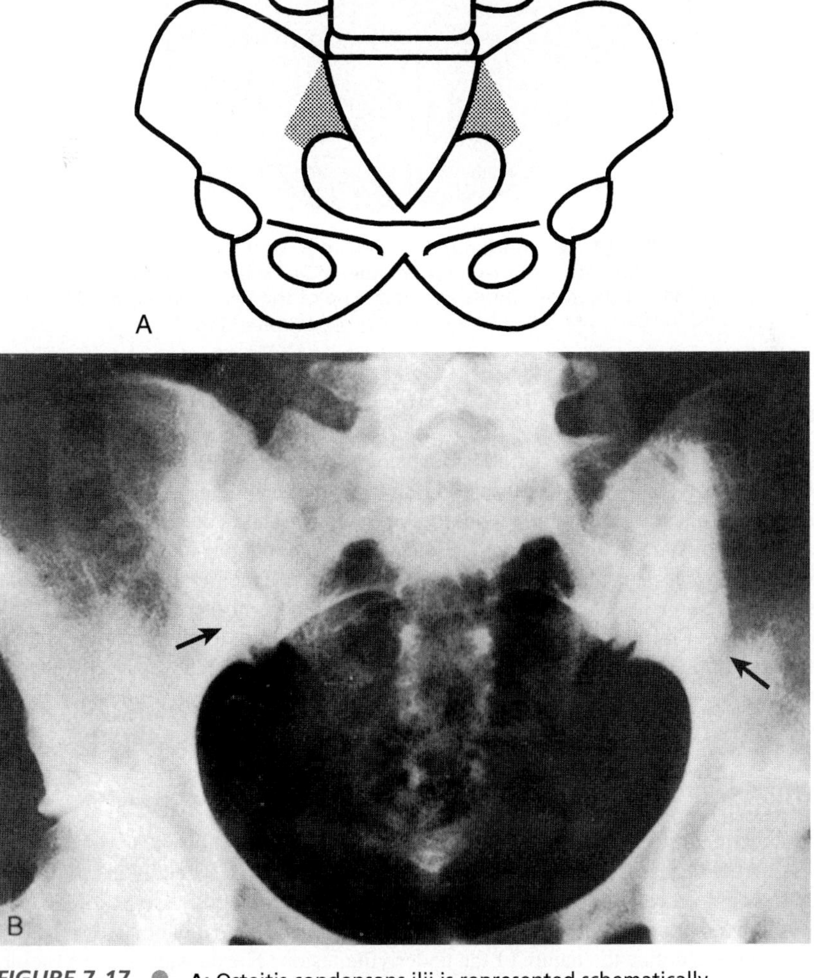

FIGURE 7-17 • **A:** Osteitis condensans ilii is represented schematically. **B:** Osteitis condensans ilii. Note that the area of bone sclerosis is confined to the iliac side of the sacroiliac joint. (From Macnab I. *Backache.* Baltimore: Williams & Wilkins; 1977:70 with permission.) *(continued)*

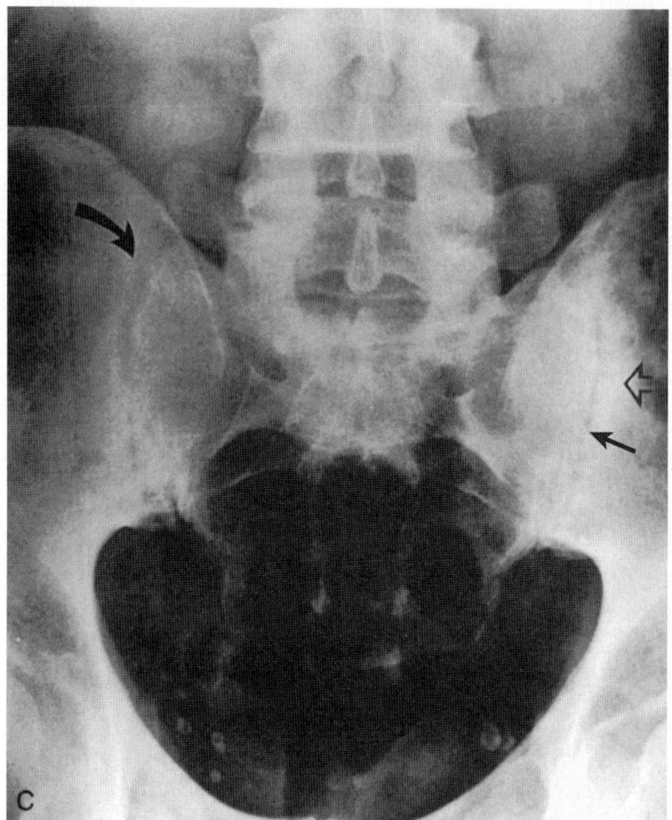

FIGURE 7-17 ● *(Continued)* **C:** In ankylosing spondylitis there are simultaneous erosions (pseudowidening of the joint) *(curved arrow),* subchondral sclerosis on each side of the joint *(open arrow),* and transarticular bony bridges (ankylosis) *(long arrow).*

SUMMARY

In summary, it is worth repeating that SI strains, apart from those following parturition, are excessively rare, although commonly diagnosed. The concept of a SI strain is yet another example of how the phenomenon of referred pain and tenderness has clouded and confused the recognition of the pathologic basis of spondylogenic pain. The SI region is a common site for referred pain and tenderness derived from segmental discogenic backache. The mere complaint of pain over the SI joint and the demonstration of local tenderness do not justify the diagnosis of a SI sprain.

After decades of injection of and manipulation of the SI joint, it is time for prospective scientific studies on the natural history, clinical presentation, and treatment of the SI joint syndrome. Failure of those practitioners in the manual therapy fields to pursue these studies will only discredit the SI sprain diagnosis.

INFECTIONS OF THE SI JOINTS

In the past, tuberculosis was the most common cause of infective arthritis of the SI joints. Recently, an increasing frequency of pyogenic involvement has been noted, especially in children. The clinical picture is unfortunately vague. There are pain and tenderness over the SI joints, and the erythrocyte sedimentation rate is raised. With pyogenic infections, the patient may be febrile, but there is very little else to define the nature of the underlying lesion. The damage to the SI joint may not be apparent for several weeks, and it is understandable that definitive diagnosis may, therefore, be delayed for a long period of time. If the clinician is very suspicious of the diagnosis, a bone scan or

MRI may be helpful. It must be remembered, however, that this area of the skeleton always takes up more technetium on a routine scan than other portions of the pelvis.

On occasion, a fluctuant abscess will form. Under such circumstances, confirmation of the diagnosis and isolation of the organism can be achieved by needle biopsy. If aspiration proves impossible, with the presumptive diagnosis provided by the overall clinical picture, the bone scan, and the CT scan, open biopsy is mandatory in order that appropriate antibiotic therapy can be instituted.

Ewing's sarcomata have a predilection for the pelvis and, when occurring adjacent to the SI joint, may mimic the radiologic appearance of destructive pyogenic arthritis. On occasion, the differentiation from septic arthritis in such instances can only be established by open biopsy.

Because of the rarity of septic arthritis of the SI joint as a cause of backache and because of the nonspecific nature of the clinical picture, the diagnosis may be missed easily.

SUMMARY

Afflictions of the SI region may present as backache. The anatomic characteristics of the joint and the natural history of ankylosis should prevent the occurrence of the so-called SI sprains.

Pelvic instability is an infrequent but definite hazard of taking a bone graft from the posterior superior iliac crest and is related to the inadvertent division of the iliolumbar ligament.

The introduction of the use of histocompatibility antigen studies may lead to a redefinition of AS as a broader disease process. At present, radiographic changes in the SI joints are essential to a firm diagnosis.

The sophistication of today's bone scanning techniques minimizes the delays in diagnosis so prevalent with infection and neoplasm involving the SI joint region.

REFERENCES

1. Goldthwaite JE. *Essentials of Body Med.* Philadelphia: JB Lippincott; 1937.
2. Little H. The natural history of ankylosing spondylitis [editorial]. *J Rheumatol.* 1988;15:1179–1180.
3. Potter NA, Rothstein JM. Intertester reliability for selected clinical tests of the sacroiliac joint. *Phys Ther.* 1985;65:1671–1675.
4. Stuvesson B, Selvik G, Uden A. Movements of the sacroiliac joints: a roentgen stereophotogrammetric analysis. *Spine.* 1989;14:162–165.
5. Walker JM. The sacroiliac joint: a critical review. *Phys Ther.* 1992;72:903–915.
6. Wilkens RF, Arnett FC, Bilter T, et al. Reiter's syndrome. Evaluation of preliminary criteria for definite disease. *Arth Rheum.* 1981;24:844–849.

CHAPTER 8

The History

"A doctor who cannot take a good history and a patient who cannot give one are in danger of giving and receiving bad treatment."

—Anonymous

When taking an adequate history, patience is not only a virtue, it is a vital necessity, as the following verbatim report of the first part of a prolonged consultation reveals:

Doctor: "Well, Mrs. Jones, what can I do to help you today?"
Patient: "I sure hope you can cure it."
Doctor: "Well, I'll try. Have you any pain?"
Patient: "Of course I have, I wouldn't be here if I didn't have any pain. I'm not the sort of person that keeps running to doctors with nothing wrong with them. I know you're all very busy and if . . ."
Doctor: "Where is the pain?"
Patient: "Haven't you looked at my radiographs?"
Doctor: "I will look at your radiographs after I have taken your history and completed an examination. Please tell me where your pain is located."
Patient: "The same place it's always been."
Doctor: "Where is that?"
Patient: "In my back, of course."
Doctor: "Where in your back—in the low back?"
Patient: "I don't know whether you would call it low or high. All I can say is it's sure a bad pain."
Doctor: "Could you point to the pain? Ah, I see. How long have you had this?"
Patient: "Ever since I tripped on the stairs."
Doctor: "When was that?"
Patient: "Didn't my doctor send you my history? His nurse promised me she'd mail it to you. Oh, this is terrible. I don't see any point in coming here if you don't know anything about me. I wonder why . . ."
Doctor: "When did you have the accident on the stairs?"
Patient: "In June."
Doctor: "What year?"
Patient: "Why, this year of course. I'm so sorry my doctor didn't send you my history!"
Doctor: "Have you had pain every day since then?"
Patient: "Sometimes."
Doctor: "You mean the pain is intermittent?"

Patient: "No. I mean sometimes I have the pain, and sometimes I don't."
Doctor: "When you have the pain, what aggravates it?"
Patient: "How do you mean aggravates?
Doctor: "Does anything make the pain worse?"
Patient: "No, it's worse all the time."
Doctor: "Does lifting make the pain more severe?"
Patient: "No."
Doctor: "You can lift anything you want without hurting your back?"
Patient: "No, I can't lift anything."
Doctor: "Why?"
Patient: "Because of my back."
Doctor: "Let's just think of some things you do in your house. Vacuum cleaning, bed making, doing the laundry; do any of these things make it worse?"
Patient: "If I could do all of those things I wouldn't be here. I don't believe in running to the doctor with the least little thing. I can take a lot of pain, more than most people. You ask my husband. I can't even sit down because of the pain."
Doctor: "Does anything relieve your back pain?"
Patient: "No."
Doctor: "What do you do when the pain is bad?"
Patient: "I lie down."
Doctor: "Does lying down make the pain better?"
Patient: "No. It's just as bad when I get up."
Doctor: "When you are actually lying down, is the pain any easier?"
Patient: "Yes, but I can't spend my life lying down."
Doctor: "Does the pain stop you from doing anything you want to do?"
Patient: "I can't play golf with my husband."
Doctor: "Do you get a lot of pain in your back every time you play golf?"
Patient: "Yes."
Doctor: "When did you last play golf?"
Patient: "Eight years ago."
Doctor: "Why haven't you tried to play golf again?"
Patient: "My doctor told me not to."

It is easy to describe a color, a sound, a taste, or a smell because these are sensations that can be shared. "I went down to the beach later that evening, when the setting sun had turned the sea into a vivid red, all that could be heard was the plaintive cry of the sea gulls and the gentle splashing of the waves against the rocks." Statements such as this make a clear impression in the mind of the listener. It is more difficult, and yet more important, to interpret the statement, "I have this uncomfortable feeling in my back—I wouldn't call it a pain really," or, "I was paralyzed with pain that felt like red hot rivers rushing down my legs." Is the second patient exaggerating, or does he or she have more serious back trouble?

When taking a history, it is not good enough to find out that patients have "back pain" or that they have pain in the right leg or left leg. It is essential to obtain a description of the pain in meticulous detail. Having obtained a clear description of the discomforts from which the patient is suffering, it is then necessary to find out as much as you can about the personality of the patient and his or her activities to try to correlate the pain to the disability about which the patient is complaining. The majority of patients do not come because of pain; they come because of the disability it produces. "I've got this backache and I can't play badminton." The patient can do everything else; he or she wants you to overcome the "disability" and make him or her able to play badminton again.

You have to obtain a clear picture of the pain. From this, you must assess the possible source of pain. You have to obtain an equally clear picture of the patient who has the pain. From these facts, you have to assess why the pain is causing the complained-of disability.

Before you go any further, remember:

1. After listening to the patient's story, there is an 80% chance you will know the diagnosis (you will improve the odds another 10% by doing the physical examination, and another 5% by ordering fancy, expensive tests).

2. If after a history, physical examination, and review of tests you are still not sure of the diagnosis, go back and repeat the history! A few minutes of good history taking can save thousands of dollars in expensive testing.

Now, you can close the book and know that all you need to do in assessing a patient with back pain (and any other complaint in most of medicine) is to listen to your patients! Can you imagine how hard it is to be a good veterinarian?

PICTURE OF THE PAIN

SITE OF THE PAIN

When patients state that they have "back pain," they may mean anywhere from the base of the neck to the buttocks. It is not good enough to ask patients where they feel the pain; they must demonstrate it. A patient's grasp of anatomy is understandably vague. When patients say that they have pain in their backs, they may be referring to the interscapular region of the back, and even when they state that they have pain in the "small of the back," they may be referring to the lumbodorsal junction. When patients describe pain in the "hip," they generally mean pain in the buttock. It is necessary always to get the patients to point to where they have the pain. Let us slip in a little word about pain over the greater trochanter, so often called "trochanteric bursitis." More often it is pain referred to the region from the lumbar area. Injecting the area with local anesthetic and cortisone can often have a placebo effect and mislead you into accepting the erroneous diagnosis of trochanteric bursitis.

The method the patient chooses to demonstrate the site of pain is instructive. The emotionally stable patient generally places the palm of the hand at the site of maximal pain and moves it across the body to demonstrate the route of radiation. The psychologically troubled patient generally points out the area of the pain with his or her thumb (Fig. 8-1). He or she never touches the painful area. The pain, so to speak, is outside his or her soma.

Spread of pain to the leg is an important symptom, and patients should be asked to demonstrate the distribution of the pain. It is important to you, as the examiner, to know what constitutes the leg (Fig. 8-2). To a patient, a leg is a leg, and most will not volunteer any information as to whether the pain radiates down to the knee or whether it goes below the knee. The examiner needs to know this when trying to determine whether the patient is suffering from referred pain or whether the pain in the leg is due to root irritation and, if so, which root. By having patients point with their fingers, the distribution of the leg pain will be clear.

Referred pain is rarely felt below the knee, whereas pain due to root irritation may spread to the calf or even into the foot. Pain resulting from compression of the third and fourth lumbar roots radiates down the front of the thigh. Pain from first and second lumbar root involvement is easily confused with hip disease because it concentrates around the groin.

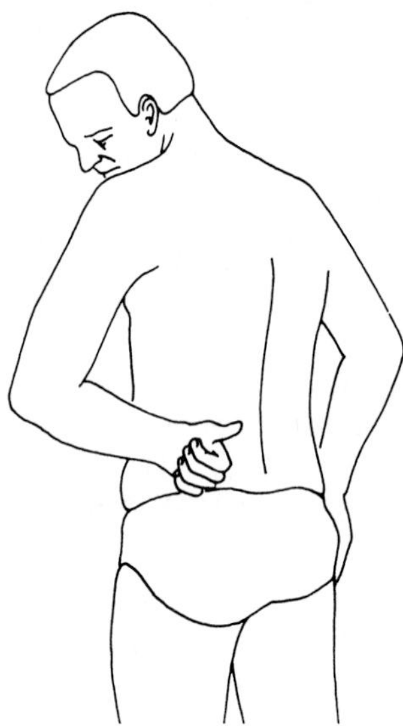

FIGURE 8-1 ● "Macnab sign." Patients who are suffering from a significant emotional overlay will frequently point to the area of pain in the lower back with their thumbs. They never actually touch their body. (From Macnab I. *Backache.* Baltimore: Williams & Wilkins; 1977:109 with permission.)

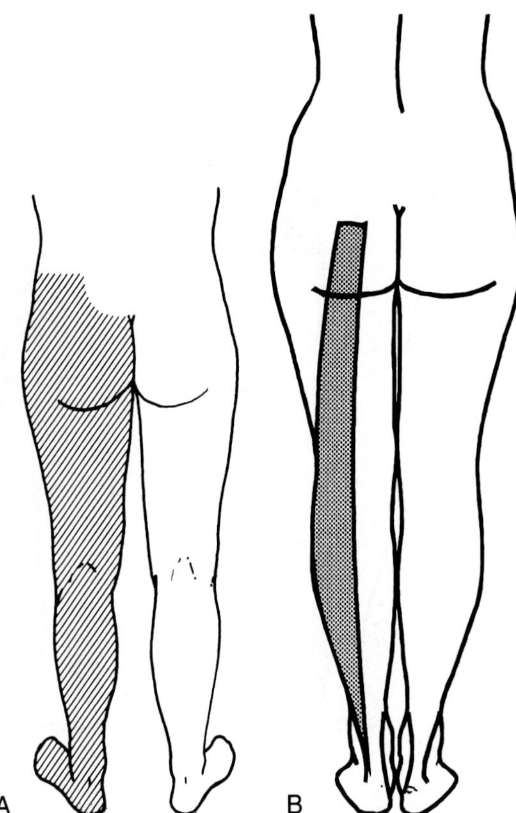

FIGURE 8-2 • **A:** The "leg" includes the buttock as its proximal extension. **B:** Radicular pain in the leg will follow a more "linear" radicular distribution.

PARESTHESIA

You are aware that the symptom of a sensory change is a paresthetic complaint, and the associated sign is numbness. Pain due to root irritation is frequently associated with a paresthetic sensation, and its location is a key to anatomic localization of root involvement. Paresthesia involving the lateral border of the foot is usually indicative of an S1 lesion, and a patient with an L5 lesion may describe numbness over the dorsum of the foot and even into the big toe. The location of the pins and needles or paresthetic discomfort in the shin indicates fourth lumbar root involvement, the kneecap location is third root involvement, and the lateral thigh represents second lumbar root involvement (Fig. 8-3).

The presence of these symptoms is helpful in making the diagnosis of root irritation and localizing the level of involvement. The patient does not usually volunteer this information; he/she must be asked for specifically. Table 8-1 outlines the two historical criteria important to the diagnosis of the acute radicular syndrome.

WHAT SYMPTOM ARE YOU HEARING?

Remember, degenerative conditions of the spine cause pain. If the patient has a history of any other symptoms, be careful. Morning stiffness is a symptom of ankylosing spondylitis and some neurologic conditions. It is also a classic symptom for lumbar degenerative disc disease. Parkinson's disease in its earliest phase may present with back stiffness, legs that do not function properly, and a diffuse aching buttocks sensation.

Is the leg symptom predominantly weakness or sensory upset? If there is sensory upset, then there is a very high likelihood that you are dealing with a neurologic disorder such as a cord myelopathy or cauda equina tumor, a neuropathy, or motor neuron disease. Lumbar spine doctors are pain doctors. Cervical spine doctors may hear about leg symptoms, but rather than symptoms of leg pain, these symptoms will be gait disturbances. The English expression for a cervical myelopathic symptom is a patient "going off their legs."

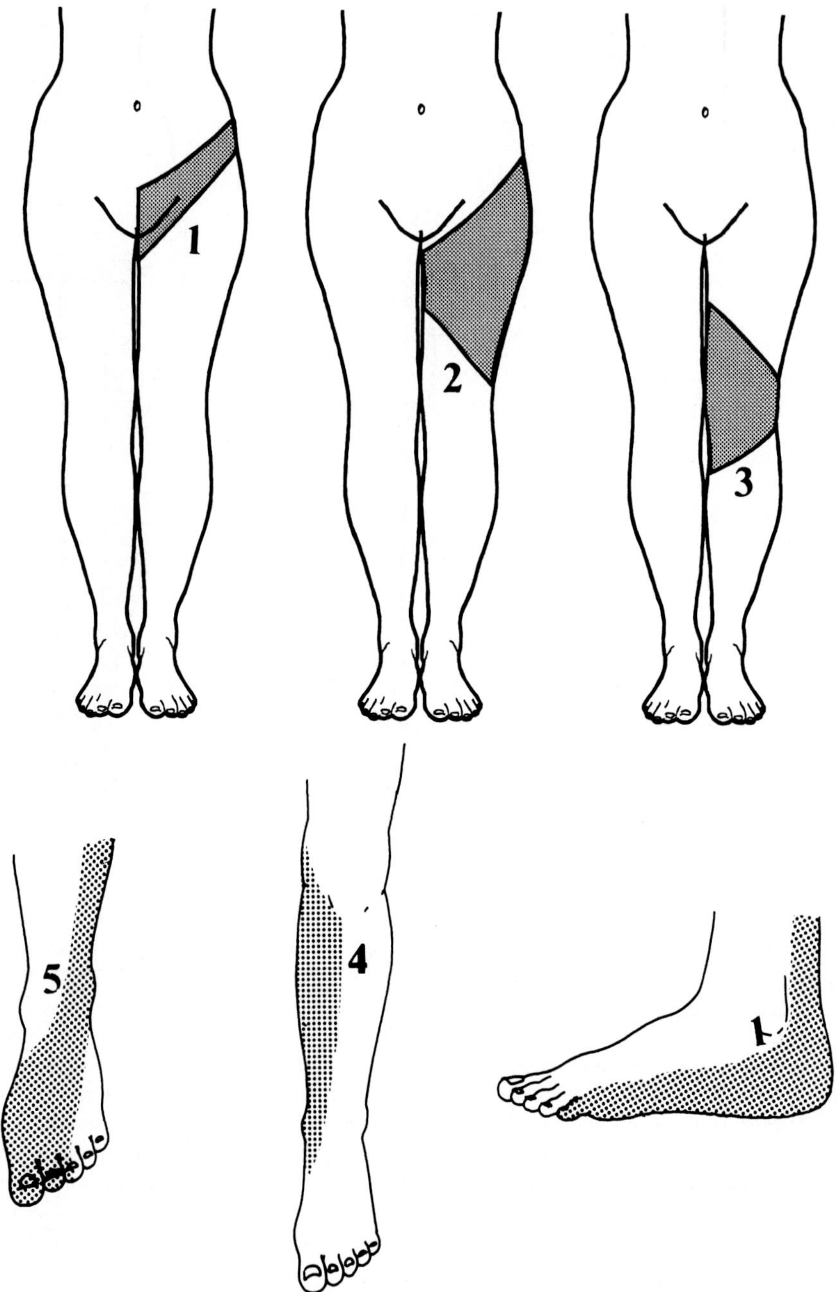

FIGURE 8-3 ● The dermatomes of L1 to S1 are outlined and numbered.

TABLE 8-1

Historical Criteria Important to the Diagnosis of an Acute Unilateral Radicular Syndrome (Usually Due to a Herniated Nucleus Pulposus)

1. Leg pain is the dominant symptom when compared in severity with the back pain.
   - It dominates at the onset of the symptoms ("I've never had any back pain.").

     Or
   - It dominates at the time of patient presentation.

     Or
   - At some time during aggravating activity, the patient states that the main complaint is leg (and buttock) pain.
2. Paresthesias (and occasionally numbness) in a typical dermatomal distribution, for example:
   - Lateral foot and heel for S1 root.
   - Lateral calf and/or dorsum of foot and/or big toe for L5 root.
   - Medial shin for L4 root.
   - Kneecap for L3 root.

Even domination of the history by pain does not ensure a diagnosis of degenerative disc or disc rupture. Tumors of bone and neurologic tissues, as well as intra-abdominal conditions, can cause pain. But the pain of these conditions is nonmechanical, that is, present at rest.

INFLUENCE OF ACTIVITIES

Specific questions must be asked to determine the factors that influence the pain. Backache due to a mechanical breakdown of the spine is almost always aggravated by general and specific activities and is relieved by rest. There are, of course, some exceptions to this general rule, but on the whole, it is fairly reliable. Backache due to a penetrating duodenal ulcer is not aggravated by activities, nor does it ease if the patient lies down. Patients with a neurofibroma involving a nerve root frequently report a history of having to get up at night to walk around to "get away" from the pain, and patients with a secondary deposit in the spine commonly report the story of sudden cramps of pain in their back even when lying down. A few patients with disc degeneration find that their pain is worse lying in bed, but this is most unusual. Patients who complain of pain in bed may sleep face downward, a position that, by extending the lumbar spine, aggravates discogenic pain. Constant pain in bed is also seen in the emotionally distraught.

When trying to find out whether activities increase pain, it is best to ask the following specific questions: "Does lifting hurt?", "Is your pain worse when you bend over the sink?", "Can you make beds?", "Can you use the vacuum cleaner?", and "Is the pain made worse by walking or climbing stairs?" Discogenic pain is frequently increased by maintaining one posture over a period of time: prolonged walking, prolonged sitting, or prolonged standing. Sudden jars to the body will aggravate any form of mechanical pain.

The history of pain shooting down the leg as a result of coughing or sneezing is highly suggestive of root compression. This is due to the Valsalva maneuver, which increases the pressure transmitted through the spinal fluid, further aggravating nerve root compression.

Many patients are confused by the question, "Is your pain better when you lie down?" They will frequently answer, "No," in the belief that the question implied that the act of lying down completely cured their backache for a period of time. They may answer, "No, it is not made better by lying down; it is just as bad as ever when I get up." It is probably better to ask them, "What do you feel like doing when the pain is very bad?" Although some patients may regard this question as being absurd, most will tell you they would like to lie down, or sit down, if they could. A classic position of comfort is lying on a hard floor with the hips and knees flexed, with the calves resting on a chair or a sofa (Fig. 8-4).

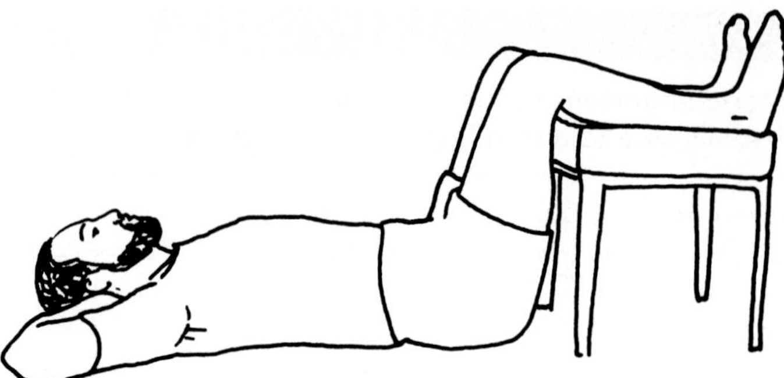

FIGURE 8-4 ● A position of comfort for a patient with sciatica is lying on the floor with his feet up on a chair or sofa.

Although it may be tedious at times, it is imperative to learn from the patient what aggravates and relieves his or her symptoms.

DURATION AND PROGRESSION OF SYMPTOMS

It is important to have a clear knowledge of the onset, duration, and progression of the symptoms. How did the pain start? Gradually, or suddenly? Spontaneously, or with an accident? If it started with an accident, is there a lawyer involved? Is there some "commercial" value to the symptoms? Did it follow provocative activity? Has the pain been continuous or intermittent?

The sudden onset of pain after provocative activity with an intermittent course subsequently is highly suggestive of a mechanical basis for the symptoms. The sudden onset of severe back pain with a simple twisting movement is very suggestive of pathologic fracture. In a man older than 50 years, this latter presentation may also be the presenting symptom in multiple myeloma.

Is the pain getting worse? If the patient feels that his or her symptoms are getting progressively worse, is this because the attacks are more frequent, more severe, and more prolonged, or is it because the patient has lost all tolerance and is fed up with this bothersome burden?

WHAT IS THE FUNCTIONAL LIMITATION?

A patient who has had to take to bed because of severe leg pain has a much different disability than the individual who cannot swing a "nine iron" because of back pain. The type of symptoms and the functional limitations allow you to decide if the disability is mild, moderate, or severe, a classification that allows for rational treatment decisions.

ARE THERE ANY ASSOCIATED SYMPTOMS?

Specifically, you are interested in whether there are any intra-abdominal symptoms that suggest a source of referred back pain. You are interested in that patient as a person. Is he or she anxious or depressed, or is the patient taking a rather belligerent or indifferent approach to his or her symptoms? Throughout this book, there is ceaseless referral to the patient with nonorganic spinal pain. There is good reason: The nonorganically disabled patient is common, and the cost of missing this diagnosis amounts to multimillions of dollars each year in misspent investigations and ill-conceived surgery. We are sorry to keep raising the issue, but once more, you should commit to reading Chapter 4.

Most important, you would like to know if there is any serious effect of the disc pathology on urinary or bowel function. Urinary retention, with or without overflow incontinence, is an ominous symptom. Even more ominous is the association of perineal numbness signifying compression of the cauda equina. Any doubt about the presence or absence of a cauda equina syndrome requires emergency investigation.

At this state of the history, it is a good time to inquire about the patient's general health through a functional inquiry, past history, and family history. In today's age of drug addiction and immunocompromised states, all kinds of unusual low back pain will present, more often than not, due to disc space infections. Watch out for peripheral neuropathy associated with diabetes.

TABLE 8-2

Conservative Treatment Modalities

Rest
- Restricted activity, brace, weight reduction, job modification

Medication
- Analgesic, anti-inflammatory, muscle relaxant

Temperature change
- Heat and cold

Exercise
- Flexion, extension, isokinetic

Manipulation

Miscellaneous
- Acupuncture, biofeedback, transcutaneous electrical nerve stimulation, relaxation therapy

Time

WHAT TREATMENT HAS BEEN ADMINISTERED?

Excluding the failed back surgery patient who is discussed in Chapter 17, what conservative treatment modalities have been tried? Table 8-2 summarizes the classes of conservative treatment commonly administered to low back pain sufferers. If a patient has tried bed rest, physical therapy, and appropriate medication, it is senseless to suggest that they all be tried again. Once adequate conservative treatment modalities have failed in a patient with a moderate or severe disability, it is time to consider surgery. The last item listed in Table 8-2 is time. Has enough time elapsed for the natural historical course of the symptoms and disease to occur? It is not necessary to rush a patient into the operating room until nature has taken its course. Obviously, bladder and bowel involvement and an advancing neurologic lesion are exceptions to this rule.

ANATOMIC BASIS OF THE PAIN

It must be remembered that back pain is a symptom and not a disease and that its source may lie outside the spine. It is essential, therefore, to include in the history a general functional inquiry. For example, the history of dorsolumbar pain relieved by the ingestion of food raises the possibility of a penetrating duodenal ulcer. The history of difficulty in micturition demands further inquiry to rule out prostatic cancer with secondary lesions in the spine. A family history of diabetes raises the possibility of diabetic neuropathy. A diabetes diathesis, by itself, markedly intensifies the pain of root compression. A chronic cough or a history of unexplained weight loss cannot be ignored.

It cannot be overemphasized that spondylogenic back pain is aggravated by general and specific activities and is relieved, to some extent, by recumbency.

CONCLUSION

Take time to listen to the patient. If you are a music lover, you will instantly recognize Beethoven's Symphony No. 5 in C Minor. Even the casual classical listener can recognize Tchaikovsky's 1812 Overture. Listening to a patient with a complaint of pain in the back presents the same opportunities for recognition.

A patient with a herniated nucleus pulposus paints a different historical picture than a patient with mechanical instability due to degenerative disc disease. A malingerer tells a classic story in a typical manner. In fact, the history is so important that most low back pain diagnoses are known before the examiner begins the physical examination.

CHAPTER 9

Examination of the Back

"More mistakes are made from want of proper examination than for any other reason."

—Russell Howard

"The examining physician often hesitates to make the necessary examination because it involves soiling the finger."

—William Mayo

The purpose of this chapter is to give a general outline of a routine clinical examination of a patient suffering from significant back pain. Specific findings are alluded to again when the examination and treatment of common clinical syndromes are discussed in later chapters. It is important to emphasize that accurate records of the history and examination should be made. These must include exact measurements and not vague terms such as "good," "poor," "limited," and so on. Good records are necessary for case analysis and comparison, and, on case reviews, for assistance to a consulting physician, and, at times, for legal purposes.

The examination of the back should be conducted in an orderly, predetermined manner. Examination of the patient should not be directed solely at eliciting signs of a specific disease suggested by the history, nor should individual systems be examined serially: neurologic examination, abdominal examination, vascular examination, and so on. The examination must be conducted in an orderly manner so that all possible physical findings may be evaluated. When you finish examining each patient, you must know as much about his or her physical state as the last patient and every patient you have seen or will see.

The first prerequisite is that the patient must be undressed. To some practitioners, this is an absurd statement, because patient undressing is a routine; to clinicians who see a lot of patients in a short amount of time, patient undressing is an inconvenience. A cursory examination is worse than no examination at all, because it may give the false hope that the lesion is minor.

STEP 1 GAIT

Watch the patient walk. Is there an antalgic gait that suggests hip or knee disease? Is there a shuffling gait that suggests a neurologic disorder of rigidity or spasticity? Does the patient walk slightly flexed, which suggests a spinal canal stenosis? Gait observation reveals a lot of secrets. Not infrequently, it is difficult to decide if a patient's back and hip pain is due to pathology in the back or in the hip. More often than not, watching the patient walk the length of the hall will make the diagnosis, especially if the patient has the spastic gait of myelopathy or the antalgic limp of hip disease.

STEP 2 SPINE CONTOURS

By looking at the patient from the side and behind, gross postural changes will be evident. It is best to think of these postural changes as being in the sagittal plane (Fig. 9-1) or the coronal or frontal plane (Fig. 9-2).

FRONTAL PLANE ASYMMETRY

There are three basic causes of frontal plane asymmetry as shown in Figure 9-2. To separate a structural scoliosis (e.g., idiopathic) from a sciatic scoliosis, make the following observations:

STRUCTURAL SCOLIOSIS

1. The curve is fixed and does not change on forward flexion.
2. The common right thoracic idiopathic curve has a rib hump that becomes more obvious on flexion.
3. The curve does not reduce on recumbency.

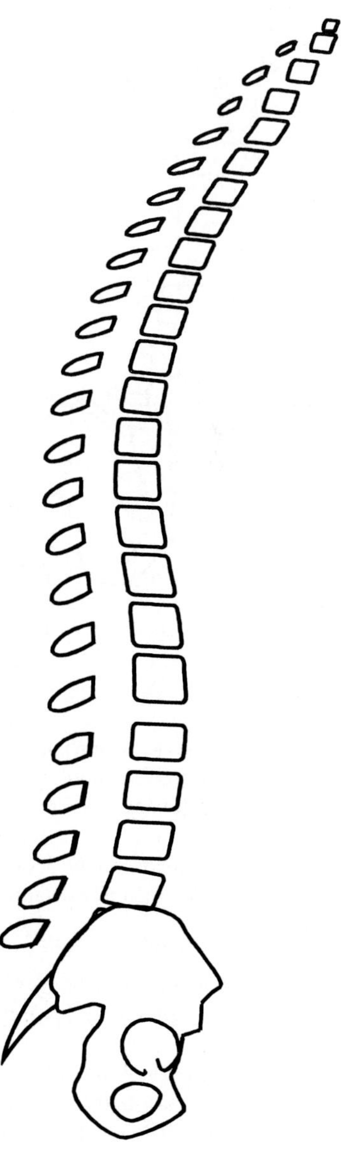

FIGURE 9-1 ● Sagittal plane malalignment: kyphosis.

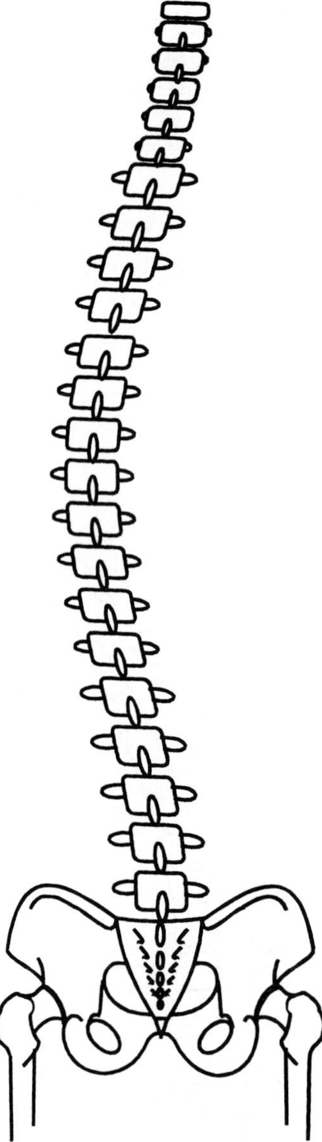

FIGURE 9-2 ● Coronal plane malalignment: scoliosis.

SCIATIC (REACTIVE) SCOLIOSIS

1. Sciatic scoliosis is a more diffuse curve that does not have a rib hump.
2. On forward flexion, the curve changes, usually becoming worse, but it may even reverse its direction.
3. Forward flexion in sciatic scoliosis is much more limited than that in structural scoliosis.
4. Sciatic scoliosis usually disappears on recumbency.

Other observations to be made when examining the patient from behind are as follows:

1. Look for skin crease changes in the lumbosacral regions that might indicate a step-off of a lytic or degenerative spondylolisthesis [see Chapter 6, "Steps" of spondylolisthesis (Fig. 9-3)].
2. Skin markings: look for café-au-lait spots, a hallmark of neurofibromatosis. Other masses such as fatty tumors or hairy patches in the lumbosacral region may indicate deeper skeletal lesions such as spina bifida with or without associated tumors of or in neurogenic tissues.

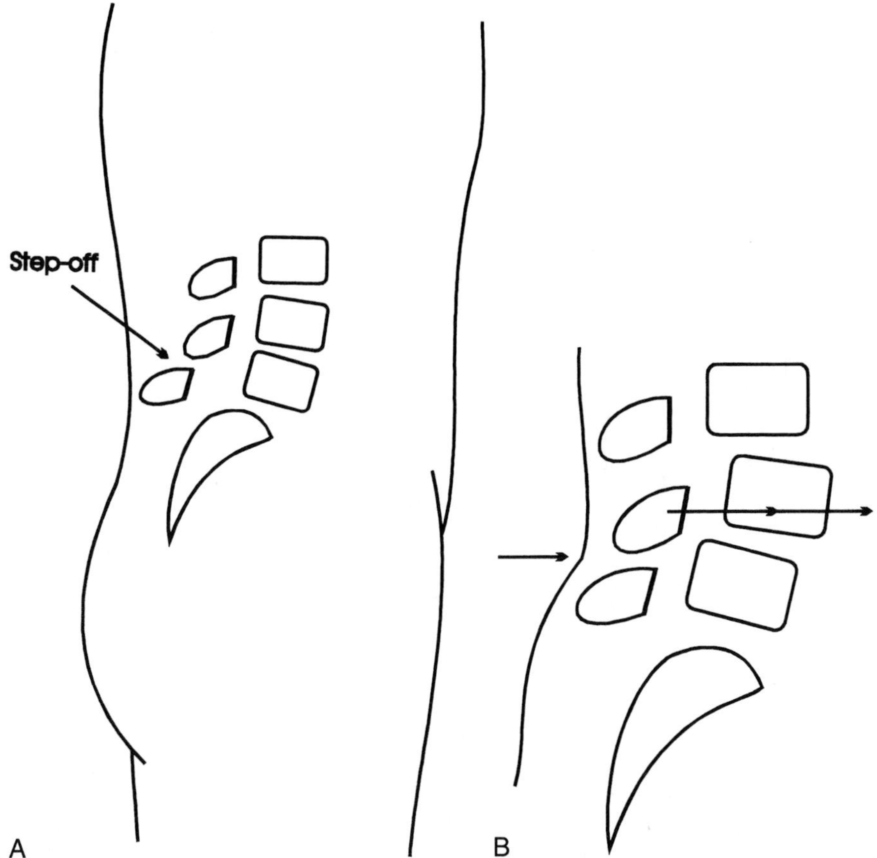

FIGURE 9-3 ● The "steps" in spondylolisthesis. **A:** In a lytic spondylolisthesis (most common at L5-S1), the spinous process of L5 is left behind, that is, the step is palpable between the L4 spinous process that has moved forward and the L5 spinous process. **B:** In a degenerative spondylolisthesis, a similar situation exists, except the slip vertebrae is one level higher, and the L5 spinous process is also left behind.

STEP 3 RANGE OF MOTION/RHYTHM

The range and rhythm of spinal movement are tested next. The range of forward flexion is recorded by noting how far the hands come toward the floor. The rhythm of forward flexion is observed by placing the fingertips on the spinous process and noting how far they separate on flexion of the spine (Fig. 9-4).

Extension is recorded by noting how far the patient can lean backward before the pelvis tilts. Lateral flexion is measured by noting how far the patient can slide the hand down the thigh toward the knee (Fig. 9-5). Rotation can be tested by getting the patient to stand with his or her feet wide apart and rotate with hands on hips (Fig. 9-6). Also, do the simulated rotation test demonstrated in Chapter 16.

During the examination, observe any specific abnormalities; for example, look for marked limitation of the range of forward flexion without lumbar movement, as occurs in root irritation due to disc herniation. These patients frequently show deviation to the painful side on forward flexion. The rigidity of the whole spine in the later stages of ankylosing spondylitis is characteristic. Reversal of normal spinal rhythm on attempting to regain the erect posture after forward flexion is characteristic of disc degeneration associated with a posterior joint lesion. To avoid putting an extension strain on the posterior joint, the patient tucks the pelvis under the spine to regain the erect position. When getting up from forward flexion, he or she will start to extend the spine, but this

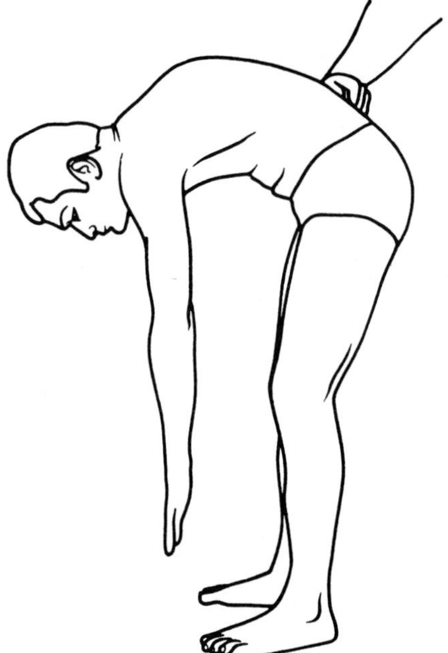

FIGURE 9-4 ● When the patient is asked to bend forward, not only should the range of movement be noted, but the ability of the spinous processes to separate should also be recorded. This is best done by placing the fingertips over the spinous processes in the lumbar spine.

movement is uncomfortable. To avoid this, he or she will slightly flex the hips and knees to tuck the pelvis under the spine and then regain the erect position by straightening the legs (Fig. 9-7).

With the patient still standing, the strength of the gastrocnemius is determined by testing the ability to stand on tiptoe (Fig. 9-8). Repetitive toe raising (fatigue testing) may bring out early changes. Lesions involving the first sacral root such as lumbosacral disc herniation may produce weakness of tiptoe raising and diminution of the ankle jerk, which can be tested with the patient kneeling on a chair. The examiner must remember that if a patient has a weak quadriceps, his or her leg will tend to buckle on attempting to rise on tiptoe. This is a diagnostic trap for the unwary.

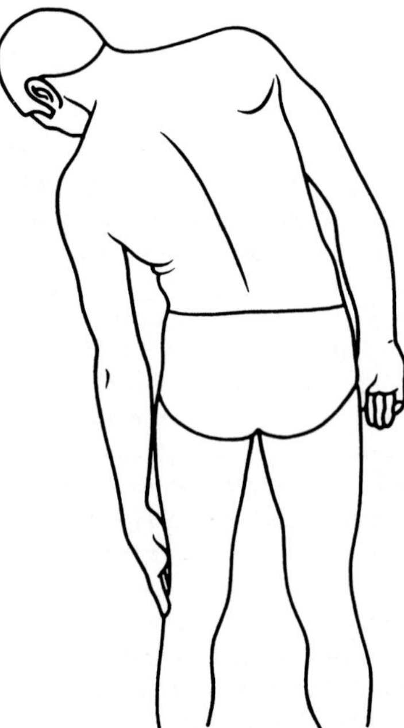

FIGURE 9-5 ● Lateral flexion is recorded by noting how far the patient can slide his or her hand down the thigh toward the knee.

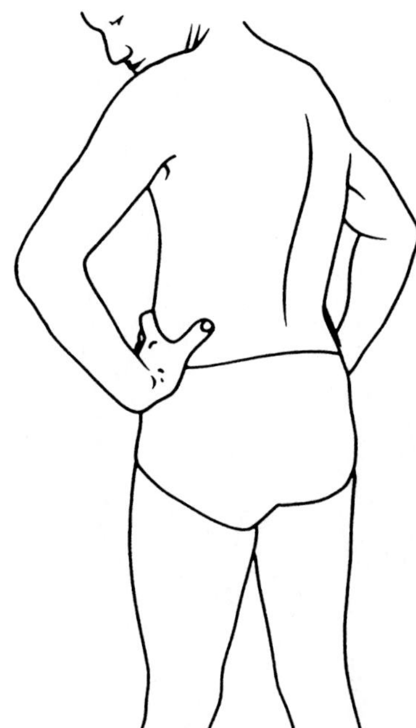

FIGURE 9-6 ● Rotation is recorded by asking the patient to place his or her hands on the hips. The elbows then act as the arms of a goniometer and the degree of rotation permitted can be measured.

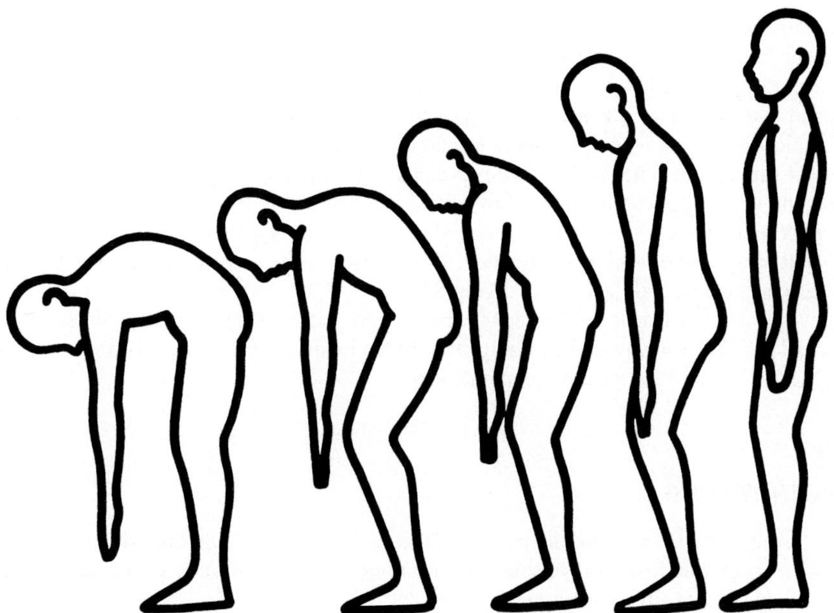

FIGURE 9-7 ● Reversal of spinal rhythm. On attempting to regain the erect position from forward flexion, the patient will bend the knees and tuck the pelvis underneath the spine to stand erect. This type of movement is very characteristic of segmental instability.

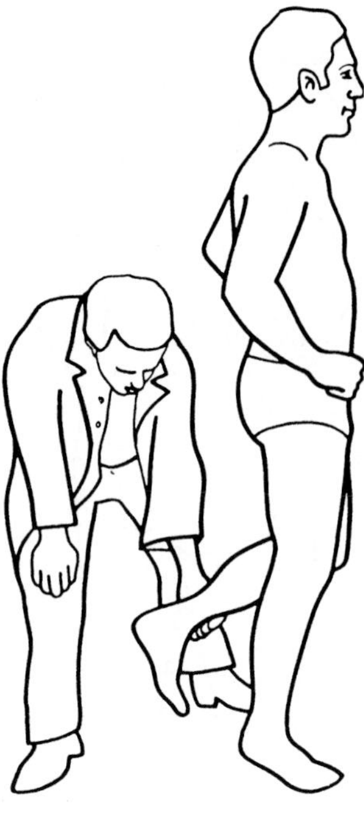

FIGURE 9-8 ● The strength of the gastrocnemius is best tested by asking the patient to rise on tiptoe repetitively and rapidly. You are looking for fatigability, and therefore the patient must be asked to rise on tiptoe a minimum of 10 times.

STEP 4

Two examinations are conducted with the patient sitting on the edge of the examining table. First, examine the knee and ankle reflexes. This is usually the most comfortable position for a back pain patient and allows for reflex examination without painful posturing, something that will distort the reflex examination. Every now and then, a patient will have such a great degree of sciatica that he or she cannot sit without lifting the buttock (and thus the painful sciatic nerve) off the bed, which may falsely suppress the knee reflex. Reflexes can also be altered by a patient visually watching the reflex examination. This can be negated by reinforcement (Fig. 9-9).

The next reflex to be tested is the superficial plantar-flexor response (see Fig. 9-9). One feature of the plantar response is a reflex contraction of the tensor fascia femoris. This portion of the withdrawal response is lost with lesions involving S1.

Oh, by the way! Go back to Figure 9-9 and observe the position of the leg during the sitting Babinski's test. This is a way of examining straight leg raising in the sitting position (the so-called flip test; see Chapter 16 for a further explanation).

STEP 5

STRENGTH TESTING

Strength testing is best done with the patient in the supine position. The dorsiflexors of the ankles may become weak with lesions involving the fifth lumbar nerve root, such as herniation of the disc between the fourth and fifth lumbar vertebra.

The strength of the dorsiflexors should not be tested with the knee extended, because if the patient has significant sciatic pain, any attempt by the patient to resist forced plantar flexion of the ankle will be painful, and a false impression of weakness may be obtained. The knee should be flexed, and full body weight pressure should be applied against the dorsum of the foot to assess the strength of the dorsiflexors (Fig. 9-10). Lesions involving the fifth lumbar root may cause weakness of the extensor hallucis longus before any significant weakness of the dorsiflexors of the ankle is apparent (Fig. 9-11). Similarly, with an S1 lesion, the flexor hallucis longus may become detectably weak before there is any noticeable weakness of the gastrocnemius. Sometimes, this can

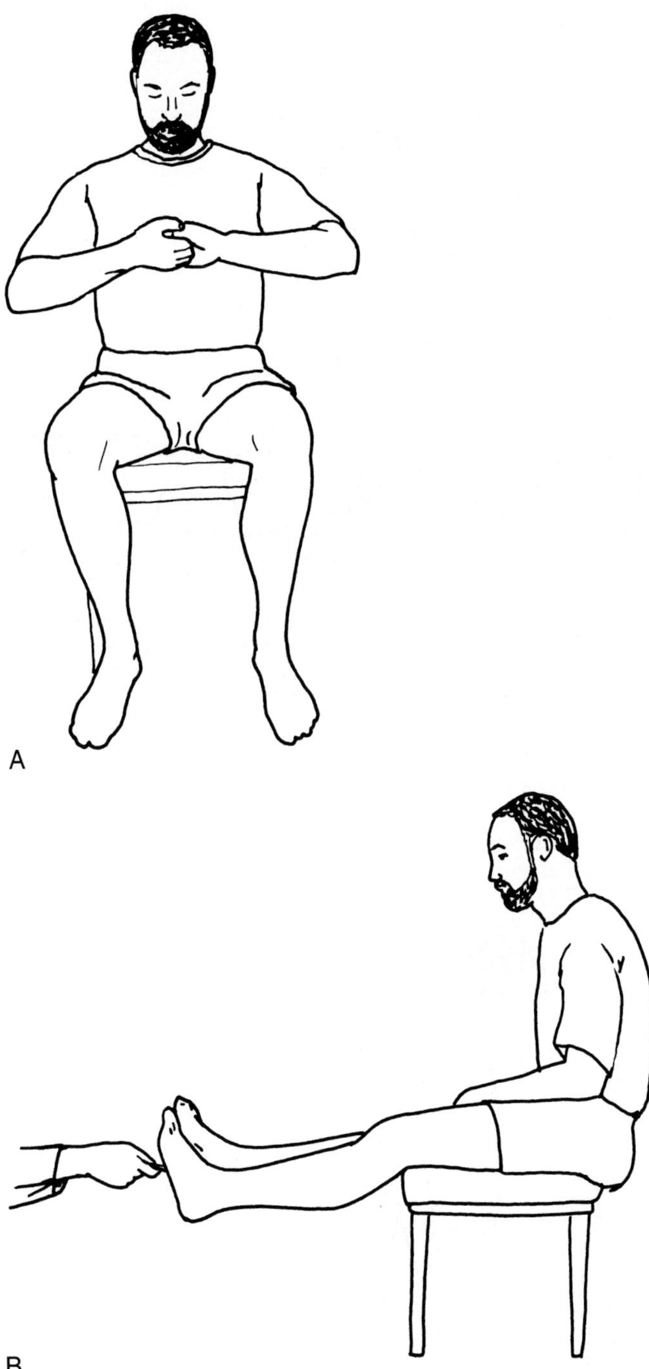

FIGURE 9-9 ● **A:** Asking the patient to grasp and pull on the hands serves as reinforcement of reflexes. **B:** Sitting Babinski's test: the straight leg raising (SLR) test can be done in the sitting position while doing other tests, such as that to test Babinski's reflexes.

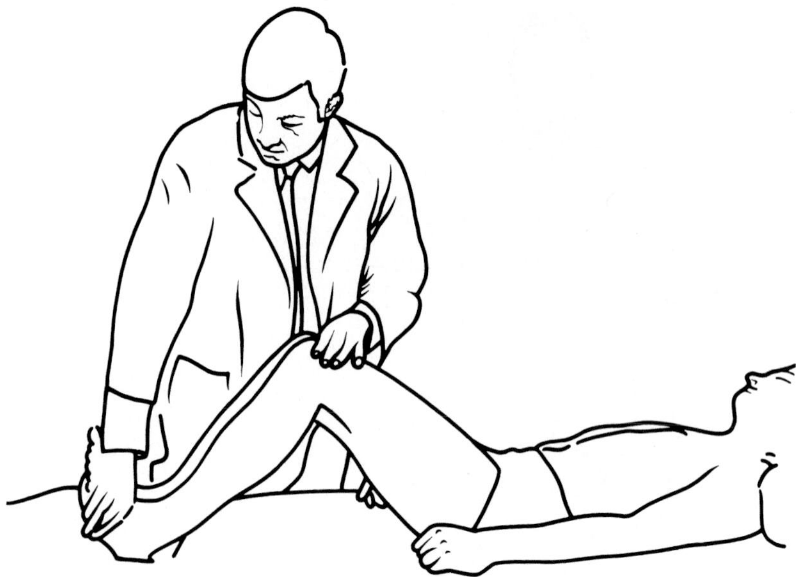

FIGURE 9-10 ● The power of the dorsiflexors of the ankle should be tested with the patient lying on his/her back, with hips and knees flexed. The patient holds the ankle in full dorsiflexion and attempts to resist the maximal force that the physician can apply to the dorsum of the foot.

be dramatically demonstrated by asking the patient to claw or flex the toes, whereupon it may be noted that the patient can flex the big toe on one side but not on the other. Many examiners use the heel-toe walking test to examine L5 and S1 root weakness (see Fig. 9-11).

The quadriceps may be weak with lesions of the third and fourth lumbar nerve root. The strength of the muscle is best tested with the patient lying on his or her back, with the hips slightly flexed

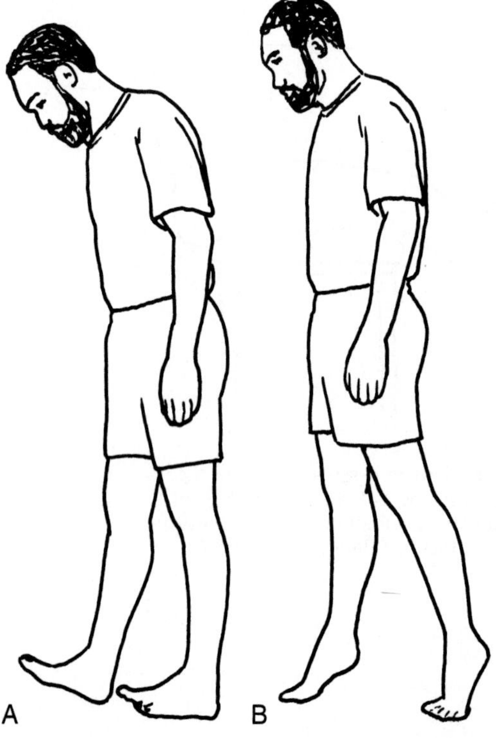

FIGURE 9-11 ● **A:** The patient is walking on the heels: tests of L5 motor function. **B:** The patient is walking on the toes: test of S1 motor function.

TABLE 9-1

Grading of Muscle Strength

0—No movement of muscle unit
1—Flicker to tendon movement
2—Some muscle/tendon movement of joint only if gravity removed
3—More movement of joint against gravity and some resistance
4—Movement against gravity with reasonable resistance, but still weakness evident
5—Normal strength

and the knee placed over the examiner's forearm. The patient then tries to extend the knee against the resistance of the examiner's other hand.

Diffuse weakness of all muscle groups, particularly the psoas, is highly suggestive of an emotional breakdown. Functional or emotional weakness is characterized by jerky relaxation of the muscles regardless of what force is applied. Quite frequently, these patients will be able to resist breakdown of a fixed position, but will be unable to initiate movement of a joint against weak resistance. This is the so-called "discrepant" motor weakness. In gross emotional disturbances, there may be diffuse, unreasonable weakness of many muscle groups. Characteristically, these patients will be unable to extend the terminal interphalangeal joint of the thumb against the slightest resistance and will not be able to hold their eyes closed tightly shut when the examiner tries to push the eyebrow up.

Muscle strength test results should be graded according to the standard method of a 0 to 5 scale (Table 9-1). The fourth grade (movement against gravity and resistance) is usually subgraded into the following levels:

- 4+ Significant weakness (but not grade 3)
- 4++ Moderate weakness
- 4+++ Almost normal but weak

At times, be cognizant of the effect pain has on the patient's ability to carry out the strength testing. Some patients have so much back or leg pain that, despite trying to cooperate with you, they cannot participate in strength testing maneuvers. Some of the patients assume the appearance of pain and inability to cooperate, but other aspects of the history and physical examination will point you toward considering the nonorganic reactions described in Chapter 16.

STEP 6

Nerve root irritation is commonly associated with specific muscle tenderness. With first sacral root irritation, the calf becomes tender. With fifth lumbar root irritation, the anterior tibial muscles become tender; with fourth lumbar root irritation, the quadriceps are tender. Tenderness over the subcutaneous surface of the tibia is seen when emotional overtones play a large part in the clinical picture. Specific muscle tenderness is a very important physical sign of root irritation.

With the patient still supine, appreciation of pinprick can be tested, thus comparing the sensibility of the same areas in both legs. Dermatome areas are well localized. S1 supplies the sole and the outer border of the leg and foot. L5 supplies the dorsum of the foot and the anterior aspect of the lower leg, L4 supplies the anteromedial aspect of the shin (Fig. 9-12); L3 supplies the kneecap region, and L2 supplies the lateral thigh. The correct evaluation of sensory appreciation demands, strangely enough, a meticulous technique. Only gross changes can be detected by the perfunctory jab of a pin. When minor changes are sought, it is important to remember that sensory appreciation is dependent on summation of stimuli. Because of this physiologic phenomenon, 10 pinpricks applied to a partially denervated area of the skin may be appreciated as readily as one or two pinpricks on the opposite leg. For accurate evaluation, the "stimulus" applied should be the same in both areas under comparison. The most tedious and uncomfortable part of the examination for the patient is being pricked with a pin (make sure it is not the same safety pin that has jabbed a

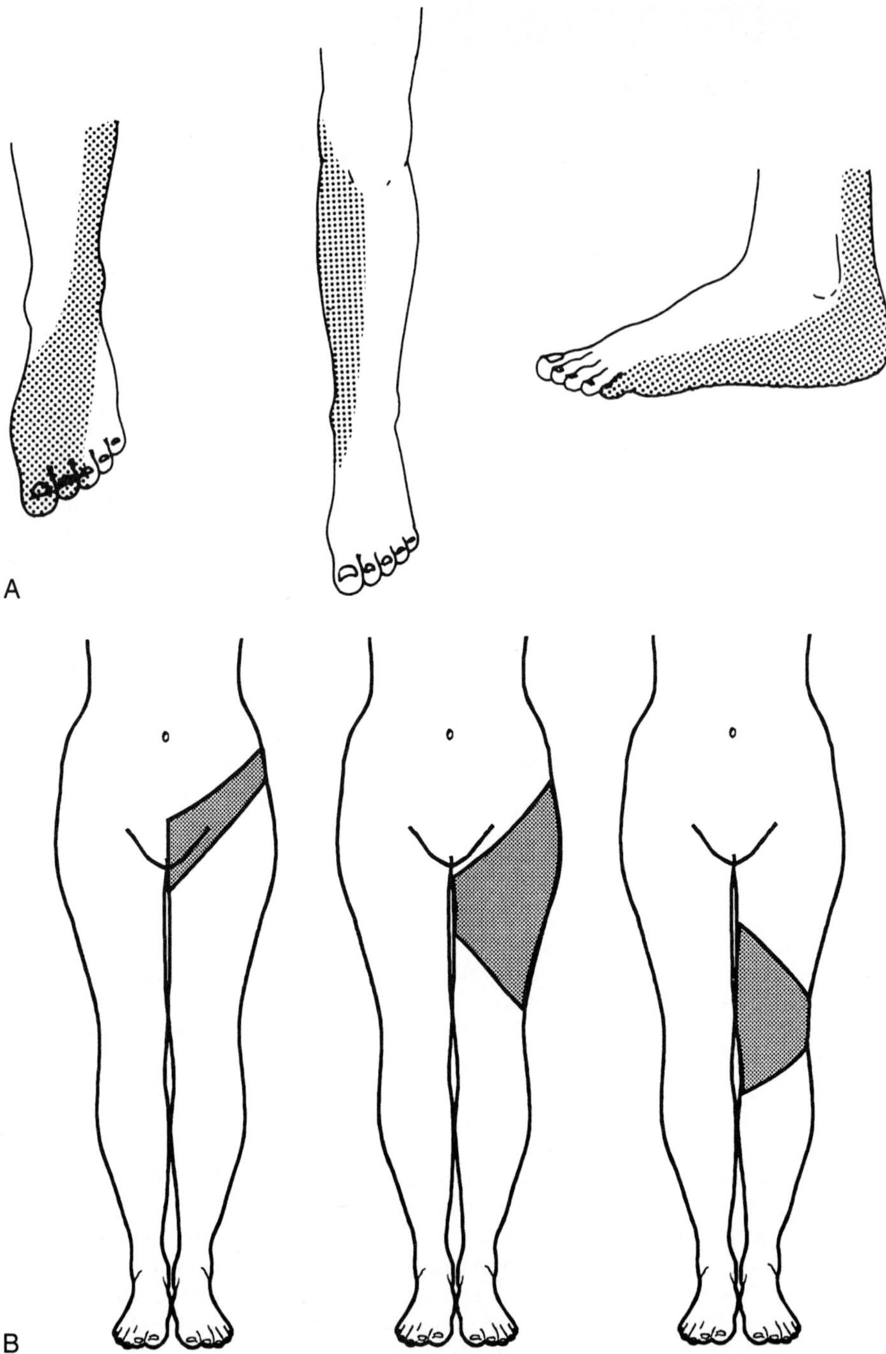

FIGURE 9-12 ● **A:** The distribution of sensory dermatomes for lumbar roots L4 and L5 and sacral root S1 (left, L5; middle, L4; right, S1). It is unusual for a sensory loss to be dense throughout the complete dermatome; rather, the deficit may appear spotty throughout the dermatome. It is not unusual, especially in younger patients, to hear a classic story of a paresthetic discomfort in a typical dermatomal distribution, yet find no numbness on physical examination. **B:** L1, L2, L3 dermatome: the stippled areas, left to right.

patient before). Patients want to get the pinprick test over with quickly and are apt to agree to any suggestion of the examiner, just to get that portion of the examination over.

Vibration sensibility below the knees is not as acute in patients more than 50 years of age, and the same applies to temperature appreciation. It must be remembered that the demonstration of a "stocking" type of diminished appreciation of pinprick does not necessarily indicate that the pain is hysterical in origin. It may merely indicate that the patient is demonstrating a hysterical exaggeration of signs derived from a significant organic lesion. The significance of such a demonstration of sensory loss must be evaluated with all other symptoms and signs presented by the patient.

STEP 7

Signs of root tension may now be evaluated. Root tension is a term reserved to denote reproduction of extremity pain by stretching a peripheral nerve. When testing the sciatic nerve, the leg must never be raised suddenly by lifting the heel, because so much pain may be evoked by this maneuver as to make all other examinations useless. The leg should be raised slowly, with the knee maintained in the fully extended position by the examiner's hands (Fig. 9-13). It is important to record the range through which the leg must be raised before leg or buttock pain is experienced. Reproduction of back pain in this manner does not necessarily indicate root tension, of course. With any painful lesion of the back associated with hamstring spasm, straight leg raising will rotate the pelvis and irritate the lumbosacral region, giving rise to pain. However, reproduction or aggravation of sciatic pain by forced dorsiflexion of the ankle at the limit of straight leg raising is highly suggestive of root tension, and this impression is confirmed if the patient admits relief on bending the knee. If a patient still has pain after the knee has been flexed, and if the pain is increased on further flexion of the hip (bent leg raising), then the examiner should be concerned that he or she is dealing with a patient suffering from a significant emotional breakdown, or else there may be a lesion of the hip joint presenting as sciatic pain.

Straight leg raising of the opposite leg, the symptom-free leg, that gives rise to an exacerbation of pain in the affected extremity is known as crossover pain and is suggestive of a disc herniation lying in the axilla or medial to the root (Fig. 9-14).

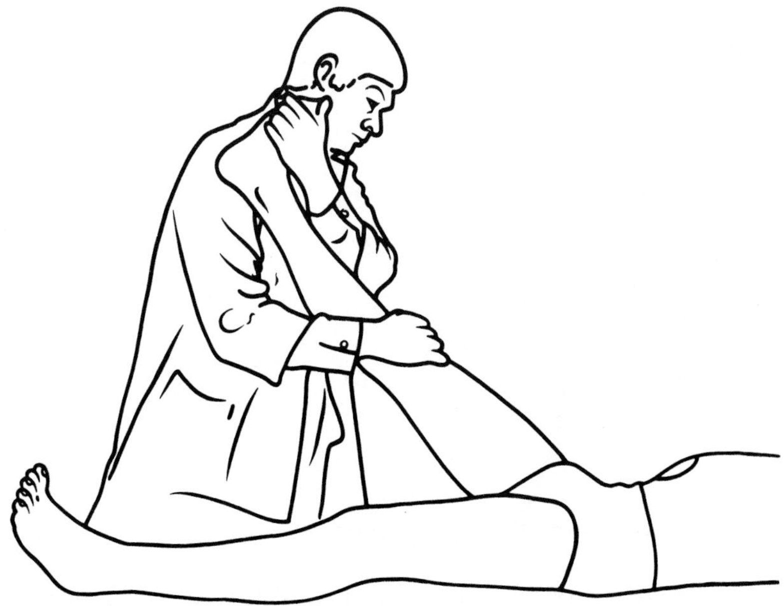

FIGURE 9-13 ● When carrying out the straight leg raising test, it is important to remember that the leg should be raised slowly, and during this movement, the knee must be maintained in the fully expended position by the examiner's hand.

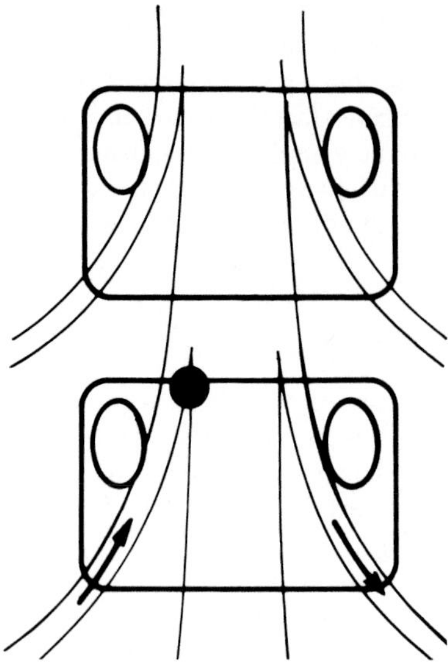

FIGURE 9-14 ● A disc herniation is present in the axilla of the right nerve root. Straight leg raising (SLR) on the left will not only move the asymptomatic left root but also pull the right root against the disc rupture. This will produce pain into the symptomatic right buttock, a phenomenon known as crossover pain.

The most reliable test of root tension is the bowstring sign. In this test, straight leg raising is carried out until pain is reproduced. At this level, the knee is slightly flexed until the pain abates. The examiner rests the limb on his or her shoulder and places the thumbs in the popliteal fossa over the sciatic nerve. If sudden firm pressure on the nerve gives rise to pain in the back or down the leg, the patient is almost certainly suffering from significant root tension (Fig. 9-15). An excellent audit of the value of this test is to use the hamstring (Fig. 9-15). Two sets of situations can exist: (a) pressure over the medial hamstring tendon causes no pain; pressure over the lateral hamstring tendon

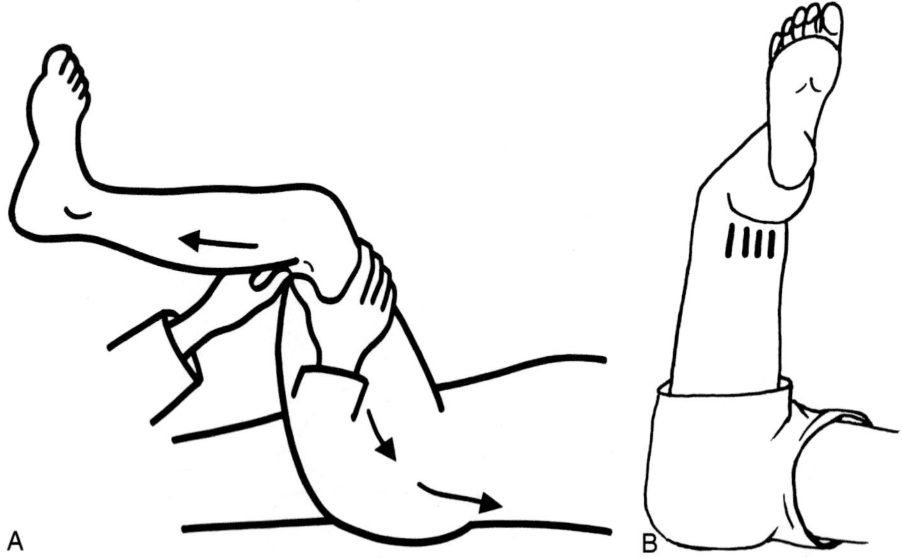

FIGURE 9-15 ● **A:** When eliciting the bowstring sign, the patient's foot should be allowed to rest on the examiner's shoulder, with the knee very slightly flexed at the limit of straight leg raising. Sudden firm pressure is then applied by the examiner's thumbs in the popliteal fossa. Radiation of pain down the leg or the production of pain in the back is pathognomonic of root tension. **B:** An audit of the bowstring test: the four "cords" behind the knee are the medial and lateral hamstrings and the tibial and peroneal nerves; the latter two will be tender. The hamstring tendon pressure should not elicit pain.

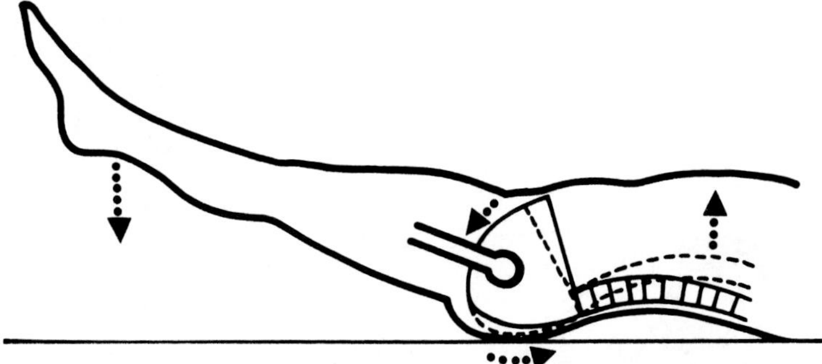

FIGURE 9-16 • When the patient carries out bilateral active straight leg raising, the weight of the leg causes the pelvis to rotate and thereby hyperextends the lumbar spine. Hyperextension of the lumbar spine in the presence of disc degeneration gives rise to pain. This is probably the most useful test to demonstrate the presence of painful segmental instability.

causes no pain; pressure over the lateral peroneal nerve causes radiating pain and (b) pressure over the medial hamstring tendon causes pain; pressure over the tibial nerve causes pain; pressure over the lateral hamstring causes pain; pressure over the lateral peroneal nerve causes pain. The patient in the first situation has an obvious organic syndrome; the patient in the second situation may be an emotional cripple.

In a patient with weak abdominal muscles and disc degeneration, attempts to perform bilateral active straight leg raising are painful because the weight of the legs rotates the pelvis, causing hyperextension of the lumbar spine (Fig. 9-16).

Flexion of the hip with the knee flexed should not aggravate a mechanical back pain, but patients with emotional breakdowns frequently complain bitterly during this maneuver.

With lesions involving the third and fourth lumbar roots, the patient will experience pain on stretching the femoral nerve. This test can be performed with the patient lying face downward. The hip is then extended, with the knee maintained in a slightly flexed position. This test is only of significance if the patient experiences pain radiating down the front of the symptomatic thigh (Fig. 9-17) and not down the thigh of the asymptomatic leg.

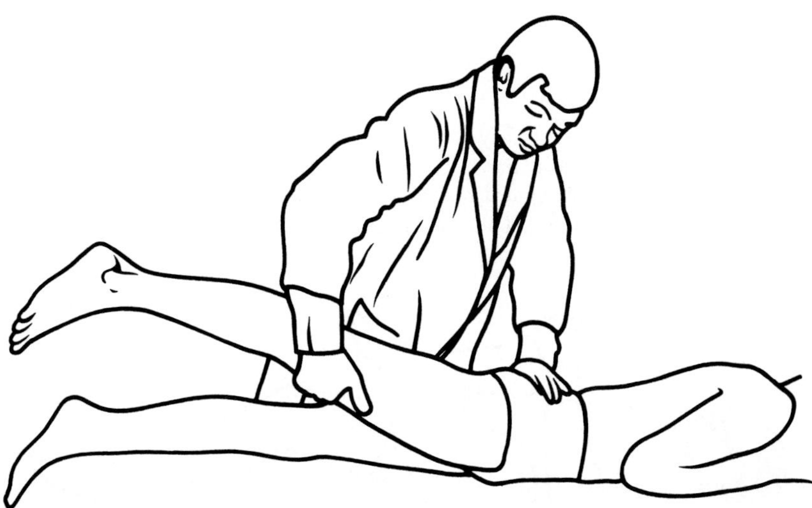

FIGURE 9-17 • When the fourth lumbar nerve root is compromised, the patient experiences pain radiating down the front of the thigh. This pain will be aggravated if the hip is extended with the knees slightly flexed. It is to be noted that this test may give rise to back pain by virtue of hyperextending the spine, but this finding is not of diagnostic significance.

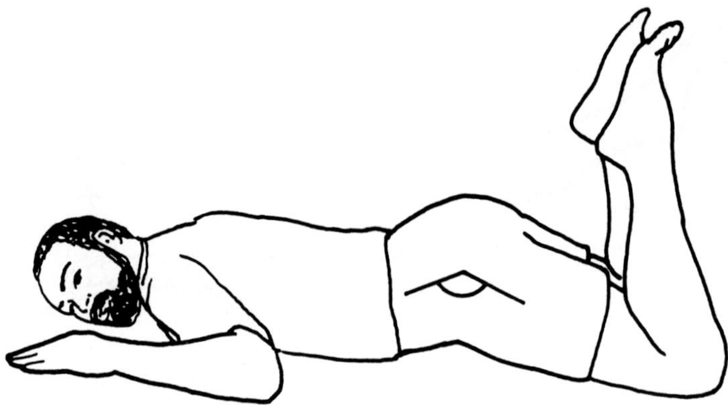

FIGURE 9-18 ● Ely's sign: In the prone position, flexion of the knees should not normally cause flexion of the hips, as in this schematic.

Care must be taken not to confuse the femoral nerve stretch test with Ely's sign (Fig. 9-18). The test for Ely's sign was designed to demonstrate contracture or shortening of the rectus femoris. The rectus femoris spans both the hip joint and the knee joint, flexing the hip and extending the knee. When the knee is fully flexed, the rectus femoris is stretched. If there is any contracture of the muscle (i.e., due to hip disease), passive stretching in this manner will cause the hip to flex. This can be easily demonstrated by fully flexing the knee with the patient lying face downward; the resulting flexion of the hip is shown by the fact that the buttock rises off the bed. This is Ely's test. This test is frequently positive in patients of mesomorphic build. In some patients suffering from fourth lumbar root irritation, this maneuver gives rise to severe quadriceps pain.

STEP 8

At this stage of the examination, the full range of hip joint movements should be assessed. Osteoarthritis of the hip joint may give rise to symptoms and signs mimicking fourth lumbar root compression: pain down the front of the thigh, weakness and atrophy of the quadriceps, tenderness on palpation of the quadriceps, and pain on the femoral nerve stretch test. This confusion arises from a perfunctory examination. Always assess hip joint motion fully by: (a) watching the patient walk, (b) testing internal rotation, and (c) assessing if there is any flexion deformity (Fig. 9-19).

STEP 9

Next, examine the peripheral pulses for signs of impairment of arterial circulation. Hair distribution and other atrophic changes, such as in the nails, will give some indication of vascular insufficiency. Impairment of venous outflow should also be noted. With the patient still supine, the abdomen is palpated for evidence of intra-abdominal masses, and the peripheral pulses are palpated for evidence of vascular insufficiency.

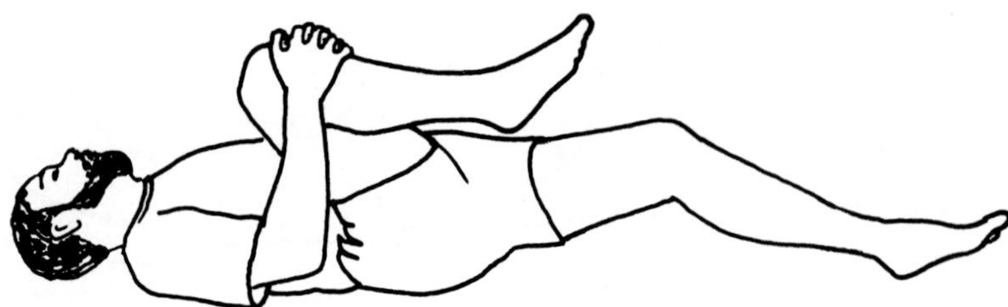

FIGURE 9-19 ● Demonstration of a flexion deformity of the hip: the patient is full flexing the right hip; a normal left hip would allow the left leg to rest flat on the bed. A flexion deformity of the left hip with this test would not allow the left leg to rest on the bed.

STEP 10

The patient is then turned on his or her side. The ability to abduct the leg against resistance is tested. When this movement is performed, the glutei must contract vigorously and should tend to pull the pelvis away from the sacrum. A patient with a sacroiliac strain or any sacroiliac disease will find this movement painful.

The sacroiliac joint can also be tested by applying a rotary strain. The unaffected hip joint is flexed, and the thigh is held firmly against the chest by the patient to lock the lumbar spine. The uppermost hip is now extended to its limit. When the hip is pushed beyond its limit of joint extension, a rotary strain is applied to the sacroiliac joint, which is a movement that causes pain when sacroiliac diseases are present (Fig. 9-20). If a sacroiliac joint lesion is present, lateral compression of the pelvis when the patient is lying on his or her side sometimes gives rise to pain.

MISCELLANEOUS STEPS

It is frequently convenient, because the patient is already on his or her side, to carry out a rectal examination at this stage. The patient is turned face downward, and the buttocks and thighs are palpated for tumors involving the sciatic nerve.

At some point during the examination leg lengths should be measured. The maximal girth of the calf is compared on the two sides, and the circumference of the thigh is measured on both sides at a fixed distance from the tibial tubercle. The patient is then asked to sit on the side of the couch so that chest expansion can be determined. A decrease in chest expansion is an early change in ankylosing spondylitis.

The patient is then asked to step down from the couch and drape himself or herself over its edge, resting the abdomen on a pillow. This position is usually comfortable and brings all the spinous processes into prominence. An area not expected to be tender is tested first. Firm pressure applied to the spine may be uncomfortable. The patient must be able to differentiate between the expected discomfort of such pressure and the abnormal discomfort when the damaged segment is palpated.

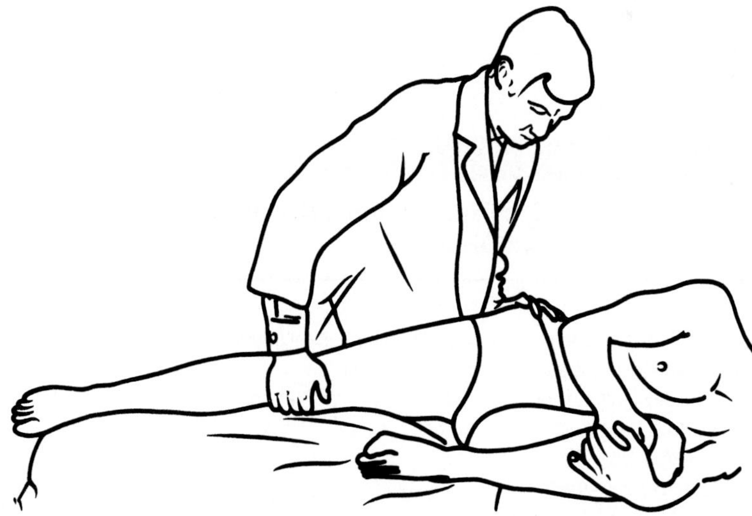

FIGURE 9-20 • Gaenslen's tests. The patient lies on his or her side and holds the lumbar spine rigid by flexing the lowermost hip and pulling the knee against the chest. The uppermost hip is now extended by the examiner. At the limit of hip joint extension, any further extension strain applies a rotary strain to the pelvis and tends to rotate one half of the ilium against the sacrum. With sacroiliac joint lesions, this maneuver is painful. This test can also be performed with the patient lying on his or her back holding the knee flexed against the chest. A hyperextension strain can be applied to the hip by allowing the leg to drop over the side of the table. (From Macnab I. *Backache.* Baltimore: Williams & Wilkins; 1977:128 with permission.)

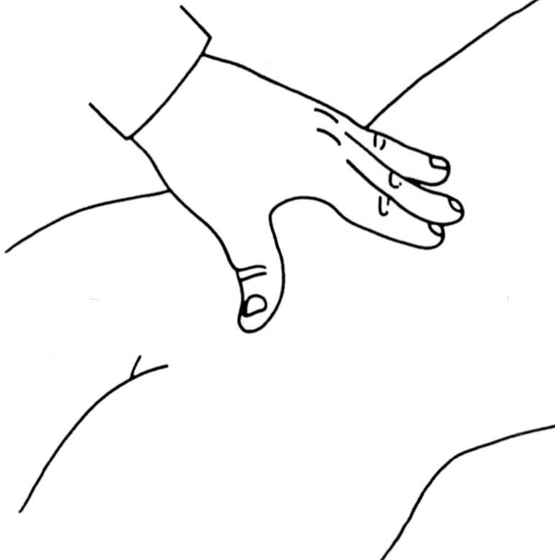

FIGURE 9-21 ● Pain on direct pressure over a spinous process may reflect nothing more than referred tenderness. More information can be obtained if the examiner places his or her thumb against the side of the spinous process and applies pressure not only in a forward direction but in a lateral direction as well, thereby applying a rotary strain to the segment. Reproduction of the clinically experienced pain by this maneuver is of great diagnostic significance. (From Macnab I. *Backache.* Baltimore: Williams & Wilkins; 1977:130 with permission.)

Each spinous process is palpated separately, with firm pressure being exerted anteriorly and in a lateral direction (Fig. 9-21). Examination of the back for tenderness is probably the most poorly administered part of the examination, mainly because the examiner fails to assess the patient for superficial tenderness and tenderness over the sacrum. Tuck this in the back of your mind because you will meet the concept again in Chapter 16.

Although the specific findings on examination of patients suffering from non-organic spinal pain are discussed in detail in Chapter 16, physical signs of emotional overtones are so commonly overlooked that they cannot be overemphasized and should be separately tabulated at this point. Table 9-2 summarizes the historical and physical characteristics that suggest a nonorganic component to the patient's disability.

TABLE 9-2

Symptoms and Signs Suggesting a Nonorganic Component to Back Disability

Symptoms

1. Pain is multifocal in distribution and nonmechanical (present at rest)
2. Entire extremity is painful, numb, and/or weak
3. Extremity gives way (as a result, the patient carries a cane)
4. Treatment response
   a. No response
   b. "Allergic" to treatment
   c. Not receiving treatment
5. Multiple crises, multiple hospital admissions/investigations, multiple donors

Signs

1. Tenderness is superficial (skin) or nonanatomic (e.g., over body of sacrum)
2. Simulated movement tests are positive
3. Distraction test is positive
4. Whole leg is weak or numb
5. "Academy Award" performance

TABLE 9-3

Potential Neurologic Findings in Root Lesions

Change	Root		
	L4	L5	S1
Motor weakness	Knee extension	Ankle dorsiflexion; EHL	Ankle plantar flexion: FHL
Sensory loss	Medial shin to knee	Dorsum of foot and lateral calf	Lateral border of foot and posterior calf
Reflex depression	Knee	Tibialis posterior	Ankle
Wasting	Thigh (no calf)	Calf (minimal thigh)	Calf (minimal thigh)

EHL, extensor hallucis longus; FHL, flexor hallucis longus.

SUMMARY

When you leave the examining room to look at the patient's radiographs (good spine clinicians will never look at radiographs before they look at the patient!), you will be able to say the following:

1. I heard the patient's story (I listened to the music of their history), and I suspected a diagnosis.
2. I not only verified the diagnosis on physical examination, I know the anatomic level of spinal involvement (Table 9-3).
3. I also know everything there is to know about the lower extremity systems other than the neurologic system, that is, the locomotor system and the vascular system.

Now I am ready to review the radiographs and verify that the structural lesion that I suspect, because of the history and physical examination, is indeed present. I will look at the radiographs and other investigations with a commitment to a perfect marriage between what I suspect on clinical assessment and what I see on radiograph. If I do not have that perfect marriage just described that results in determining not only the structural lesion but also the anatomic level, then I have made a mistake. Either my history and physical examination are in error or my interpretation of the investigation is wrong. It is then time to return to the drawing board of medicine, the patient's bedside, and start over.

CHAPTER 10

Disc Degeneration Without Root Irritation: Acute and Chronic Low Back Pain

"It is easy to get a thousand prescriptions but hard to get a single remedy."

—Anonymous

Low back pain is a symptom not a diagnosis. It is a very common symptom, affecting 80% of individuals during their lifetime (17). It is an expensive symptom with direct costs (for treatment) and indirect costs (due to lost time) totaling up to $50 billion a year in the United States.

DISC FUNCTION AND DYSFUNCTION

To understand the phenomenon of disc degeneration, you need an understanding of disc function and how disease causes the disc to dysfunction.

DISC FUNCTION

Two balances occur within the disc:

1. Swelling pressure balance (Fig. 10-1) or chemical balance.
   The nucleus of the disc is composed of collagen fibers woven throughout a proteoglycan gel. The proteoglycans imbibe water and swell while the collagen tissues resist that swelling. The swelling pressure balance obviously is the contest between swelling proteoglycans and the resisting collagen fibers.
2. Mechanical balance.
   When mechanical loads are applied to the disc, the nucleus absorbs the force and in turn transfers the force to the annulus. The ability of the nucleus to dissipate these forces depends on its ability to imbibe and release water—that is, its swelling pressure. If the nuclear/annular complex starts to degenerate, the swelling pressure balance is upset and the ability of the disc to absorb forces is reduced—that is, disc mechanics are no longer balanced (24).

DISC DYSFUNCTION

Lumbar disc degeneration (dysfunction) is the result of deterioration of the mechanical and chemical properties of the disc. The cause is the universal phenomenon of the aging process and aggravated by environmental factors such as trauma, high-impact activity, type of work, and smoking. Genetics with a predisposition also plays a role. The deterioration in physical and chemical properties leads to the loss of low back function manifest as mechanical disorders ("my back hurts when I bend and lift") and/or neurologic compressive disorders ["my leg(s) hurt(s) when I sit or walk"]. We

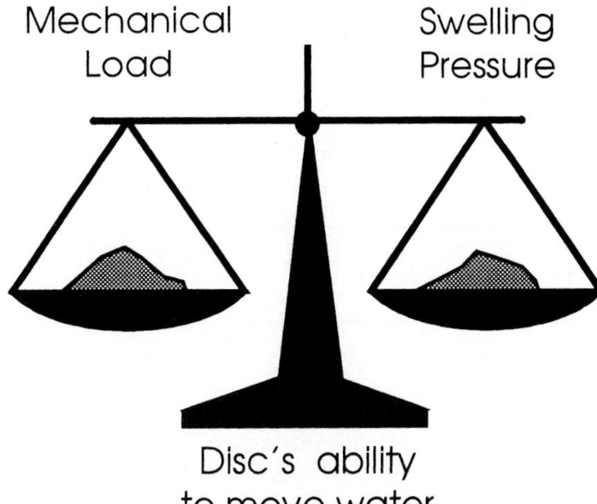

FIGURE 10-1 ● Swelling pressure balance of a disc depends on the movement of water in and out of the nucleus; as the mechanical load increases, water moves out of the nucleus to decrease the swelling pressure to help absorb the load.

all get older and by default we all deteriorate our discs yet we are not all symptomatic (6). It is a constant theme throughout this book that degenerative disc disease routinely occurs without symptoms, or when it does become symptomatic there is a powerful natural tendency toward self-healing.

The actual physical and chemical changes that occur with aging are loss of water in the nucleus and the annulus (the conversion of a grape to a raisin!), the end stage of which is intradiscal fibrosis. The body does an autofusion with fibrous tissue replacing the nucleus and annulus reducing movement in the segment. This explains why we get stiffer as we get older and why the vast majority of individuals grow older without back pain.

The reason for these chemical changes centers around an understanding of disc nutrition (Fig. 10-2). The intervertebral disc is avascular after age 8 years and receives its nutrition through transport across the cartilaginous endplate and through the annulus. With aging these vascular channels start to fail and diffusion of nutrients decreases. The result is a decrease in the number of fibroblasts and chondrocytes and a decrease in formation of collagen and proteoglycans. The end result is failure of the disc to absorb mechanical forces because of failure of the swelling pressure balance.

THE STAGES OF DISC DYSFUNCTION

Kirkaldy-Willis and Farfan (31) described three phases of disc degeneration (Fig. 10-3).

Phase 1 Disc Dysfunction

In this phase, the ability of the disc to exchange water and balance the swelling pressure starts to deteriorate. With microtrauma, annular tears appear and facet cartilaginous fissures develop, along with increased secretion of synovial fluid into the irritated facet joints.

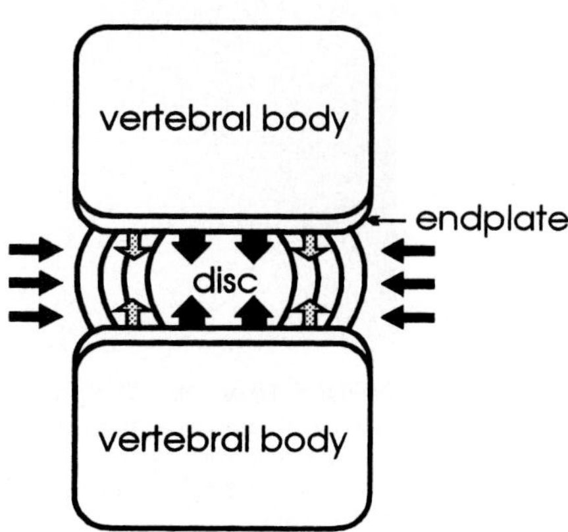

FIGURE 10-2 ● Disc nutrition is by diffusion of nutrients across the endplate and through the annulus.

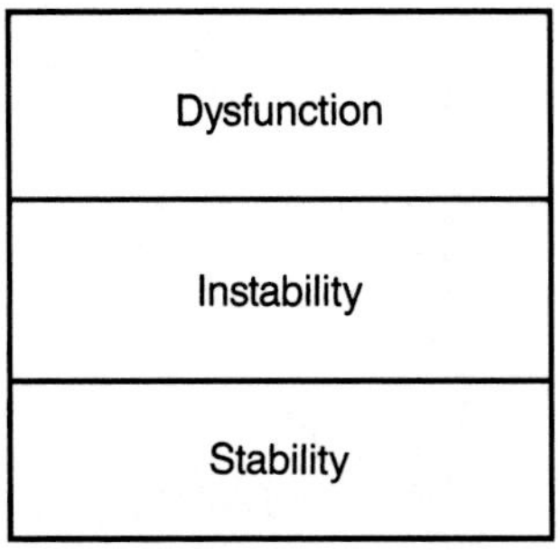

Dysfunction
Instability
Stability

FIGURE 10-3 ● The three stages of disc degeneration.

Phase 2 Instability

In this phase, disc height is decreased, ligaments become lax, and osteophytes form in an attempt to restabilize the functional spinal unit (FSU) (Fig. 10-4). The narrowed disc height and instability result in uneven and unstable facet articulation. Facet joint changes include degeneration of the cartilage and laxity of the capsule.

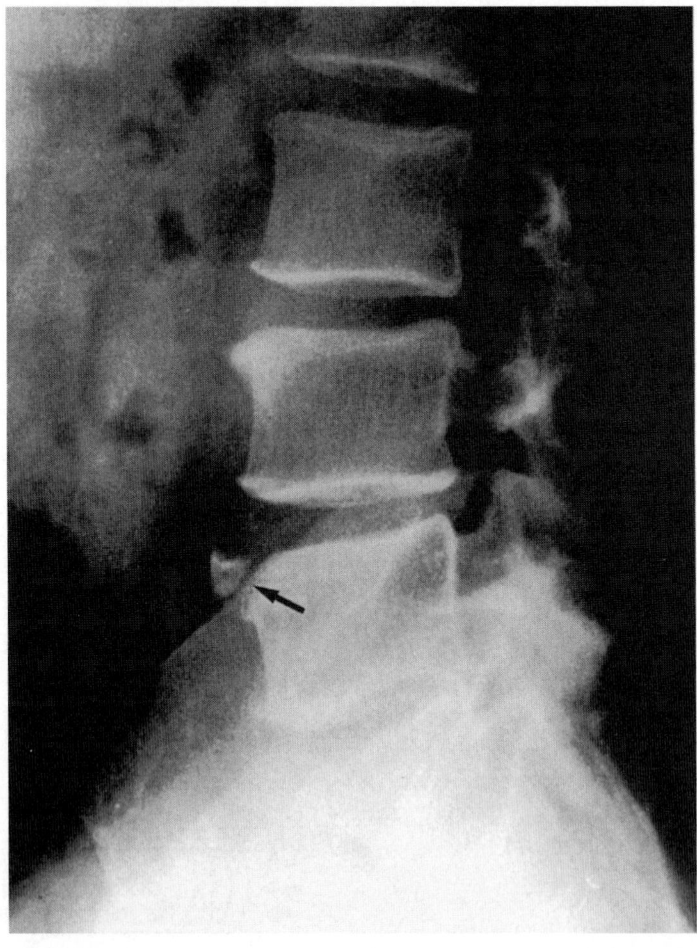

FIGURE 10-4 ● The phase of instability: the L4-L5 disc space is narrowed, and an early retrospondylolisthesis is present. The L3-L4 space is also narrowed, and osteophytes are forming anteriorly. Note the limbus vertebrae *(arrow)* that is a variant of Schmorl's node; it is not a fracture.

Phase 3 Stability

In this phase, the FSU restabilizes itself. Within the disc space, disc narrowing and fibrosis do the trick while osteophytes (Fig. 10-5) stabilize the periphery of the disc space. In the facet joint, subluxation (Fig. 10-5) and capsular fibrosis further stabilize the FSU. Unfortunately, the stabilizing osteophytes may encroach on nerve roots and interfere with root function (see Chapter 12).

WHICH TISSUES ARE THE SOURCE OF PAIN?

Kuslich and coworkers (32) have carried out the best clinical work in this field. While doing microdiscectomies for disc ruptures under local anesthesia in more than 700 patients, these researchers took the opportunity to stimulate various tissues and record the patient's response. They found that muscle, fascia, and bone were largely insensitive structures, whereas the facet joint capsule was painful in half of the patients. The outer annulus was the most consistent structure to produce back pain when stimulated. The inner annulus and nucleus were largely insensitive structures. The surgery for the patients in this study was being done for the symptom of sciatica and the disease of disc rupture. The researchers found that stretching the already stretched, compressed, and inflamed nerve root reproduced or exacerbated the patients' leg pain.

PROOF OF INSTABILITY

Instability may be demonstrated on flexion/extension lateral x-rays (Figs. 10-6 and 10-7). In those patients in whom instability cannot be demonstrated on radiograph, some investigators have used provocative/ablation testing. Examples of the latter are bracing or the external fixator (11,43) to see if back pain can be decreased. Bracing does not work because to immobilize the lower lumbar

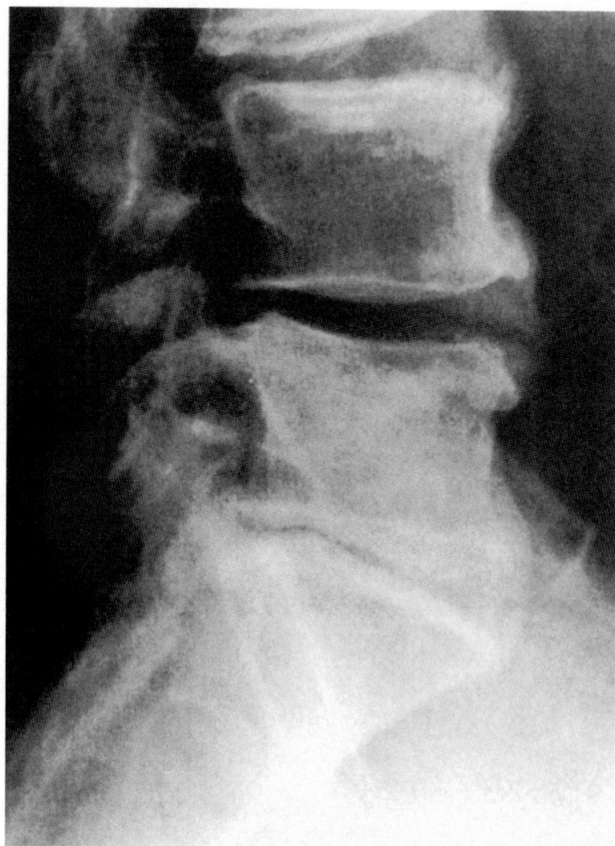

FIGURE 10-5 • A well-stabilized L5-S1 disc with osteophytes. The same osteophytic stabilization is occurring at the L4-L5 and L3-L4 levels.

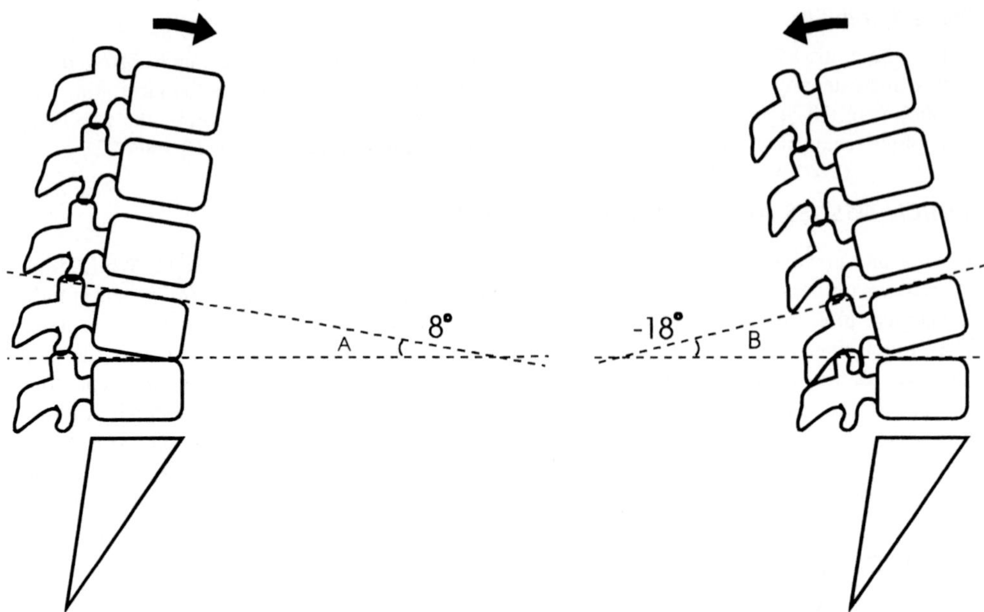

FIGURE 10-6 ● On flexion-extension (schematic drawn from a radiograph), angulation goes from 8 degrees to –18 degrees, a change of 26 degrees, which is by definition an unstable segment.

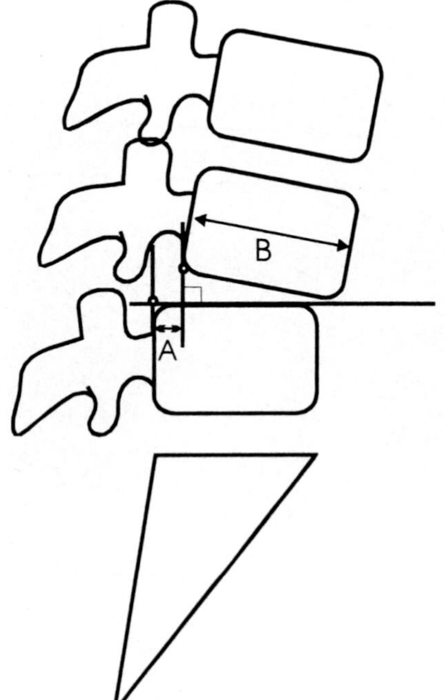

FIGURE 10-7 ● A schematic of a degenerative spondylolisthesis showing angulation of more than 10 degrees and forward subluxation of L4 on L5 of more than 4 mm.

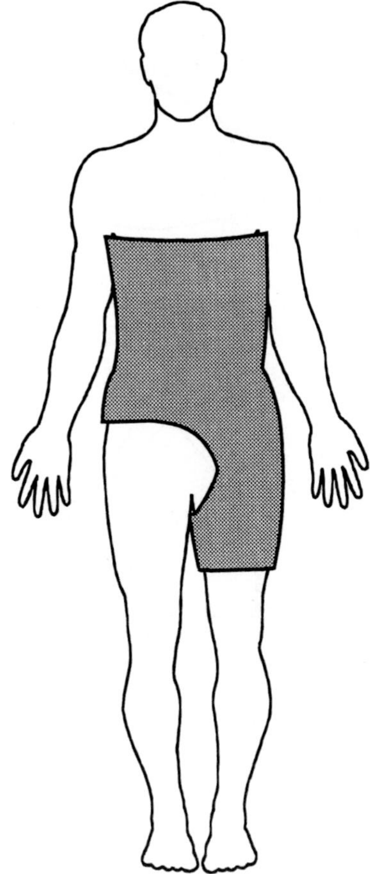

FIGURE 10-8 ● A brace or cast that holds onto the rib cage and one thigh.

spine, where most instability occurs, the thigh must be included in the brace (Fig. 10-8), which severely strains patient compliance. There is controversy about the usefulness of this test in identifying the source of low back pain.

An example of provocative testing is lumbar discography, a discussion of which splits the orthopedic community into naysayers and enthusiasts. For most neurosurgeons performing spine surgery there is no controversy: discography is a useless test (26).

DISCOGRAPHY

Discography involves introducing a needle under radiographic control into the nucleus of an intervertebral disc and injecting contrast material. The approach used most widely is the posterolateral or lateral approach (36) (Fig. 10-9). The exact site of the tip of the needle is identified by radiographs taken in two planes. To test the integrity of the disc, a water-soluble contrast material, or water itself, can be injected. If the disc is normal, the injected contrast material is confined to the nucleus (Fig. 10-10). Although a normal disc offers considerable resistance to the injection, the resulting distention does not evoke a painful response. In the presence of disc degeneration, on the other hand, there is little or no resistance to the injection, the dye spreads diffusely through the disc, and the patient may experience pain. There are four parameters to assess in discography (Table 10-1).

No statement can be made that the demonstration of morphologic abnormality indicates that the disc injected is the source of symptoms.

Injection into a normal disc is painless. Injection into a degenerate disc may also be painless (54), but if the degenerative changes are symptomatic, distention of the disc may or may not reproduce the patient's clinically experienced symptoms (47). The presence or absence of pain on distention of the disc may be the important finding.

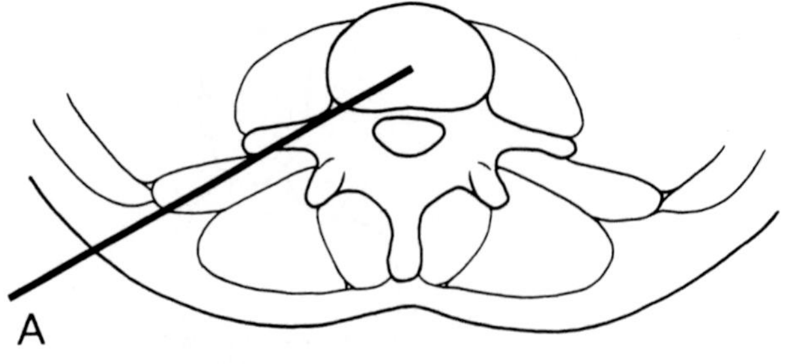

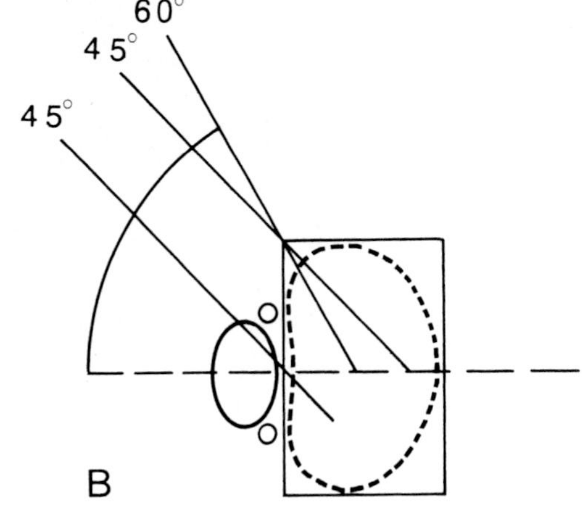

FIGURE 10-9 ● **A:** The posterolateral approach to disc penetration. **B:** The various angles and distances from the midline. Ideal is 8 to 10 cm from the midline and 60-degree angulation into the disc.

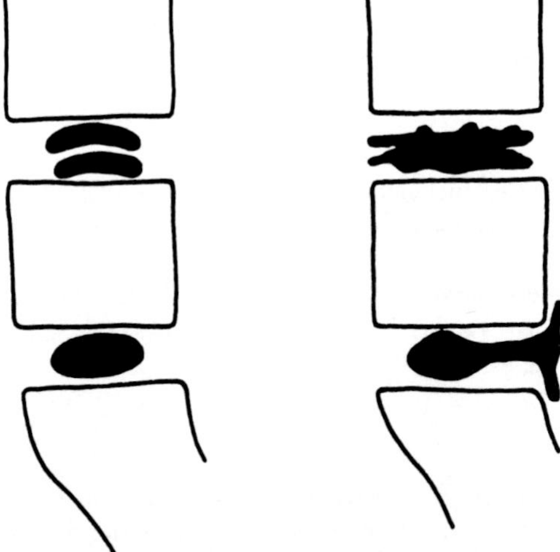

FIGURE 10-10 ● Discography. With normal discs, the injected dye remains confined within the nucleus. The dye may present a spherical or bilobular appearance. When degenerative changes have taken place, the injected dye spreads throughout the disc and into the annulus. On occasion, the dye may be seen to spread posteriorly and run vertically underneath the posterior longitudinal ligament. This latter appearance, however, does not denote the presence of a disc rupture.

TABLE 10-1

Parameters to Assess in Discography

	Normal Disc	Disc Degeneration
1. Volume of test material	Limited (1–2 mL)	More than 4 mL
2. Resistance	Firm endpoint	Significant decrease in resistance
3. Pain reproduction	None	Often painful
4. Pattern of contrast material	Round ball (Fig. 10-10)	Diffuse (Fig. 10-10)

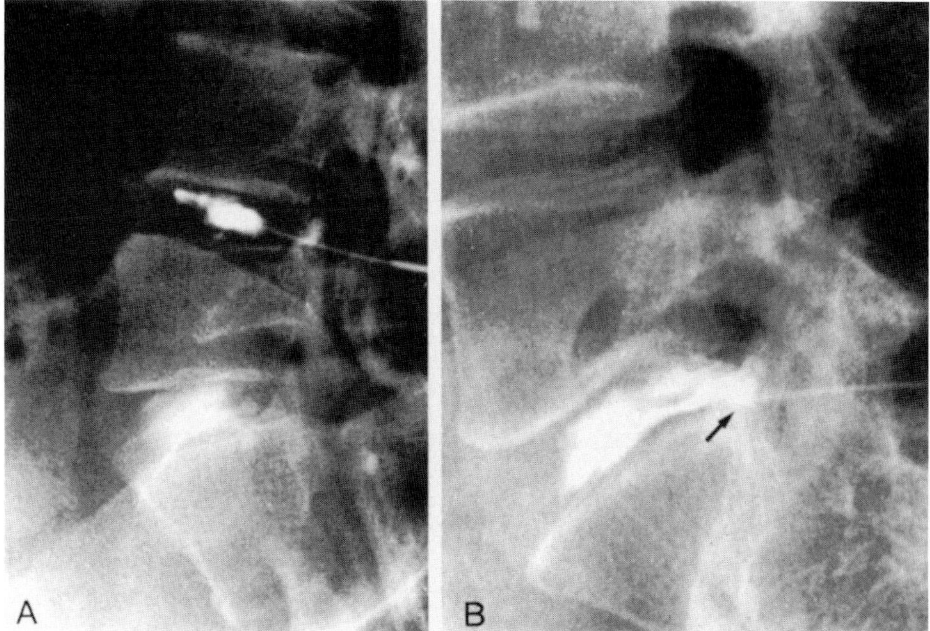

FIGURE 10-11 • **A:** Abnormal discogram, L4-L5, with contrast (dye) leaking to back of disc space *(arrow)*. At L-S1 the needle has been withdrawn, but the dye pattern reveals a normal disc. **B:** Abnormal discogram, L5-S1 *(arrow)*.

The injection of contrast material is an important part of the procedure (Fig. 10-11). A very small quantity (0.5 mL) may be injected after the insertion of the needle to confirm the fact that the point of the needle is, indeed, lying in the center of the nucleus. At the conclusion of the procedure dye may be injected to demonstrate the morphologic pattern of the disc, thereby providing documentary evidence of a normal disc or a painless disc degeneration.

Correlation of discogram findings with magnetic resonance imaging (MRI) findings is also recommended.

ACCEPTABLE STATEMENTS ABOUT DISCOGRAPHY

Most scientists, aware of the pros and cons of discography, would agree on the following points:

1. Unlike computed tomography (CT) and MRI, discography is an invasive test. It is painful to patients and carries with it the risk of disc space infection (1%–4%) (15).
2. Most discographers would agree that it is necessary to evaluate both the appearance of contrast on radiographs (variously described as morphology and/or nucleogram) and the patient's pain response to the injection (48).
3. Discography for the evaluation of cervical or lumbar radicular pain has largely been abandoned because (28) (a) it has never been proven of value and (b) CT and MRI are so much more accurate in the assessment of radicular pain. Discography is now used primarily in the assessment of axial (back) pain.
4. Discography, for the assessment of back pain, should only be used after the decision has been made to operate, that is, to do a fusion (52). Its sole purpose is to assist the surgeon in deciding on what levels to include in the fusion. This is a conclusion that has never been tested in a prospective scientific study.

The other two parameters of discography, namely volume of test material and the pressure of injections, have largely been abandoned.

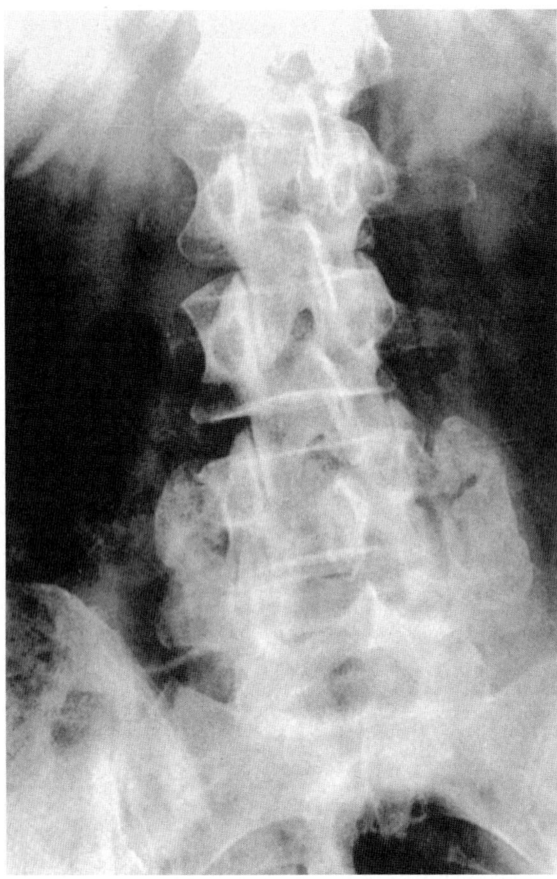

FIGURE 10-12 ● An L4-L5 lumbar fusion in the intertransverse interval.

THE TREATMENT OF BACK PAIN (INSTABILITY) ASSOCIATED WITH DISC DEGENERATION

Like anything else, the choices for treatment of instability causing back pain are either conservative or surgical. Conservative measures include short terms of bed rest, anti-inflammatories, modification of activity, exercise, and back school.

Surgical methods to stabilize the spine are most commonly accomplished by fusion (Fig. 10-12). Artificial discs are an alternative to fusions in select patients.

THE NATURAL HISTORY OF DEGENERATIVE DISC DISEASE

When deciding on treatment for back pain it is important to keep in mind the natural history of lumbar degenerative disc disease. Many studies have shown that with time, most patients' symptoms will settle and interfere little with their function. Before getting too aggressive with surgery, too prolonged with conservative treatment efforts, and too enthusiastic about your claims to cure back pain, it is best to pay homage to the natural ability of the body to stiffen an unstable motion segment and ameliorate pain.

Another fundamental understanding necessary to grasp in treating a patient with low back pain is that there is often no relationship between the patient's symptoms and what is seen on radiograph (Fig. 10-13).

With these concepts in mind let us discuss some of the clinical presentations of low back pain.

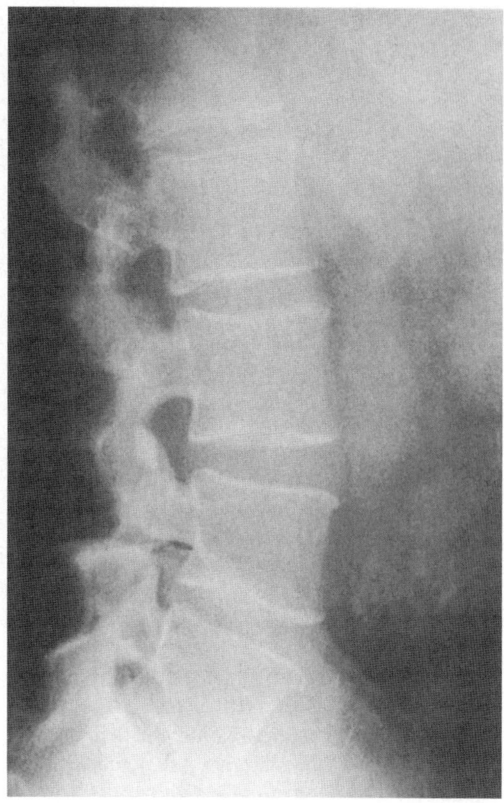

FIGURE 10-13 • A lateral plain film of a patient with severe back pain. Note two things: (a) the normal lumbar spine, except for degenerative disc disease at L5-S1, and (b) the large aortic aneurysm!

ACUTE INCAPACITATING BACKACHE: THE ACUTE BACK STRAIN

There are not many people who have lived for a half century who have not, at some time in their lives, been smitten by an acute episode of incapacitating backache. Perversely, this is encouraging. These people do not remain incapacitated: they get better, perhaps despite treatment rather than because of it. They are visiting with Kirkaldy-Willis and Farfan's (31) Phase 1 of spinal dysfunction.

Characteristically, the patient, while engaged in some trivial activity, is suddenly seized with back pain and cannot move. "I was paralyzed with pain." The lumbar spine is splinted rigidly and the patient can only move with painful caution, clutching his or her back and walking with the trunk leaning forward, keeping the hips and knees slightly bent.

Examination reveals that all movements of the spine are limited by pain and muscle spasm, but there is no evidence of root tension, irritation, or compression. In some of these patients, there is so much back spasm and muscle splinting that attempting to perform the straight leg raising (SLR) test will cause back pain and leave the examiner with the false impression that a disc rupture may be present. A useful examination is the sitting SLR test. Most of these patients can sit in a few moments of comfort; in this sitting position, gentle SLR testing (Fig. 10-14) will reveal good SLR.

The clinical picture is explosively dramatic and threatening to the patient, if he or she has not been through a previous episode. The physician must not overreact. The physician must constantly remind himself or herself that even if the elected treatment involved rubbing peanut butter on each of the patient's buttocks, in the balance of probabilities, the patient would get well fairly quickly.

In the majority of such cases the patient is suffering from painful dysfunction of the disc space or a "sprain" of one of the zygapophyseal joints. When trying to rationalize treatment, one should compare the lesion with a severely sprained ankle in a patient who has only one leg and who is unable to wear a prosthesis. There is only one way to treat a severely sprained ankle in such a patient: the patient has to be put to bed. Theoretically, the patient with an acute severe low back strain should also be considered for bed rest. However, theoretical treatment must be tempered by reason. If your patient is a young married woman who is responsible for care of the children and getting

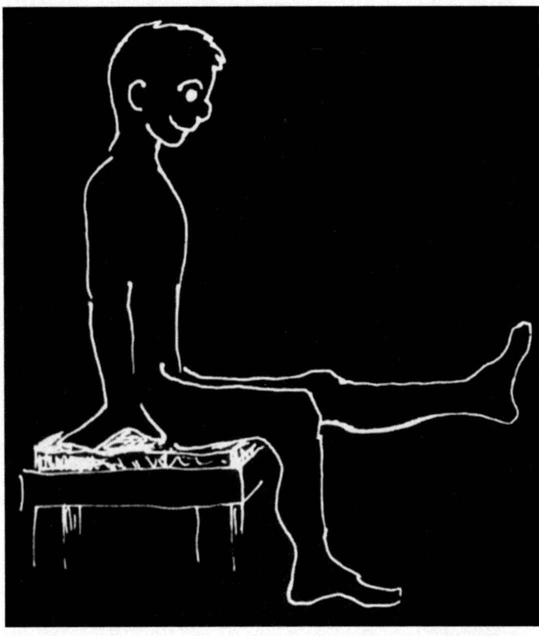

FIGURE 10-14 ● The sitting straight leg raising test. If a patient with acute back pain can sit in this position, the ability to raise each straight leg to 90 degrees, as shown, tends to rule out a herniated nucleus pulposus.

the meals, how are these responsibilities going to be met? What about the responsibilities of functioning in the office for the dentist with acute back pain?

Let us repeat: you are treating a patient and not a spine, and the experience of the lay world is that many, in fact, the majority, will get better by just creeping around, with their pain mollified by analgesics.

Some patients, however, cannot cope. The pain is too severe. In such instances, if they cannot do their normal daily work, they should be sent to bed. A patient with pneumonia is ill and may feel defeated; that person is happy to go to bed. A patient with severe low back pain feels well except for his or her back and does not want to go to bed. This patient is hopping mad at the affliction, and your insistence on bed rest will increase the frustration, unless you take care and time to explain in detail the purpose of this apparently neglectful form of management. It is advisable to give the low back pain patient some literature explaining in detail the probable underlying pathology and the rationale of

TABLE 10-2

Instructions for Patients on the Purpose of Bed Rest

- Many patients with an acute incapacitating back pain are surprised when they are told that the only significant form of treatment is complete bed rest. This does not appear to be treatment at all. It almost seems like neglectful indifference on the part of the physician.
- You must remember that the spine is a column made of blocks of bone connected together by small joints and that an acute mechanical backache is in reality simply a severely sprained joint. It gives rise to pain in the same way that a severe sprain of the ankle gives rise to pain. With a sprained ankle, however, you can limp and continue to get around by taking the weight off the injured joint, while putting most of your weight on the other leg.
- However, if a patient with only one leg sprains his or her ankle, he or she cannot limp. The patient cannot take the weight off the injured foot. He or she cannot walk around. He or she must go to bed until the "inflammation" of the sprain settles down.
- The same applies to the spine. You have only one spine, and when you severely sprain the joints in your spine, the only way to take the weight and strain of activities away from the spinal canal is to lie down.
- Therefore, bed rest is rational treatment. It is the quickest way to recovery.
- Prolonged bed rest (beyond a few days) is not good for your bone strength and muscle strength. Prolonged bed rest will lead both to weaken, and extend your recovery.

treatment by bed rest (Table 10-2). You must advise the patient regarding the use of toilet facilities. Using a bedpan at home is impractical. The use of crutches makes it easier for the patient to get to the bathroom, and the purchase of a high toilet seat is sometimes essential.

Although analgesics are rarely needed once the patient is in bed, in the majority, sedatives such as tranquilizers are essential. At present there is no specific medication to speed the resolution of the symptoms, although anti-inflammatory drugs may help some patients (3).

The question of the role of manipulation is always raised. The "locking" of the back by spasm of the paraspinal muscles may tend to perpetuate the problem, and gentle flexion of the spine into the fetal position of rest appears to release the muscle by hyperactivity. This is best accomplished initially by getting the patient to flex the knees and hips and then use the hands to pull the knees against the chest repetitively (Fig. 10-15). Later, a passive flexion manipulation can be carried out. The patient lies on his or her back with hips and knees flexed. The heels are grasped so that feet point toward the ceiling. The feet are then pushed gently over the patient's head. The movement is repeated slowly and rhythmically. This repetitive rocking must be carried out with slow, simple harmonic motion with each swing of the legs flexing the spine a little further. This rhythmical swinging is continued for approximately 2 minutes (Fig. 10-16). This is a much more effective maneuver for the occasional manipulator than the specific manipulation of spinous processes or the commonly employed flexion rotation manipulation of the lumbosacral joint.

To be effective, however, this manipulative therapy must continue on a daily basis and, therefore, the patient must learn how to perform these maneuvers independently. The patient should be taught specific steps. The manipulation exercises are carried out on a bed, not on the floor. The neck is kept slightly flexed by a pillow to minimize the effects of the inevitable contraction of the sternomastoids when the patient first makes an attempt to kick his or her feet up in the air.

The hips and knees are first flexed to a right angle. The legs are then raised toward the ceiling, keeping the knees slightly bent. The feet are then moved over the patient's head. This movement must not be in the form of a sudden kick. The buttocks must be raised slowly and smoothly off the bed by contraction of the trunk flexors and then, just as slowly, the legs are lowered. This movement is repeated several times, each time lowering the legs just to the starting position with the hips flexed at 90 degrees. The legs must not be lowered to the bed.

After five "kickups," the patient rests by lowering his or her legs, with the knees fully flexed, thereby putting the feet onto the bed, soles first (Fig. 10-17). This routine, at this stage in the treatment of an acute back pain, is not designed to be an exercise program. It is really an active flexion manipulation of the spine. The duration of these flexion manipulations should be restricted to 10 kickups only and these should be repeated three times a day.

If you are uncomfortable describing this regime to the patient and you think the patient can be driven to a professional's office, refer them to a skilled practitioner of the manipulative arts. Chiropractors are the most skilled, and many osteopaths are pursuing more "traditional" methods of medical care. Some physical therapists also include manipulation (in addition to mobilization) in their armamentarium (19).

Bed rest should be continued until the patient can make journeys to the toilet in relative comfort without the aid of crutches (usually no more than a few days). After this period of time, the patient

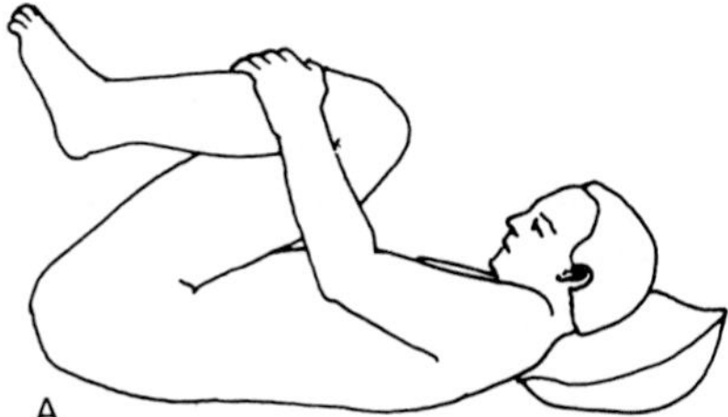

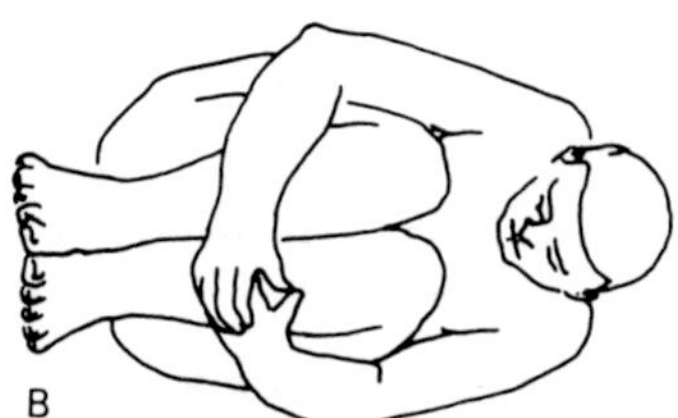

FIGURE 10-15 • A patient may abort an acute episode of low back pain by lying on the back and pulling the knees slowly up to the chest **(A)**. He should maintain this position for 5 minutes. In very acute attacks with severe pain, the patient may find it easier to assume the same position lying on the side **(B)**.

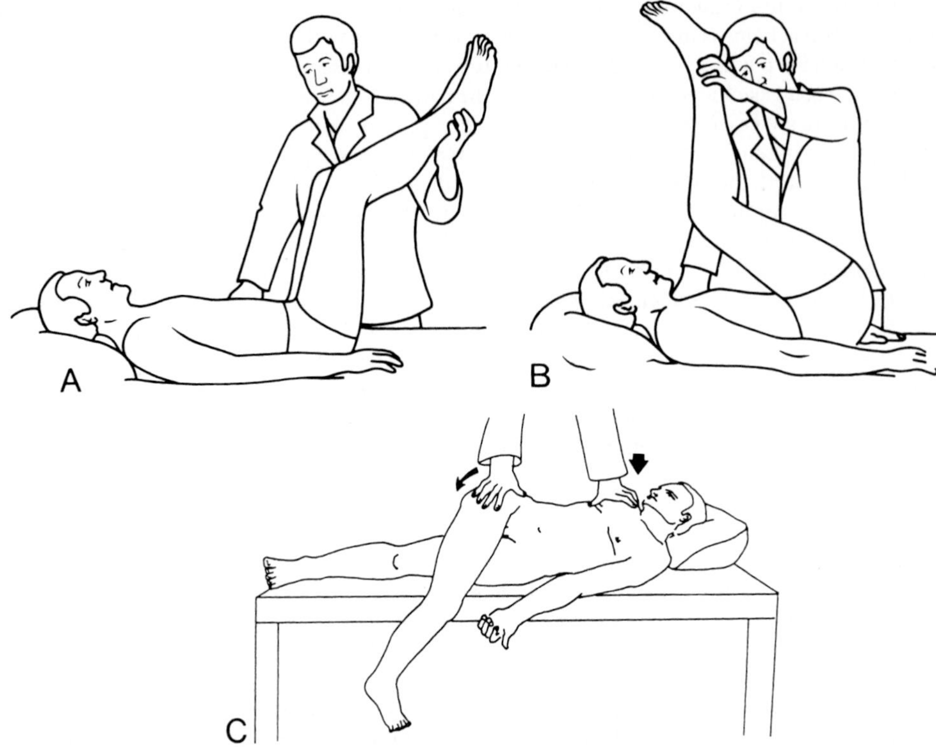

FIGURE 10-16 ● If, on clinical examination, there is no evidence of root compression, resolution of symptoms may be speeded by a flexion manipulation. The patient lies on the back, and the physician raises the patient's legs, maintaining the knees in flexion **(A).** By applying pressure to the heels, the physician then pushes the patient's knees toward the shoulders **(B).** This movement is done very slowly, and the degree of flexion obtained is determined by the discomfort the patient experiences. This movement is then repeated slowly and rhythmically over a period of 5 minutes. In the majority of instances, the range of movement that can be achieved by this passive manipulation gradually increases. At the conclusion of the manipulation, the patient is instructed to flex his knees fully and allow his feet to come down to the bed, soles first. **C:** Rotation manipulation.

gradually increases activities within the limits set by his or her own tolerance of decreasing discomforts. The time of return to work is determined largely by the demands made on the patient's need to return to the job.

Well-designed braces and corsets may also be helpful during the active phase. When considering a brace, remember that most of these patients will be better in a few days, and a brace is not indicated thereafter.

The treatment program previously described has been officially blessed by the Agency for Health Care Policy and Research (5), an arm of the American Government (U.S. Department of Health and Human Services). The agency has, with great fanfare including media exposure, recommended a few days of bed rest, nonsteroidal anti-inflammatory drugs (NSAIDs), a brace for return to work, physical therapy, and manipulation for acute low back pain of less than 3 months' duration. They did not recommend acupuncture, transcutaneous electrical stimulation, trigger point injections, epidural injections, or traction.

Prevention of Further Episodes

Regardless of how you treat these patients, they will get better. Your value as a health care professional is to attempt to prevent further attacks. Exercise in moderation on a regular basis is the most important step. It is prudent to discuss lifestyle factors that are detrimental to overall good health such as smoking and obesity.

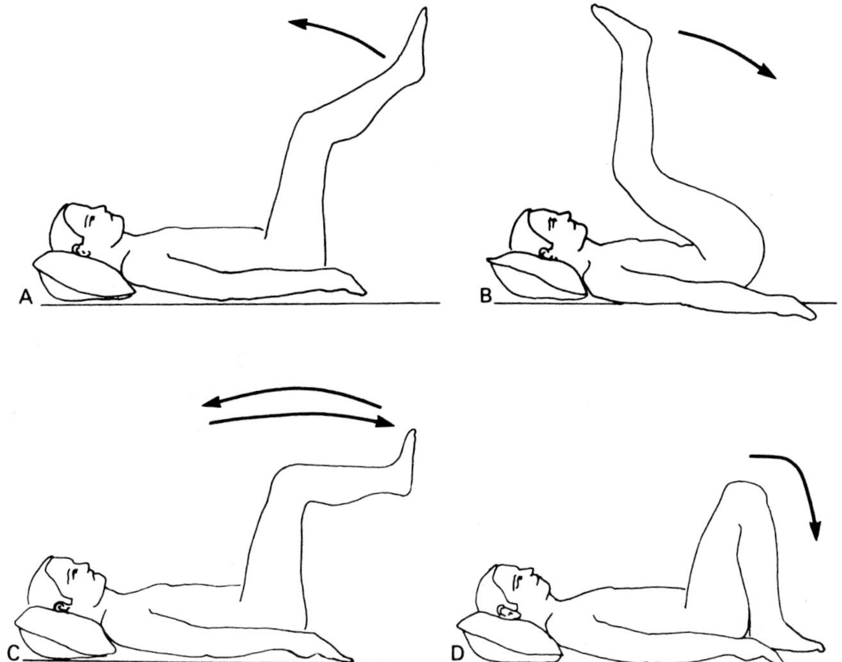

FIGURE 10-17 • Flexion exercise manipulation of the lumbar spine. The patient lies on the bed with the head supported by a pillow. The hips are flexed to 90 degrees, and the knees are slightly flexed **(A).** The patient now attempts to kick the feet over the head, raising the buttocks approximately 6 inches off the bed **(B).** After each "kickup," the patient returns to the starting position **(C).** After five kickups, the patient rests by lowering the legs with the knees fully flexed, thereby putting the feet on the bed, soles first **(D).** It is very important not to lower the legs with the knees fully extended, because this places a painful hyperextension strain on the spine.

Return to Function

Within a few days to a week most of these patients are back to work, within or outside of home. Hopefully you have them on a path of exercise and a healthier lifestyle to lessen the chance of further episodes.

RECURRENT AGGRAVATING BACKACHE

This is probably the most common manifestation of disc degeneration and is the phase leading from dysfunction to instability. Rowe (45,46), studying the incidence of low back pain in workers at the Kodak Company, found that 85% of the patients with backache had intermittent attacks of disabling pain every 3 months to 3 years, each attack lasting 3 days to 3 weeks. Between the attacks, the patients were relatively free from backache. The posterior joints are vulnerable to extension strains because degenerative changes in one or more discs may give rise to segmental hyperextension or persistent posterior joint subluxation. The facets of the involved segment or segments in these conditions are held at the extreme limit of extension; they have no safety factor of movement. A simple analogy can be drawn with the wrist. If a moderate blow is applied to the palm of the hand with the wrist in the neutral position, no pain results because the force of the blow is absorbed by the movement that occurs. If, however, the hand is hit with the same force, with the wrist in full extension, then this is painful because there is no safety factor of movement and the full brunt of the injury is transmitted to the capsule of the wrist (Fig. 10-18).

The same mechanical principle applies to the spine. In the neutral position moderate extension strains are not painful, but if a segment is held in hyperextension, there is no safety factor

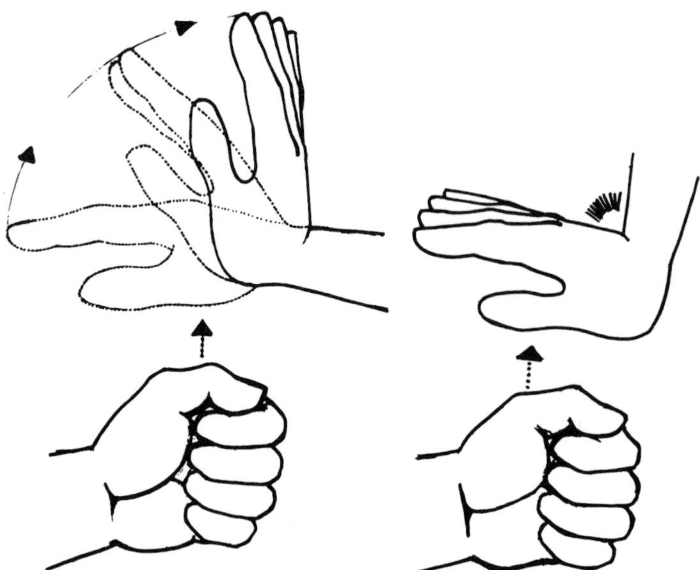

FIGURE 10-18 ● The safety factor of movement. When a blow is applied to a wrist in the neutral position, the force of the blow is absorbed by the movement that occurs. When the same force is applied to the wrist in dorsiflexion, pain results because there is no safety factor of movement, and the full force of the blow is felt by the capsule of the wrist joint.

in movement and the extension strains of everyday living give rise to painful capsular lesions. The significance of extension strains is noted both in the history and examination of the patient.

Working with the hands above the head, such as in hanging up laundry, reaching, and so on, applies extension strains to the back and is painful. When the forward stooped position is maintained, the sacrospinales have to contract to hold the spine. With an unstable lumbar disc segment in this position, the sacrospinales act as a bowstring producing hyperextension at the involved segment (Fig. 10-19). These patients complain of pain on stooping over the wash basin in the morning and when maintaining the bent forward position, as when making beds, and so on.

Sitting in a soft chair will allow the lumbar spine to become concertina-like and sag into hyperlordosis. These patients find it more comfortable to sit on a hard seat. Sitting in a theater with the knees out straight and the floor sloping away will apply a significant extension strain to the spine, and the patients tend to irritate the patrons in the row in front by putting their feet on the back of their seat to keep knees and hips flexed. Similarly, sitting in a car with the knees held straight hyperextends the spine and makes prolonged driving uncomfortable.

When these patients stand for long periods of time, the lumbar spine sags into extension, and the patients automatically try to flatten the lumbar spine by flexing one hip and knee, as in the act of putting one foot on the seat of a chair or on a bar rail. Emotional tensions and frustrations will make the patient adopt the fight position, tightening up the sacrospinales. This posture will aggravate the pain, and the patient's increase in pain will aggravate his or her frustrations.

The pain experienced is commonly localized to the lumbosacral junction radiating out to one or both sacroiliac joints. If the pain intensifies it may radiate down one or both posterior thighs as far as the knee, which may be confused with sciatica. On occasion, the pain may radiate into the groin and can be mistaken for hip disease.

On examination, the patients may demonstrate an increase in the normal lumbar lordosis, but more commonly they do not demonstrate any postural spinal abnormalities. They may, however, show many mechanical features that tend to aggravate hyperextension of the lumbar spine.

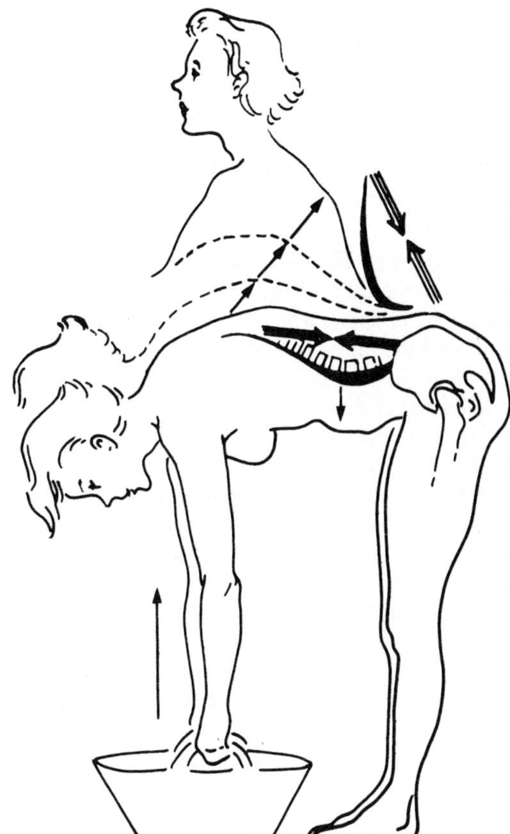

FIGURE 10-19 ● When a patient bends forward with the knees straight and then tries to lift, the sacrospinales, when contracting, act as a bowstring and hyperextend the lumbar spine.

Weak Abdominal Muscles

These patients have difficulty in doing situps with their hips and knees bent and the palms of the hands clasped behind their heads. Because of the weakness of the abdominal muscles, when they lift both legs off the couch (bilateral SLR) the weight of the legs tends to rotate the pelvis, hyperextending the spine and producing pain in the back (Fig. 10-20). Back pain reproduced by bilateral active SLR is probably the best demonstration of the instability phase of lumbar disc degeneration aggravated by weak abdominal muscles.

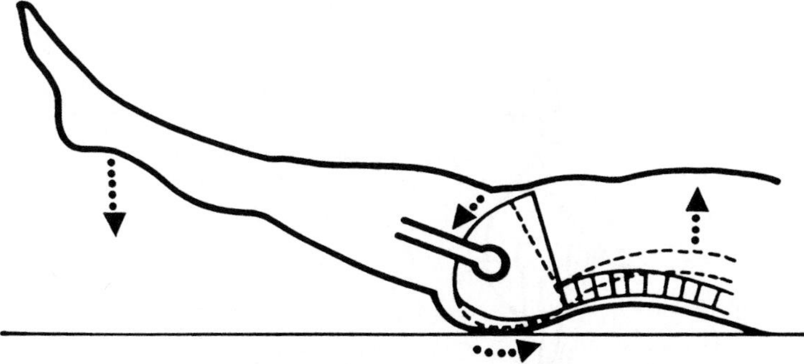

FIGURE 10-20 ● When the patient carries out bilateral active straight leg raising, the weight of the leg causes the pelvis to rotate and thereby hyperextends the lumbar spine. Hyperextension of the lumbar spine in the presence of disc degeneration gives rise to pain. This is probably the most useful test to demonstrate the presence of painful segmental instability and facet pain.

Obesity

Excessive weight loading hyperextends the lumbar spine. This is particularly apparent in the patient who has a "politician's pouch" (a protuberant fat abdomen). With the center of gravity anterior to the spine, the patient has to hyperextend his back to stand erect.

Tensor Fascia Femoris Contracture

Some patients, especially those with a mesomorphic build, have a tight tensor fascia femoris that tilts the pelvis forward (Fig. 10-21). With the pelvis fixed in this position, the lumbar spine must hyperextend to allow the spinal column to remain erect. When these patients stand against the wall with the back of the head, chest, buttocks, and heels touching the wall, they cannot flatten their lumbar spine. The only way they can flatten their backs against a wall is to step forward and bend their hips and knees, thereby relaxing the tensor fascia femoris and allowing the pelvis to rotate. On examination, adduction of the hip is markedly limited when the hip is internally rotated and extended at the same time.

Special note, then, is made of these aggravating factors: abdominal weakness, weight, and tightness of the tensor fascia femoris.

The physical findings in this stage of chronic degenerative disc disease are not very dramatic. If the patient is seen after the acute attack has subsided, movements of the lumbar spine may not be significantly limited. If muscle spasm is still present there may be maintenance of lumbar lordosis on forward flexion. On extending from the forward flexed position, however, the patient generally shows reversal of normal spinal rhythm. After starting to extend their backs, they will bend their knees and hips to tuck their pelvis under the spine to regain the erect position (Fig. 10-22). Extension in the erect position usually is limited and painful. If the examiner places his fingers on the anterior and posterior superior spines of the pelvis and then asks the patient to bend backward, the pelvis can be felt to rotate after approximately 20 degrees extension, and any further extension is painful.

Reversal of spinal rhythm on extending from the forward flexed position, pain on extension from the erect position, and pain on bilateral SLR are common and, indeed, characteristic findings in chronic symptomatic degenerative disc disease. The demonstration of tenderness is not of significant diagnostic value and its distribution may be confusing. The injection of an irritating solution into the supraspinous ligament of L5 and S1 may give rise to local pain and also to pain referred to the sacroiliac joints and the buttocks or down the back of the thigh. Not only is pain referred in this distribution, but there may also be "referred tenderness." The upper outer quadrant of the buttock is normally tender on deep pressure. After the injection of hypertonic saline into the supraspinous ligament between L5 and S1, the upper outer quadrant of buttock becomes extremely tender and this form of "central irritation" may produce tenderness over the sacroiliac joints and tenderness on pressure over the back of the thigh. The physician must not allow himself to be led to believe that the demonstration of a point of tenderness indicates that the pathol-

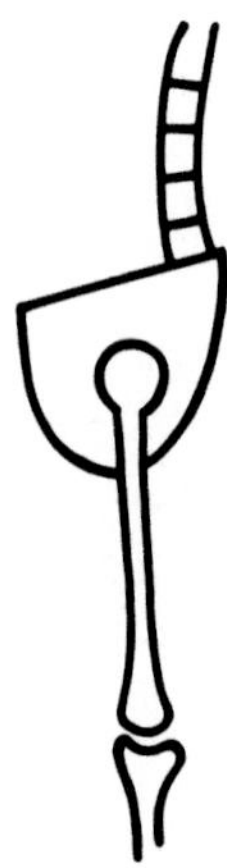

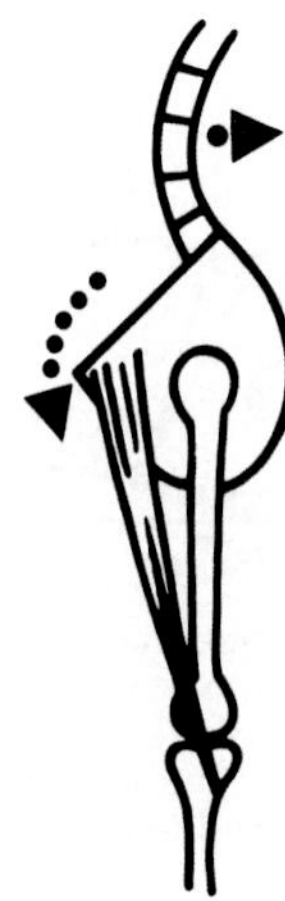

FIGURE 10-21 ● A tight tensor fascia femoris, by rotating the pelvis anteriorly, produces hyperextension of the lumbar spine.

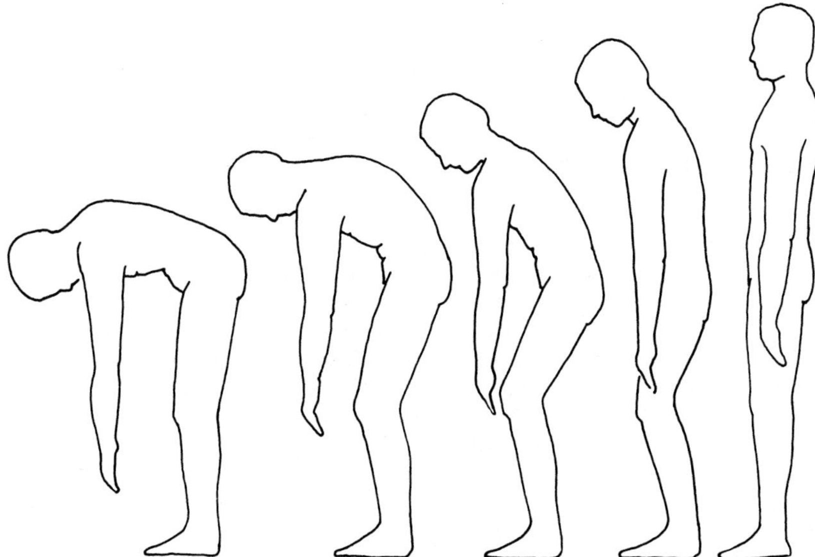

FIGURE 10-22 • With segmental instability, the patient will present reversal of normal spinal rhythm on extending from the forward flexed position.

ogy lies deep to this area. It was because of this common zone of tenderness over the sacroiliac joints associated with degenerative disc disease that the diagnosis of sacroiliac joint lesions became so popular about a half century ago.

Treatment of the Instability Phase

In the treatment of recurrent aggravating discogenic back pain, the same general principles are employed as in the management of the acute incapacitating backache during its convalescent phase. Greater emphasis, of course, must be placed on the flexion exercise program and on general physical training.

With recurrent episodes of back pain of an aggravating rather than incapacitating nature, a sense of frustration on the part of the physician may result in the patient being thrown into the garbage dump of undirected physical therapy. If you are going to employ the services of a physical therapist, you must do so with reason and purpose. Physical therapy should never be employed as a form of entertainment until such time as nature cures the symptoms. Heat by itself and in whatever modality employed, although making the patient feel better temporarily, does little to speed the resolution of the symptoms. To request massage is no more than using the physical therapy department as a medically approved body rub parlor.

Physical therapists can be sensibly and usefully employed to teach patients how to carry out an exercise program and supervise their initial progress. Some patients lack musculoskeletal skills. When trying to follow instructions on kickup exercises, these patients look like a butterfly having an epileptic fit. These patients need help and direction. Rotation exercises may place undue stress on the discs and the posterior joints and should only be undertaken by the very physically fit. Diverse corporal contortions may be inflicted on your patient and, although splendid in their place, such exercises should be kept in their place and reserved for the time when the patient has been symptom free for many months.

Discuss the exercise program you want with your physical therapist, so that, for better or for worse, you will know what exercises your patients are doing. Some patients need instruction in muscular relaxation far more than they need instruction in muscular contraction. Probably one of the most useful roles of the physical therapist is to teach the patient the technique of voluntary muscular relaxation. Probably the most important instructions the patient will receive from the therapist will be advice on how to pursue activities of daily living without reaggravating symptoms.

Your job is to emphasize the role of exercise in controlling symptoms and the negative impact smoking and obesity have on recurrent episodes of back pain. This is not a group of patients in whom you want to introduce the "crutch of bracing" and it is very important that you avoid long-term use of narcotics and mood-altering drugs.

CHRONIC PERSISTENT BACKACHE

The *bête noire* of orthopedic surgeons is the syndrome of chronic, persistent discogenic low back pain, easily made intolerable by modest activity. These patients are in the midst of chronic spinal instability and have yet to advance into Kirkaldy-Willis's third phase of spontaneous stabilization.

Patients with a chronic persistent daily backache generally report a history of having been plagued by intermittent episodes of back pain for several years. Eventually, they reach the stage when the back pain never really leaves them. By pushing themselves, they may get through the average day with barely tolerable nagging discomfort in their backs. They are very vulnerable to the traumatic insults of everyday life and, on minimal provocation, may get a "flare-up" of back pain. They have to be careful about everything they do and gradually, almost imperceptibly, their activities grind to a halt. They become the subjects of spinal rule, with their spine acting as a malevolent dictator, determining what they can do and what they cannot do. These patients then report the history of a back pain that seriously interferes with their ability to do their work and their capacity to enjoy themselves in their leisure hours.

When assessing such patients, it must be remembered that, although a chronic back pain may make the patient's life very miserable, persistent incapacitating back pain is most unusual. For example, if a woman presents with these complaints, the first question that the physician has to ask is "Why is this patient so disabled by the back pain she experiences?" It must be remembered that pain and disability are not synonymous. "The pain in my back is so severe I can't stoop to make the beds." This seems to be a perfectly reasonable complaint, but, nevertheless, it must be remembered that the patient is not describing the pain: she is describing her own reaction to the pain. Her next-door neighbor with the same degree of pain may be out playing tennis. In chronic depressive states when the patient's emotional state is affected, the patient may describe an obviously unreasonable decrease of activities: "For the last 2 years the pain has been so bad that I have had to use two canes to get around the house, and I haven't slept for more than 1 or 2 hours any night," "I got a sudden severe attack of pain in the middle of the symphony concert and they had to carry me out on a stretcher." This grossly exaggerated degree of disability is obviously divorced from reality. Discogenic back pain never gives rise to this degree of physical impairment for this length of time. The magnification of the disability may be less bizarre. "I spend at least half the day lying down." "I can't walk a block."

Emotional problems commonly play a significant role in the disability resulting from chronic persistent low back pain. A patient with an hysterical personality tends to react hysterically to any pain, including a backache, but the histrionics generally subside as the pain abates. When the disability represents just one small facet of a general emotional breakdown, the symptoms will be intensified and perpetuated if too much attention is paid to them and too little attention is paid to the patient as a whole.

In the management of these patients, then, the important questions to answer are: "Why is this patient so disabled by the pain he or she experiences?" "Where has the breakdown occurred: in the patient, or in the spine, or in both?"

Examination of the spine will reveal the features described in patients suffering from recurrent back pain due to segmental instability: pain on extension of the spine, reversal of normal spinal rhythm, pain on bilateral active SLR, and tenderness on palpation and manipulation of the lower lumbar spinous processes. It is frequently observed that the lower lumbar spine moves very little on forward flexion, a fact that can be measured by noting that the spinous processes do not separate very much on forward flexion. There are no signs of root tension, root irritation, or root compression.

Other factors contributing to the persistence of the pain may be noted: excessive weight, flabby abdominal muscles, a tight tensor fascia femoris. Radiographs will show the stigmata of degenerative disc disease at one or more segments (Fig. 10-23).

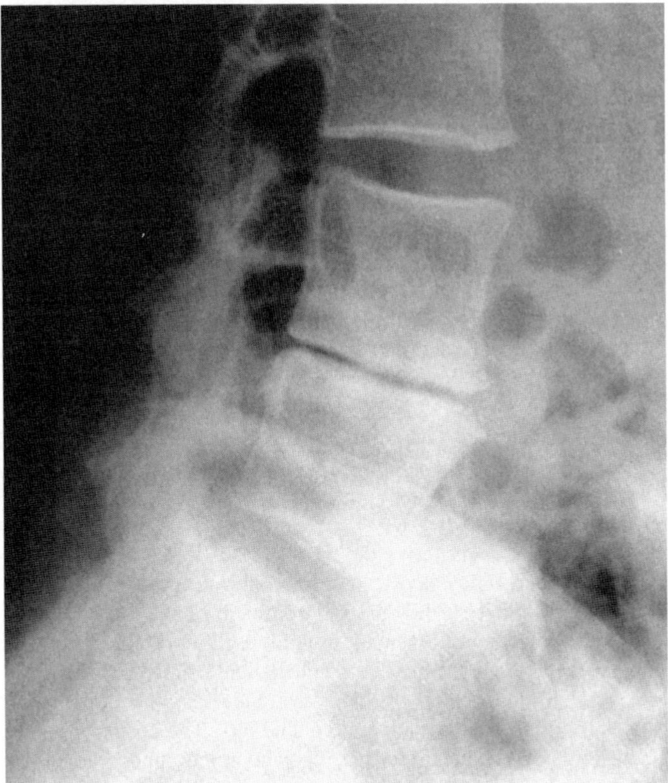

FIGURE 10-23 ● A plain radiograph showing severe degenerative disc disease at L4-L5. You will meet this type of degenerative disc disease later in the chapter. Read on!

TREATMENT

No form of therapy will alter the degenerative changes that have occurred. Manipulation of the spine may result in a short-lived amelioration of symptoms but rarely, if ever, gives rise to permanent relief. Manipulation is most useful to break the pain cycle and allow a patient to pursue an appropriate exercise program.

In trying to outline a rational form of management of these patients, the following points must be remembered: (a) the natural tendency of the disease is eventually toward subsidence of symptoms and, occasionally, recovery; (b) no specific treatment alters the changes in the disc; and (c) treatment perforce must be directed at making the patient comfortable while nature affects the control of symptoms by stabilizing the painful motion segment.

When considering the means to make the patient comfortable, it must be remembered that (a) the pain is relieved by lying down, by unloading the spine, and (b) any activity that puts an extension strain on the spine increases the pain. Bearing these two points in mind, patients can be managed by unloading the spine in the following manner:

1. Losing weight, where indicated.
2. Wearing a corset with a strong abdominal binder to increase intra-abdominal pressure and bring the center of gravity nearer the spine. This should be seen by the doctor and the patient as a temporary step.
3. Changing occupation. This course of action, although undesirable, may on occasion be the only realistic form of treatment. It most certainly must be considered before a spinal fusion for all workers engaged in heavy work.

4. Teaching the patient to guard his or her spine against the extension strains of everyday living. The symptom of chronic persistent discogenic low back pain is almost invariably associated with fixed hyperextension of the zygapophysial joints resulting either from segmental hyperextension or from disc narrowing with posterior subluxation. The posterior joints are maintained at the limit of extension and any further attempt at extension is painful.

Extension strains are common: reaching, pushing, sitting with the legs out straight, prolonged standing, walking with big strides, and so on. In the act of lifting with the knees straight, the sacrospinales act as a bowstring and extend the spine (Fig. 10-19).

The patients must be taught to modify activities and assume postures that maintain the lumbar spine in the neutral position. They must be given written instructions in this regard (Table 10-3).

Extension strains are more liable to occur if the trunk flexors are weak, and a prolonged program to build up the trunk flexors is an essential part of treatment. The kickup exercise-manipulation program is the simplest to learn and the one most readily accomplished and persevered with by the patient.

A corset should not be prescribed early in treatment. Flexion exercises and the flexion routine should be tried first and, as long as the patient shows some measure of improvement, they should be continued. If the patient reaches a plateau in recovery and is still plagued by back pain, a corset should be ordered (Fig. 10-24).

As mentioned previously, patients derive the most benefit from a corset with a strong abdominal binder worn tightly, but a simple canvas corset cannot produce significant compression of the abdomen in thin patients, especially if they have a prominent rib cage. The most that can be done for these patients is to try to restrict movement to some extent with a high thoracolumbar brace (TLSO) (1). The upper part of the brace must grasp the patient firmly around the lower rib cage and the pelvic band must fit snugly just below the iliac crest. Side and posterior steel supports will protect the patient, to some extent, against sudden jolts and jars. The posterior steel supports should not be curved in but should run in a straight line. The abdominal binder should be padded so that some pressure can be exerted against the abdominal wall (Fig. 10-25).

Once the back pain is under some control an increase in daily physical activities is an essential part of treatment.

We encourage our patients to join a health club and work out on a regular (three to four times per week) basis. We instruct our patients to avoid impact/contact and lifting. The impact sports that should be avoided are running, skipping, stair-stepper, and volleyball. Basketball is a particularly poor choice for these patients because of both contact and impact. Our instructions on lifting are to never use two legs in the same moment of activity (Fig. 10-26). To be really effective, the progress of the patient must be checked regularly by the physician or by the physical therapist for a year. The treatment of a chronic, grumbling persistent back pain is like the treatment of a chronic alcoholic: nothing can be achieved during a single 15-minute consultation. If you are willing to follow through with these patients, or get a team to do this, in the well-motivated patient the result will be worth the effort.

Exercises: Flexion Versus Extension

Much of human low back pain is ascribed to the fact that we walk upright instead of on all fours, which in turn causes lumbar lordosis and extension strains. Over the years, much of our treatment has been directed at reducing the natural lordotic curve with Williams' flexion exercises (53). More recently, McKenzie (37) has popularized the extension school and others have taken the best of both programs, combined with isokinetic theories of exercise, and spawned the exercise cult that is sweeping America with posh clubs containing expensive Cybex and Nautilus equipment. Some therapists believe that relaxation and stretching exercises are equally as important as flexion, extension, and/or isokinetic exercises. As a fifth option, most patients will choose the laissez-faire approach of exercising when they want and how they want: "walk a little, swim a little, and so on."

The basis of encouraging patients to consider exercises is (a) numerous studies have shown that a fit patient is less likely to end up with low back pain as a consequence of occupation (8) and (b) a fit person recovers faster and stays better longer after an episode of low back pain (4,38).

Which exercise is best to help rehabilitate the patient is unknown. What is important is that the doctor recognize the patient who will respond to exercise therapy, and the therapist, familiar with all theories and techniques, knows "when" to intervene with "what" technique. If the response

TABLE 10-3

Instructions for Patients on Flexion Routine

General Observations

Whenever possible, sit down. Sit with the knees higher than the hips. The best way of doing this is to sit with the feet on a footstool. If no footstool is available, cross the legs. Never sit with the legs out straight.

- Do not reach.
- Do not lift weights above the head or out in front of you.
- Do not stoop.
- Do not move furniture by pulling it in front of you.
- Do not push windows up.
- Do not put on weight.
- Do not get overtired.
- Do not maintain any one position for a prolonged period.

Sleeping

The mattress should be firm. If the mattress is soft, a board should be placed underneath it. Sleep on your side with your hips and knees bent.

Sitting

When driving a car, the seat should be as close to the steering wheel as possible, thereby flexing the knees and hips. When riding in a car, you should put a pillow behind your back so that you sit forward in the seat, again flexing the knees and hips. Whenever possible throughout the day, you should sit down with your knees higher than your hips in the "lazy boy" position.

Getting up from sitting

It is important not to arch the back on the act of getting up from sitting. Move to the front of the chair and stand up, keeping your back straight. Use your hands to help you if necessary.

Standing

The best way to stand is to adopt the posture commonly seen in a hotel bar: one foot on the ground and one foot on the brass rail. When the brass rail is not available, get one foot on any raised object: the bottom of a desk or the seat of a chair. NEVER maintain a stooped forward position when standing.

Lifting

Ideally, you should not lift anything heavier than 15 lb while your back is sore, and ideally you should not lift anything heavier than 50 lb for 6 months. When lifting something off the floor, bend the hips and knees, keeping the spine straight.

- NEVER bend over to lift something off the ground with the knees straight.
- NEVER hold anything weighing more than 15 lb more than 1 ft from the body.
- NEVER lift anything over 20 lb above the shoulder level.

Housework

Equipment. All equipment should have long handles so that you do not have to stoop too much.

Vacuuming. The vacuum should be pushed with short sweeps rather than long lunges. Do not try to vacuum the whole house at once.

Kitchen. Never reach for objects from high shelves. Rearrange your kitchen so that articles in daily use are on the first shelf above counter level. When you have to stand for any length of time (ironing or at the kitchen sink), stand with one foot on a box 9 inches high. Use the box as a step to reach for articles above shoulder level. When getting articles from cupboards underneath the counter level, bend your hips and knees and squat down, keeping your back straight. Never bend forward with the knees straight to reach for anything from these low cupboards.

Laundry. When carrying laundry, it is best to carry the clothes in a small basket held against one side. Never carry a heavy laundry basket in front of you. It is better to make several trips than to stagger once under an enormous load.

Stairs. Avoid, as far as possible, going up and down stairs. Do all the housework you have to do upstairs and then leave the rest of the housework downstairs for another day.

Bedmaking. You have to bend forward when tucking in sheets, and this will aggravate your back pain. When your back pain is severe, if you cannot persuade some other member of the family to do this chore, the only way you can tuck in the sheets in comfort is to get on your hands and knees.

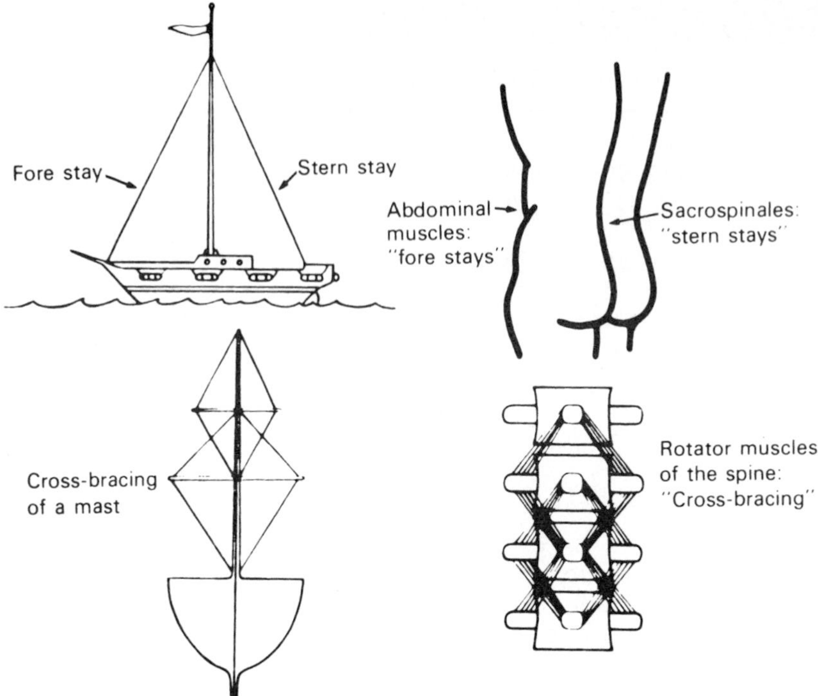

FIGURE 10-24 ● It is interesting to note the similarity between the bracing used to support the mast of a ship and the muscular bracing of the human spine.

desired is not being achieved, then the patient, therapist, and doctor should each be prepared to accept the limitations of exercise and either discontinue the exercise or change its nature.

Other Conservative Treatment Options

The most important treatment you offer a patient with mechanical low back pain is the passage of time, during which most disabilities will resolve (3). Next in its effectiveness is the use of various forms of rest (bed, corset, weight loss, job modification) and the use of anti-inflammatory and/or analgesic medication. Short of these measures, there is very little else one can do to positively affect

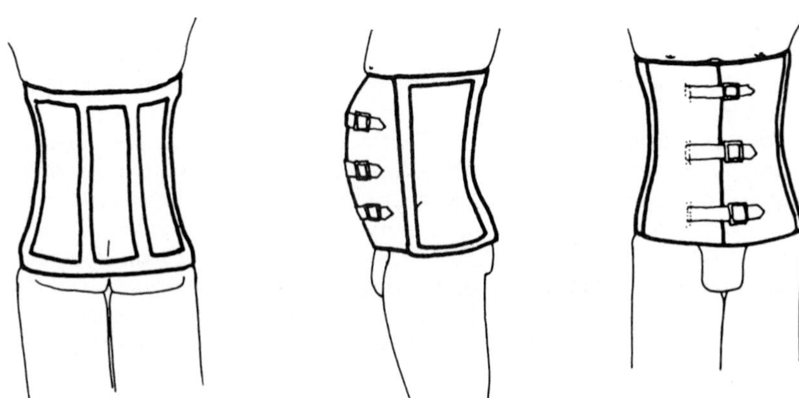

FIGURE 10-25 ● A rigid spinal brace with posterior and side steels and a firm abdominal binder.

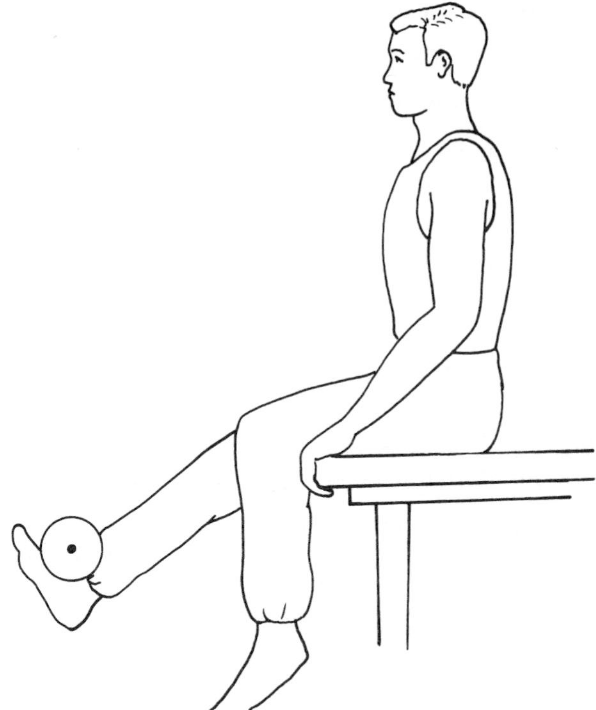

FIGURE 10-26 • Always use one leg at a time when working with a back pain patient. The use of two legs at the same time for weight lifting will immediately transfer forces to the back.

the natural course of the disease. We have discussed other treatments in other chapters, such as medications, braces, and exercises, and allow that they each have their own limitations.

Other Modalities

Heat, ice, short-wave diathermy, ultrasound. There is no scientific proof that the use of these modalities by themselves affect the natural course of low back disability, but they may bring short-term relief.

Manipulation. The self-administered manipulative exercises previously described may be of some benefit to the patient. Even better, is short-term chiropractic manipulation. However, the institution of long-term treatment and preventative manipulation programs have no scientific basis for support (19).

Education. Patient education is an important aspect of treatment in many diseases. Providing a patient is receptive to this approach, attendance at back school (51) will help the patient understand "what went wrong" and hopefully encourage habits that will lower the incidence of recurrence of the disability. The school, generally directed by a therapist, will involve the patient in treatment and place the responsibility for improvement on the patient (22). Patients need to understand that disc degeneration is not a traditional disease.

Injections. There is no scientific support for anything beyond placebo effect for injections into muscle, ligaments, trigger points, or facet joints. To some patients and some doctors, the occasional use of this placebo effect is beneficial. To make extensive use of these injections, although beneficial to the remunerative aspects of doctoring, is frustrating to the advancement of the science of low back pain. Epidural steroids may give short-term relief but will not affect long-term outcome.

Miscellaneous efforts. The use of transcutaneous nerve stimulation, behavior modification, biofeedback, and psychotherapy are treatment efforts used in the management of chronic pain syndromes.

DEGENERATIVE DISC DISEASE WITH SPECIAL STATUS

There are five separate conditions we can lump in this group, including:

1. Isolated disc resorption
2. Degenerative scoliosis
3. The facet joint syndrome
4. Internal disc disruption
5. Cervicolumbar syndrome

Isolated Disc Resorption

This is the easiest of the five special status conditions to deal with because it is easily recognized and easily treated. To "cut to the quick" of the subject, the patients are usually women; they have backache that totally dominates their life; they have the radiographic studies shown in Figure 10-30; they rarely get better with conservative treatment once they become symptomatic; and they should have surgery if conservative treatment has failed. You might find this position a little dogmatic, so let us explore further.

In 1970, this condition was first described by Crock (9,10,50), who stressed three features.

1. The dominance of back pain (we agree).
2. The presence of bilateral leg pain due to nerve root encroachment in the foramen (we disagree) (Fig. 10-28).
3. The condition is more common than the ruptured disc (we disagree).

By definition, the term "isolated disc resorption" means the condition is isolated to one disc, whereas adjacent discs are normal. The usual involvement is L5-S1, although a few patients have L4-L5 involvement (Fig. 10-23). Only when the disc is completely resorbed (Figs. 10-27

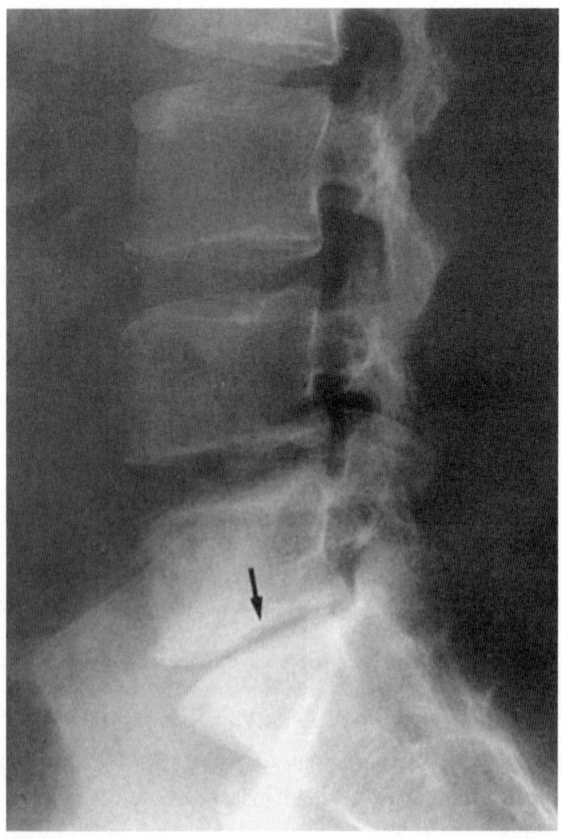

FIGURE 10-27 ● Plain radiograph showing isolated disc resorption at L5-S1. Look back at Figure 10-23.

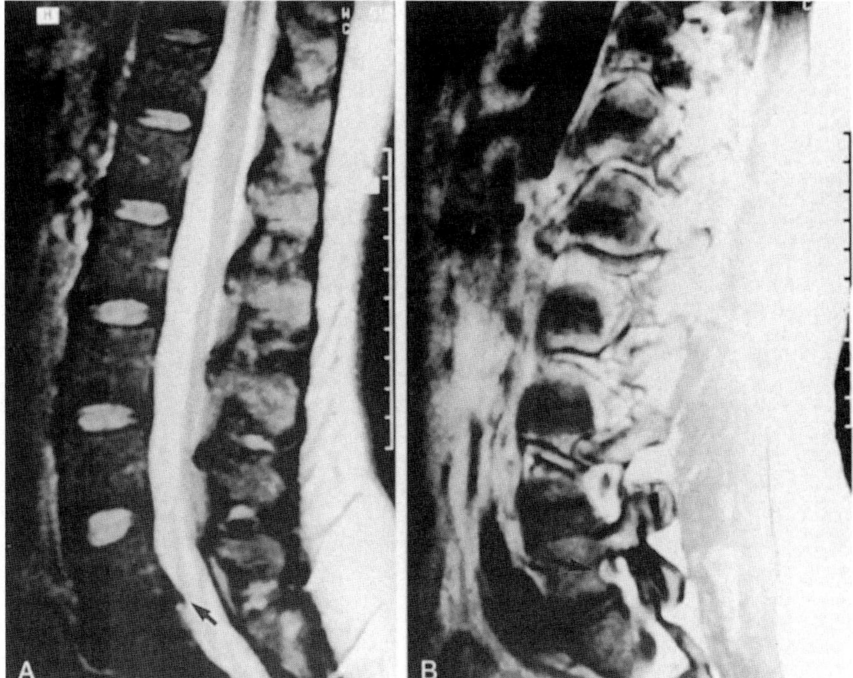

FIGURE 10-28 • **A:** Sagittal MRI (T2 weighted) showing isolated disc resorption at L5-S1 (the black disc, *arrow*). The rest of the discs have a high water content (bright signal). **B:** Parasagittal cuts showing the foramen at L5 to be wide open *(arrow).*

and 10-28) has the definition of isolated disc resorption been fulfilled. Some degree of disc degeneration affecting multiple segments is simply degenerative disc disease and does not qualify for special status.

The patients are usually women, who have borne children and who may or may not recall a significant back injury many years earlier. They start with the usual history of intermittent episodes of back pain, and within 1 or 2 years, their disc space collapses, and they end up with constant back pain that totally dominates their life. They are unable to do any activity other than rest in bed or stand and walk upright. As soon as they try to bend or lift, they develop significant back pain that takes hours of bed rest to settle. This is a combined picture of instability and inflammation. They are unstable in that the slightest level of activity triggers their back pain, yet on flexion-extension radiographs there is no instability demonstrated. The disc inflammation component is manifested by the persistent pain despite bed rest and the erosions in the endplate seen on plain radiographs (Figs. 10-23 and 10-27). The radiographic appearance is so unsettling that many of these patients undergo extensive investigation, including a CT-guided biopsy, despite the fact that there is no systemic or laboratory evidence of infection.

After months of failed, yet excellent conservative care, these patients present with the dominant symptom of back pain. Aside from some minor referred leg pain, there is no historical or physical evidence of radicular involvement. Crock originally stressed foraminal nerve root compression, but MRI (Fig. 10-28) shows that this is not present. The patients have a very stiff back and fail to reverse lumbar lordosis on forward flexion, yet often can reach the floor with their fingertips because of hip flexion.

Investigation is straightforward. The patients are usually young to middle-aged women in whom associated debilitating diseases (e.g., diabetes or immunocompromise) are not suspect. All you have to do is show that there is no fever and the white blood cell count and erythrocyte sedimentation rate (ESR) are normal; no other investigation is needed. It is necessary to do an MRI with T2 sagittals (Fig. 10-29) to verify that the disc involvement is isolated, the adjacent discs are normal, and the foramen are open.

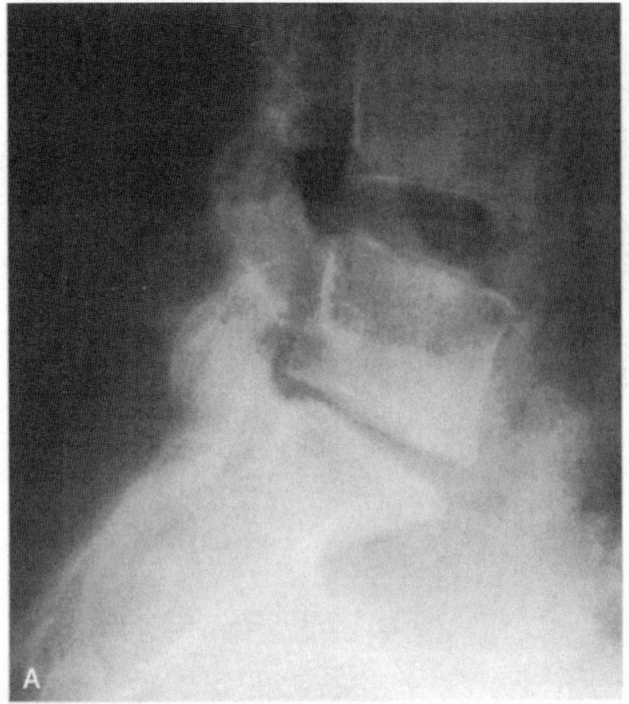

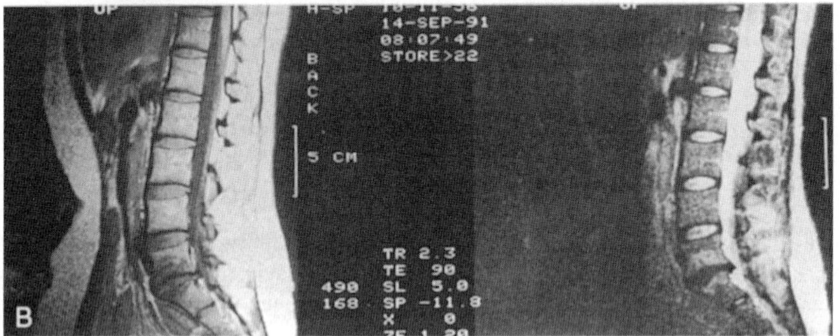

FIGURE 10-29 ● **A:** Plain radiograph showing isolated disc resorption at L5-S1. **B:** Sagittal MRI. **Left:** T1 weighted. **Right:** T2 weighted showing the black disc.

The pathology of this lesion is not understood. The condition is not unlike spondylodiscitis seen in ankylosing spondylitis and rheumatoid arthritis. Crock (10) has biopsied these discs at the time of surgery and has concluded the cause is a very active chemical process leading to degradation of the nuclear and annular portions of the intervertebral disc. The last phase of disc destruction is necrosis of the cartilaginous endplate, which leaves behind the worrisome cortical erosions seen on radiograph.

Treatment. These patients almost always fail conservative treatment efforts and do very well with a limited lumbar fusion (Fig. 10-30).

Degenerative (Adult Onset) Scoliosis

Scoliosis (a frontal/coronal plain curve) is to be distinguished from a sagittal plain (kyphosis) malalignment (Fig. 10-31).

Adult onset scoliosis occurs in the older patient (older than 50 years) and is secondary to degenerative disc and/or facet joint disease. It is present in 5% of patients older than 50 years and is most often symptomatic in the female osteoporotic patient (female-to-male ratio is at least 2:1).

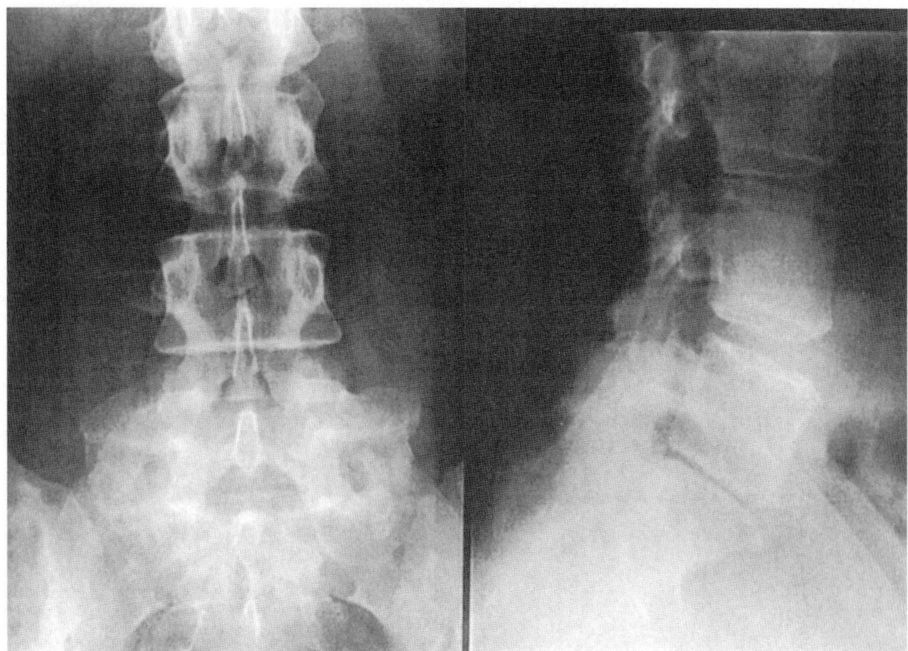

FIGURE 10-30 ● A "limited" exposure for an L5–S1 uninstrumented fusion **(left)** for isolated disc resorption **(right)**.

Etiology. Degenerative facet and disc disease is universal. Degenerative scoliosis as a variety of degenerative disc disease develops because one facet joint wears and subluxes more than its mate (Fig. 10-32), which leads to a lateral subluxation and the subsequent development of the scoliosis (44). Asymmetric disc space narrowing is also present (Fig. 10-32), either as a cause or a result. Osteoporosis is a common feature in women who, in turn, usually have worse curves and more pain than men. A history of previous laminectomy, especially with loss of a facet joint, will accelerate the scoliosis.

Clinical presentation. The most common presentation is low back pain (21). At least 50% of the patients will have neurologic involvement, either in the form of monoradicular pain or claudicant leg pain due to spinal canal stenosis.

These patients all present with a long history of back pain, increasing in severity as the curve progresses. Curve progression may be up to 3 degrees per year and is more apt to occur in the following:

Women
Individuals with osteoporosis
Individuals with right-sided curves
Individuals with shorter-segment curves
Individuals with high Cobb angles (more than 30 degrees) on presentation
Individuals with a rotation of Grade 2 or more (Fig. 10-33)
Individuals with a high L5-S1 junction (Fig. 10-34)
Individuals with significant lateral subluxation (Fig. 10-35)

On examination, patients will have an obvious lumbar curve. They usually stand in a forward flexed position with a loss of lumbar lordosis (the flat back). At least half of the patients will have decompensation (Fig. 10-36). Neurologic examination will determine mono- or multiradicular involvement.

Curve characteristics. The curvature of adult onset scoliosis is most typically lumbar, which is another feature that distinguishes this condition from that of children (Table 10-4).

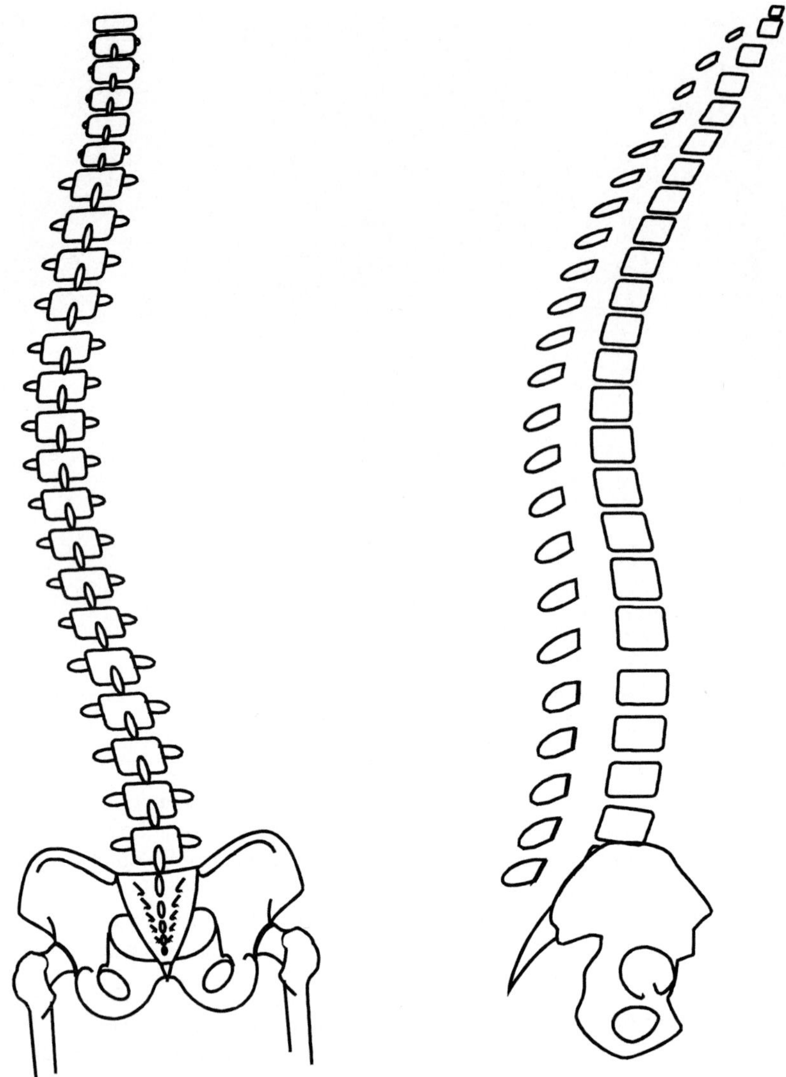

FIGURE 10-31 ● Scoliosis, convex left, on the left; kyphosis on the right.

Right-sided curves are equally as common as left, and usually no more than six vertebrae (average four) are included in the curve (Fig. 10-35). Curves with a Cobb angle greater than 60 degrees are unusual, with most of these curves lying between 20 degrees and 30 degrees on patient presentation.

The apex of the curve is most often at L3. An apex at L2 will shift the curve into the low thoracic region and often be associated with a secondary curve just above the pelvis (Fig. 10-37). Some curves may be associated with rotary lateral listhesis.

Treatment. These patients are incredibly difficult to treat because of many factors:

They are older (more concurrent medical problems).
They are osteoporotic.
They have often had previous surgery.
They all have significant back pain.

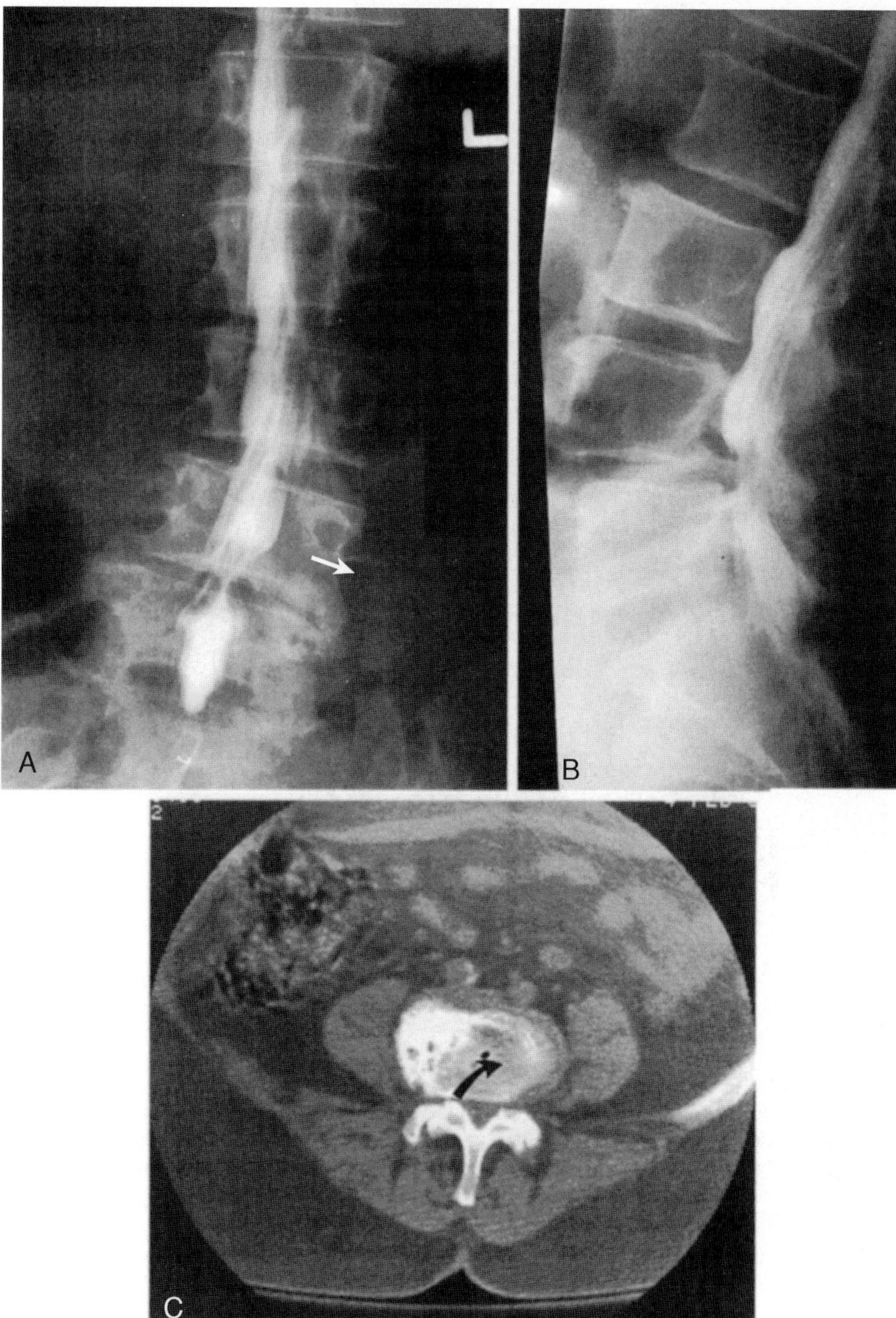

FIGURE 10-32 ● **A:** A left lumbar degenerative scoliosis; the lateral spondylolisthesis of L4 on L5 *(arrow)*. **B:** There is also a forward slip of L4 on L5. **C:** Note the facet joint subluxation, more on the right *(arrow)* than the left.

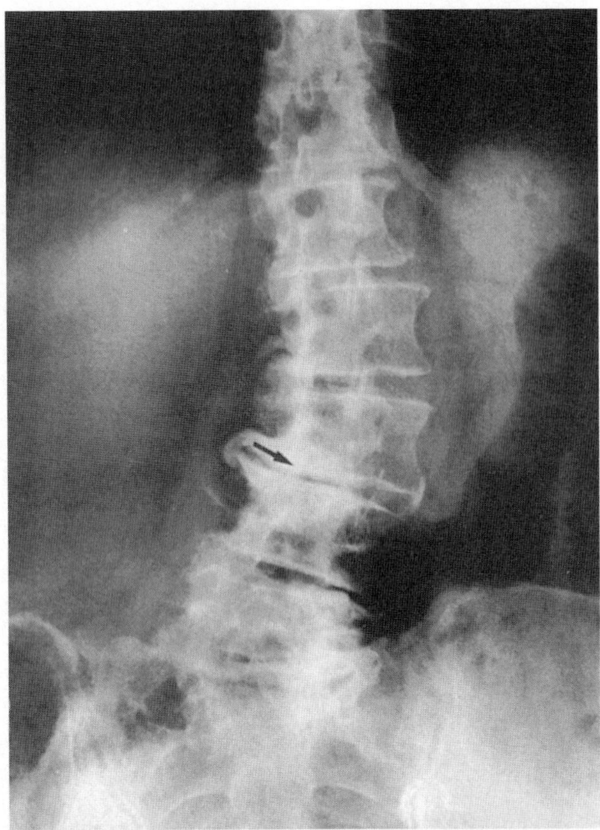

FIGURE 10-33 ● Degenerative scoliosis showing significant rotation of spinous process *(arrow).*

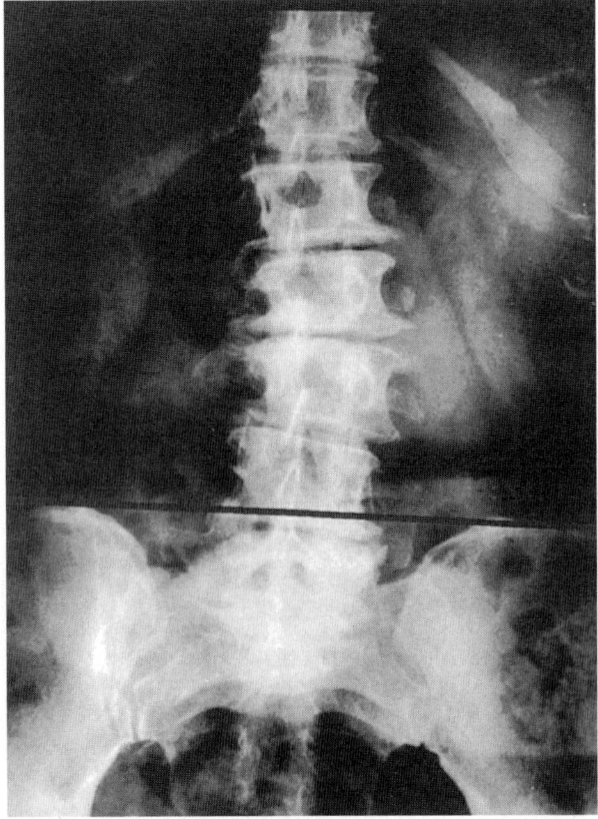

FIGURE 10-34 ● Degenerative scoliosis with the intercrestal line through the L4-L5 disc space, which is considered to be a higher than normal lumbosacral junction.

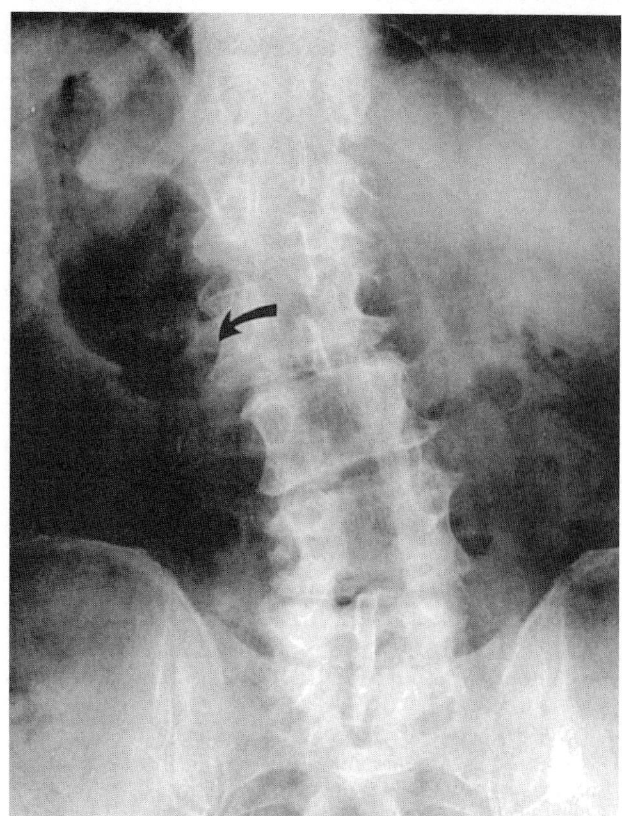

FIGURE 10-35 • Degenerative scoliosis with lateral subluxation of L2 (*arrow,* above a midline decompression at L3 and L4).

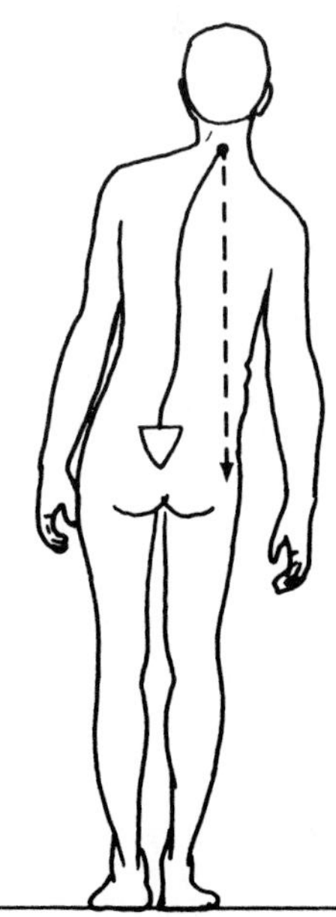

FIGURE 10-36 • Degenerative scoliosis with decompensation, that is, the upper torso is not centered on the sacrum.

TABLE 10-4

Characteristics of Scoliosis in the Young and Old

	Idiopathic Adolescent Scoliosis	Adult Onset Degenerative Scoliosis
Age	<20y	>50 y
Sex	F > M	F > M
Location	Thoracic or thoracolumbar	Lumbar
Side	L > R	L = R
Length	Longer curves	Average 4 vertebral segments in curve
Severity	Can be more than 60 degrees	Rarely more than 60 degrees
Vertebral deformity	Common (vertebral wedging and laminar changes)	Uncommon (degenerative changes on concavity)
Presentation	Deformity ± pain	Pain
Neurologic involvement	Rare	Common

This has led most surgeons to the use of instrumentation to correct and stabilize the curve (Fig. 10-38), which seems to be a fine concept except that a segment of the spine is rigidly immobilized, stressing the segments above (Fig. 10-39). Over time, these unfused segments are likely to deteriorate.

Do everything you can to treat these patients conservatively. Use physical therapy, bracing, epidural cortisone, and any other placebo-inducing treatment you can come up with. Above all, be open and honest with the patients when proposing surgery.

Surgery for adult degenerative scoliosis. The aim of surgery is to relieve neurologic compression, fuse to relieve back pain, and obtain some (50%) curve correction. This is impossible without instrumentation. Because lamina have to be removed to accomplish the neurologic decompression, the only viable instrumentation system is pedicle fixation (35). Attempts should be made to avoid fusing to the sacrum; remember to build in some lumbar lordosis.

Surgery for monoradicular pain can be a limited microdecompression for root involvement.

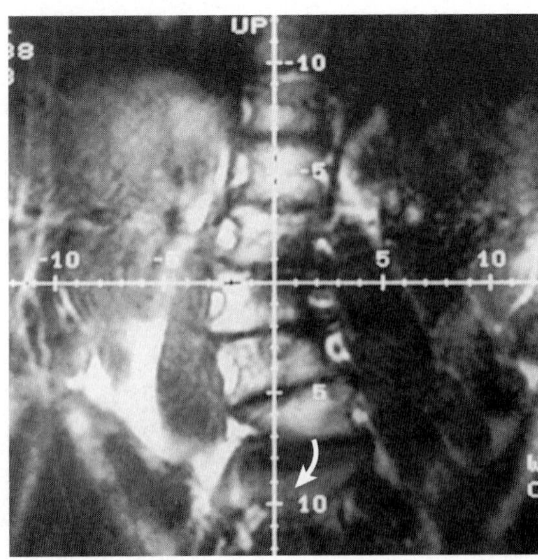

FIGURE 10-37 ● A degenerative scoliosis on the MRI scout film. The root encroachment will be most severe in the "cross hairs" of the grid. Note the secondary curve heading toward the pelvis *(arrow).*

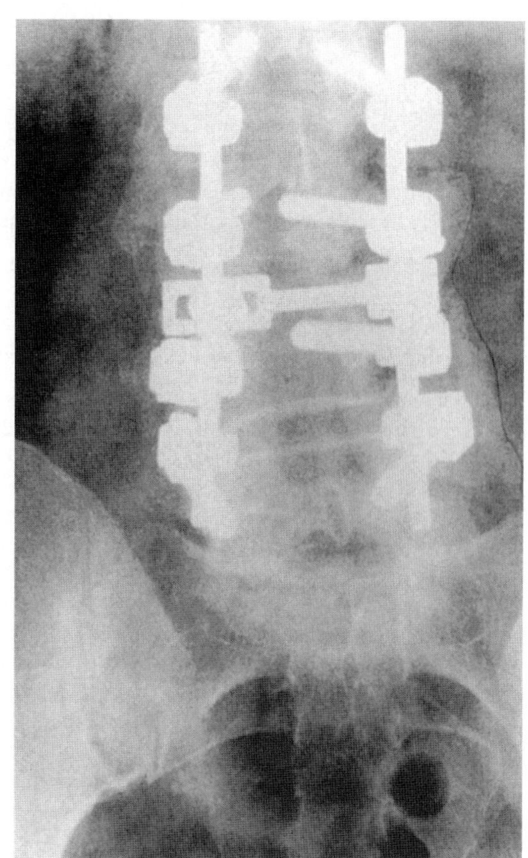

FIGURE 10-38 ● Instrumentation for degenerative scoliosis.

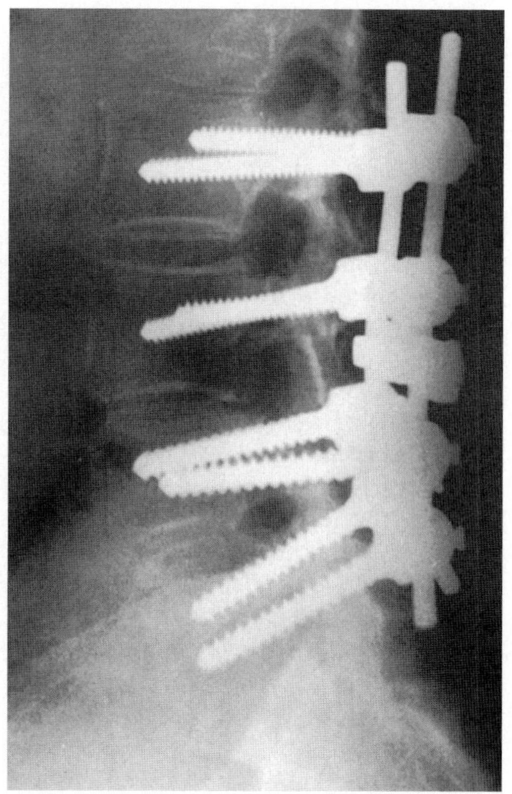

FIGURE 10-39 ● The segment above the instrumented fusion is developing degenerative changes.

The Facet Joint Syndrome

In 1933, Ghormley (18) introduced the possibility that lumbar facet joints were a source of low back pain. A year later, his study was eclipsed by the report of Mixter and Barr (39) of the ruptured disc. Sixty-three years later, we still do not know what the facet joint syndrome is!

It is easy to postulate that the facet joints are a source of pain:

1. They are synovial joints, paired at each level, lined by hyaline cartilage, and encased in a capsule: they are a miniaturized version of a knee joint.
2. They are innervated by the medial branch of the posterior primary ramus.
3. They degenerate in concert with the disc space (Fig. 10-40).

Yet numerous, recent, well-controlled studies suggest that directing treatment (facet joint blocks) at the facet joints is largely a waste of time (27,29).

Biomechanically, the facet joints share the load in each spinal motion segment. Their primary function is to protect the disc space from shear and rotational (torsion) forces. Their secondary role is to share a portion of the axial load when a person is standing (they share 0% of the axial load on the spine when you are sitting). When degenerative changes develop in the disc space, the facet joints share even more of the load.

There is no question that facet joints degenerate, just like knee joints degenerate. The work of Fairbank et al. (13) and Mooney and Robertson (41) showed that the facet joints can be painful when appropriate stimulation is applied to the joint. Pathology, in the form of typical osteoarthritic changes, has been demonstrated in facet joints removed at surgery (2).

So with the stress and strains on the facet joints, with the anatomy and innervation described, and with the degenerative changes that develop, why should not the facet joints be a source of low back pain, just as Ghormley proposed 73 years ago?

The patient complains of increased pain with extension activities that include standing, working overhead, using the sweeper, pulling, and so on. The pain is not aggravated by and/or is relieved by sitting, walking, and lying down. Often, there will be a stiffness in the back on arising in the morning.

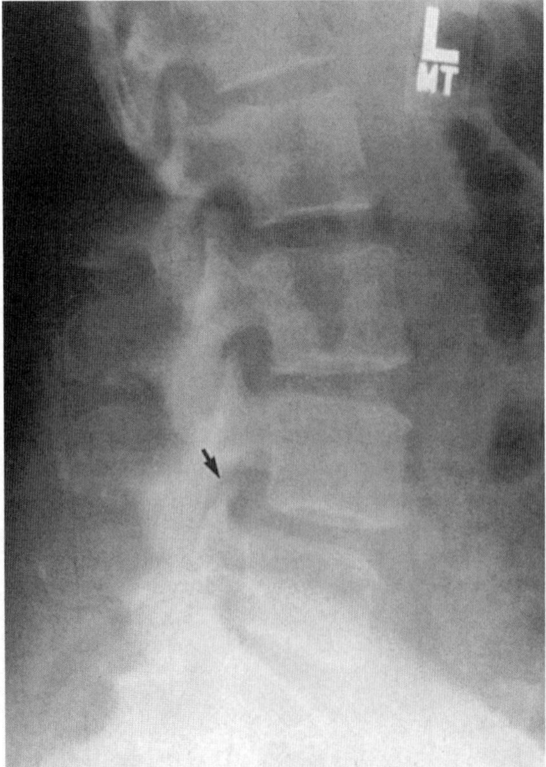

FIGURE 10-40 ● A lateral plain film showing degenerative disc disease at L4-L5, with a degenerative spondylolisthesis. Note the associated facet joint changes, including the characteristic lipping of the tip of the superior facet *(arrow).*

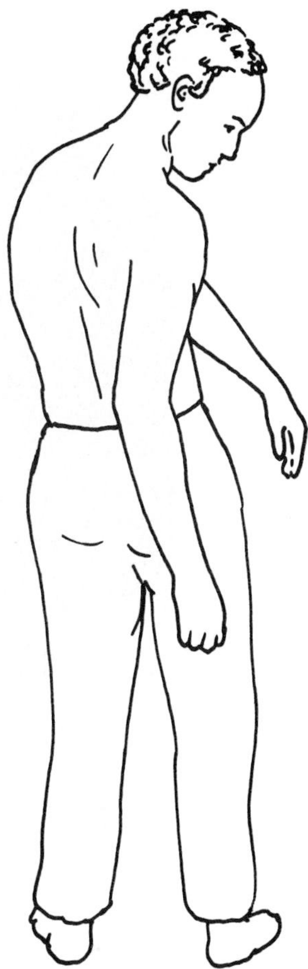

FIGURE 10-41 ● Extension and lateral flexion will often increase pain arising from the facet joint.

On physical examination, there is some stiffness to flexion and often increased pain on extension, especially into the lateral position (Fig. 10-41). Obviously, there will be no signs of root tension, irritation, or compression on examination of the lower extremities.

Fairbank et al. (13) and Mooney and Robertson (41) have shown that pain can be reproduced and then diminished with facet joint injections of local anesthetics. The addition of steroids follows the same principles as injection of a knee joint for degenerative changes. The procedure is known as a facet joint block and should be done bilaterally. Because facet joint degenerative disease advances in concert with the aging changes in the lumbar spine, it affects multiple levels, and thus multilevel facet joint injections (usually L3-L4, L4-L5, and L5-S1) are required.

Treatment of the facet degenerative syndrome. If you suspect the facet joints as the source of pain, a useful treatment modality is the multilevel, bilateral facet joint block (Fig. 10-42). A significant number of patients will be relieved of their symptoms in the long term, but a number will experience recurrent symptoms in a few days to a few months of injection. For all of these patients, a general fitness program of flexion-type exercises is indicated. For these patients, a facet joint rhizolysis (Fig. 10-43) can be considered, but like all denervation procedures for arthritic joints, it is of limited usefulness. It is unusual that the facet joint syndrome would be severe enough to merit a decision to fuse the involved motion segments.

Cervicolumbar Syndrome

Symptomatic degenerative disc changes are most commonly seen in the lower lumbar spine. Often, the changes are multisegmental and involve the whole lumbar spine, and on occasion the changes are multifocal, involving both the lumbar and cervical spine. It is to this latter group that the term

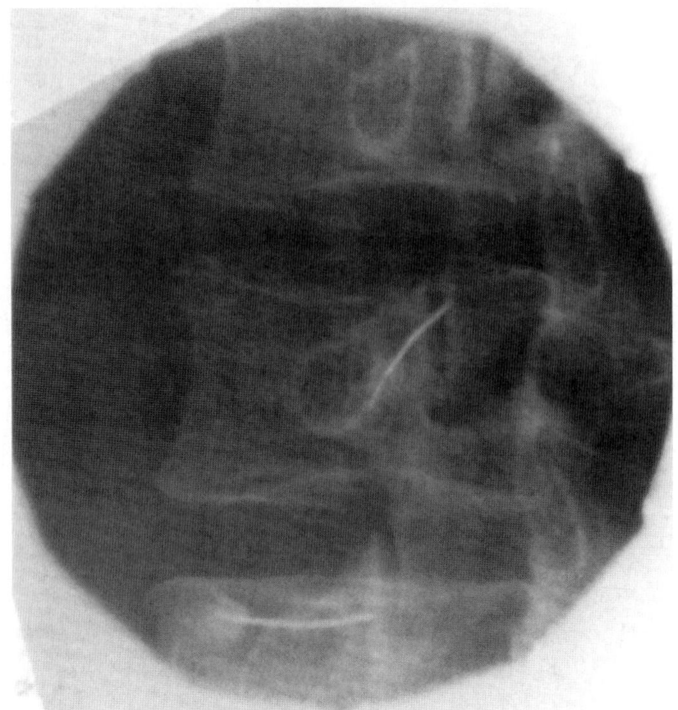

FIGURE 10-42 ● Fine needles in the facet joints for the purpose of a block.

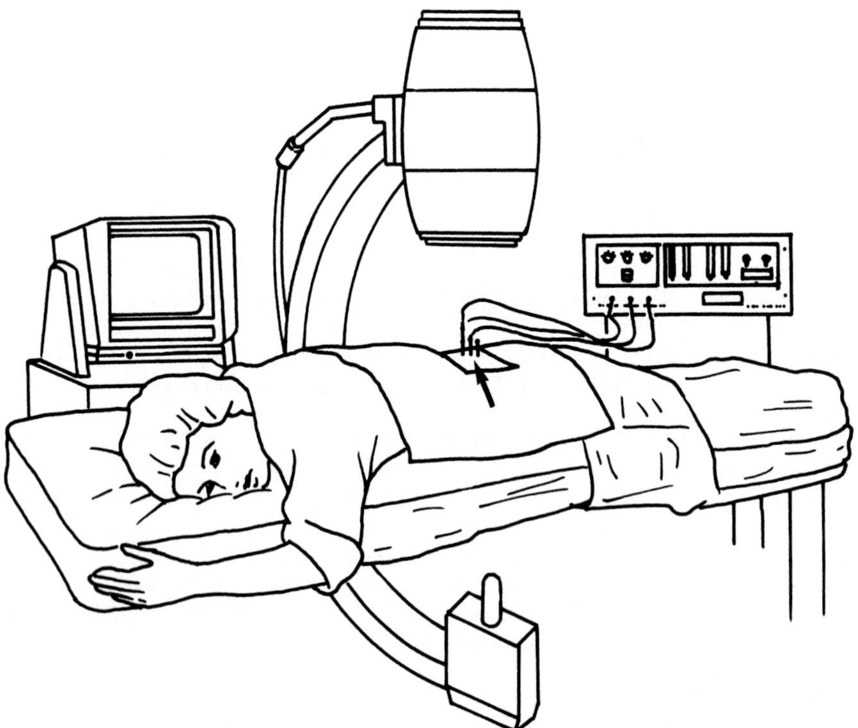

FIGURE 10-43 ● A facet joint rhizolysis, with the patient prone and image intensifier control to guide placement of the probes *(arrow).* The radiofrequency generator is in the background on the right.

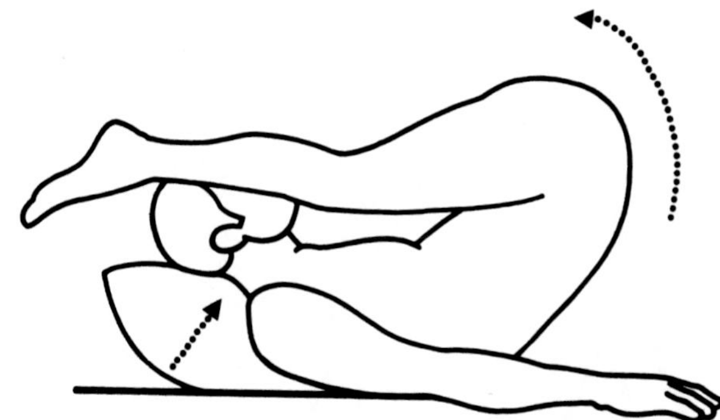

FIGURE 10-44 ● With kickup exercises, the patient may put a severe flexion strain on the neck, particularly if the neck is not supported by a pillow.

"cervicocolumbar syndrome" has been applied. Commonly, the degenerative changes in the cervical spine are not symptomatic at the time that the patient is seen about low back pain, or else the symptoms are relatively minor, and the patient does not believe them worthy of mention. As part of conservative treatment, the patient may be given situp or kickup exercises. Situp exercises can place a severe extension strain on the neck, and in kickup exercises the patient may injure the neck by straining or overflexing (Fig. 10-44). As a result of the exercise program, the previously asymptomatic disc changes in the neck may become painful and may indeed constitute a significant continuing disability.

If a lumbosacral fusion is undertaken in such a patient, the hyperextended, rotated position of the neck adopted during the course of surgery may leave the patient with intractable cervicobrachial pain.

If, when the patient is first seen, symptoms are derived from the degenerative changes in both the cervical and lumbar spines, the patient presents the almost unbelievable picture of "total body pain," pain in the neck radiating to the occiput, to both shoulders, and maybe down the arms. In addition, these patients may have pain radiating to the chest. The lumbar disc changes result in low back pain frequently associated with referred pain to one or both legs (Fig. 10-45). It is little wonder, when confronted with such a picture, that the physician is defeated, and examination and treatment tend to be perfunctory.

An awareness of this syndrome is important to the physician. Before suggesting situp or kickup exercises for the treatment of low back pain, the patient should be specifically asked if he/she has any pain in the neck, shoulders, or arms. The neck should be examined carefully, with particular attention being paid to the first sign of symptomatic cervical disc degeneration, namely, painful limitation of extension of the neck. If there is any suggestion of cervical disc degenerative changes in such patients, the exercise program should be conducted with the patient's neck protected in a cervical collar.

When the patient complains of what appears to be total body pain, the possibility of a cervicolumbar syndrome should be considered, and its probability should be assessed by careful examination of both the cervical and lumbar spines. Admittedly, many of these patients are emotionally disturbed, but the emotional disturbance may be secondary to this irksome burden of pain. It is often wise to put the patient on a short course of adequate analgesia with mild sedation for a week, allow the discomfort to subside, and then re-examine the patient's clinical picture. There is no reason why simultaneous treatment for both the cervical and lumbar disc changes should not be performed.

TREATMENT OF SYMPTOMATIC LUMBAR DEGENERATIVE DISC DISEASE

We hope that you have the message by now! Most patients with axial (midline back) pain will respond to conservative care and the passage of time. Because these conditions are chronic, we advise against the use of narcotics and other mood-altering drugs. The treatment should be confined to physical measures.

The choices are as follows:

1. Rest
2. Mobilization/exercise

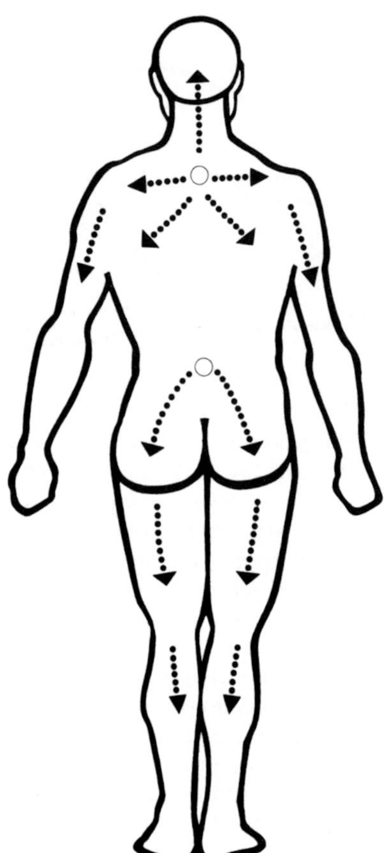

FIGURE 10-45 ● Diagram to show the distribution of pain when symptoms are derived from degenerative disc disease in the cervical spine and the lumbar spine simultaneously. This gives rise to the unbelievable picture of total body pain.

Rest

Certainly, bed rest has little role to play in the treatment of chronic low back pain. Occasionally, an acute episode will be so severe that a few days of bed rest is required. Most often bed rest is detrimental to these patients, reinforcing the idea that they have a serious problem and adversely affecting bone and muscle mass as well as disc and cartilage nutrition. We have the same feelings about a brace except in (a) severe pain in a patient who must be ambulating and (b) an older patient who cannot be treated in any other way because of comorbid medical problems.

There are other forms of rest such as job or activity modification and weight loss that are worthwhile efforts.

Mobilization/Exercise

The management of chronic (axial) low back pain centers around the concepts of mobilization and exercise. The aim of this approach is to improve functional capacity, while encouraging the patient to take an active role and begin to cope with the pain. Letting the patient use the back pain as a barometer for activity will fail. Rather, set down a mobilization/exercise program and encourage the patient to follow that plan, regardless of the pain.

OPERATIVE TREATMENT

It seems only reasonable to conclude that if mechanical low back pain is related to instability of a lumbar spine segment, stabilization (fusion) of that segment(s) will rid the patient of the wretched complaint (33). Spine fusion as treatment of low back pain is rarely indicated. Nearly every back pain due to degenerative disc disease will settle to a tolerable level if the stress is taken off the spine by weight loss, strengthening of the abdominal muscles, the occasional use of temporary spinal support, and modification of activities that sometimes necessitates a change of employment.

A spinal fusion may be considered in those instances in which an emotionally stable patient is unable, or unwilling, to restrict work and pleasure activities or, despite doing so, is still disabled by recurrent episodes or persistence of incapacitating low back pain. The word "considered" is used advisedly. Before admission to the hospital, two things must be assessed in greater detail: first, the patient who has the backache and, second, the backache the patient has.

In the natural history of degenerative disc disease, the L5-S1 disc is usually the first to be involved, followed subsequently by changes in the L4-L5 disc. Clinical experience has shown that the degenerative changes in the lumbosacral disc are self-limiting and rarely give rise to prolonged symptoms. The L4-L5 disc is the "backache disc," and a single segment L4-L5 fusion is rarely indicated, except for isolated disc resorption. This means that most patients are faced with the requirement of at least a two-level fusion. That makes sense because the aging process is universal. As we get older, we wrinkle our skin, gray our hair, and wear out our discs. Doing a two-level fusion (L4 to sacrum) does not stop the aging process at L3-L4, especially if it is established at the time of the fusion. Let us repeat: Spine fusion as a treatment of low back pain is rarely indicated.

SURGICAL OPTIONS

Let us assume that you have that rare indication for a primary fusion for the treatment of discogenic low back pain. What are your options?

Surgical Approach

Primary fusions may be done posteriorly, anteriorly, or combined (the so-called 360-degree fusion). Artificial discs are done for patients with early painful disc degeneration without facet involvement.

TECHNIQUE OF SPINE FUSION

Operative techniques are the concern of the individual surgeon and are not dealt with here in any detail. Certain principles, however, are briefly discussed.

Posterior Lumbar Intertransverse Fusion

Para-articular or intertransverse fusions present several advantages:

1. There is a continuous bed to which the graft may be applied (Fig. 10-46).
2. The technique permits intra-articular fusion or facet fusion. It has long been established that the achievement of facet fusion is mandatory for the success of the extensive fusions performed for

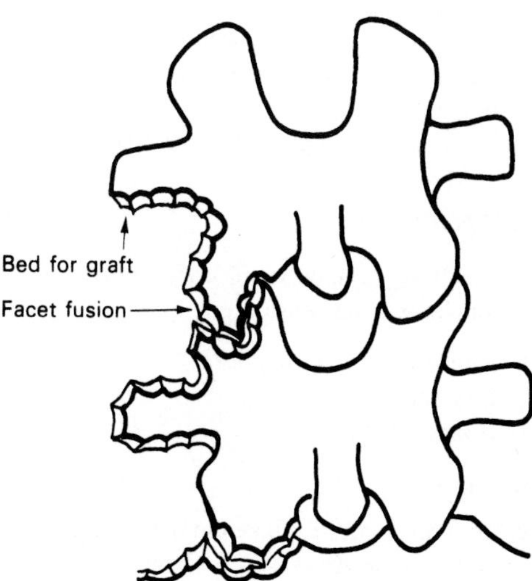

FIGURE 10-46 ● When an intertransverse fusion is performed, there is a continuous bed of cancellous bone to which the bone graft can be applied. In addition to this, the intertransverse fusion can be combined with a facet fusion.

adolescent scoliosis. We believe that facet fusion is just as important in fusions for degenerative spine conditions.

3. The fusion mass lies nearer the axis of movement.
4. The graft does not extend medial to the facets, and the danger of an iatrogenic spinal stenosis, seen on occasion with routine posterior fusions, is thereby obviated.

BONE GRAFT CHOICES: BASIC CONSIDERATIONS

The aim of bone grafting in lumbar degenerative disc disease is to get osteogenesis to occur. To achieve this, one needs to attend to two basic factors.

1. Stimulus. There must be a stimulus to the body to want to form bone, and that stimulus is in the form of the operative injury with the placement of the appropriate cells to form bone.
2. Environment. The host environment has to be inducive to the formation of new bone.

Each of these basic considerations are covered in this chapter.

ALTERNATIVES IN BONE GRAFTING

Various options are open when selecting material for a bone graft. At one time or another, the following choices need to be considered:

1. Genetic: autograft, allograft, xenograft
2. Composition: cancellous, cortical
3. Anatomic: size, shape, origin
4. Method: vascularized, nonvascularized
5. Preservation
   a. Physical alteration: fresh, frozen, freeze-dried, irradiated, autoclaved
   b. Chemical alteration: ethylene oxide, deproteinization, decalcification
6. Substitutes
   a. Cellular: marrow
   b. Scaffolding: coral hydroxyapatite, hydroxyapatite, tricalcium phosphate (TCP), collagen fiber, biodegradable polymers (polyglycolic acid)
7. Stimulation: electrical
8. Growth factors—bone morphogenic protein

IDEAL BONE GRAFT

The ideal bone graft material is as follows:

1. Readily available
2. Biologically inert and/or biodegradable
3. Of the shape and size required
4. In enough quantity
5. Has a large enough surface (porosity) to be replaced by host bone

FACTORS

When trying to understand bone grafting and arrive at the appropriate choice of materials, three factors have to be considered.

1. Biology
2. Immunology
3. Biomechanics

Biology

When a bone graft is placed in the lumbar spine, it is incorporated through healing by regeneration and not by scar. Any insult in tissues can heal by scar, and there is nothing the surgeon can do about this phenomenon. However, to get bone tissue to heal by regeneration takes much in the way of extra effort. Despite this extra effort, a number of bone grafts necrose, which accounts for the high nonunion rate in fusions for lumbar disc disease, especially intradiscal fusions. To prevent this, it is essential to understand the biologic healing of a bone graft so that the surgeon can take steps to optimize the conditions for bone graft incorporation and achieve a solid fusion.

The standard for bone grafting in degenerative disc disease is fresh, cancellous, autogenous bone, in enough quantity, laid in a good vascular bed with no extenuating circumstances such as nutritional depletion of the patient or scarring of the bed (Table 10-5). Any condition less than this optimal situation is going to increase the rate of nonunion/pseudarthrosis. Almost all of the following discussion centers on the fresh cancellous autogenous bone graft as being the only logical choice for grafting in lumbar degenerative disc disease.

Stages of incorporation. The five stages of incorporation of a fresh cancellous nonvascularized autograft are described in the following sections.

Stage I: Clot and Inflammation. Within minutes to hours of the wound and the placement of the bone graft, hemorrhage occurs, which then is followed by the standard stages of inflammation, including clot and exudation (invasion of the area by inflammatory cells). The initial inflammatory cellular invasion is comprised of acute inflammatory cells (neutrophils), followed by chronic inflammatory cells (lymphocytes and macrophages).

Stage II: Revascularization or Osteoprogenitor Stage. Within days of the wound, granulation tissue appears. The fibrous granulation tissue, in the form of blood vessels on a scaffolding, invades the graft as the inflammatory cellular exudate decreases. Along with blood vessels, the following appear:

1. Osteoblasts to clean up the bone debris.
2. Macrophages to clean up the cellular debris.
3. Osteoprogenitor cells (mesenchymal cells): the source of the mesenchymal cell is the host, and these cells will only appear if an appropriate bed has been laid for the bone graft.

If cancellous bone has been the grafting material, then this stage of revascularization is completed within 2 weeks (7). Cortical bone takes much longer for this stage to be completed because the cortical bone has to be resorbed through osteoclastic activity before any vascular invasion can occur. Up to this stage, there is not much difference between an autograft and an allograft. However, in the next stage the body's immune system will be stimulated if the grafting material is foreign to the body.

TABLE 10-5

Technical Factors Contributing to a High Rate of Fusion

Donor Factors
The best bone is:
Autogenous
Freshly harvested
Cancellous
Great quantities
Recipient (Bed) Factors
A nutritionally intact patient (no excessive alcohol or smoking)
A bed with a good blood supply (no scarring)
A bed free of contamination (no tumor or infection)
A firm bed (no excessive tissue dissection)

Stage III: Osteoinductive Stage. This is the most vital stage with regard to bone graft incorporation (7). The mesenchymal cells differentiate into osteogenic cells (osteoblasts). This is the most important source of osteogenic cells, although there are, in all, four sources of osteogenic cells:

1. Cells of the graft. A fresh cancellous bone graft will contain osteoblasts that will survive.
2. Cells from the host.
   a. The cambrial layer of the periosteum is a source of osteoblasts, especially in children.
   b. Cortical elements are probably the least important source of osteoblasts.
   c. The endosteum and marrow are the most important source of mesenchymal cells, with equal contribution from each one. It is these mesenchymal cells that ultimately contribute the most to new bone formation in the adult patient undergoing a fusion for lumbar degenerative disc disease.

There are two theories to explain why osteoinduction occurs.

1. The first theory states that the formation of bone is entirely due to the cells in the area stimulated by the injury of muscle dissection and decortication. It is simply the presence of osteogenic cells in the area that results in the formation of bone.
2. A more complicated theory is based on bone morphogenic protein (BMP). It is thought that BMP exists in the bone matrix and leads to the enhancement or the redirection of mesenchymal cells to form bone (49). It is also thought to be the basis of ectopic and excessive bone formation in myositis ossificans around total hip revision, in paraplegia, and in ankylosing spondylitis.

This osteogenic or osteoinductive phase is well established within 1 month, and the majority of a cancellous bone graft is replaced within 3 months. Because of this timing, it is important to support a patient's back postoperatively with some form of bracing, waiting for this first stage of osteogenesis to occur. Sometime between 1 and 3 months, when osteogenesis is well established and the majority of the bone graft is replaced, it is important to stimulate the wound so that further new bone formation occurs on the basis of Wolff's law (14).

As previously mentioned, it is at the stage of osteogenesis or osteoinduction that the antigen antibodies will affect the ultimate outcome if the grafting material is recognized as foreign (16).

Stage IV: Osteoconductive Stage. This stage is closely entwined with the osteoinductive stage, occurring over the same period of weeks to months. It is based on the fact that the grafting material serves as a passive template for the ingrowth of vascular and cellular activity. If a template is not present, then the osteoinductive stage cannot spread its wings, and a large enough fusion mass cannot occur. It is essential to this stage that the grafting material is in close contact with, as well as almost under compression with, the host bed. The one thing that will stop the osteoconductive phase is the formation of fibrous tissue, or the presence of fibrous tissue, between the graft and host bed. For this reason, it is futile to lay a bone graft in a scarred field because of the resultant inability of the host to bridge the gap between the scar tissue and the passive template of the bone graft.

Stage V: Incorporation and Remodeling. If the stages just described have followed their normal course of events, and if enough bone has been formed, the body will remodel the graft to perform the mechanical function demanded of the graft. It is during this stage that stabilization of the motion segment is achieved, and backache decreases. This is facilitated by an increased activity program at approximately 2 or 3 months, which stimulates further new bone formation and remodeling on the basis of Wolff's law (14). The final stage in remodeling is the accumulation of hemopoietic cells within the transplanted bone to form a marrow cavity. In an intertransverse graft, this is minimal, and in intradiscal and posterior grafts, it is almost nonexistent.

Dynamics of the stages. It is important to recognize that these stages of bone graft incorporation are not sequential but are, instead, closely entwined. There is a delicate balance between each of the stages, just as there is for a great classical music piece. Just because the violins start to play does not mean that the trumpets cease to be involved in the score. This delicate balance between osteoinduction and osteoconduction can be easily upset. Perhaps the most important thing that upsets this delicate balance is the body's immunologic reaction to anything that is recognized as foreign (16). This reaction results in slowing down of the osteoinductive stage, which, in turn, results in the breakdown of the scaffolding for osteoconduction. This accounts for the high failure rate in anything but fresh autogenous cancellous bone.

Creeping substitution. A cancellous bone graft is replaced by creeping substitution. New tissue invades along the channels made by the invading blood vessels or along pre-existing channels in the cancellous transplanted bone. Leading this invasion are the osteoblasts, which lay down viable new bone on top of the necrotic old bone. The old bone is subsequently resorbed, and more new bone is laid down. The phenomenon of osteoblasts laying new bone on old bone, accompanied by the subsequent resorption of the old bone, is known as creeping substitution.

Cortical bone requires the reverse of creeping substitution for incorporation. First, cortical bone is in need of osteoclastic resorption of the bone before new bone can be laid down by osteoblasts. The phenomenon of creeping substitution is one of the major advantages of cancellous bone for grafting material. In addition, cancellous bone is revascularized in a broader and quicker fashion than cortical bone, which allows for an early and wide distribution to the phenomenon of creeping substitution. Finally, all cancellous bone is eventually replaced by new bone, which does not occur with cortical bone grafting. In cortical bone grafting, there is always some cortical bone that is never incorporated. It is unusual for much in the way of cortical bone to be used in bone grafting in lumbar degenerative disc disease, which is fortunate. Unfortunately, most of the bone removed at the time of a decompression for lumbar degenerative disc disease is cortical in nature, and this explains the very poor success rate when the bone removed at the time of surgery is used in an attempt to accomplish the fusion.

FAILURE OF THE BONE GRAFT

There are many fusions in lumbar degenerative disc disease that are not successful. The reasons are given in the following sections.

Local Causes of Failure

The Bed

1. If the bed is poorly vascularized through previous insult, such as surgery or radiotherapy, then there is no hope for the bone graft to be incorporated. Next to "fresh cancellous autogenous bone in great quantities," this is the most significant factor in successful bone grafting.
2. Site: In an intertransverse fusion, it is very important to save the intertransverse ligament and the decorticated transverse processes so that there is a firm bed for the bone-grafting material. Breaking off the transverse processes or destroying the intertransverse ligament takes away the foundation (bed) for the bone graft and introduces a degree of mobility that is bad for the bone graft.
3. Infection: Obviously, infection will interfere with incorporation of a bone graft.
4. Foreign objects (e.g., bone cement) will interfere with bone graft incorporation.
5. Local bone disorders such as tumors will also interfere with bone graft incorporation.

Graft Material

1. Volume: If a less-than-optimal volume of bone grafting material is placed in the wound, then a strong fusion will not be achieved. The basic rule is that you can never have too much bone packed into the intertransverse or the intradiscal interval to achieve solid grafting.
2. Local disorders within the graft. Not unlike the bed, it is important that grafting material be uninfected and/or free of tumor cells.

General conditions. Poor general patient conditions (such as infection and nutritional deprivation) and the use of drugs (such as steroids and antimetabolites) will interfere with incorporation of the bone graft. The most significant general factor in bone graft incorporation is immunity. If the graft is recognized by the body as "non-self," the immunologic reaction will be provoked, with detrimental effects on incorporation of the graft.

Failure. If failure is to occur, there results a nonunion and resorption of the bone graft. It is a most frustrating experience when the patients return for their postoperative visits and are still complaining of pain a number of months after the fusion while radiographs show a poor fusion mass with pseudarthrosis.

Immunology

Problems with autografting. Although the best source of grafting material is the fresh cancellous autograft, it does introduce problems. The autograft requires a second incision with its associated time restraints. It introduces a second set of complications in the donor site, such as infection and pain. If a large mass of bone is required, then enough bone often cannot be obtained from the donor site. These problems have led to attempts to circumvent the use of autograft bone, largely in the form of allografting. This introduces a high risk of failure to the bone graft and, to this day, is not a suitable option for intertransverse or intradiscal fusions.

The two directions of circumvention are as follows:

1. Allografting bone. Today, this is the most frequent direction the surgeon takes to avoid the problems of autografting. There are renewed attempts to improve allografting by altering the allograft, histocompatibility matching, suppression of the immune response (20), and vascularization of the graft immediately on placement.
2. Bone substitutes or composite grafts (40).

Allografting (The Immunology of Bone Grafting). The greatest concern with allografting is the immunologic reaction that interferes with satisfactory incorporation of the graft. In today's world, the transmission of disease, such as hepatitis and acquired immunodeficiency syndrome, is offering even further barriers to the use of allografting material. This aspect of disease transmission are not discussed in this section; that is not to say that it is unimportant, but it is beyond the scope of this discussion.

Allograft and xenograft bone are recognized as nonself. This provokes the immunologic reaction and results in rejection of the graft.

Antigenic (non-self) components of bone. The antigenic components of bone are as follows:

1. Cells. The cells of bone are the most significant source of antigens. Any cell, such as an osteogenic cell, a fibrous cell, or a cartilaginous cell, will contain proteins or glycoproteins on its cell surface that are noncompatible with the host.
2. Matrix. The proteoglycans of the matrix have antigenic characteristics that can invoke the immunologic reaction.
3. Collagen. This is the least important source of antigens, but it is still a source of antigenic protein that can be recognized as non-self.

Histology of rejection. By the end of the second week, the immune response has started, and mononuclear cells invade the graft. This is at the end of the osteoprogenitor stage and at the beginning of the osteoinductive stage. It is the osteoinductive stage that is delayed by the appearance of immune cells.

The rejection histology is as follows: The inflammatory process soon includes lymphocytes. There is disruption of the vessels of the granulation tissue that are invading the graft. Eventually, the graft itself is encapsulated with a fibrouslike material, and the peripheral portion of the graft is resorbed. This breaks down the callus bridging between the host and the graft and ultimately results in failure of the graft with nonunion.

Through the work of many investigators, attempts have been made to reduce this rejection phenomenon. They are as follows:

1. Altering the allograft. The most effective method of altering the allograft appears to be freeze-drying of the grafting material. Other alterations that are less effective are freezing, decalcification, and deproteinization.
2. Histocompatibility matching.
3. Immunosuppression (20).
4. Immediate vascularization.

Despite these efforts to reduce the rejection phenomenon, it is still the general experience that at least 25% of allograft material fails to incorporate (16). This is a guaranteed failure rate that is too high to be acceptable for grafting in intertransverse and intradiscal fusions. For this reason, we do not recommend the use of allograft material.

Xenografts are mentioned only to be condemned. They provoke an even more profound immunologic reaction than allografts, and eventually all xenograft material ends up as a sequestered fibrous-enveloped dead piece of bone. The immunologic reaction occurs early in the osteoprogenitor stage. The more porous the implant, the more profound the inflammatory response. This is a strong position to take, but we think it is time for everyone to seriously look at the fusion rate in xenograft material and admit that there is an extremely high failure rate.

The only xenograft material used today is Kiel bone (Surgibone). This is partly deproteinized bone from freshly killed calves. Immediately after death of the calf, the bone is harvested, washed in water, and then bathed in hydrogen peroxide. It is then passed through a fat solvent stage and subsequently dried with acetone. Sterilization is accomplished in the United States by use of ethylene dioxide and in Europe by use of gamma radiation.

Numerous other attempts at xenografts in the form of Boplant bone, which is freeze-dried calf bone, Oswestry bone, and Kobe bone, have been attempted. All of these xenograft materials provoke a significant immunologic reaction and are associated with a very high pseudarthrosis rate. In the authors' practice, they are unacceptable materials.

Biomechanics

In lumbar degenerative disc disease surgery, the biomechanical properties of the bone graft initially are not that important. In the end, one is trying to achieve a solid fusion and stabilization of a motion segment, and thus, biomechanics becomes more significant. Some surgeons feel that immediate stabilization is important, which is why they use rigid internal fixation with pedicle screws, plates, rods, and other devices. It is important in grafting for lumbar degenerative disc disease that one initiates the appropriate osteoprogenitor, osteoinductive, and osteoconductive stages. The earliest these phenomena are well established is sometime around 2 months. Before 2 months, it is imperative that the patient's back is protected (rest, corset support, and activity limitations). After that, you can mobilize the patient in a hope of invoking Wolff's law and stimulating the biomechanical aspects of the fusion mass.

Bone Substitutes

Because of the problems with allograft bone, attempts have been made to find bone substitutes (25). The earliest attempt was the sprinkling of inorganic calcium in the area. It was initially thought that the excess of the calcium ion would stimulate mineral deposition. This was a failure.

Ceramics (calcium phosphate ceramics). Calcium phosphate biomaterials can be fused at high temperatures to form ceramics (23). These can be composed of hydroxyapatite or tricalcium phosphate (TCP). These products have a high degree of biocompatibility. Although both products are biocompatible, only TCP is biodegradable. These products can be used in the form of granular particles, porous intact implants, or dense intact implants. They must have an appropriate pore size between 100 and 400 t, and, as such, they serve only as an osteoconductive mechanism.

There are drawbacks to the use of these ceramics, including their very brittle nature and the fact that they easily fracture. Sometimes the matrices do not get oriented in the correct direction and thus, retard remodeling. The use of ceramics requires a very stable interface between the living tissue and the biodegradable graft. If this does not occur, then a fibrous tissue membrane forms between the host and the graft and interferes with incorporation.

The future. It would appear that substitution for autogenous bone grafting will be directed away from allografting and toward composite grafting. A proposed composite graft would be as follows:

1. Marrow cells to introduce the osteogenic requirements
2. Bone Morphogenic Protein (BMP) to introduce the osteoinductive requirements (49)
3. Hydroxyapatite to introduce the osteoconductive requirements

Obviously, this combination or composite graft will have to be laid in a good bed with (a) a good blood supply, (b) appropriate decortication, (c) appropriate immobilization, and (d) the absence of any soft tissue interposition. In addition, these materials will need to be placed in a patient that has the general conditions to incorporate the graft: good nutrition, the absence of steroid or antimetabolite drugs, the absence of excessive alcohol ingestion, and the absence of disease processes such as diabetes.

Conclusion. If allografting is so unacceptable, then why does allografting work well in cervical fusions? A number of investigators are suggesting that you do not need any bone in an anterior cervical disc excision to obtain a fusion. Perhaps this accounts for the high fusion rate with allografting, that is, no grafting is necessary to achieve a solid cervical fusion.

If allografting is so poor for intertransverse fusions, then why does it work so well in scoliosis surgery? There are a number of reasons for this. Most scoliosis surgery, in which allografting is being used, occurs in the younger patient population who have great healing potential. The allografting material is often mixed with autograft and laid on a very large bed of decorticated interlaminar bone. This solid bed is a great source of mesenchymal cells. Finally, there is usually rigid internal fixation placed at the time of scoliosis surgery. Thus, there are many factors present in scoliosis surgery that are conducive to allograft bone incorporation that are not present when doing intradiscal or intertransverse surgery. It is a mistake to transfer the concepts of allograft bone in scoliosis surgery to any use in intertransverse/intradiscal surgery. Stick with sufficient volume of fresh cancellous autograft to obtain your best results. In the future, look to composite grafting, not allografting, to resolve the problems in bone grafting.

Harvesting Autogenous Bone Graft

By way of introduction, let us state that the requirement for a separate incision to harvest autogenous bone will be unnecessary once bone substitutes are available. Although osteoconductive material such as coral (hydroxyapatite) is available, it is missing the osteogenic (cells) and osteoinductive components necessary for a viable solid fusion. Osteoinductive chemicals such as BMP have been successfully used in animals and are just starting into clinical trials. There is reason to believe that by the time the next edition of this book is written, we can drop this section on the harvesting of autogenous bone graft because of the usefulness of bone substitutes.

Technique. Because the patient is usually in a prone (kneeling) position for posterior lumbar surgery, the posterior iliac crest (Fig. 10-47) is the natural choice for donor bone. We routinely use the right iliac crest and take the bone graft while standing on the opposite side of the operating table. An incision approximately 4 to 5 cm long is started at the posterior superior iliac spine (Fig. 10-48). Do not extend the incision more than one hand's breadth away from the midline because you will cut the cluneal nerves, leading to an immediate postoperative numb buttock and later a neuroma. Alternately, the crest may be reached through the interfascial plane from the midline incision.

Expose the outer aspect of the iliac crest subperiosteally, and place a bone graft retractor.

Save the entire thickness of the pelvic cortex, and start by taking slices of cortical cancellous bone from the outer table. Your first cut with the osteotome should be the distal cut; this is designed to avoid the sciatic notch (Figs. 10-48 and 10-49). Entering the sciatic notch with an osteotome may sever the superior gluteal artery and cause the loss of a considerable amount of blood. The sciatic nerve is also in the notch, and damage to it will be noticeable as soon as the patient awakens.

It is very important not to cross the inner cortex and damage the sacroiliac joint (Fig. 10-50). Harvest as much bone as you can, and remember the two admonitions about bone grafting:

You never have too much bone.
When you think you have enough bone, take a little more.

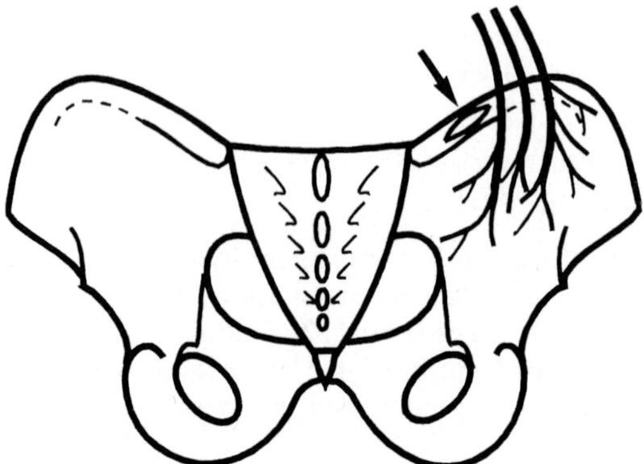

FIGURE 10-47 ● The pelvis from behind showing the incision for a bone graft *(arrow)*: keep it small, and keep it medial to the cluneal nerves.

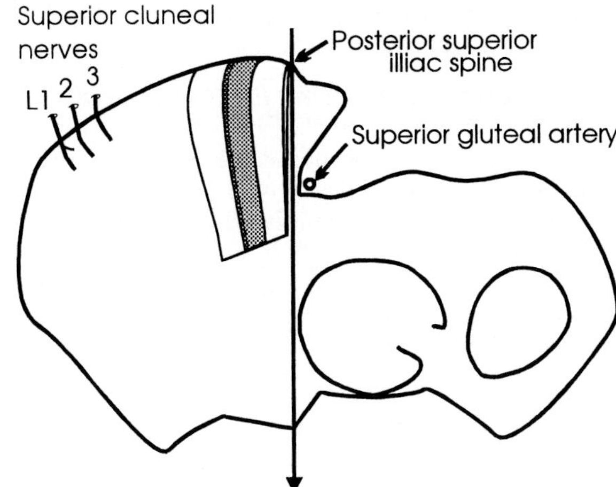

FIGURE 10-48 ● The patient's hemipelvis as it appears on the operating room table. The cortex has been cut with an osteotome to allow for three cortical slabs of bone. As much cancellous bone as possible is removed deep to these cuts.

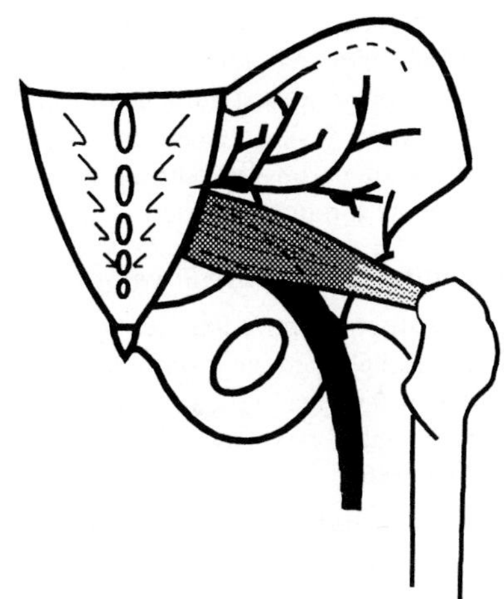

FIGURE 10-49 ● The sciatic notch contains the gluteal arteries (above the piriformis) and the sciatic nerve inferior to the piriformis.

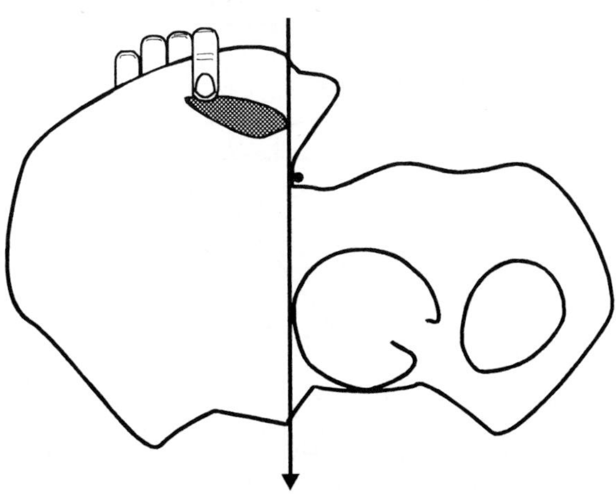

FIGURE 10-50 ● Missing the sacroiliac joint: identify it by insertion of your fingertip to the proximal interphalangeal joint at a level just anterior to the posterior superior iliac spine.

Closure is after you are satisfied the bleeding cancellous surfaces are controlled; this is accomplished with a tight closure.

Complications Of Posterior Iliac Crest Harvest. Complications of this procedure should be rare. The intraoperative complications of entering the sciatic notch and damaging the sacroiliac joint have already been mentioned. The minor but very annoying complication of cluneal nerve damage is easily avoided (Fig. 10-48).

In the immediate postoperative course, hematoma formation and/or infection are to be watched for. Each is an avoidable complication.

Donor site pain. This is the most common complication of autogenous bone grafting and is very common in anterior iliac crest sites. It is less common, but troubling in posterior iliac crest sites and is prevented by the following:

1. Making a short incision
2. Reserving the posterior cortex
3. Avoiding the cluneal nerves
4. Avoiding a postoperative hematoma or infection

The Placement of the Posterior Bone Graft

To obtain a fusion, posterior bone grafting can be done in the midline or in the intertransverse interval or as an interbody fusion (Fig. 10-51). Almost no one does a midline posterior fusion today. Most surgeons prefer the intertransverse position, and some surgeons prefer the interbody position. Today, almost all posterior interbody fusions are combined with instrumentation and an intertransverse fusion. Except in revision surgery, we would not recommend this approach. For a primary single-level posterior fusion, we recommend the intertransverse fusion (Fig. 10-52). This is done through a limited posterior subperiosteal soft tissue envelope (Fig. 10-53).

The Limited Soft Tissue Envelope

Fracture surgeons have long recognized that extensive soft tissue damage interferes with fracture healing. It makes eminent sense that extensive soft tissue dissection in the intertransverse interval devitalizes the area and can lead to a poor fusion rate. It is on the basis of this fracture healing observation that we recommend the limited soft tissue envelope (Fig. 10-53) as the preparation for the bone graft.

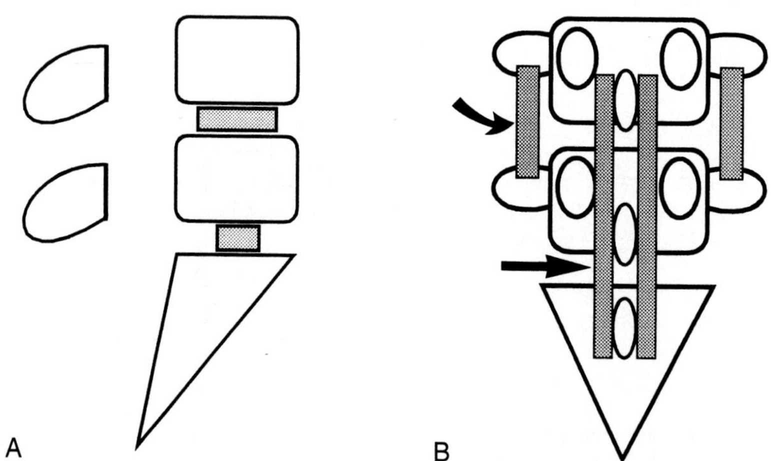

FIGURE 10-51 ● Bone graft can be placed in **(B)** the midline *(arrow),* intertransverse interval *(curved arrow),* or **(A)** interbody. A small graft, not completely filling the intradiscal space, is shown at L5-S1; this is a bone graft that is likely to fail. The graft size at L4-L5 is more conducive to a solid interbody fusion.

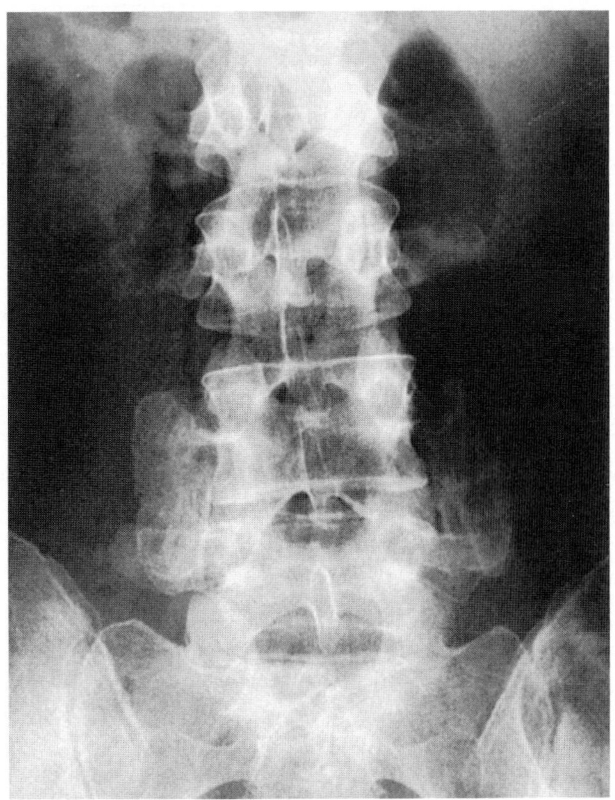

FIGURE 10-52 ● A "floating" L4–L5 fusion for degenerative disc disease.

This limited soft tissue dissection has the added benefit of more rigidly immobilizing the bone graft and enhancing healing (Fig. 10-53).

Complications of Pedicle Screw Instrumentation Systems

Perhaps the best way to appreciate the resistance to pedicle screw systems is to look at the complications associated with their use (12).

Screw malpositioning. Placing a screw down the center of the pedicle is technically demanding. The screw may exit the pedicle and cause nerve root damage (Fig. 10-54) that can be permanent. This problem gets more serious the higher in the lumbar spine that screws are inserted. Screws may also break the pedicle and in turn damage nerve roots.

Implant failure. Screws break (Fig. 10-55), and the screw-rod-plate-rod junction can separate (Fig. 10-56). In osteoporotic bone the rigid nature of the construct may lead to screw pull out or the "windshield washer" phenomenon of screw loosening (Fig. 10-57).

Infection. Pedicle screw instrumentation and fusion are long, tough cases. They require many members of the staff to assist (cell saver technician, radiographic technologist, spinal cord monitoring personnel, and so on). Because of the wide dissection needed to insert the instrumentation, more dead space and hematoma are left behind on closure. It is only reasonable to conclude that the postoperative infection rate will be high (up to 10% in some series).

The potential for infection may be further enhanced by the fact that you are often dealing with an older patient who has somewhat impaired wound healing and a foreign (avascular) mass of instrumentation and bone graft (that can easily die instead of heal). Obviously, these infections are difficult (and expensive) to treat.

Pseudarthrosis with instrumentation. The instrumentation systems have enjoyed wide support among spine surgeons because they decrease the pseudarthrosis rate (34, 55). It is still

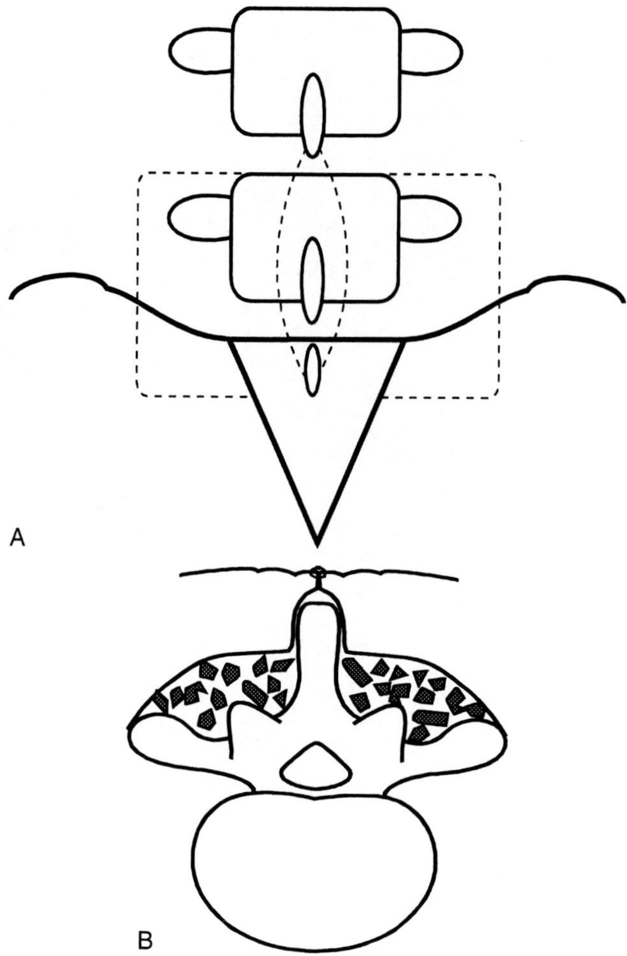

FIGURE 10-53 ● **A:** The limited soft tissue envelope at L5-S1 is depicted as separate fascial incisions *(dotted lines)* for each side and limited soft tissue elevation as shown within the rectangular dotted line. **B:** An axial view of the limited soft tissue envelope, wherein the muscle serves as a firm cover for the bone graft.

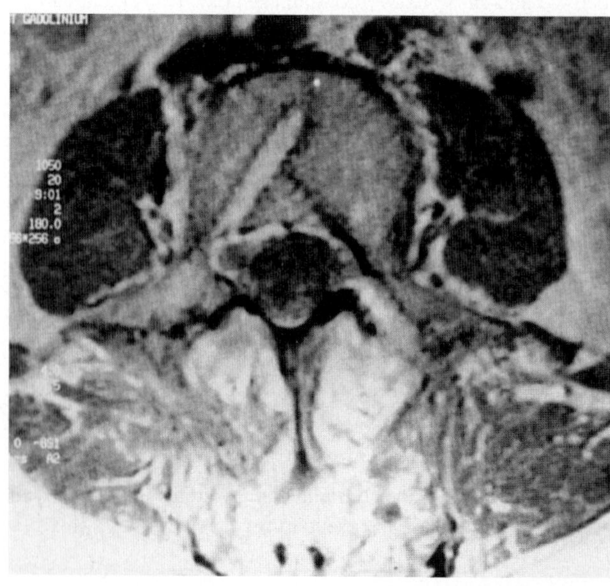

FIGURE 10-54 ● An MRI (after pedicle screw removal) showing that the path of the screw was close to nerve roots on both sides.

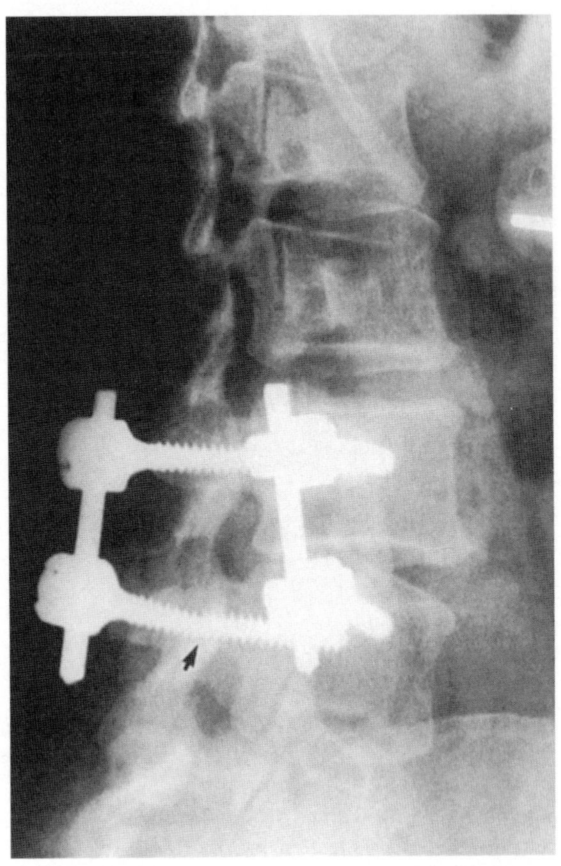

FIGURE 10-55 • Screw breakage *(arrow).*

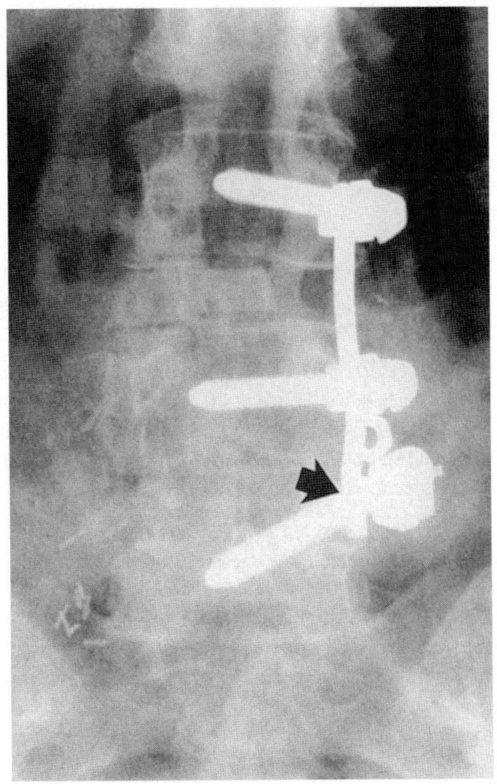

FIGURE 10-56 • Screw-rod separation *(arrow).*

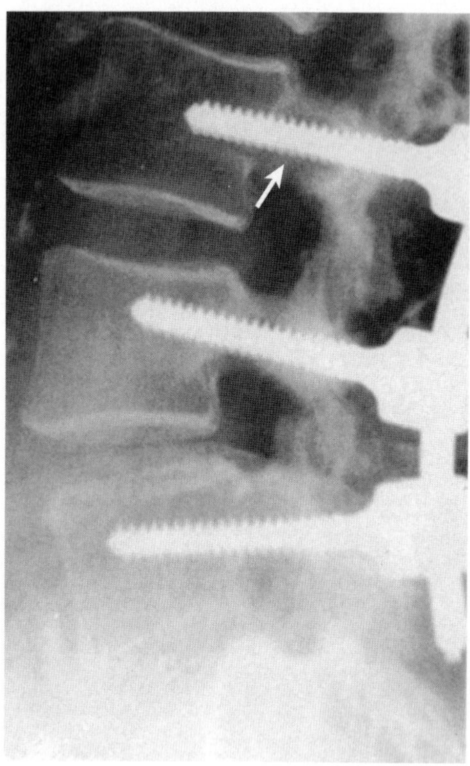

FIGURE 10-57 ● The "windshield washer" phenomenon of screw loosening *(arrow).*

possible to end up with a pseudarthrosis in an instrumented fusion, which may be very hard to demonstrate on investigation and requires re-exploration of the fusion mass. When you combine a pseudarthrosis with one of the complications previously mentioned, you have a very difficult clinical problem, which often results in permanent long-term problems that are difficult to treat even with repeat surgery. Because of this possibility, a number of spine surgeons use these systems sparingly, or not at all.

Painful hardware. In some patients, an apparently solid fusion may continue to be painful. In approximately 50% of these patients, removal of the hardware will result in relief of a significant amount of pain.

Degenerative changes at the motion segment above the fusion. The instrumentation system's greatest advantage is the rigid immobilization of the instrumented segments and the higher successful fusion rates (34). At the same time, this presents a disadvantage to the motion segment above the instrumentation, which becomes more mobile. This is apt to lead to degenerative changes that may become very symptomatic.

Miscellaneous complications. There are a number of miscellaneous complications such as screw perforation of a vessel anteriorly (Fig. 10-58) and damage to adjacent facet joints. These should not occur in skilled hands, but nevertheless they are complications associated with pedicle instrumentation, and not the uninstrumented intertransverse fusion. An allergy to the metal implant, although rare, has been reported.

General complications. Long, tough surgeries, with prolonged patient positioning on the operating table, are associated with higher complication rates (12) (Table 10-6).

The Biomechanical Principle of Stress Risers

Raising stress on spinal motion segments has the potential for increasing degeneration in those FSUs. Instrumented fusions are rigid constructs that raise stresses on adjacent motion segments (Fig. 10-59). The transfer of forces is most pronounced at the adjacent higher levels, and over the long haul, this transfer can lead to degeneration and symptoms at these unfused levels. This takes

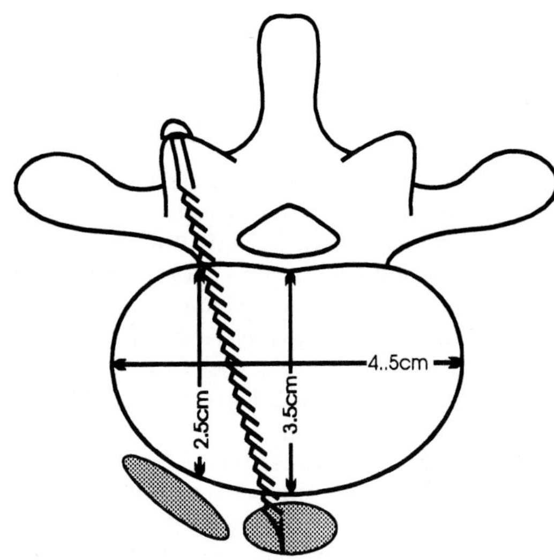

FIGURE 10-58 • Screw penetration of a vessel (aorta) anteriorly.

TABLE 10-6

Complications of Prolonged Operating Table Positioning

Pressure complications (eyes, ulnar and other peripheral nerves, and so on)
Phlebitis and pulmonary embolism
Atelectasis ± pneumonia
Urinary tract infection

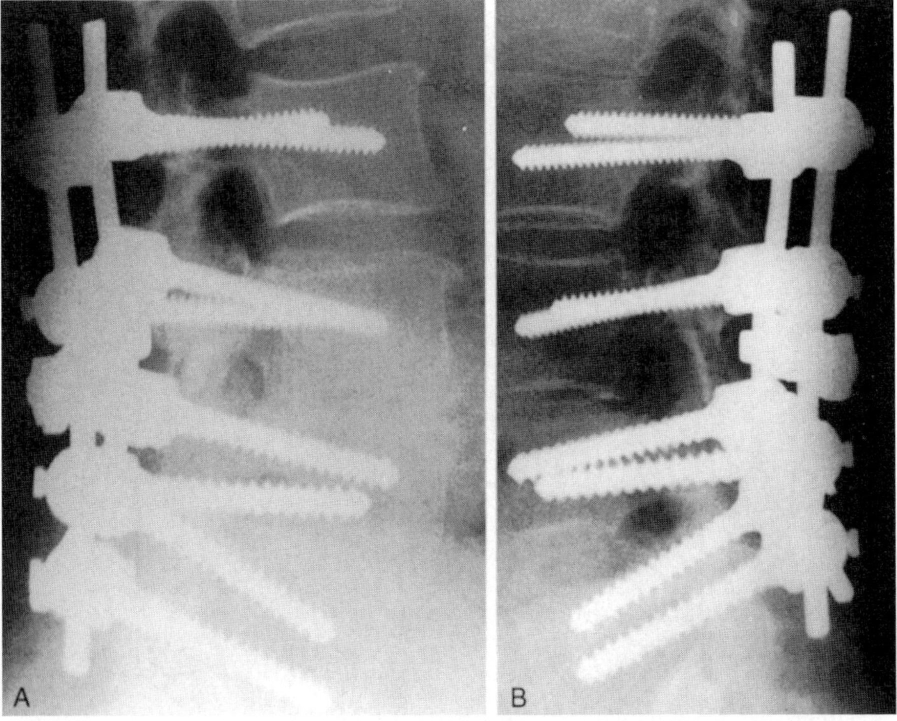

FIGURE 10-59 • The stress riser above a fusion. **A:** A normal L1-L2 disc above a three-level instrumented fusion. **B:** Degenerative changes have started to develop at L1-L2.

time (years) to develop, but it is our prediction that this will become the single biggest problem attendant on the use of spinal instrumentation for degenerative spinal conditions.

THE USE OF ELECTRICAL STIMULATION TO AUGMENT FUSION

It has been long established by research in fracture healing that stresses in the area of active bone formation produce electrically negative signals. Less active areas of bone turnover were also noted to be electropositive. By the mid 1950s, researchers noted increased bone formation around the negative lead (cathode) in long bone healing. Although most of the investigation on electrical stimulation has centered around long bone healing, there have been published studies suggesting electrical stimulation may enhance the fusion rate in lumbar spine surgery. The fact that we are 40 years down the research road on electrical stimulation of spinal bone grafts without clear evidence of clinical efficacy should tell you how tenuous the claims are for improved lumbar fusion rates using electrical stimulation.

The theoretical foundation for electrical stimulation is based on good scientific evidence. A negatively charged electrode in an area of bone healing will consume oxygen and increase the pH, which is beneficial to bone formation. There may also be a direct stimulation of cells to increase their osteogenic activity. Kahanovitz (30) has shown that direct current stimulation of facet joint fusions in adult mongrel dogs increases the fusion rate to 100%. The problem has been to extend these excellent basic science works into the clinical realm to show efficacy. To date, there are as many clinical studies showing usefulness and uselessness.

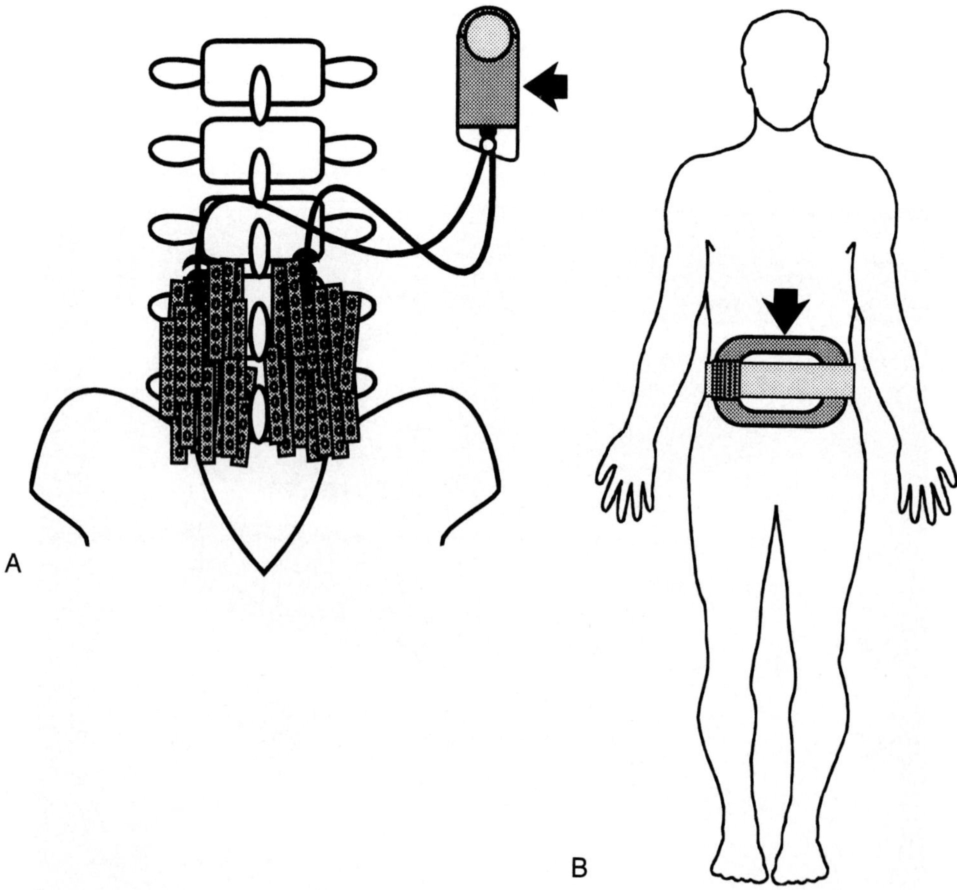

FIGURE 10-60 **A:** Electrical stimulation: internal battery pack *(arrow)* implanted in muscle. **B:** Electrical stimulation: external brace *(arrow)* creating pulsed electromagnetic fields.

Technique

There are two methods of applying electrical stimulation to lumbar fusions.

1. Implantable electrodes that apply direct current to the fusion site (Fig. 10-60).
2. Pulsed electromagnetic fields, worn in a brace (Fig. 10-61B), that apply indirect current to the area of fusion.

Both mechanisms are safe. The direct current stimulation applies 5 to 20 microamperes constantly to the field, over a minimum of 20 weeks, through two to four electrodes. After 6 months, the subcutaneous battery pack is surgically removed, and the electrodes are left in place. To date, there have been no reports of adverse affects from this approach. The external electrical stimulator is inserted in a brace, and patients are instructed to wear the cumbersome apparatus 8 to 10 hours per day. The hope is that they will wear their stimulator at least 4 hours per day, but patient compliance has been a major problem in all research studies.

The authors' opinion is that properly selected patients, undergoing single-level fusions, and living up to the criteria outlined in Table 10-5, do not need electrical stimulation to achieve a solid fusion. Using the limited soft tissue envelope to create the primary fusion bed is the most important of these principles. The use of electrical stimulation has led surgeons to extend their indications for fusions to patients who are undergoing multiple-level fusions, patients who are undergoing revision of failed fusions, smokers, and the malnourished. Further studies in this group of patients will show the futility of even operating on these patients, let alone adding the expense of electrical stimulation.

Postoperative Care of the Fused Lumbar Spine

It is essential that, before any fusion, the patient be made fully aware of the prolonged nature of the convalescence. The graft is rarely fully incorporated in under 9 months. Sedentary workers and

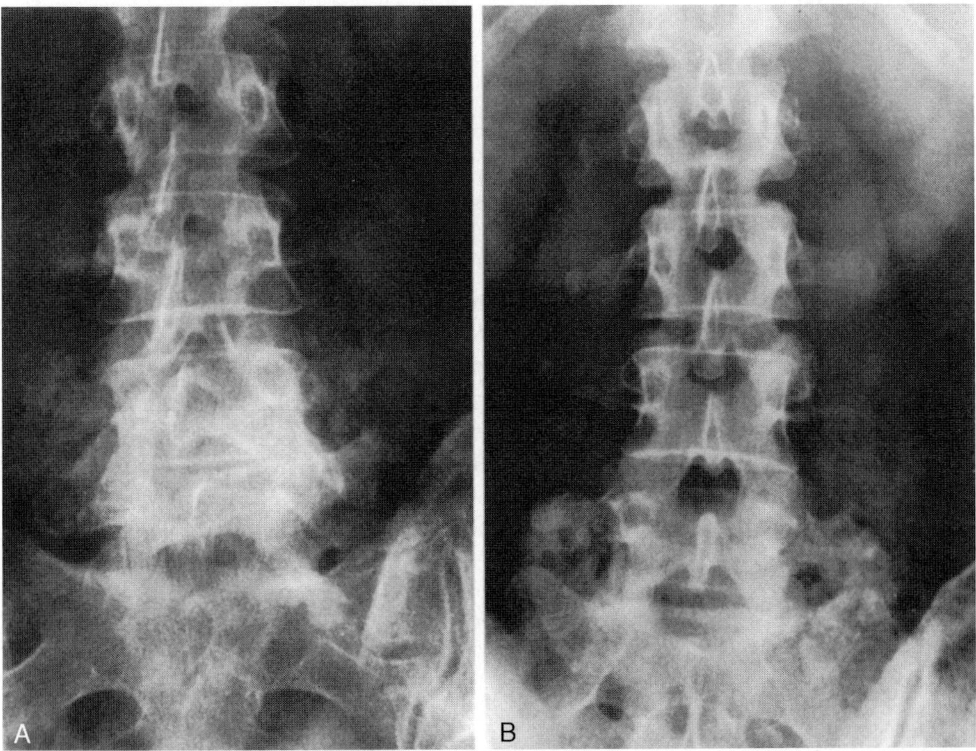

FIGURE 10-61 • **A:** A poor fusion mass (L4-L5, i.e., last mobile level) at 6 weeks: The patient was kept in a brace and then went on to undergo a solid fusion. **B:** A good fusion mass (L5-S1) at 6 weeks.

housewives may return to their duties with some persistent discomfort in 2 to 3 months. Patients whose jobs require prolonged standing, climbing stairs, walking, repetitive bending, and stooping rarely return to work in under 6 months. Patients engaged in heavy work will take 1 year to return to work. None will really experience the full benefit of the operative procedure until approximately 1 year to 18 months after surgery. Unless the patient is fully aware of the time involved and is prepared for it, the operation may lead to financial disaster. These points are particularly applicable when spinal fusion is considered for the injured workman.

It is our routine to brace all patients for a minimum of 6 to 8 weeks postoperatively. The choice of a brace is not important. We use a simple corset for single-level fusions simply to remind the patient to keep the trunk straight and not bent. We avoid multilevel fusions for degenerative disc disease and thus avoid the requirement for a more rigid corset. We do not use corsets or braces with external electrical stimulators because we have not seen any scientific studies to support their usefulness.

All patients are instructed to supplement their daily diet with 1500 mg of extra calcium per day, along with multivitamins with iron.

From day 1 of surgery, we encourage our patients to walk. On their first postoperative visit, we would like them to be walking up to 2 to 3 miles per day. Obviously, they are in their brace for this exercise. No other exercises are prescribed until the fusion mass shows signs of maturation.

The first postoperative visit is 6 to 8 weeks after surgery. At this time, radiographs and the patient's symptoms determine the need for further bracing for another 6 to 8 weeks. Patients with continuing back pain requiring analgesia and/or patients with less-than-optimal fusion mass (Fig. 10-61) are kept in their braces. A patient who is withdrawn from analgesic medication because of a reasonable comfort level and who shows signs of a good fusion mass (Fig. 10-61) is weaned from the brace and stepped up in activity.

For at least 3 months, patients are not allowed to smoke, drink excessively, or use NSAIDs or aspirinlike products. They are asked to "treat themselves well," that is, lots of rest, limited sitting, and no work for at least 6 to 8 weeks.

CONCLUSION

The classic disease model on which medicine is founded is known as the Sydenham model:

1. Signs and symptoms, when added together, suggest a pathology (etiology).
2. The diagnosis can be proved with appropriate tests.
3. There is a clearly prescribed treatment protocol that consistently alters the symptoms and signs (hopefully making them disappear, i.e., cure).

The lumbar disc rupture, causing sciatica, fits this disease model. Lumbar degenerative disc disease does not.

In the mid 1800s, the building of the railroad was an important part of the industrial revolution. Laborers and passengers started to show up with low back pain. Legislation was enacted enshrining the concept that all back pain arose from injury and was due some sort of financial reward. Since the introduction of these laws, back pain has become as much a societal phenomenon as a medical problem (42). It has become complicated by emotions, feelings about one's job or mate, financial reward, and so on. To step in with the simplistic concept of seeking the "pain generator" with both discography and the abolishing movement with an instrumented spinal fusion has caused considerable consternation for many health care professionals, insurers, and federal and state governments.

It is best to remember our admonitions throughout this chapter: Spinal fusion for disc degeneration is not commonly indicated. The emotionally stable, intelligent patient can usually keep this self-limiting condition under control with slight modification of daily activities, and the emotionally fragile are rarely helped by this surgical exercise.

REFERENCES

1. Axelsson P, Johnsson R, Stromquist B. Effect of lumbar orthosis on intervertebral mobility. *Spine.* 1992;17:678–681.
2. Beaman DN, Graziano GP, Glover RA, et al. Substance P innervation of lumbar spinal facets. *Spine.* 1993;18:1044–1049.
3. Bell GR, Rothman RH. The conservative treatment of sciatica. *Spine.* 1984;9:54–56.

4. Biering-Sorensen F. Physical measurements as risk indicators for low-back trouble over a one year period. *Spine.* 1984;9:106–119.
5. Bigos S, Bowyer O, Braen G, et al. *Acute Low Back Problems in Adults.* Clinical Practice Guideline, Quick Reference Guide Number 14. Rockville, MD: US Department of Health and Human Services, Public Health Service, Agency for Health Care Policy and Research, AHCPR Pub No. 95-0643, December 1994.
6. Boden SD, Davis DO, et al. Abnormal magnetic resonance scans of the lumbar spine in asymptomatic patients. *J Bone Joint Surg Am.* 1990;72:403–408.
7. Burwell RG. Studies in the transplantation of bone. *J Bone Joint Surg Br.* 1966;48:532–566.
8. Cady LD, Bischoff DP, O'Connell ER, et al. Strength and fitness and subsequent back injuries in firefighters. *J Occup Med.* 1979;21:169–272.
9. Crock HV. Isolated lumbar disc resorption as a cause of nerve root canal stenosis. *Clin Orthop.* 1976;115: 109–115.
10. Crock HV. Isolated disc resorption. In: Frymoyer, JW, ed. *The Adult Spine.* New York: Raven Press; 1991.
11. Esses SI, Botsford DJ, Kostuik JP. The role of external spinal skeletal fixation in the assessment of low-back disorders. *Spine.* 1989;14:594–601.
12. Esses SI, Sachs BL, Dreyzin V. Complications associated with the technique of pedicle screw fixation. A selected survey of ABS members. *Spine.* 1993;18:2231–2239.
13. Fairbank JCT, Park WM, McCall IW, O'Brien JP. Apophyseal injection of local anesthetic as a diagnostic aid in primary low back pain syndromes. *Spine.* 1981;6:598–605.
14. Forrester JC, Zederfeldt BH, Hayes TL, Hunt TK. Wolff's law in relation to the healing skin wound. *J Trauma.* 1970;10:770–779.
15. Fraser RD, Osti OL, Vernon-Roberts B. Discitis after discography. *J Bone Joint Surg Br.* 1987;69:26–35.
16. Friedlaender GE, Strong DM, Sell KW. Studies on the antigenicity of bone. *J Bone Joint Surg Am.* 1984;66:107–112.
17. Frymoyer JW, Cats-Baril WL. An overview of the incidences and costs of low back pain. *Orthop Clin North Am.* 1991;22:263–271.
18. Ghormley RK. Low back pain with special reference to the articular facets, with presentation of an operative procedure. *JAMA.* 1933;101:1773–1777.
19. Godfrey CM, Morgan PP, Schatzker J. A randomized trial of manipulation for low-back pain in a medical setting. *Spine.* 1984;9:301–304.
20. Goldberg VM, Bos GD, Heiple KG, et al. Improved acceptance of frozen bone allograft in genetically mismatched dogs by immunosuppression. *J Bone Joint Surg Am.* 1984;66:937–950.
21. Grubb SA, Lipscomb HJ, Conrad RW. Degenerative adult onset scoliosis. *Spine.* 1988;13:241–245.
22. Hazard RG, Fenwick JW, Kalisch SM, et al. Functional restoration with behavioral support: a one year prospective study of patients with chronic low back pain. *Spine.* 1989;14:157–161.
23. Heiple KG, Chase SW, Herndon CH. A comparative study of the healing process following different types of bone transplantation. *J Bone Joint Surg Am.* 1963;45:1593–1616.
24. Holm S. Pathophysiology of disc degeneration. *Acta Orthop Scand.* 1993;64(suppl 251):13–15.
25. Holmes RE, Salyer KF. Bone regeneration in coralline hydroxyapatite implant. *Surg Forum.* 1978;24: 611–616.
26. Hudgins WR. Diagnostic accuracy of lumbar discography. *Spine.* 1977;2:305–309.
27. Jackson RP. The facet syndrome: myth or reality? *Clin Orthop.* 1992;279:110–121.
28. Jackson RP, Cain JE, et al. The neuroradiographic diagnosis of lumbar herniated nucleus pulposus. *Spine.* 1989;14:1356–1361.
29. Jackson RP, Jacobs RR, Montesano PX. Facet joint injections in low-back pain. A prospective statistical study. *Spine.* 1988;13:966–971.
30. Kahanovitz N. Electrical Stimulation of Spinal Fusion. In: Herkowitz H, Garfin S, et al., eds. Rothman-Simeone *The Spine* 5th ed. Philadelphia: Saunders Elsevier; 2006.
31. Kirkaldy-Willis WH, Farfan HE. Instability of the lumbar spine. *Clin Orthop.* 1982;165:110–123.
32. Kuslich SD, Ulstrom CL, Michael CJ. The tissue of origin of low back pain and sciatica: a report of pain response to tissue stimulation during operations on the lumbar spine using local anesthesia. *Orthop Clin North Am.* 1991;22:181–187.
33. Lee CK, Langrana NA. Lumbosacral spinal fusion. A biomechanical study. *Spine.* 1984;9:574–581.
34. Lorenz M, et al. A comparison of single-level fusions with and without hardware. *Spine.* 1991;16:S455–S458.
35. Marchesi DG, Aebi M. Pedicle fixation devices in the treatment of adult lumbar scoliosis. *Spine.* 1992;17:5304–S309.
36. McCulloch JA, Waddell G. Lateral lumbar discography. *Br J Radiol.* 1978;51:498–502.
37. McKenzie RA. *The Lumbar Spine. Mechanical Diagnosis and Therapy.* Waikanae, New Zealand: Spinal Publications, Limited; 1981.
38. Mitchell RI, Carmen GM. Results of multicenter trial using an intensive active exercise program for the treatment of acute soft tissue and back injuries. *Spine.* 1990;15:514–521.
39. Mixter WJ, Barr JS. Rupture of the intervertebral disc with involvement of the spinal canal. *N Engl J Med.* 1934;211:210–215.
40. Mooney V, Derian C. Synthetic bone graft. In: White AH, Rothman RH, Ray CD, eds. *Lumbar Spine Surgery.* St. Louis, Mo: CV Mosby; 1987:471–482.
41. Mooney V, Robertson J. The facet syndrome. *Clin Orthop.* 1976;115:149–156.
42. Nachemson A. Work for all. For those with low back pain as well. *Clin Orthop.* 1983;179:77–85.
43. Ordeberg G, Enskog J, Sjostrom L. Diagnostic external fixation of the lumbar spine. *Acta Orthop Scand.* 1993;64(suppl 251):94–96.

44. Pope MH, Frymoyer JW, Krag MH. Diagnosing instability. *Clin Orthop.* 1992;279:60–67.
45. Rowe ML. Preliminary statistical study of low back pain. *J Occup Med.* 1963;5:336–341.
46. Rowe ML. Low back pain in industry. A position paper. *J Occup Med.* 1969;11:161–169.
47. Shinomiya K, Nakao K, et al. Evaluation of cervical discography in pain origin and provocation. *J Spinal Disorders.* 1993;6:422–426.
48. Simmons JW, Emery S, et al. Awake discography. A comparison study with magnetic resonance imaging. *Spine.* 1991;165:S216–S221.
49. Urist MR, Dawson E. Intertransverse process fusion with the aid of chemosterilized autolyzed antigen-extracted allogenic (AAA) bone. *Clin Orthop.* 1981;154:97–113.
50. Venner RM, Crock AU. Clinical studies of isolated disc resorption in the lumbar spine. *J Bone Joint Surg Br.* 1981;63:491–494.
51. White AH. *Back School and Other Conservative Approaches to Low Back Pain.* St. Louis, MO: CV Mosby; 1983.
52. Wiley JJ, Macnab I, Wortzman G. Lumbar discography and its clinical applications. *Can J Surg.* 1968;11: 280–289.
53. Williams PC. Examination and conservative treatment for disc lesions of the lower lumbar spine. *Clin Orthop.* 1955;5:28–35.
54. Yasuma T, Ohno R, Yamauchi Y. False-negative lumbar discograms. *J Bone Joint Surg.* 1988;70:1279–1290.
55. Yuan HA, Garfin SR, Dickman CA, Mardjetko SM. A historical cohort study of pedicle screw fixation in thoracic, lumbar and sacral spine fusions. *Spine.* 1994;19:2279S–2296S.

CHAPTER 11

Disc Degeneration with Root Irritation: Disc Ruptures

"Thou cold sciatica, cripple our senators and make their limbs halt as lamely as their manners."

—W. Shakespeare

A patient with a mechanical compression of a lumbar nerve root will present with the complaint of leg (radicular) pain with or without associated pain in the back. However, it cannot be too strongly emphasized that the mere complaint of pain in the leg does not indicate, by itself, root irritation or root compression. Any painful lesion on the lumbosacral region may give rise to pain referred down the leg in a sciatic distribution. Diabetes can affect peripheral nerves and mimic sciatica due to a disc rupture (6,18).

Referred or "reflex" pain has the same neurophysiologic basis as the referred pain to the shoulder associated with gallbladder disease and the referred pain down the arm associated with myocardial infarcts.

Referred leg pain derived from mechanical insufficiency of the lumbar spine is rarely experienced below the knee: it is not associated with paresthesia, and there is no evidence of root tension, as reflected by limitation of straight leg raising (SLR) or the presence of a positive bowstring sign.

DISC RUPTURES (HERNIATED NUCLEUS PULPOSUS)

To understand the clinical syndrome of lumbar root irritation and compression due to a disc rupture is to take the most important step in understanding all of low back pain. Although there is tremendous variation in the presentation of a patient with a disc rupture causing sciatica, there is a common thread of historical and physical features that allows for a fairly accurate clinical diagnosis.

CLINICAL PICTURE

History

Onset. It is fairly constant that a patient who has radicular pain due to a disc rupture has, or had, back pain in their history. The exception to this is the younger patient who may manifest only leg pain as a symptom of the disc rupture and at no time will have had back pain. However, most patients with a disc rupture will have experienced some degree of prodromal back pain for varying lengths of time (from minutes to years). It may be intermittent in its occurrence and extended over a considerable period of time, representing the instability phase that Kirkaldy-Willis et al. (31) has described. It may be acute, followed soon after by the onset of leg pain.

Approximately half of the patients will attribute their back pain to various forms of traumatic experience. This is especially prevalent in the litigation and compensation population but, in fact, is retrograde rationalization on the part of many patients. Experimental studies and careful statistical analysis of case histories (30) do not support the concept that direct trauma or sudden weight loading of the spine are the causal agents of disc rupture, although they may aggravate a preexisting asymptomatic degenerative condition.

Either in a gradual or sudden fashion, the pain will lateralize to the hip or leg. This moment of lateralization heralds the contact of the ruptured disc with the nerve root and may or may not be precipitated by a simple traumatic event, such as bending over in the shower to pick up the soap.

Location of pain. Various combinations of back, hip, and leg pain present. When trying to understand sciatica, think of five different areas: the back, the buttock, the thigh, the leg, and the foot. There may be symptoms in all five areas or only in a few of these areas.

The back. Back pain is considered to be pain localized to the midline lumbosacral region. Any radiation of pain from this area should most likely be considered lateralization of discomfort, and except for the vague referred pain, possibly indicative of radicular involvement. This is a rather controversial statement, but we think that as one gains more experience with radicular involvement, this historical feature will become more evident. Radiation to such areas as the sacroiliac joint region, the high iliac crest region, and the coccygeal region is more indicative of dural irritation than the commonly believed notion that the pain radiation represents muscular splinting of the back with referred pain. This is especially true if this referral is associated with leg pain characteristics as follows:

The buttock. In essence, the buttock is the proximal part of the leg (Fig. 11-1). The younger the patient, the more likely sciatica will be limited to the buttock and more proximal lower extremity. The nature of the pain in the buttock is usually one of a deep-seated, sometimes cramping pain that is especially aggravated by sitting.

The thigh. Pain in this area tends to be the sharpest component of sciatica and sometimes is described as having an associated superficial "burning-sensitive" feeling. For both L5 and S1 root involvement, it is located in the posterolateral or posterior thigh and not the lateral thigh. For higher lumbar root involvement, the sharp pain will be in the anterior thigh. Unless the patient has a very sensitive bowstring sign, pain is usually absent from the popliteal fossa.

The leg. The sensation in this area can be mixed. For L5 to S1 root compression, the prevailing discomfort is a cramp and almost viselike feeling in the belly of the gastrocsoleus or peroneal muscles. In addition, the patient may report a paresthetic discomfort in the lateral calf (fifth root) or back of the calf (first root). Most but not all adult patients with sciatica due to a herniated nucleus pulposus (HNP) will have pain below the knee. Again, the younger patient can be a trap, in that he

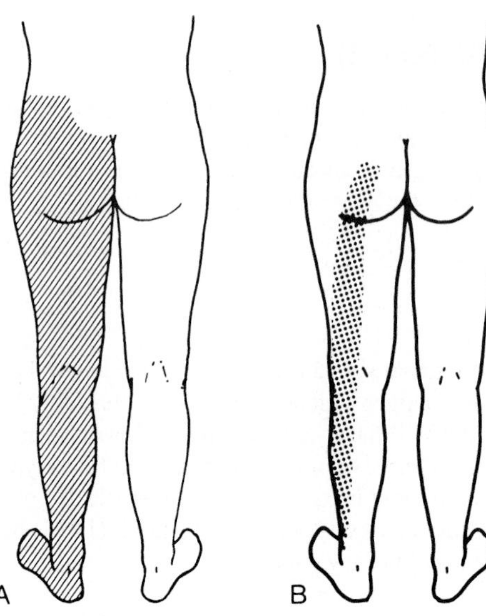

FIGURE 11-1 ● **A:** The proximal part of the leg is the buttock. Pain in the buttock is considered leg pain. **B:** Radicular pain will be confined to a nerve root distribution in the leg.

or she may have pain only in the high iliac crest region, the proximal buttock, and/or thigh. Although rare, this does occur, and offers much confusion in the assessment of the young patient with a disc rupture.

Higher lumbar root lesions (L2, L3, L4) will have no pain below the knee. In L4 root involvement, the patient will often describe a paresthetic discomfort down the medial shin (below the knee), but not pain.

The foot. Unlike the calf, the most common symptom in the foot is paresthesia rather than pain. The lateral border of undersurface of the foot is often, but not always, involved with 1st sacral root compression, whereas the dorsum of the foot may be affected with fifth lumbar root involvement. It is unusual that the patient will complain of pain in the foot.

The term sciatica implies that the patient has leg pain. The younger the patient with a disc rupture, the more likely the sciatic pain will dominate the history. It is a good general rule that, regardless of age, if the radiating hip and leg pain is, at all times, less significant to the patient than the complaint of back pain, the sciatica is not likely due to a disc rupture.

In general, pain derived from the L5 to S1 root involvement courses down the posterior aspect of the leg, whereas lesions of the second, third, and fourth lumbar roots give rise to pain on the anterior part of the thigh (39). It is routine for sciatic pain due to fifth and first root compression to radiate below the knee but, as often mentioned, the younger patient may not have this more distal radiation of discomfort. It is safe to teach that most sciatic pain due to root compression radiates below the knee, but there are exceptions to every generalization in medicine.

Paresthesia in the form of tingling, pins and needles, or numbness is of great value in localizing the level of root compression (29), and the more distal its location, the more reliable it is in helping with root localization. If a patient can volunteer that the paresthetic discomfort is along the lateral border of the foot into the little toe or up the back of the calf, one can assume that the most likely nerve root involved is S_1. Similarly, paresthetic discomfort over the dorsum of the foot or lateral calf implicates the fifth lumbar nerve root; paresthesia over the medial shin indicates fourth lumbar root involvement. Similarly, paresthetic discomfort centered around the knee indicates third root involvement, and lateral thigh pins and needles indicates second root involvement. If the paresthetic discomfort or numbness is vaguely described and has a stocking-and-glove-like distribution, it is not indicative of radicular involvement and is more suggestive of a neuropathy or psychogenic pain. Rarely, motor symptoms predominate and are more disabling to the patient. In such instances, the clinician has to beware of the presence of a spinal tumor or a peripheral neuropathy. When trying to determine the localization of leg pain, have the patient put his/her foot up on a chair and then draw the location of their symptoms (Fig. 11-2).

Aggravation. Back and sciatic discomfort is spondylogenic in nature. That is to say, the pain is aggravated by general and specific activities and relieved by rest. Bending, stooping, lifting, coughing, sneezing, and straining at stool will intensify the pain. Which particular activity bothers a patient varies from patient to patient. Most patients with sciatica find difficulty in sitting, especially in a soft lounge chair, including most automobile seats. Standing and walking, although not comfortable, are usually more tolerable. Some patients may find other forms of activity aggravating, but a constant thread throughout the history of sciatica is the fact that some activity bothers the patient. The corollary is also true; if a patient with sciatica rests long enough, or gets into the proper position, some relief of the leg pain will ensue. Aggravation of sciatic discomfort by coughing and sneezing is one of the most commonly mentioned symptoms in textbooks. Although rather specific for radicular involvement, aggravation of pain due to coughing and sneezing is absent often enough from the history to be considered insensitive as a symptom.

Relief. Most patients get some relief from lying in the hip-knee flexed position (Fig. 11-2B). Sleeping is a more comfortable position for most patients when it is done with a pillow under the knees (Fig. 11-2C) or on the asymptomatic side in the fetal position. Some patients have so much sciatic discomfort that there is no position of comfort. This is especially true for the high lumbar root lesions.

Unusual referral patterns of pain. On occasion, unusual referral patterns of pain may occur, such as perineal or testicular discomfort and lower abdominal discomfort. Waddell and Main (55,56) have stated that referral of pain to the low sacrococcygeal region is suggestive of nonorganic involvement. We believe that just the opposite is true, in that patients with midline dural irritation will often refer discomfort to the lower sacrococcygeal region. Testicular pain is also common and somewhat

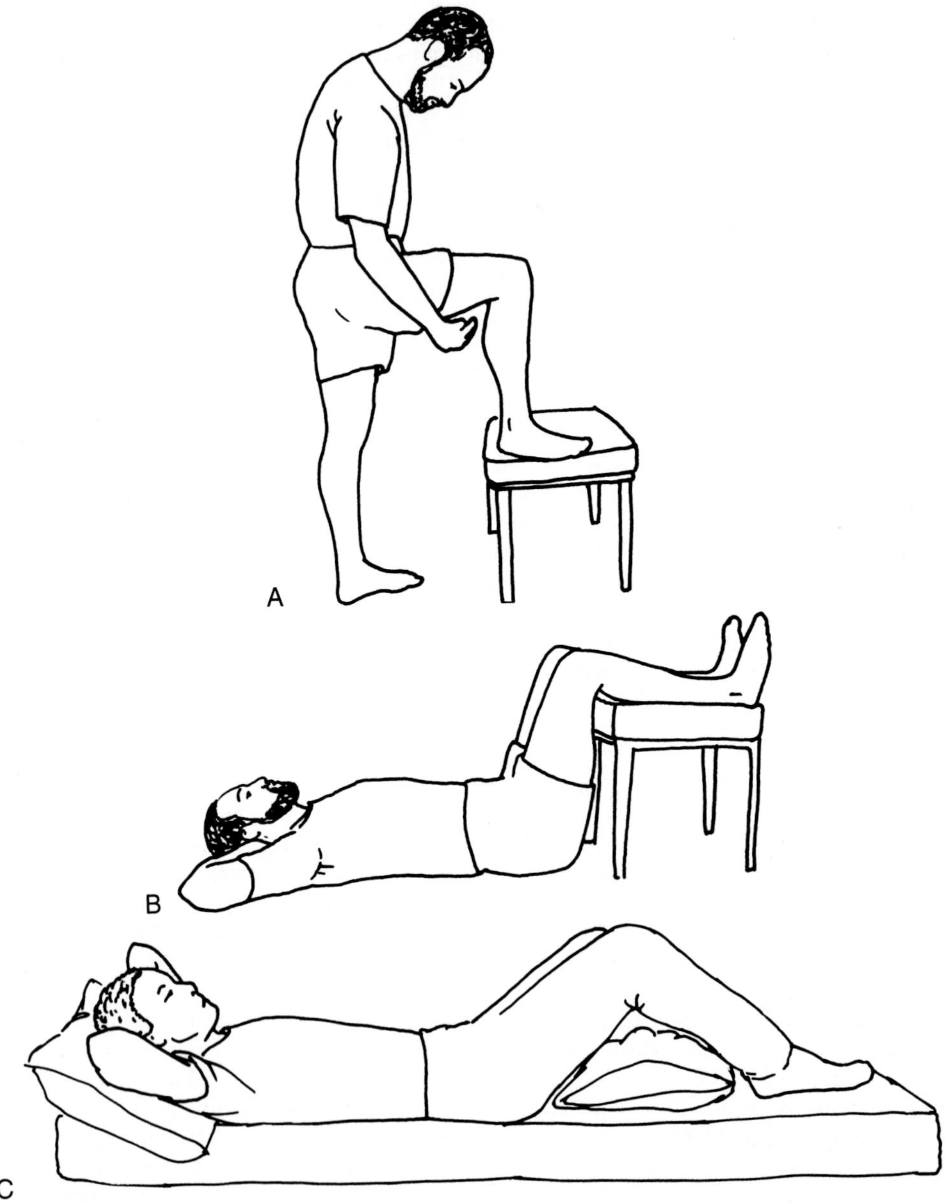

FIGURE 11-2 ● **A:** Ask the patient to put the symptomatic foot up on a chair and draw the distribution of the leg pain. If he or she draws a line in a radicular distribution with one finger, you not only have the diagnosis of radicular syndrome—you can usually figure out which root is involved. **B:** Most patients with sciatica will have figured out that the fastest way to relief of some leg pain, when they get home from work, is to assume this position. **C:** The position of comfort when in bed (the semi-Fowler position).

confusing. Obviously, anyone with testicular pain needs to evaluated for a local testicular cause of their discomfort. In some cases, this referral to the testicular region, or perineum in women, is again due to irritation of the midline sacral nerve roots. On a rare occasion, it is indicative of a higher lumbar disc lesion and represents the dermatomal radicular distribution of pain (L1 root).

Severe sciatica. On occasion, you will encounter a patient who has so much leg pain that he or she will not be able to localize the symptoms. These are the patients who say either, "fix my leg pain or amputate my leg." To persist in trying to get them to localize their leg pain or their paresthesias is fruitless. Get on with the examination and the diagnosis!

PHYSICAL EXAMINATION

The physical examination of a patient with sciatica due to a disc rupture is so variable as to be confusing. Some patients present with little in the way of back findings, with all of their findings confined to the lower extremities, whereas others present with incapacitating back spasm, sciatic scoliosis, and are significantly disabled. The common thread through this variable presentation is the fact that the majority of objective findings in a patient with sciatica due to a disc rupture will be in the lower extremity rather than the back.

The Back

The posture is characteristic. The lumbar spine is flattened and slightly flexed. The patient often leans away from the side of pain, and this sciatic scoliosis become more obvious on bending forward. The patient is more comfortable standing with the affected hip and knee slightly flexed, a manner accentuated by asking the patient to flex forward (Fig. 11-3). In the very acute phase, these patients will walk in obvious discomfort, sometimes holding their loins with the hands. The gait is slow and deliberate and is designed to avoid any unnecessary movement of the spine. With gross tension on the nerve root, the patient may not be able to put the heel to the floor and walks slowly and painfully on tip-toe. On rare occasion, this reaction may extend to needing crutches for ambulation.

Forward flexion may be permitted so the hands reach the knees by virtue of flexion of the hip joint. If the examiner keeps his/her fingertips on the spinous processes, it can be felt that the lumbar spine moves little because of splinting. Limitation of flexion in such instances is, therefore, the result of root tension and is due to the increase in leg pain. The degree of flexion should be recorded by measuring the distance between the fingertips and the floor.

Extension is also limited, although to a lesser degree than flexion, and in most instances the pelvis starts to rotate as soon as the patient attempts to lean backward. The complaint on extension is usually back pain, but at times the patient may feel leg pain. It is our impression that the complaint of leg pain on extension is indicative of an extruded or sequestered disc.

Lateral flexion can be full and free to one side, but usually lateral flexion toward the concavity of the sciatic curve (side of sciatica) is limited. The phenomenon of sciatic scoliosis and the relief of aggravation of pain on lateral flexion have been attributed to the position of the protrusion in relation to the nerve root (Fig. 11-4). However, this may be a simplistic explanation in view of the fact

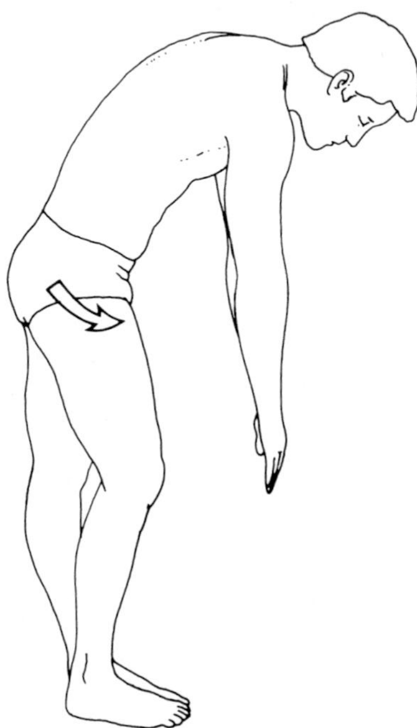

FIGURE 11-3 ● The classic posture in sciatica on forward flexion; the knee of the affected leg flexes while the hip rotates forward (external rotation of hip to relax pyriformis).

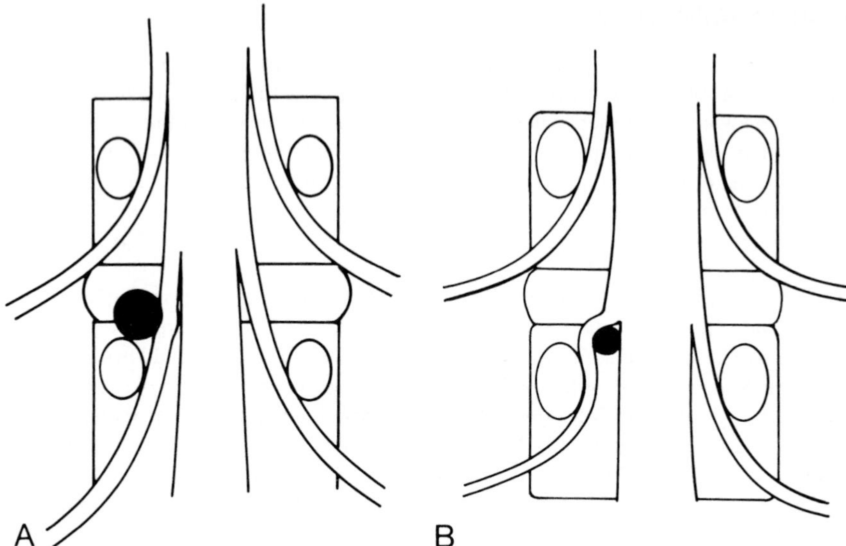

FIGURE 11-4 ● **A:** A disc herniation lateral to the nerve root. Theoretically, lateral flexion to the same side would increase the pain. **B:** An axillary disc herniation. Theoretically, lateral flexion to the opposite side increases the pain.

that the sciatic scoliosis disappears on recumbency. This observation, the loss of lateral curvature of the lumbar spine on recumbency, differentiates the sciatic list from a fixed structural scoliosis.

Tenderness and Muscle Spasm

In the standing position, especially in the presence of scoliosis, muscle spasm can be observed. However, at rest, the spasm often subsides, and there is little tenderness to be found on examination. Selectively palpating and applying a lateral thrust to the spinous process may cause some back pain and, on the rare occasion, produce leg pain. The patient with sciatica due to a HNP, at complete rest in the prone position on the examining table, has little symptoms to be found in the back. The patient's major complaint is leg pain, and the majority of physical findings are in the extremity.

The Extremities

The cardinal signs of lumbar root compromise are root tension, root irritation, and root compression.

Root tension and irritation. The term "root tension" denotes distortion of the emerging nerve root by an extradural lesion. The two most useful tests for the presence of root tension are limitation of SLR and the bowstring sign, the latter also arising in part from root irritation.

When testing SLR, it is important not to hurt the patient. Never jerk the leg up in the air suddenly. The knee must be kept fully extended by firm pressure exerted by the examiner's hand, while the hip is slightly internally rotated and adducted. With the other hand under the heel, the examiner slowly raises the leg until leg pain is produced (Fig. 11-5). Two additional maneuvers are of vital importance to add significance to the finding of limitation of SLR:

1. Aggravation of pain by forced dorsiflexion of the ankle at the limit of SLR (a variation of Lasegue's sign) (52,58)
2. Relief of pain by flexion of the knee and hip

Physiogenic sciatic pain due to nerve root tension is always relieved by flexion of the knee and hip. Further flexion of the patient's hip with the knee bent does not reproduce and aggravate sciatic pain (Fig. 11-5). This phenomenon is only seen in the emotionally destroyed.

If SLR is permissible to 60 to 70 degrees before leg pain is produced, the finding is equivocal for an HNP. Below this level, the reproduction of pain on SLR, aggravated by dorsiflexion of the

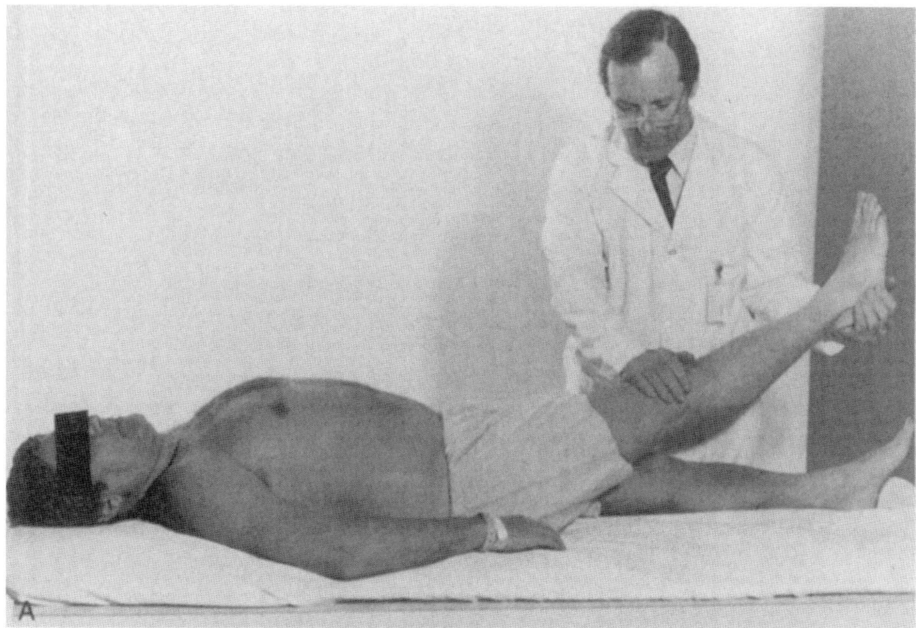

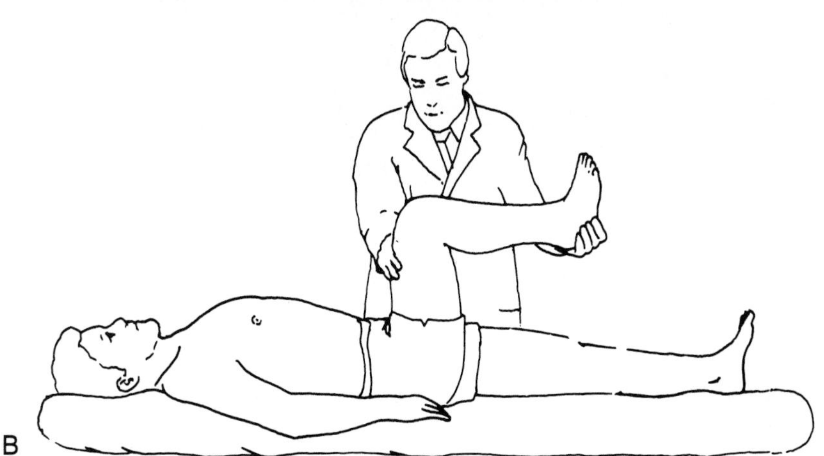

FIGURE 11-5 ● **A:** The standard for the straight leg raising (SLR) test: knee straight, hip neutral or slight internal rotation, and slow lifting of the leg by the heel. **B:** Hip and knee flexion should relieve the pain of radicular origin.

ankle and relieved by flexion of the knee, is strongly suggestive of tension on the fifth lumbar or first sacral root. In patients in whom paresthesia in the foot is a predominant symptom, repetitive SLR, that is, "pumping of the leg," frequently intensifies the sensation of numbness.

Location of pain on SLR. The examiner is seeking to reproduce leg (buttock, thigh, and/or calf) pain when doing the SLR test. Reproduction of back pain, especially in the high ranges of SLR testing, is usually not indicative of root tension. However, there is one exception that is discussed later in this chapter under midline disc herniation.

False-positive SLR test. Hamstring tightness may cloud the assessment of the SLR test. Patients with hamstring tightness have a generally tight body build (e.g., inability to fully extend the elbow) and plenty of room between the wrist flexed, thumb abducted position, and the volar surface of the forearm (Fig. 11-6). Hamstring tightness should be bilateral, and the discomfort the patient experiences is distal in the thigh, in the region of the hamstring tendons. Hamstring tightness

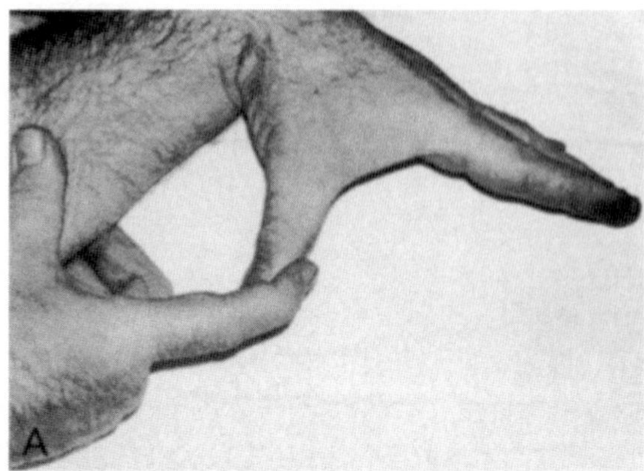

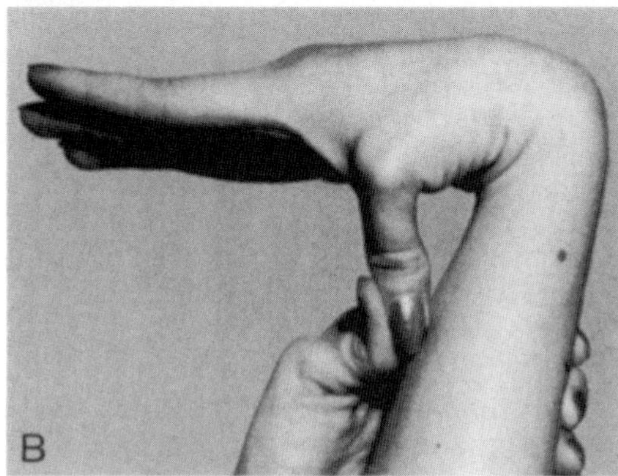

FIGURE 11-6 ● **A:** A tight-jointed individual with limited abduction of thumb. **B:** A loose-jointed individual with much greater passive abduction ability.

does not radiate below the knee. Finally, other physical findings of root irritation and compression are absent in hamstring tightness.

False-negative SLR test. On occasion, you will encounter a loose-jointed individual with sciatica due to an HNP. On SLR testing, you may not be impressed with the degree of impaired SLR until you examine the unaffected leg and see the individual's ability to straight leg raise well beyond 90 degrees.

Bowstring sign. The bowstring sign (7) is an important indication of root tension or irritation. The examiner carries out SLR to the point at which the patient experiences some discomfort in the distribution of the sciatic nerve. At this level, the knee is allowed to flex, and the patient's foot is allowed to rest on the examiner's shoulder (Fig. 11-7). The test demands sudden, firm pressure applied to the popliteal nerve in the popliteal fossa. The action may startle the patient enough to make him or her jump, and this jump may hurt. To prevent this, first of all, tell the patient that you are just going to press firmly on the back of the knee and that it may hurt. Apply firm pressure to the hamstrings; this will not hurt. Then, move your thumbs over to the popliteal nerve. A positive bowstring test is reproduction of radiating leg discomfort. Most commonly, the radiating discomfort is pain felt proximally in the thigh and even into the back. Less commonly, radiating discomfort will travel distally, and this discomfort is more often paresthetic in nature than painful. If the test produces only local pain in the popliteal fossa, it is of no significance. This demonstration of root irritation is probably the single most important sign in the diagnosis of tension and irritation of a nerve root caused by a ruptured intervertebral disc.

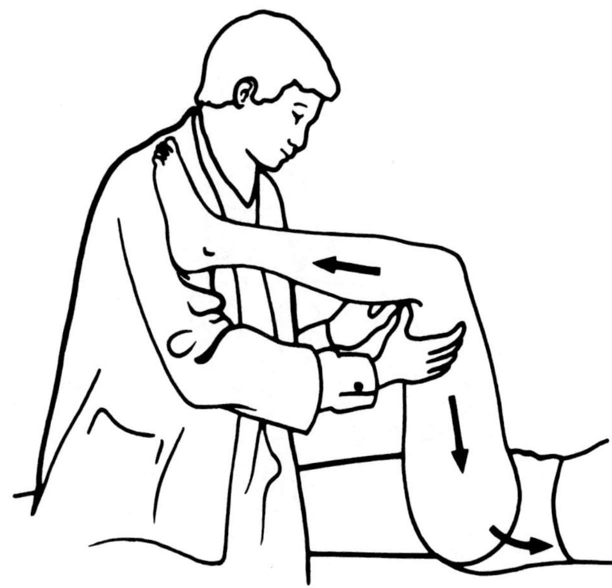

FIGURE 11-7 ● The bowstring test.

Tests to verify SLR reduction. When the patient sits with knees dangling over the side of the bed, the hip and knee are both flexed at 90 degrees. If the knee is now extended fully, the position assumed by the leg is equivalent to 90 degrees of SLR (Fig. 11-8). If the patient is suffering from root compromise, this will cause sudden, severe pain, and the patient will throw his or her trunk backward to avoid tension on the nerve. This is commonly referred to as the "positive flip test." With the psychogenic regional pain syndrome, the patient will permit the examiner to extend the knee of the painful leg without showing any response at all.

Crossover pain (Well-Leg Raising Sign). There is some confusion as to what constitutes a positive crossed SLR test (61). Some have stated that a positive crossed SLR test occurs when you lift the symptomatic leg and produce pain in the asymptomatic leg. Historically, the original description of crossover pain was the reverse; that is, when lifting the well leg, pain crosses over into the symptomatic hip. Most people would agree that a positive crossed SLR test occurs when the well leg is lifted and the opposite symptomatic side becomes more painful. This is indicative of a disc herniation lying medial to the nerve root, either in the axilla of the nerve root or in a midline position.

A variation in the crossover pain test is the sitting SLR test. If in the sitting position, SLR of the well leg crosses pain over to the symptomatic hip, this is pathognomonic of an HNP. This test is valuable in assessing a patient with combined organic and nonorganic features. It is of value in assessing patients with acute back conditions who have significant back pain in the supine position on SLR tests. Some of them may be able to sit, and it is in this position that SLR testing can be done, with crossover pain being an early sign of an HNP, and the absence of SLR reduction or crossover pain indicating acute back muscle strain only.

Nonorganic Pain. If the patient complains of severe sciatic pain when attempting to bend forward, and there is a suspicion that there may be a significant degree of functional overlay, the patient should be asked to kneel on a chair. This will relax the hamstrings and reduce the tension of the sciatic nerve. In this position, the patient is asked to bend forward. With a physiogenic source of pain, the patient will be able to bend the spine and let his or her fingertips go below the level of the seat. In the nonorganic pain phenomenon, even with the knees flexed and the patient kneeling on a chair, he or she will not allow the spine to bend (Fig. 11-9).

Nerve root pain is probably the result of a combination of pressure and an inflammatory response to the prolapsed disc material. This "inflammatory response," or "radiculitis," has been loosely termed "root irritation." Root irritation is an important factor in the demonstrated limitation of SLR, and it would appear to be productive of peripheral muscle tenderness. Such tenderness is not always present,

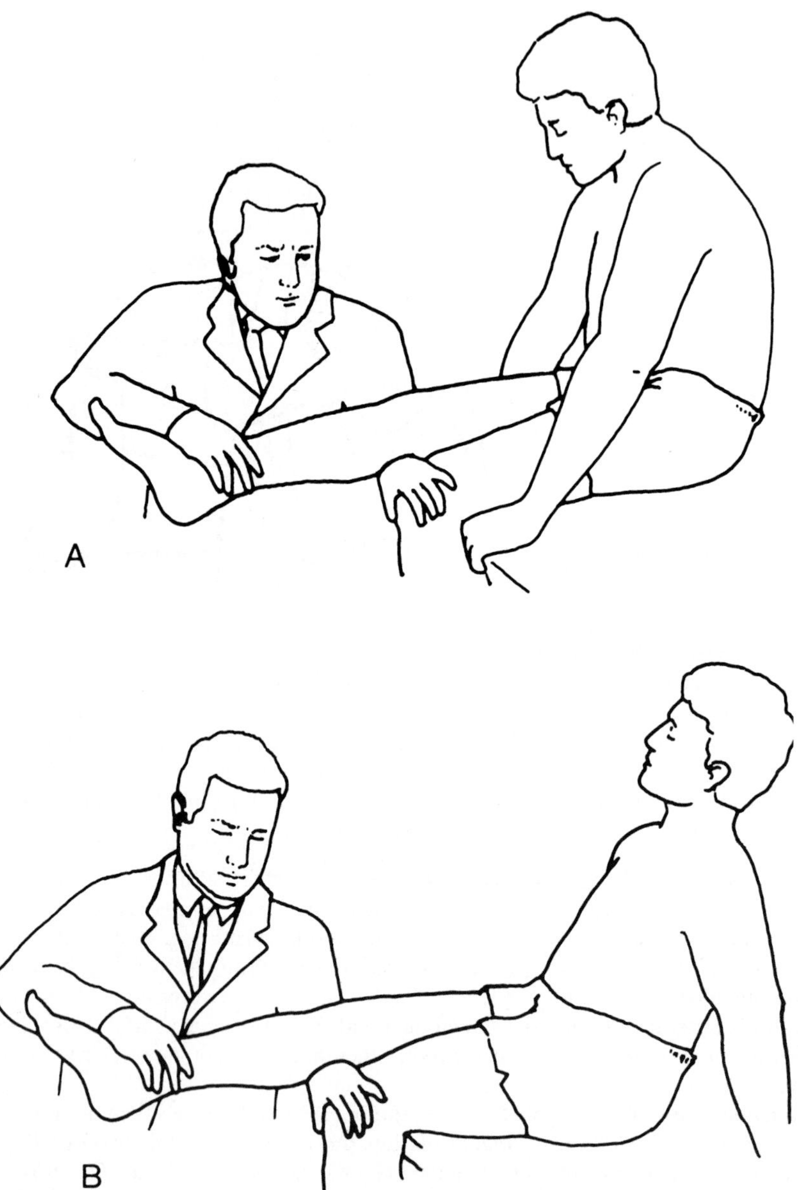

FIGURE 11-8 ● The flip test (staged). **A:** Negative. No backward flip on 90 degrees of straight leg raising (SLR) because there is no root tension. **B:** Positive. Physical root tension (SLR test) causes patient to flip posteriorly when straight leg is raised.

but, if demonstrable, it is of value in localizing the level of root involvement (15,51). Frequently, the calf is tender with S1 root lesions, the anterior tibial compartment is tender with L5 root involvement, and the quadriceps is tender when the fourth lumbar nerve root has been compromised.

The shin is the body image of the leg, and very marked tenderness on palpating the subcutaneous surface of the tibia should warn the clinician that the patient has a large emotional content in this total disability. In the psychogenic regional pain syndromes, the patient frequently presents skin tenderness with pain on merely pinching the skin. Obviously, no meaningful statement can be made about the presence of deep muscle tenderness unless skin tenderness has been tested first. This is a trap for the unwary.

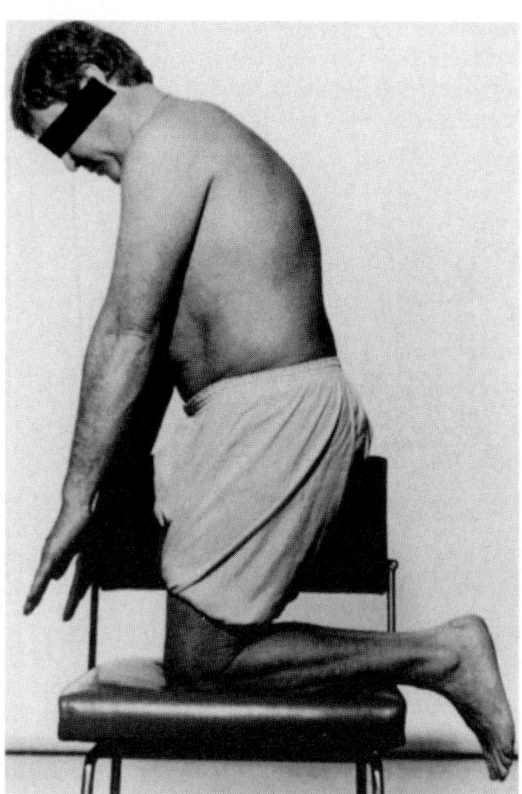

FIGURE 11-9 ● Nonorganic reaction. The patient will not permit any flexion of spine despite relaxation of hamstrings.

It should be noted that the upper quadrant of the buttock is a tender area in most people, with or without backache, and this area becomes increasingly tender in the presence of root irritation at any segment. The demonstration of this tenderness is of no localizing value. Patients with discogenic back pain with root irritation may also present tenderness over the sacroiliac joints and down the course of the sciatic nerve. This referred tenderness over the sacroiliac joint has given rise to confusion in the past, which results in the diagnosis of "sacroiliac strain" without any other clinical or radiologic evidence of damage to the sacroiliac joint.

Femoral nerve stretch. Figure 11-10 shows the femoral nerve stretch test. It is not nearly as satisfactory a test as is the SLR test but is considered positive when unilateral thigh pain is produced and aggravated by knee flexion (9), and it indicates tension on the second, third, or fourth lumbar roots. It is difficult to interpret in the presence of hip and/or knee pathology.

Impairment of root conduction (Root Compression). The diagnosis of disc rupture is in no way exclusively dependent on the demonstration of root impairment as reflected by signs of motor weakness, changes in sensory appreciation, or reflex activity. However, the presence of such changes reinforces the diagnosis (20,53). The common neurologic changes are documented in Table 11-1.

Changes in reflex activity. The ankle jerk may be diminished or absent with an S1 lesion. This is tested with the patient kneeling on a chair or sitting comfortably. If a patient's sciatica is so bad that he or she cannot sit with comfort, do not test any reflex in the sitting position, as the subconscious guarding and posturing required of the patient to become less uncomfortable will upset the assessment of reflexes. This guarding and posturing explains the occasional depression of a knee reflex seen in the presence of sciatica due to an L5–S1 disc protrusion. If the patient has suffered from a previous attack of sciatic pain with significant compression of the first sacral nerve to obliterate the ankle jerk, this may not return to normal. The absence of an ankle jerk, therefore, may merely be a stigma of a previous episode of disc rupture, and the present attack may be due to a disc rupture at another level. Scratching the sole of the foot, as in the plantar

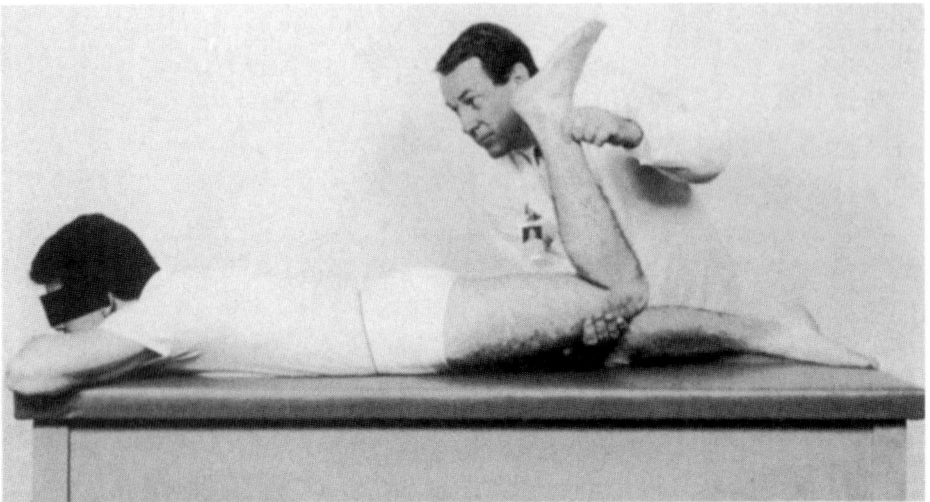

FIGURE 11-10 ● The femoral nerve stretch test.

response, produces a reflex contraction of the tensor fascia femoris. This little-known reflex is often lost with an S1 lesion.

With an L5 root compression, the tibialis posterior reflex (obtained by striking the tendon of the tibialis posterior near its point of insertion) may be absent. This is a pure L5 response. The clinician has to practice obtaining this reflex because it is not easy to elicit. Diminution of the lateral hamstring jerk is also seen on occasion with an L5 root compromise, but multiple innervation of this muscle group makes this an unreliable reflex. With L4 and L3 lesions, the knee jerk may be diminished.

Wasting. Muscle wasting is rarely seen unless the symptoms have been present for more than 3 weeks. Very marked wasting is more suggestive of an extradural tumor than a disc rupture.

The girths of the thigh and calf can be measured. This will act as a baseline, on occasion, to assess the progress of the lesion. It must be remembered that if there is gross weakness of the gastrocnemius, the main venous pump of the affected extremity is no longer working, and these patients may, indeed, show some measure of ankle edema. The combination of calf tenderness due to S1 root irritation and the observation of a swollen ankle may give rise to the erroneous diagnosis of a thrombophlebitis.

TABLE 11-1

Common Neurologic Changes in Herniated Nucleus Pulposus (HNP)

	Root		
	L4	L5	S1
Change			
Motor weakness	Knee extension, ankle dorsiflexion	Ankle[a] dorsiflexion EHL	Ankle plantar flexion FHL
Sensory loss	Medial shin below knee	Dorsum of foot and lateral calf	Lateral border of foot and posterior calf
Reflex depression	Knee	Tibialis posterior, lateral hamstrings	Ankle
Wasting	Thigh (no calf)	Calf (minimal thigh)	Calf (no thigh)

EHL, extensor hallucis longus; FHL, flexor hallucis longus.

[a]To separate peroneal nerve palsy from L5 root, examine tibialis posterior (inversion/plantar flexion), which will be weak in latter and not in former.

Motor Loss. The weakness of the gastrocnemii is best demonstrated by getting the patient to rise on tiptoe five or six times (Fig. 11-11). The patient is asked if it requires more effort to rise on tiptoe on the affected extremity. If the quadriceps are weak, the physician must be wary of this before ascribing the difficulty of tiptoe rising to weakness of the calf muscles. If sciatic pain is severe, the test cannot be performed by the patient. Jumping on tiptoe may be painful, and it is not a good method of examination, although slight weakness may be assessed by asking the patient to walk backward and forward across the length of the examining room on tiptoes to find out whether the gastrocnemii tire more easily.

The power of ankle dorsiflexion is best tested by applying your full body weight to the dorsiflexed ankle (Fig. 11-11). Testing the dorsiflexor by asking the patient to walk on his/her heels will only demonstrate marked weakness in this muscle group. Weakness of the flexor hallucis longus (S1) or weakness of the extensor hallucis longus (L5) is often the first evidence of motor involvement. The evertors of the foot may be weak with an L5 lesion. The gluteus maximus may become weak with lesions involving the 1st sacral nerve root, and this weakness may be demonstrated by the sagging of one buttock crease when the patient stands (Fig. 11-12). Weakness of the gluteus medius is seen with an L5 lesion and occasionally is marked enough to produce a Trendelenburg's lurch, particularly noticeable when the patient is tired. When the gluteus medius is involved, there is frequently marked tenderness on pressure over the muscle near its point of insertion, and this may be confused with a trochanteric bursitis or with gluteal tendinitis.

Quadriceps weakness is seen with an L4 and L3 lesion and can be assessed by the examiner placing his arm under the patient's knee and asking the patient to extend the knee against the resistance of the examiner's hand. However, this maneuver may produce pain, and a false impression of weakness is obtained. In such instances, it is better to have the patient lying face downward and flexing his or her knees to 90 degrees and then assessing the power to fully extend the knee from this position (Fig. 11-13).

Sensory Impairment. The regions of sensory loss are reasonably constant (Fig. 11-14). Within each dermatome, there appear to be areas more vulnerable to sensory loss that others. Loss of appreciation of pinprick is first noted in an S1 lesion below and behind the lateral malleolus and in an L5 lesion in the cleft between the first and second toes. Sensory appreciation is a subjective

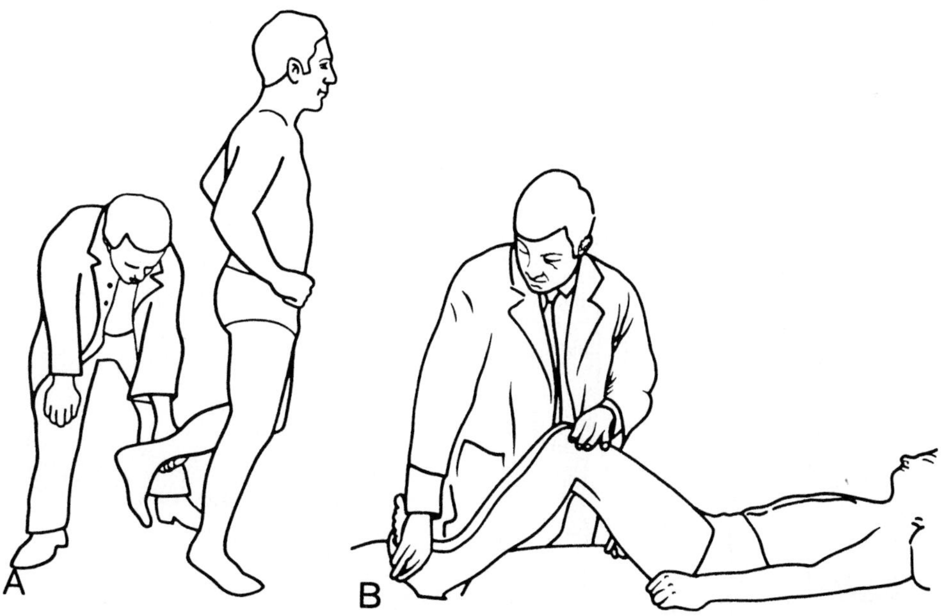

FIGURE 11-11 • **A:** It is important to recognize the fact that when trying to assess the strength of the gastrocnemius by asking the patient to rise on tiptoe, this action must be carried out repetitively and rapidly. The examiner is really attempting to assess fatigability of the muscle. **B:** Ankle dorsiflexion (L4 and L5 roots) is best tested in this position of comfort.

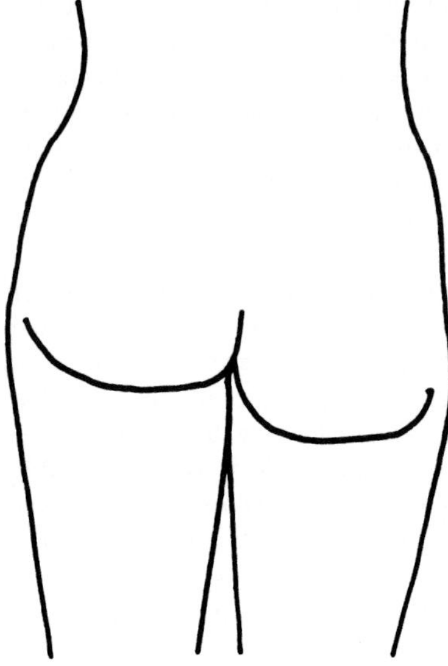

FIGURE 11-12 ● The gluteus maximus is supplied mostly by S1. Lesions involving the first sacral root may cause weakness of the gluteus maximus, which is apparent on examination by the sagging of one buttock crease.

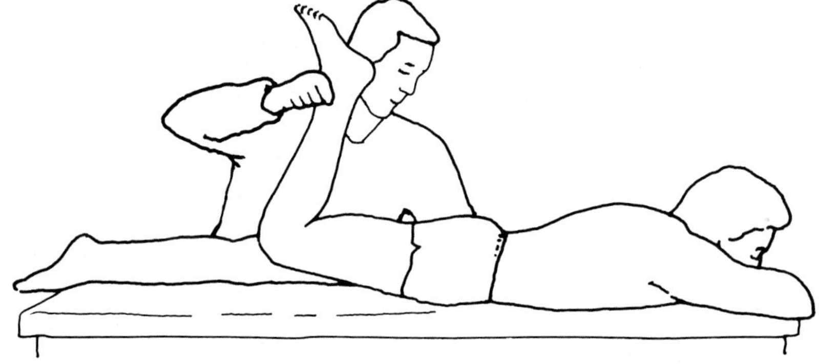

FIGURE 11-13 ● Prone position for testing quadriceps strength.

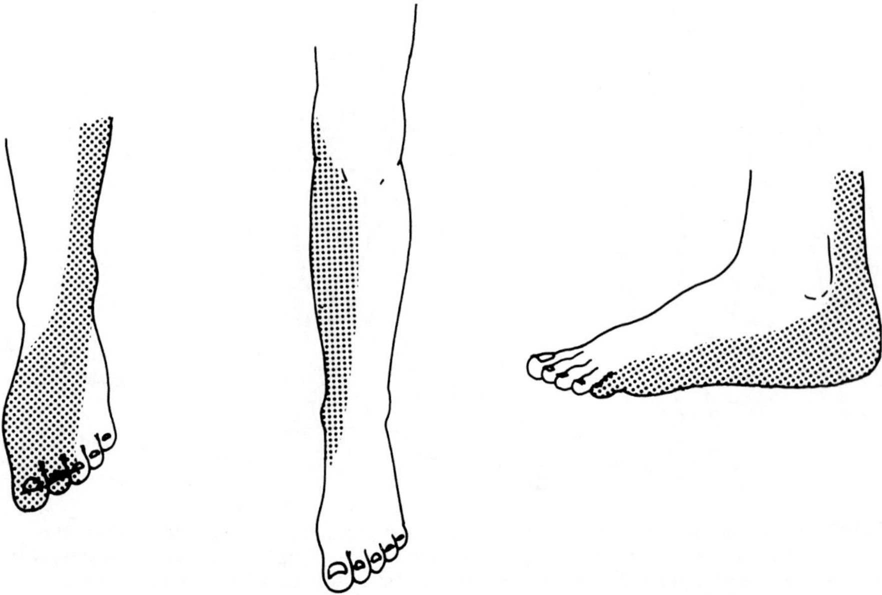

FIGURE 11-14 ● The dermatomal areas supplied by each root where a sensory loss may be detected (**left,** L5; ***middle,*** L4; **right,** S1).

response and, as such, may at times be difficult to assess. Certain precautions must be followed. Sensibility varies in different parts of the limb. Identical areas in each limb must be tested consecutively. The examination must be carried out as expeditiously as compatible with accuracy, because the patient will soon tire of this form of examination, and answers may not be accurate. When the skin is pricked with a pin, the physiologic principle of recruitment is present. The overall sensory appreciation is dependent then not only on the action of the pinprick but also on the number of pinpricks experienced.

A sensory examination is only interpreted as positive for a radicular lesion when the sensory loss approximates one dermatomal distribution, and the loss is not present in the adjacent ipsilateral dermatomes or the same contralateral dermatome.

AGE DIFFERENCE IN THE PRESENTATION OF A "DISC RUPTURE CAUSING THE ACUTE RADICULAR SYNDROME"

Throughout this discussion we have often referred to the different types of presentation for the acute radicular syndrome in young patients. In fact, the acute radicular syndrome from a disc rupture tends to have a characteristic presentation in the three age groups as outlined in Table 11-2.

High Lumbar Root Lesions

Higher lumbar root lesions (i.e., L2, L3, L4) are a different breed (2,16)! First lumbar root lesions also occur, but they are extremely rare. High lumbar root lesions are frequently missed, so let us try to prevent this by drawing all the historical and physical features together in point form.

1. High lumbar root lesions are almost always due to a disc herniation and rarely are caused by bony encroachment. Therefore, they present as an acute, rather than chronic, radicular syndrome.
2. They are difficult to diagnose because they are rare (5% of disc ruptures) and carry with them a significant differential diagnostic challenge. The most common condition confused with a high lumbar root lesion from a disc herniation is a diabetic femoral neuropathy (6,18).
3. These disc ruptures/root lesions usually occur in the older patient population (50+ years).
4. They are extremely painful, producing severe discomfort in the anterior thigh. The patients usually volunteer that they have so much pain that they are unable to sleep at night.
5. They almost all have a very positive femoral nerve stretch test (see Fig. 11-10).

TABLE 11-2

Clinical Picture of Sciatica in Different Age Groups

Symptom	Adolescent (<25 years)	Adult (26–50 years)	Senior Adult (51–80 years)
Pain	Typical radicular pattern, may not be below knee	Typical radicular pattern, almost always below knee	Typical radicular pattern, most severe below the knee
Paresthesia	50% chance of being present	Common	Most common
SLR reduction	Profound	Less than 50% of normal	Most often >50% of normal
Neurologic signs	>50% chance of being absent	>50% chance of being present	Most often present
Associated degenerative changes (spinal stenosis)	Rare	Occasional	Common
Response to conservative care	Recurrence rate of symptoms very high	Good response to conservative care	Limited tolerance for prolonged care
Protrusion/extrusion	Protrusions very common	Protrusions less common	Protrusions rare

TABLE 11-3

Neurologic Changes in High Lumbar Disc Ruptures

	L2	L3	L4
Motor weakness	Hip flexors[a]	Knee extensors[a]	Knee extensors[a]
Sensory loss	Lateral thigh	Patellar region	Medial shin
Reflex depression	0	Knee	Knee
Wasting	Thigh (minor)	Thigh	Thigh

[a]To separate pure femoral neuropathy (e.g., diabetes) from root lesion, examine hip abductors, which are spared in the former and weakened in the latter.

6. They almost always have neurologic changes (Table 11-3).
7. The best clinical clue as to the root involved usually comes from a very careful sensory history and sensory physical examination.
8. The lesions are very resistant to conservative care and are more likely to require surgical intervention.
9. At least 50% of high lumbar disc herniations occur in the foramen (35) and may be missed by the radiologist (Fig. 11-15).

The Cauda Equina Syndrome

This is the third time that you have met the cauda equina syndrome (if you have been brave enough to read the book from the beginning!). The syndrome is a true spine surgical emergency that is often missed (14,36). The reason it is missed or there is a delay in diagnosis is that it is such a rare occurrence (less than four cases per year in a busy spine surgery practice), and the much more common presentation of a disc rupture causing sciatica is never an emergency. There is considerable evidence supporting immediate surgical intervention as the best way to relieve the syndrome.

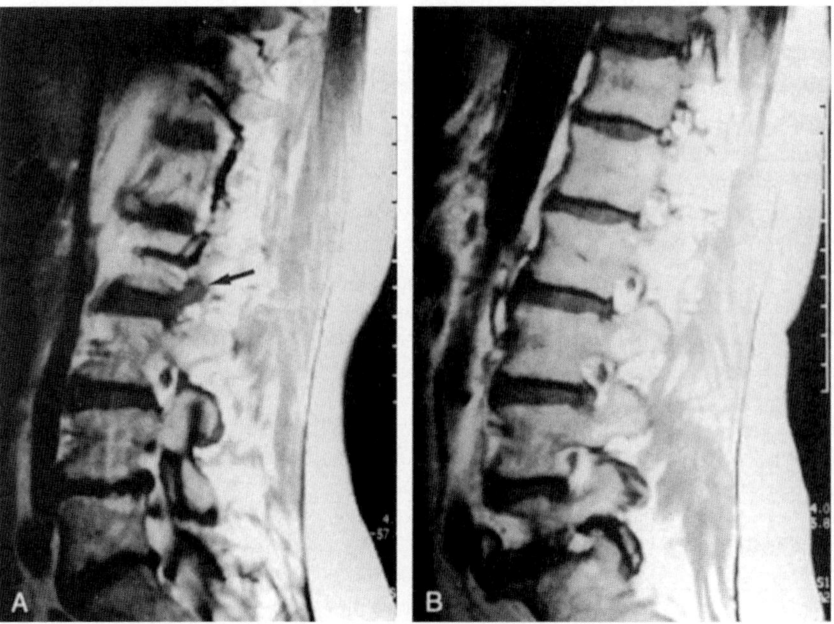

FIGURE 11-15 ● **A:** An L2 foraminal disc *(arrow)* that would be easily missed on MRI. Compare the foramen on the opposite side **(B)**.

A delay in diagnosis with a poor outcome is often cause for a malpractice suit against everyone who missed the diagnosis.

The presentation is fairly classic. The patient usually has a prodromal stage of back pain and some leg symptoms. The leg symptoms are rarely severe in the prodrome, and it is rare that they have led to much in the way of treatment or even a magnetic resonance image (MRI). Without much in the way of intervening trauma, there is a dramatic increase in back pain and the occurrence of bilateral leg pain and perineal numbness. The numbness usually extends to the penis in men. The patient then notices an inability to void because of the paralysis of the S2, 3, and 4 roots in the cauda equina.

The condition is usually caused by a massive midline disc sequestration into the spinal canal, usually at L4–L5 but also at L5–S1 and L3–L4. (19). Higher disc ruptures are a rare cause of this syndrome.

If you are seeing the patient early in the presentation, there will be marked reduction in SLR; numbness to pinprick in the perineal region (S2, 3, 4 dermatomes); and weakness corresponding to the level of the disc rupture. Reflexes will usually be depressed (e.g., bilateral ankle reflex depression with either an L4–L5 or L5–S1 sequestered disc). The bladder will be full to palpation/percussion, and any passage of urine will be due to involuntary overflow incontinence. It is essential to do a rectal examination, at which time decreased tone in the external sphincter will be noted.

It is best to consider a cauda equina syndrome an all or nothing diagnosis (i.e., there is no such thing as a partial cauda equina syndrome that can wait until morning for reassessment). If there is any suspicion at all that bladder and bowel function are impaired, in a back pain patient, an immediate diagnostic study is indicated (10,41,42). Our choice is for an emergency MRI (Fig. 11-16).

Double Root Involvement

Exclusive of the cauda equina syndrome, most patients you see with the acute radicular syndrome have single root involvement. The reason is obvious: most symptomatic disc herniations are single-level lesions. In fact, if you are reading an article on anything to do with disc ruptures, especially surgical treatment, and you see a high incidence of two level disc involvement (over 10%), you know the author has lost his or her way!

But double root involvement does occur in the occasional patient. Figure 11-17 shows how this occurs:

1. A disc rupture that migrates medially (usually L4–L5) so that L5 and S1 root impairment is evident on physical examination (see Fig. 11-17).
2. Any disc rupture that migrates cephalad and laterally. At the L5–S1 level, this would present as S1 and L5 root involvement, and an L4–L5 disc, migrating in this fashion, would present as L5 and L4 root involvement (Fig. 11-17).
3. A disc rupture that migrates cephalad and medially (Fig. 11-17).
4. A foraminal L4 disc rupture may present clinically as an apparent L4 and L5 root involvement because of the furcal nerve. This is discussed in greater detail in the next chapter.
5. A rare double disc herniation.
6. A conjoined nerve root (Fig. 11-17) (38)

Remember one important rule about double root involvement: the densest neurologic lesion determines the disc rupture level; for example, in Figure 11-17, the double root lesion was L5 and S1; the greater neurologic lesion was S1 (the lesser, L5); thus, the HNP had to be L5–S1.

CONCLUSION

There is nothing more constant in degenerative conditions of the lumbar spine than the many faces of presentation in a ruptured disc (20). Although there is a multiplicity of clinical presentations, there is a common thread of some degree of back pain, the dominance of leg pain, the significant root tension and irritation findings, and the variability in neurologic findings. Recognizing these variations, and yet their constancy, allows one to be fairly accurate with a clinical diagnosis (1). In fact, the patient with classical sciatica due to a disc rupture is one of the most obvious diagnoses in

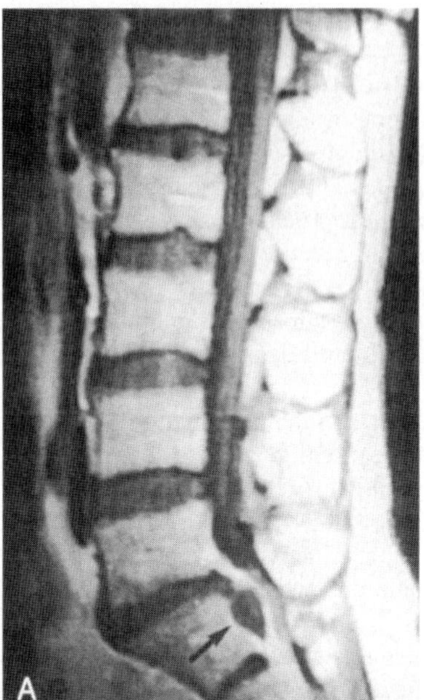

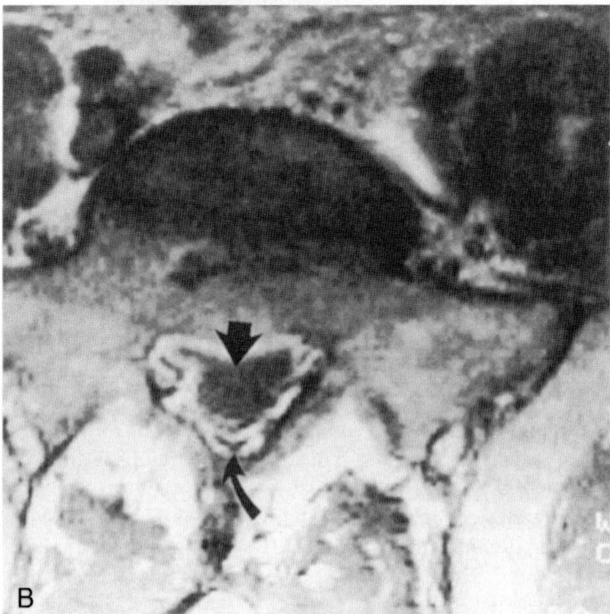

FIGURE 11-16 ● **A:** Sagittal T MRI with a large herniated nucleus pulposus (HNP) at L5–S1 causing complete obliteration of thecal sac *(arrow)*. **B:** Axial T1 MRI showing the large HNP (big arrow) and the thinned residual of a common dural sac *(curved arrow)*.

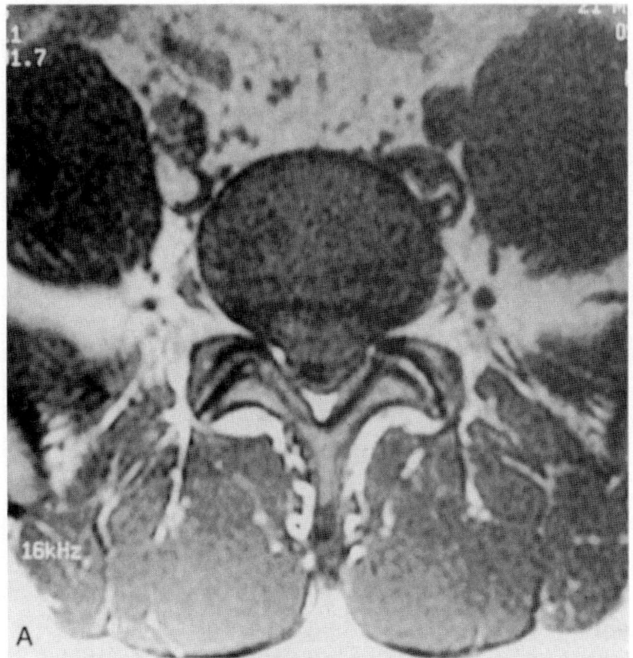

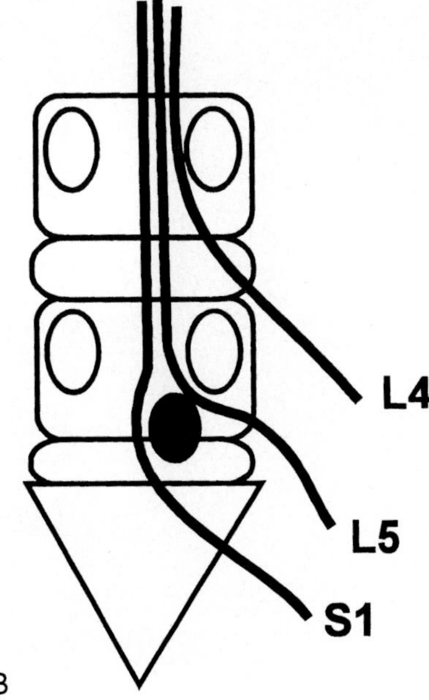

FIGURE 11-17 ● **A:** Medial migration of a disc rupture at L4–L5; the patient had L5 and S1 root symptoms. **B:** Cephalad migration of an L5–S1 disc rupture on schematic impacting on the L5 and S1 roots. *(continues)*

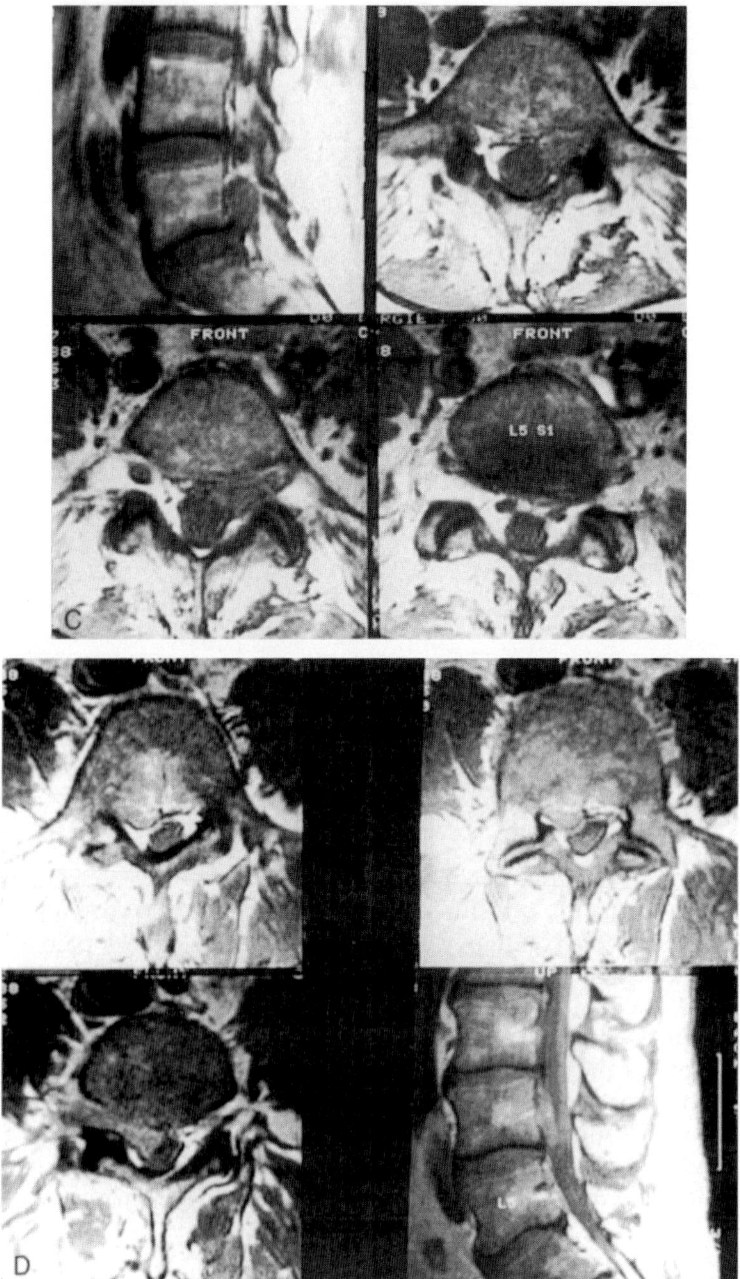

FIGURE 11-17 ● *(Continued)* **C:** An MRI of schematic in **B. D:** Cephalad and medial migration of a disc rupture at L4–L5 presenting as L4 and L5 root involvement.

TABLE 11-4

Criteria for the Diagnosis of the Acute Radicular Syndrome (Sciatica Due to a Herniated Nucleus Pulposus)[a]

1. Leg pain (including buttock) is the dominant complaint when compared with back pain
2. Neurologic symptoms that are specific (e.g., paresthesia in a typical dermatomal distribution)
3. Significant SLR changes
   - SLR less than 50% of normal
   - Bowstring discomfort
   - Crossover pain

   } any one or a combination of these
4. Neurologic signs: weakness, wasting, sensory loss, or reflex alteration (at least two of four)

[a]Three of four of these criteria must be present, the only exception being young patients who are very resistant to the effects of nerve root compression and thus may not have neurologic symptoms (criteria 2) or signs (criteria 4).

degenerative conditions of the lumbar spine and often can be made within a few moments of talking to the patient (Table 11-4). From an understanding of the patient with sciatica due to a disc rupture flows an understanding of patients with lateral zone stenosis, central canal stenosis, and the more elusive mechanical low back pain conditions with referred leg pain.

CONSERVATIVE TREATMENT

Once the clinical diagnosis of an acute radicular syndrome is made, a treatment regimen has to be designed to fit the patient's degree of disability and lifestyle. This can usually be done before extensive, expensive investigation, such as MRI or computed tomography (CT) scan. As mentioned in Chapter 13 on Investigation, the acute radicular syndrome due to a disc rupture is a diagnosis based on history and physical examination. Only when conservative treatment has failed and surgery is being considered should an MRI be ordered. An MRI can also mislead you, showing multiple changes such as disc space narrowing and annular bulging at many levels that are all clinically insignificant (5). A disc rupture causing sciatica is not a "blip" on MRI; it is a patient with lots of leg pain and positive physical findings.

Almost every episode of sciatica can be made better with conservative treatment (32). At issue are the following:

1. How long will conservative care take relative to the demands of daily living?
2. What residual neurologic deficit will be left (11)?
3. What if conservative treatment does not relieve the pain (3,4)?

Conservative treatment for an HNP is no different than for that for degenerative disc disease (DDD), the cornerstone being rest and time with appropriate medication support. The use of other treatment modalities are questionable in their effect. When conservative treatment fails, surgery is indicated.

BED REST

Most experts would agree that the maximal time in bed that a surgeon can demand from a patient who has shown no improvement whatsoever is 2 to 3 days (32). If a patient has shown no improvement in both sciatic pain and SLR ability, it is unlikely that further bed rest will make a lasting difference. If a patient does not get better with time and conservative treatment, consideration must be given to operative intervention.

EXERCISE

Patients with the acute radicular syndromes should all go on the McKenzie exercise routine.

MEDICATION

Obviously, anti-inflammatory, analgesic, and, on some rare occasions, muscle relaxant medication will help the patient comply with the prescription for bed rest.

EPIDURAL STEROIDS

There has been no scientific support for the use of epidural steroids in the treatment of an acute disc rupture (4). Occasionally, a situation presents where more aggressive treatment is indicated, but circumstances prohibit such a step. These include a pregnant woman with sciatica, a student heading into a few weeks of examinations, an elderly patient who wishes to avoid surgery, and a key athlete entering into a key game. In these situations, epidural cortisone injection might settle symptoms to a tolerable level. Except for pregnancy, epidural cortisone injection can be preceded by a 5-day course of oral steroids (e.g., prednisone in a decreasing dose), provided there are no contraindications. It is likely that epidural injections of cortisone will offer short-term relief, with recurrence of symptoms probable, and a more definitive surgical decision will be required.

MISCELLANEOUS FORMS OF TREATMENT

Traction

Used as a method of holding the patient to the bed, traction is useful; used as a method to distract the disc, create negative pressure, and thus suck the ruptured disc back into place, it is useless.

Manipulation

It is unwise to forcibly manipulate the spine of a patient with a disc rupture for fear of further disc displacement and more compromise of neurologic tissue.

INVESTIGATION OF A PATIENT WITH A DISC RUPTURE

Chapter 13 presents an in-depth discussion on investigation of patients with low back pain. Let us review some of the salient points relative to low back pain patients with a disc rupture.

1. Boden et al. (5) have clearly established the fact that asymptomatic individuals can have MRI and CT scans showing abnormalities (including disc ruptures). To further confuse the issue, many authors have shown that patients with MRI/CT documented disc herniations causing sciatica, who lose their sciatic symptoms with conservative or surgical intervention, often have persistent defects shown on posttreatment scans that are little different from the pretreatment scans. Remember, what you see on MRI or CT scanning may not explain the patient's symptoms.
2. The diagnosis of a disc rupture causing sciatica is a clinical diagnosis. It is made after a history and physical examination and before expensive testing such as MR imaging. Only when a patient fails to respond to conservative care or presents with severe neurologic compromise is it time to start investigating.
3. The investigation of choice for any patient suspected of having a disc rupture and who has failed to respond to conservative care is an MRI. The advantages of MRI over myelography, CT/myelography, CT/discography, electromyelography, and thermography (Table 11-5) are so great that the discussion only flourishes in those jurisdictions that do not have MRI readily available (Fig. 11-18).
4. For an MRI to be interpreted as positive for a ruptured disc, it has to show a focal disc protrusion (see Fig. 11-18) and not a diffuse annular bulge. The focal disc protrusion must be at a level and side that fits the patient's symptoms and neurologic findings.
5. Remember the classification of disc ruptures—contained versus noncontained (Fig. 11-19).
6. Viewing of the sagittal cuts will give you a clue as to whether or not a disc is contained or noncontained (Fig. 11-20).
7. Remember that disc herniations can migrate (Fig. 11-21).

TABLE 11-5

Advantages of MRI in the Investigation of a Patient with a Ruptured Disc

Tissue chemistry (with T1, T2 weighted images) is clearly demonstrated.
Two images, at right angles, are available (sagittal and axial).
The conus is viewed on sagittal cuts.
The foramina are more readily examined.
Greater tissue contrast sensitivity helps with the differential diagnosis of infection, tumor, and scarring.
Gadolinium enhancement adds a whole new dimension not available in other investigations.

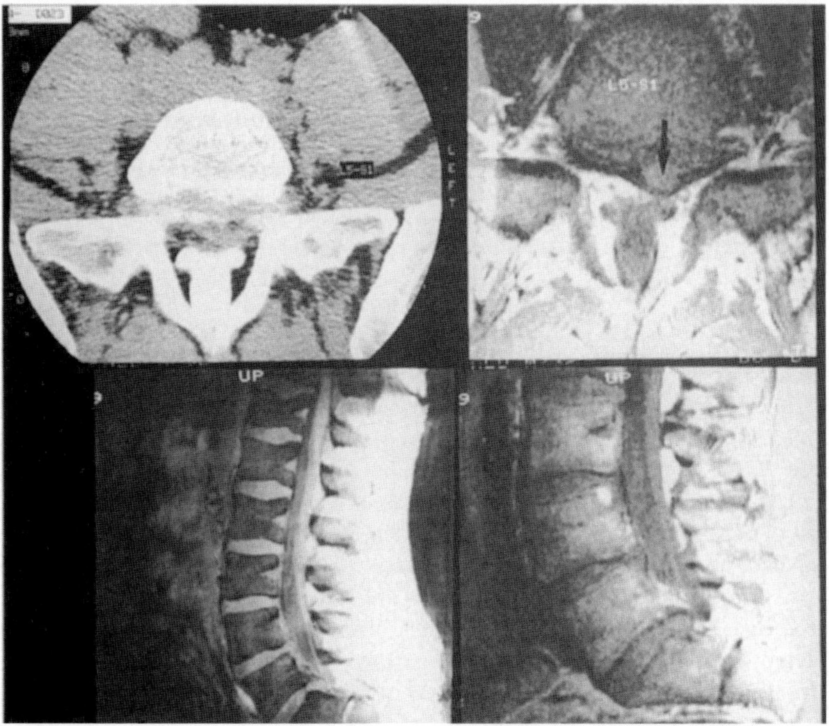

FIGURE 11-18 ● A focal disc protrusion on MRI (T_1) arrow was present on CT **(upper left)** but was much more obvious on the sagittal **(bottom)** and axial MRI.

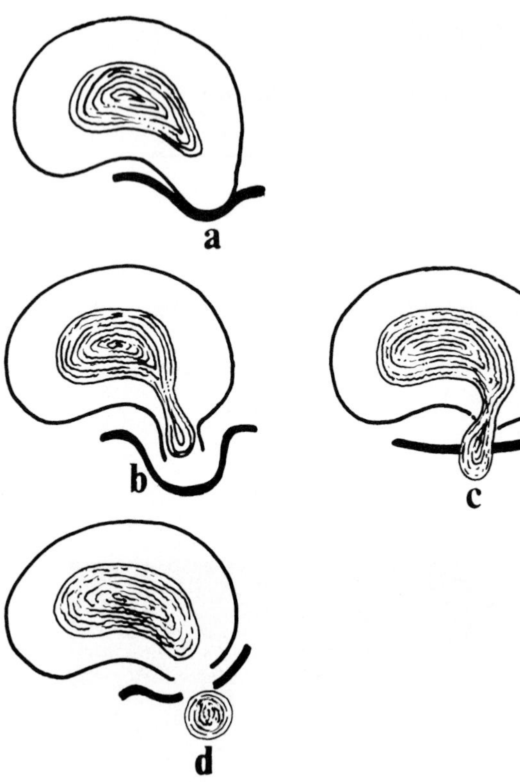

FIGURE 11-19 ● Classification of disc ruptures: contained versus noncontained: (a) contained protrusion, (b) contained extrusion (subannular), (c) noncontained extrusion (transannular), (d) noncontained sequestration.

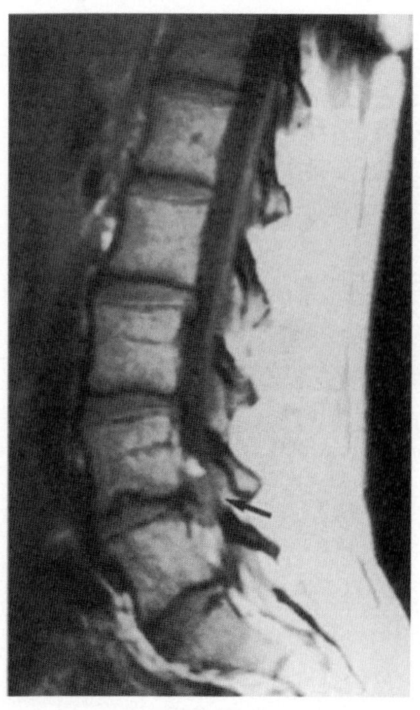

FIGURE 11-20 ● A sagittal (T1) MRI with a fuzzy margin to the disc herniation *(arrow)* (likely noncontained).

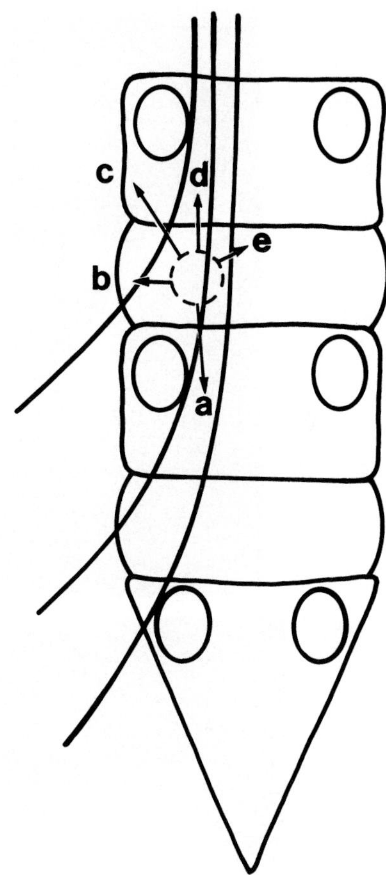

FIGURE 11-21 • Migratory patterns of disc ruptures.

8. The differential diagnosis of a mass of material interfering with nerve root territory includes (Fig. 11-22):
   a. An HNP.
   b. An osteophyte (Fig. 11-22A) (arrow) on CT, with an HNP.
   c. An epidural hematoma or abscess (Fig. 11-22B).
   d. A neoplasm (neurofibroma) (Fig. 11-22C).
   e. Meningocele/Tarlov cyst.
   f. Synovial cyst (Fig. 11-22D).
   g. Scar.

INDICATIONS FOR SURGERY

A GENERAL STATEMENT

One only has to review the natural history of lumbar disc disease to realize that spinal surgeons play a palliative role in the management of most disc herniations. An oft-cited study on the natural history of lumbar disc disease was done by Weber (57). He randomly assigned groups of patients with definite signs of a disc herniation to surgical and nonsurgical groups. Weber concluded that, although surgery initially increases the yields of good results, its advantages disappear on longer follow-up. Weber's data has been recently revisited because of concerns of how crossover patients were handled in the statistical analysis (3,4). Patients initially randomized to non-surgical treatment, but who crossed over and had surgery with good results were considered by Weber as good results under the *nonsurgical group* as this is where they were initially randomized. If these crossover patients are considered failures of nonsurgical treatment (as they eventually had to have surgery), then the statistical analysis indicates that surgical treatment still continues to do better at

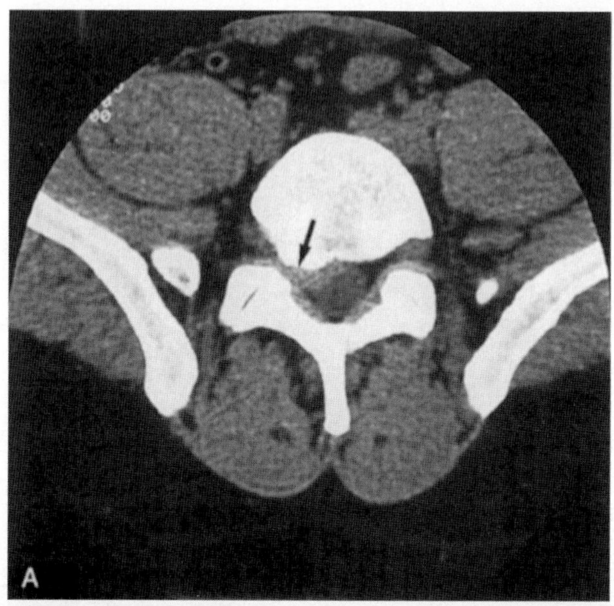

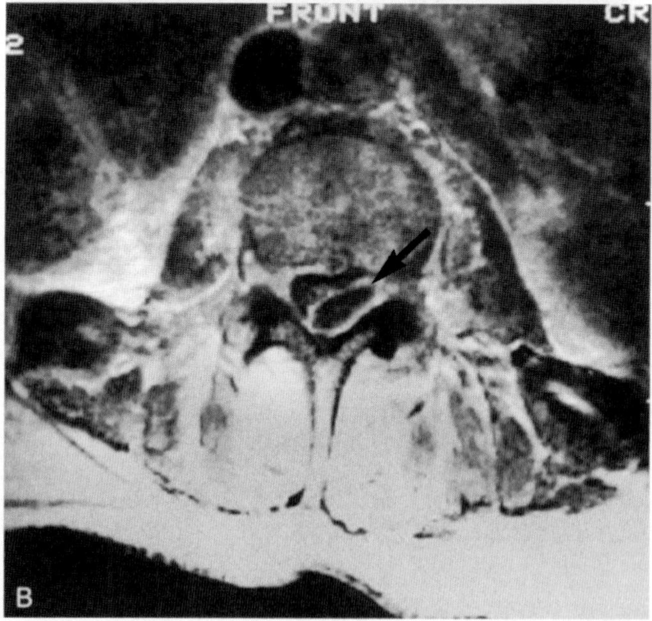

FIGURE 11-22 ● **A:** Patient with recurrent sciatica had an osteophyte *(arrow)* as a source of symptoms. **B:** An epidural abscess *(arrow)* (in a diabetic patient). *(continues)*

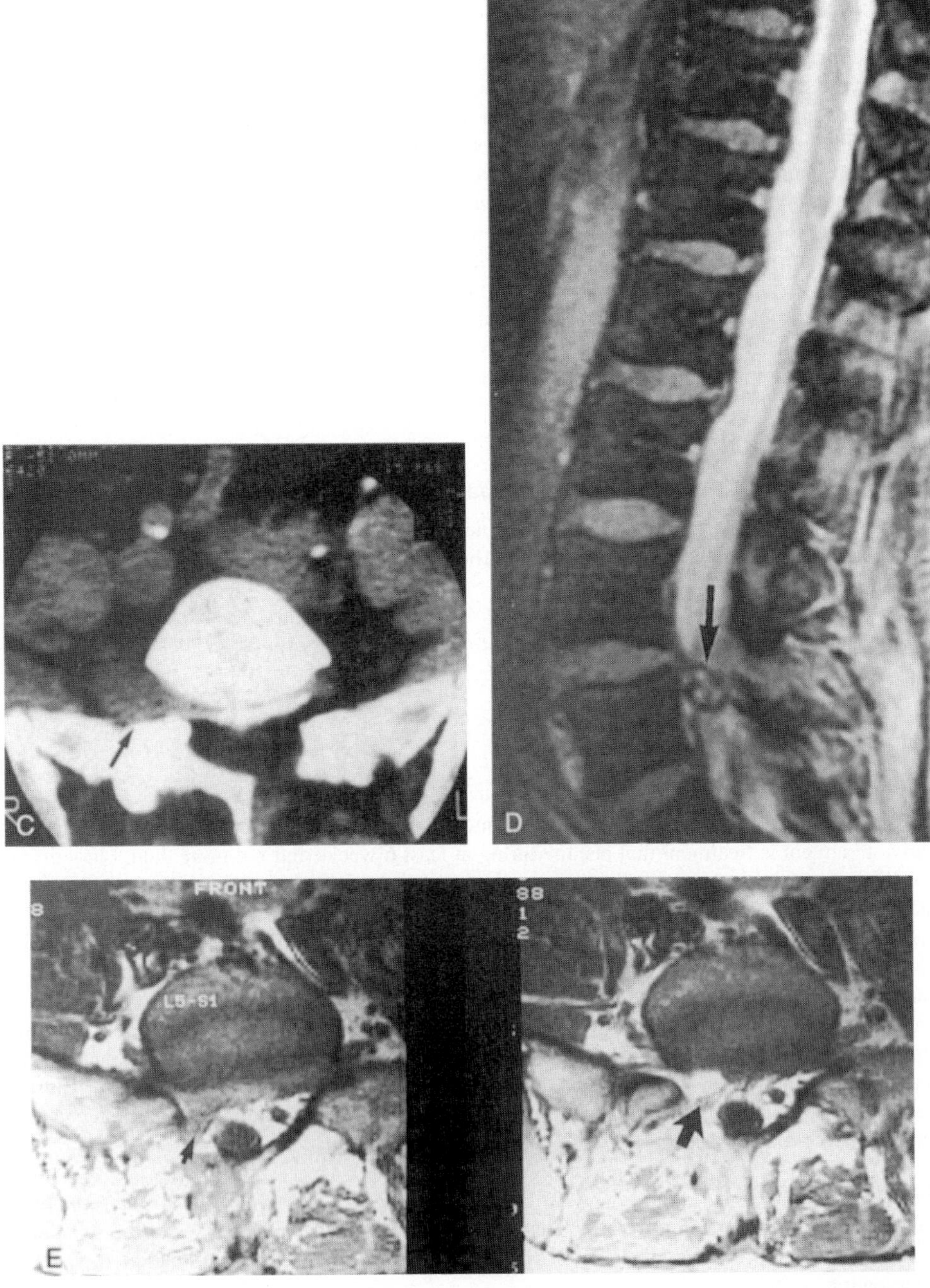

FIGURE 11-22 ● *(Continued)* **C:** Patient presented with right sciatica. The diagnosis: secondary carcinoma (primary lung). Note the bony erosions on the anterior aspect of the facet joint and ala of the sacrum *(arrow)*. **D:** A synovial cyst *(arrow)*. **E:** Scar on gadolinium-enhanced MRI: what looks like a recurrent disc herniation *(left arrow)* is all scar with injection of gadolinium *(heavy right arrow)*.

10-year follow-up. However, overall clinical improvement was seen in both the surgical and nonsurgical groups.

Hakelius (17) also completed a retrospective study of 583 patients with unilateral sciatica. His results were similar to Weber's in that the surgically treated patients initially had a better result, but by 6 months, there was no difference between the two groups of patients. He did show that on a 7-year follow-up, the conservatively treated group had somewhat more low back pain, more sciatic discomfort, more recurrences, and more lost time from work.

One can only conclude from these and other studies on the natural history of sciatica due to a disc herniation that it is a transient, self-limiting condition. Satisfactory resolution over time is likely to occur in most patients, regardless of the method of treatment intervention, be it surgery or conservative treatment. If one is proposing surgical intervention (45), it becomes essential to prove that surgery carries with it a high rate of initial success with limited risk to the patient and at the least expense possible to the payers for the service.

The following is an enumeration of indications for surgery in HNP.

ABSOLUTE INDICATIONS

Bladder and Bowel Involvement: The Cauda Equina Syndrome

The acute massive disc herniation that causes bladder and bowel paralysis is usually a sequestered disc that requires immediate surgical excision for the best prognosis (20).

Increasing Neurologic Deficit

In the face of progressing weakness, it is wise to intervene early with surgical excision of the disc rupture.

RELATIVE INDICATIONS

Failure of Conservative Treatment

This is the most common reason for surgical intervention in the presence of a HNP. Ideal conservative treatment is treatment that occurs during at least 6 weeks and not more than 3 months and results in improvement in the patient's symptoms and signs. During that time, the amount of complete bed rest that should be prescribed is 2 to 3 days. Other conservative measures (3,4) such as medication (analgesic, anti-inflammatory, muscle relaxant); modalities (heat and cold); and exercises may be used. The key to measuring the success of conservative treatment is not only the patient's relief of pain but also the improvement in SLR ability. If a patient goes to bed with appropriate medication for 2 to 3 days and there is no improvement in sciatic discomfort or in SLR ability, it is likely that the patient is going to follow a protracted conservative course, and surgical intervention is indicated. It is proposed that surgical intervention in the acute radicular syndrome occur before 3 months of symptoms to try and avoid the chronic pathologic changes that can occur within a nerve root.

Recurrent Sciatica

Conservative treatment can also fail in that the patient experiences recurrences of the sciatic syndrome. Table 11-6 outlines the use of "recurrences of sciatica" as an indication for surgical intervention.

Significant Neurologic Deficit with Significant SLR Reduction

This is a relative indication for surgical intervention for an HNP. Again, Weber (57) has shown that these patients eventually recovered just as well with nonsurgical intervention. These patients are in extreme pain and often cannot wait for the benefits of conservative care. On the rare occasion, these patients present with severe pain that has resolved as the neurologic deficit has increased; they also should go to surgery when the MRI demonstrates a large HNP.

A Disc Rupture into a Stenotic Canal

We are quick to intervene surgically when the neurologic deficit is shown on MRI to be associated with a narrowed spinal canal such as acquired canal stenosis or subarticular stenosis or congenital stenosis.

TABLE 11-6

Recurring Sciatica[a]: Indications for Surgery

Episode of Sciatica	Prognosis
First	90% of patients will get better and stay better with conservative care.
Second	90% of patients will get better, but 50% of the patients will have a recurrence of symptoms. Consider surgery.
Third	90% of the patients will get better, but almost all will have recurrent episodes of sciatica. Propose surgery.

[a] This condition is to be distinguished from recurrent herniated nucleus pulposus (disc herniation recurring after previous surgery).

Recurrent Neurologic Deficit

If a patient with sciatica and a neurologic deficit has been successfully treated with conservative care, only to have a neurologic deficit reappear with recurrent symptoms, operate.

CONTRAINDICATIONS TO SURGICAL INTERVENTION

Before intervening surgically for the acute radicular syndrome due to a lumbar disc herniation, it is essential to have an accurate clinical diagnosis of the cause of the sciatica (Table 11-7), an anatomic level of the lesion, and support for both clinical impressions by some form of investigation. If there is not a perfect marriage between the patient's clinical presentation, the anatomic level, and the

TABLE 11-7

Differential Diagnosis of Sciatica

- Intraspinal causes
- Proximal to disc: conus and cauda equina lesions (e.g., neurofibroma, ependymoma)
- Disc level
  - Herniated nucleus pulposus
  - Stenosis (canal or recess)
  - Infection: osteomyelitis or discitis (with nerve root pressure)
  - Inflammation: arachnoiditis
  - Neoplasm: benign or malignant with nerve root pressure
- Extraspinal causes
  - Pelvis
  - Cardiovascular conditions (e.g., peripheral vascular disease)
  - Gynecologic conditions
  - Orthopedic conditions (e.g., osteoarthritis of hip)
  - Sacroiliac joint disease
  - Neoplasms (invading or compressing lumbosacral plexus)
- Peripheral nerve lesions
  - Neuropathy (diabetic, tumor, alcohol)
  - Local sciatic nerve conditions (trauma, tumor)
  - Inflammation (herpes zoster)

TABLE 11-8

Contraindications to Surgery for a Herniated Nucleus Pulposus (HNP)

- Wrong patient (poor potential for recovery, e.g., workmen's compensation patient off work for more than 2 years)
- Wrong diagnosis, for example, other pathology causing the leg symptoms (see Table 11-7)
- Wrong level (see Chapter 17)
- A painless HNP (do not operate for primary complaint of weakness or paresthesia, in absence of pain)
- An inexperienced surgeon applying poor technical skills
- Lack of adequate instruments

structural lesion as demonstrated on myelography, CT scanning, or MRI, the potential for a poor result increases dramatically.

Patients with a significant nonorganic component to their disability are usually a contraindication to surgical intervention. The presence of a nonorganic component to a disability does not immunize a patient from having a disc herniation. On the other hand, few patients with a significant nonorganic component to their disability do, indeed, have a disc rupture as part of their causative pathology.

Further contraindications to surgical intervention for a lumbar disc herniation are listed in Table 11-8.

TREATMENT OPTIONS

Before considering surgical intervention, remember: Successful surgical outcomes depend 90% on proper patient selection and 10% on surgical technique.

The principle of surgical intervention is to relieve neural compression without complications and, specifically, without creating instability. Surgery for a disc rupture is nerve root surgery not disc surgery. Obviously, you need to remove offending disc material, but when you are finished, you must leave the nerve root free and mobile. The treatment choices include the following:

1. Chemonucleolysis
2. Surgery
   a. Posterior approaches
      - Standard laminectomy
      - Microlaminectomy: posterior
      - Microlaminectomy: lateral

   b. Anterior approach

   c. Percutaneous discectomy approach

CHEMONUCLEOLYSIS

Since it was first isolated by Jansen and Balls (24) in 1941, chymopapain has followed a checkered course to clinical acceptance. After 1964, when Smith (46) first reported its clinical use in the treatment of lumbar disc herniations, chymopapain was widely used in Canada, Great Britain, France, Germany, and the United States. However, a U.S. double-blind study published in 1976 (44) led to the withdrawal of chymopapain from clinical use in the United States. Subsequent double-blind studies by Fraser (13), Smith Laboratories (47–50), and Travenol Laboratories (54) led the United States Food and Drug Administration (FDA) to reconsider chymopapain's position, and this agent was again released for general use in 1982. Surgeons accustomed to surgically excising space-occupying pathology were reluctant to embrace the concept of injecting a disc with chymopapain, a constituent of meat tenderizer. Further, six deaths and 37 serious neurologic complications (47) had occurred in the United States in approximately 80,000 injections done during a time span of 18 months (ending in 1984). Unfortunately, these events have served to undermine chymopapain as a clinical tool.

TABLE 11-9

Follow-up of Patients Undergoing Microsurgery for Lumbar Disc Disease[a]

Number of patients operated on	257
Average length to follow-up	19 months
Number of patients followed up	249 (97%)
Case distribution	
Virgin HNP	119
Lateral zone stenosis	24
Previous procedure	
Chymopapain	70
Laminectomy	10
Fusion added to microdiscectomy	26
	249

HNP, herniated nucleus pulposus.
[a]Personal series of senior author of the third edition (John McCulloch).

RESULTS OF POSTERIOR MICRODISCECTOMY

A study of 257 patients undergoing microsurgery for lumbar disc disease (12) (Table 11-9) revealed an 84% success rate and a 95% return to work rate in patients undergoing surgery for virgin lumbar disc herniations. Less successful but acceptable results were obtained in patients with compensation claims who had HNP and patients with previous spine surgery procedure (Table 11-10). Analysis of a complication rate of 10% (Table 11-11) revealed relative minor problems that did not affect outcomes, and a decreasing incidence of complications as experience with the procedure grew. The short-term success rate in this series compared favorably with standard laminectomy-discectomy. Along with the reduction of hospital stay (average, 2.3 days in this series), microsurgery delivered acceptable results in patients with lumbar disc herniation. With increasing confidence in the procedure, a majority of microdiscectomies are now done on an outpatient basis.

COMPLICATIONS OF MICROSURGERY FOR LUMBAR HNP

There is more to learn from complications than from successes. Although there are many surgeons using microsurgical intervention for lumbar disc disease, there are many critics who believe that microsurgery is associated with several disadvantages and many additional risks. A major criticism is that inherent in the procedure are inadequate exposure of the nerve root and incomplete decompression of the encroachment pathology. Table 11-12 lists the complications experienced in a series of 257 microsurgical procedures done McCulloch.

TABLE 11-10

Results in Compensation Patients and Patients with Previous Surgery

	Compensation	Previous Surgery[a]
Satisfactory	66% (27)	69.7% (46)
Unsatisfactory	34% (14)	30.3% (20)
Total	(100%) 41	(100%) 66

[a]Excluding those patients with lateral zone stenosis.

TABLE 11-11

Complications of Microsurgery for Lumbar Herniated Nucleus Pulposus (HNP)[a]

Condition	No. of Patients (%)	Results
Dural tear (minor)	6 (2.70)	Only 1 required repair, no problems
Wrong level exploration	6 (2.70)	Recognized and corrected at time of surgery
Hemorrhage requiring transfusion	3 (1.35)	Poor patient positioning and technique
Superficial wound infection	2 (0.90)	Resolved on antibiotics
Disc space infection	2 (0.90)	Resolved on antibiotics
Increased neurodeficit	2 (0.90)	Recovered quickly
Hematoma	1 (0.45)	Resolved spontaneously
Gastritis	1 (0.45)	Resolved
Urinary retention	1 (0.45)	Resolved
Total	24 (10.8)	

[a]First 257 microdiscectomy procedures of the senior author of the third edition (John McCulloch).

A general review of the literature reveals complications associated with any spine invasive procedure, as listed in Table 11-13.

There are some complications that are specific to microsurgical intervention.

Wrong Level

Anyone doing any volume of microsurgery will admit that at one time or another, they have exposed the wrong level. The North American Spine Society (NASS) has developed the "Sign, Mark and X-Ray" (SMaX) program as a systems intervention to help prevent this problem (60).

Missed Pathology

Many critics of microsurgery state that because of the limited operative field, it is easy to miss a fragment of disc material that has migrated away from the disc space or miss bony encroachment (43). Microsurgery for lumbar disc disease is not seek-and-find surgery; rather, by careful examination of the preoperative investigation, including the MRI or CT scan, the surgeon will know exactly what pathology is causing the symptoms and where the pathology is located.

TABLE 11-12

Complications of Microsurgery for Lumbar Herniated Nucleus Pulposus (HNP)

Condition	No. of Patients (%)	Results
Dural tear (minor)	6 (2.70)	Only 1 required repair, no problems
Wrong level exploration	6 (2.70)	Recognized and corrected at time of surgery
Hemorrhage requiring transfusion	3 (1.35)	Poor patient positioning and technique
Superficial wound infection	2 (0.90)	Resolved on antibiotics
Disc space infection	2 (0.90)	Resolved on antibiotics
Increased neurodeficit	2 (0.90)	Recovered quickly
Hematoma	1 (0.45)	Resolved spontaneously
Gastritis	1 (0.45)	Resolved
Urinary retention	1 (0.45)	Resolved
Total	24 (10.8)	

TABLE 11-13

Complications of Lumbar Spine Surgery

Neurologic damage with increased neurologic deficit
Wound infection
  Superficial
  Deep
  CSF fistula
Hematoma with or without cauda equina compression
Fatalities
  Pulmonary embolus
  Great vessel injury
Late complications
  Spinal stenosis
  Instability resulting in vertebral body translation
  Scarring, with or without arachnoiditis

CSF, cerebrospinal fluid.
From Mayfield FH. Complications of laminectomy. *Clin Neurosurg.* 1976:23:435–439 with permission.

Intraoperative Bleeding

Because of the very small incision and the limited operative field, a small amount of bleeding under the microscope appears as a major hemorrhage. It is important to take steps to prevent excessive bleeding during microsurgery, such as withdrawing patients from anti-inflammatory medications before surgery, positioning the patient properly on the table so there is no abdominal compression, and using hypotensive anesthesia. During the surgical exercise, all bleeders should be stopped the moment they occur; regular cautery should be used outside the spinal canal and bipolar cautery within the spinal canal.

Dural Injury

The inexperienced surgeon with poor equipment is the one who causes neurologic damage during microsurgical intervention. It is essential to train oneself in the technique and to have the proper instrumentation available to reduce dural injury to a minimum. In fact, under the microscope, the nerve root can be seen so well that an experienced microsurgeon is going to have less of a neurologic complication rate than someone using a standard laminectomy approach without magnification.

Disc Space Infection

Wilson and Harbaugh (59) have reported an increased incidence of disc space infection after microsurgery. These researchers proposed that manipulation of the microscope over the wound was the source of this increased infection rate. This occurred despite surgical draping of the microscope, which leaves exposed eyepieces that are not sterile. This has led to the use of prophylactic antibiotics and the proposal that manipulation of the microscope over the open wound should be kept to a minimum. Unrecognized disc space infections can quickly lead to disasters (23).

LAMINECTOMY

Almost all of this section on surgical intervention has been about microsurgical intervention. There are still many surgeons who prefer the standard laminectomy/discectomy exposure, with or without loupe magnification. It really does not matter what technique you use to decompress the nerve root; if you fail to fully decompress the nerve root or introduce a complication to the equation, you have failed to serve the patient.

SPECIAL SITUATION WITH AN HNP

Disc herniations do not always occur in simple, uncompromised situations. Following are some unique situations relative to an HNP causing sciatica.

HNP with Spondylolisthesis

Patients with a spondylolisthesis may suffer from a disc rupture, which causes an acute radicular syndrome. Most of these will occur at the level above the spondylolisthesis (Fig. 11-23). A disc herniation at the same level of the slip usually occurs into the foramen (Fig. 11-23). For the former situation, simple disc excision or chemonucleolysis is all that is required; for the latter (disc excision at the slip level), discectomy should be accompanied by a stabilization procedure.

HNP in Spinal Stenosis

Spinal stenosis can occur in the central canal or lateral zones. It can be an asymptomatic or a mildly symptomatic condition that can suddenly convert to a significant disability when a disc herniation occurs. Investigation in these patients is somewhat inconclusive because the stenosis does not allow for a clear depiction of the disc rupture. It is only when the presenting symptoms are analyzed and the dominance of the leg pain is ascertained that one will suspect a small disc herniation in the presence of a stenotic canal or lateral zone stenosis. Simple microscopic removal of the disc herniation along with a local decompression of the stenotic segment is the proposed method of treatment. If, on history, the stenotic component was significantly symptomatic before the occurrence of the HNP, a wider decompression is needed to treat both the stenosis and the HNP.

HNP in Instability

Patients with a long history of back pain and significant DDD revealed on plain radiograph may suffer from a disc herniation at the degenerative level. Whether or not this instability should be treated at the time of the disc excision is a difficult question to answer. We feel that if the disc degeneration and HNP are confined to one level, it is reasonable to consider fusion. If the disc degeneration is present at multiple levels, either on plain radiograph, discography, or MRI, simple disc excision is the best choice.

HNP in the Adolescent Patient

The younger patient with a disc herniation is a special problem. As outlined in DeOrio and Bianco's (8) series from the Mayo Clinic, a number of these patients go on to repeat surgical procedures after their initial surgical intervention. Because of the high incidence of protrusions rather than disc extrusions, it is proposed that in this age group the optimal treatment is chemonucleolysis rather than surgical intervention (33).

Recurrent HNP (After Discectomy)

Reherniation of discal material occurs in approximately 2% to 5% of patients. The recurrence may occur at any interval after surgery (days to years) and is most often at the same level/same side. If the recurrence is at the same level/opposite side or another level, it can be considered a virgin HNP, and the principles discussed earlier in this chapter apply. Unfortunately, most recurrences are same level/same side, and scar tissue from the previous surgery introduces a whole new element to diagnosis and treatment.

ANTERIOR APPROACH

The anterior (through the abdomen) approach is mentioned only to state that the authors believe the needle, percutaneous, and microsurgical approaches are superior. The anterior discectomy (and fusion) technique should be reserved for the patient in need of salvage surgery, and it is too major an operative procedure for primary intervention for an HNP.

PERCUTANEOUS LUMBAR DISC SURGERY

There is no question that surgery in general is moving toward least invasive/same day surgery procedures. For lumbar disc herniation, chemonucleolysis was one of those procedures. But as

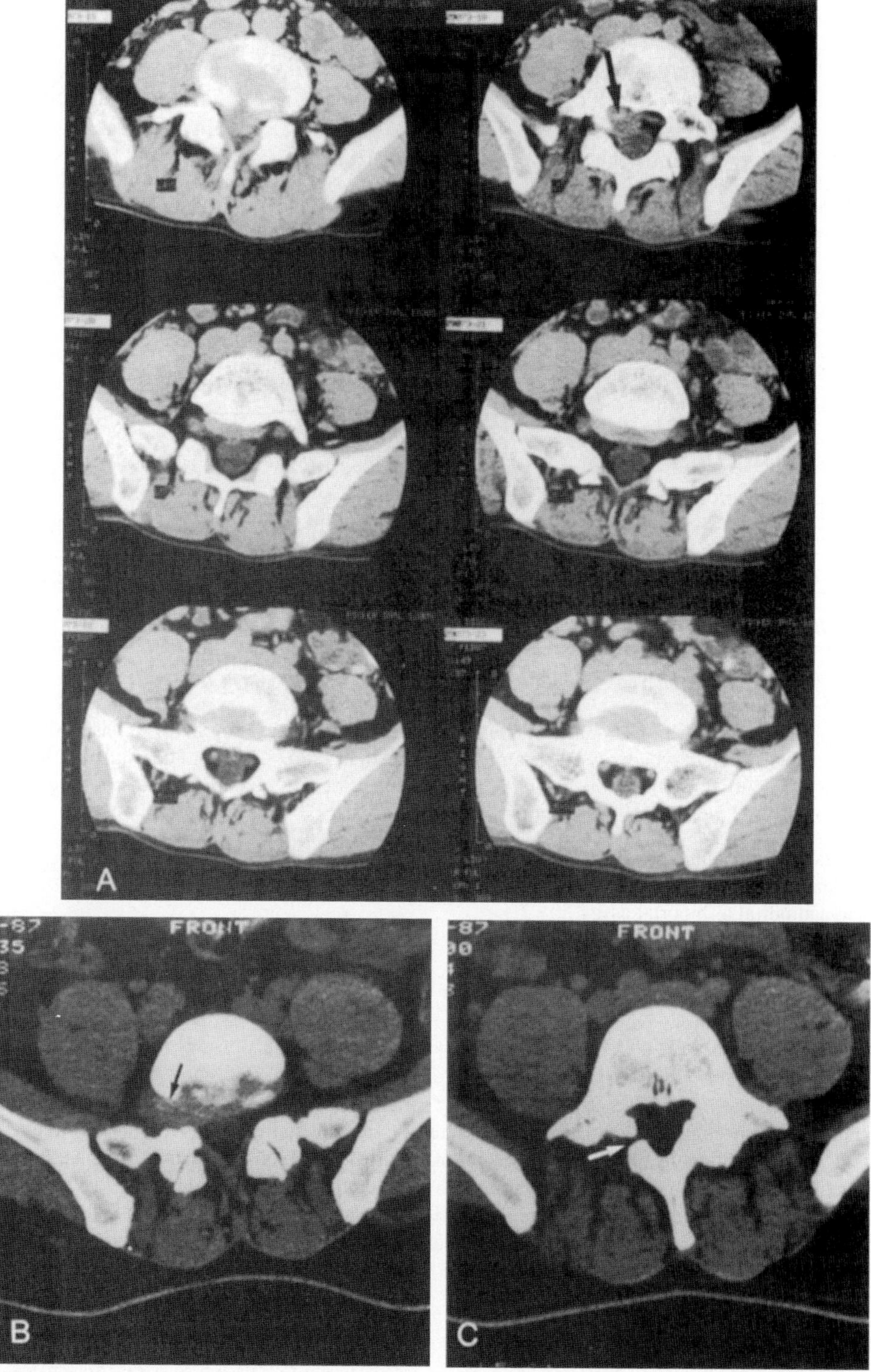

FIGURE 11-23 ● Lytic spondylolisthesis with HNP on axial cut. **A:** Herniated nucleus pulposus (HNP) above spondylolysis at L4–L5, right *(arrow).* **B:** HNP (at slip level), that is, below lysis, L5–S1, right *(arrow).* **C:** The spondylolysis, L5, of patient in **A** *(arrow).*

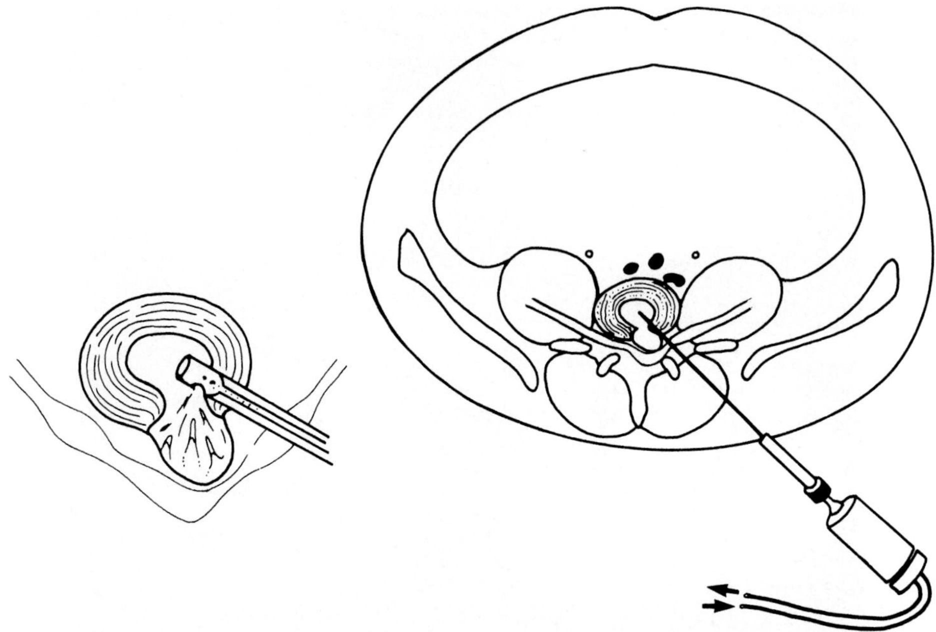

FIGURE 11-24 ● The approach to percutaneous discectomy. The small diagram **(left)** represents the probe tip in the disc space, which sucks out the nuclear material.

chymopapain complications mounted, other researchers developed yet more less invasive disc procedures, the second of which was percutaneous manual discectomy (21,22). Subsequently, Kambin (25–28) and Onik (34,40) weighed in with their particular brand of percutaneous discectomy so that today we have as options the following:

1. Automated percutaneous lumbar discectomy (APLD) (Fig. 11-24)
2. Manual percutaneous lumbar discectomy (MPLD) with:
   a. Uniportal or biportal assist
   b. Laser assist
   c. Working channel endoscope
3. Laparoscopic and thoracoscopic approaches

CONCLUSION

Since Mixter and Barr introduced us to the disc rupture causing sciatica (37), the acute radicular syndrome has become an easy condition to diagnose, most often responds to conservative treatment, and when that fails, it yields good results after surgery. For spine practitioners, and especially surgeons, this condition is a winner, gratifying to both the patient and the doctor.

The bony root entrapment syndromes and lateral zone disc herniations discussed in the next chapter are more difficult to diagnose and treat and thus have the potential for delivering less than satisfactory results to treatment intervention.

REFERENCES

1. Armstrong JR. Lumbar disc lesions. *Pathogenesis and Treatment of Low Back Pain and Sciatica.* Baltimore: Williams & Wilkins; 1965.
2. Aronson HA, Dunsmore RH. Herniated upper lumbar discs. *J Bone Joint Surg Am.* 1963;45:311–317.
3. Bell GR. Conservative vs. surgical management of lumbar disc herniation: Is outcome following conservative treatment equal to surgical management. In: Bell GR, ed. *Contemporary Issues in Spine Surgery.* Rosemont, IL: AAOS; 1999:3–7.
4. Bell GR, Rothman RH. The conservative treatment of sciatica. *Spine.* 1984;9:54–56.

5. Boden SD, Davis DO, Dina TS, et al. Abnormal magnetic resonance scans of the lumbar spine in asymptomatic subjects. *J Bone Joint Surg.* 1990;72:403–408.
6. Chokroverty S, Reyers MG, Rubino FA, et al. The syndrome of diabetic amyotrophy. *Ann Neurol.* 1977;2:181–194.
7. Cram RH. A sign of nerve root pressure. *J Bone Joint Surg Br.* 1953;35:192–195.
8. DeOrio JK, Bianco AJ. Lumbar disc excision in children and adolescents. *J Bone Joint Surg Am.* 1982;64:991–996.
9. Dyck P. The femoral nerve traction test with lumbar disc protrusions. *Surg Neurol.* 1976;6:163–166.
10. Emmett JL, Love JG. Urinary retention in women caused by asymptomatic protruded lumbar disk: report of 5 cases. *J Urol.* 1968;99:597–606.
11. Fager CA. Observations on spontaneous recovery from intervertebral disc herniation. *Surg Neurol.* 1994;42:282–286.
12. Feldman R, McCulloch JA. Microsurgery for lumbar disc disease. In: McCulloch JA, ed. *Principles of Microsurgery for Lumbar Disc Disease.* New York: Raven Press; 1989.
13. Fraser RD. Chymopapain for the treatment of intervertebral disc herniation. *Spine.* 1982;7:608.
14. Graf CJ, Hamby WB. Paraplegia in lumbar intervertebral disk protrusion, with remarks on high lumbar disk protrusion. *NY Med J.* 1953;53:2346–2348.
15. Gunn CC, Chir B, Milbrand WE. Tenderness at motor points; a diagnostic and prognostic aid to low back injury. *J Bone Joint Surg Am.* 1976;58:815–825.
16. Gutterman P, Shenkin JA. Syndromes associated with protrusion of upper lumbar intervertebral disc. *J Neurosurg.* 1973;38:499–503.
17. Hakelius A. Prognosis in sciatica: a clinical follow-up of surgical and non-surgical treatment. *Acta Orthop Scand.* 1970;129(suppl):1–76.
18. Harati Y. Diabetic peripheral neuropathies. *Ann Intern Med.* 1987;107:546–559.
19. Hardy RW Jr, David HR Jr. Extradural cauda equina and nerve root compression from benign lesions of the lumbar spine. In: Youmans JR, ed. *Neurological Surgery.* Philadelphia: WB Saunders; 1996:2357–2374.
20. Hardy RW Jr, Plank NM. Clinical diagnosis of herniated lumbar disc. In: Hardy RW Jr, ed. *Lumbar Disc Disease.* New York: Raven Press; 1982:17–28.
21. Hijikata S. Percutaneous nucleotomy. A new concept technique and 12 years' experience. *Clin Orthop.* 1989;238:9–23.
22. Hijikata A, Yamagishi M, Nakayama T, et al. Percutaneous nucleotomy: a new treatment method for lumbar disc herniation. *J Toden Hosp.* 1975;5:39.
23. Hlavin ML, Kaminski HL, Ross JS, et al. Spinal epidural abscess: a ten year perspective. *Neurosurgery.* 1990;27:177–184.
24. Jansen EF, Balls AK. Chymopapain: new crystalline proteinase from papaya latex. *J Biol Chem.* 1941;137:459–460.
25. Kambin P, Brager MD. Percutaneous posterolateral discectomy. Anatomy and mechanism. *Clin Orthop.* 1987;223:145–154.
26. Kambin P, Gellman H. Percutaneous lateral discectomy of the lumbar spine—a preliminary report. *Clin Orthop.* 1983;174:127–132.
27. Kambin P, Sampson S. Posterolateral percutaneous suction-excision of herniated lumbar intervertebral discs. Report of interim results. *Clin Orthop.* 1986;207:37–43.
28. Kambin P, Schaffer JL. Percutaneous lumbar discectomy. Review of 100 patients and current practice. *Clin Orthop.* 1989;238:24–34.
29. Keegan J. Dermatome hypalgesia associated with herniation of intervertebral disk. *Arch Neurol Psychiatry* 1943;50:67–83.
30. Kelsey JL. An epidemiological study of acute herniated lumbar intervertebral disc. *Rheumatol Rehabil.* 1975;14:144–159.
31. Kirkaldy-Willis WH, Wedge JH, Yong-Hing K, Reilly J. Pathology and pathogenesis of lumbar spondylosis and stenosis. *Spine.* 1978;3:319–328.
32. Lahad A, Malter AD, Berg AO, Deyo RA. The effectiveness of four interventions for the prevention of low back pain. *JAMA.* 1994;272:1286–1291.
33. Lorenz M, McCulloch JA. Chemonucleolysis for herniated nucleus pulposus in adolescents. *J Bone Joint Surg Am.* 1985;67:1402–1404.
34. Maroon JC, Onik G. Percutaneous automated discectomy: a new method for lumbar disc removal. Technical note. *J Neurosurg.* 1987;66:143–146.
35. Maroon JC, Schulhof LA, Kopitnik TA. Diagnosis and microsurgical approach to far lateral disc herniation in the lumbar spine. *J Neurosurg.* 1990;72:382–387.
36. McLaren AC, Bailey SI. Cauda equina syndrome: a complication of lumbar discectomy. *Clin Orthop.* 1986;204:143–149.
37. Mixter WJ, Barr JS. Rupture of the intervertebral disc with involvement of the spinal canal. *N Engl J Med.* 1934;211:210–215.
38. Neidre AN, Macnab I. Anomalies of the lumbosacral nerve roots. Review of 16 cases and classification. *Spine.* 1983;8:294–299.
39. Norlen G. On the value of neurological symptoms in sciatica for localization of a lumbar disc herniation. *Acta Chir Scand.* 1944;95(suppl):7–95.
40. Onik G, Helms CA, Ginsburg L, et al. Percutaneous lumbar diskectomy using a new aspiration probe. *AJR.* 1985;144:1137–1140.

41. Rosomoff HL, Johnston JDH, Gallo AE, et al. Cystometry as an adjunct in the evaluation of lumbar disc syndromes. *J Neurosurg.* 1970;33:67–74.
42. Ross JC, Jameson RM. Vesical dysfunction due to prolapsed disc. *Br Med J.* 1971;3:752–754.
43. Rothman RH, Simeone FA, Bernini PM. Lumbar disc disease. In: Rothman RH, Simeone FA, eds. *The Spine.* Philadelphia: WB Saunders; 1982:508–645.
44. Schwetschenau PR, Ramirez A, Johnston J, et al. Double-blind evaluations of intradiscal chymopapain for herniated lumbar discs. Early results. *J Neurosurg.* 1976;45:622.
45. Scoville WB, Corkilig G. Lumbar disc surgery: technique of radical removal and early mobilization. *J Neurosurg.* 1973;39:265–269.
46. Smith L. Enzyme dissolution of nucleus pulposus in humans. JAMA. 1964;187:137.
47. Smith Laboratories, Inc, Northbrook, Ill. Data from post-marketing surveillance, 1985.
48. Smith Laboratories, Inc, Northbrook, Ill. Product brochure 3.
49. Smith Laboratories, Inc, Northbrook, Ill. Product brochure 4.
50. Smith Laboratories, Inc, Northbrook, Ill. Product information letter, July 1984.
51. Smyth MJ, Wright V. Sciatica and the intervertebral disc. An experimental study. *J Bone Joint Surg Am.* 1958;40:1401–1418.
52. Spangfort E. Lasegue's sign in patients with lumbar disc herniation. *Acta Orthop Scand.* 1971;42:459–460.
53. Spurling RG, Grantham EG. Neurologic picture of herniations of the nucleus pulposus in the lower part of the lumbar region. *Arch Surg.* 1940;40:375–388.
54. Travenol Laboratories, Inc. New Drug Application 18-625. (Submitted to United States Food and Drug Administration on April 24, 1981.)
55. Waddell G, Main C. Assessment of severity in low-back disorders. *Spine.* 1984;9:204–208.
56. Waddell G, Main CJ, Morris EW, et al. Chronic low back pain, psychological distress and illness behavior. *Spine.* 1984;9:209–213.
57. Weber H. Lumbar disc herniation: a controlled prospective study with ten years of observation. *Spine.* 1983;8:131–140.
58. Wilkins RH, Brody IA. Lasegue's sign. *Arch Neurol.* 1969;21:219–221.
59. Wilson D, Harbaugh R. Microsurgical and standard removal of protruded lumbar disc. A comparative study. *Neurosurgery.* 1981;8:422–427.
60. Wong D, Mayer T, Watters W, et al. *Sign Mark and X-Ray (SMaX): A NASS Patient Safety Program.* LaGrange IL: North American Spine Society; 2001.
61. Woodhall B, Hayes GJ. The well-leg raising test of Fajersztajn in the diagnosis of ruptured lumbar intervertebral disc. *J Bone Joint Surg Am.* 1950;32:786–792.

CHAPTER 12

Disc Degeneration with Root Irritation: Spinal Canal Stenosis

"The loss of youth is melancholy enough: but to enter into old age through the gate of infirmity, most disheartening."

—Horace Walpole, 1765

Stenosis is defined as a narrowing or constriction of a passage or canal. When the term is applied to those changes that occur within the spinal canal, the additional connotations of irreversible and progressive narrowing of the canal are implied. Such irreversible narrowing is in contrast to the often waxing and waning symptoms of encroachment occurring with a herniated nucleus pulposus (HNP). Although both conditions are mechanical in nature, that is, aggravation with activity, relief with rest, there are often gaps of days to months in the history of patients with an HNP, during which time they function reasonably well. There are no gaps in the history of patients with spinal canal stenosis (SCS) except early in the disease.

The term claudication means "limp." Often, patients with spinal stenosis experience claudication or "limping," after walking. The lameness is thought to be caused by an upset in neurologic function, thus, the term neurogenic claudication. Infrequently, patients with spinal stenosis have more radicular symptoms than the typical picture of neurogenic claudication. However, claudication is prevalent enough that it forms the foundation of the definition of SCS: (a) claudicant limitation of leg(s) function, (b) clinical evidence of chronic nerve root compression with the presence of, (c) a stenotic spinal canal lesion on imaging and, (d) in the absence of vascular impairment to the lower extremities.

Neurogenic claudication is generally defined as calf discomfort (pain, numbness, paresthesia, weakness, tiredness, heaviness), that is aggravated by both walking and standing and is relieved only after many minutes of resting in the flexed (sitting) lumbar spine position. The posterior and occasionally anterior thigh can also be involved.

CLASSIFICATION AND DESCRIPTION

The standard classification of SCS is outlined in Table 12-1 (1). This classification and the term spinal stenosis are used by most authors to describe narrowing of the central spinal canal as well as "lateral recess" narrowing in the subarticular and foraminal area. Although the central and lateral recess division helps in understanding the pathoanatomy of the two conditions, it is an artificial separation that often does not stand the test of clinical medicine, in which the two conditions so often coexist (8).

The most common stenotic conditions are acquired: stenosis due to degenerative changes in the central spinal canal including bulging or herniation of the disc, osteophyte formation and buckling of an hypertrophied ligamentum flavum. An element of stenosis may be associated with a degenerative spondylolisthesis. On occasion, these acquired conditions occur along with developmental

TABLE 12-1

Classification of Spinal Canal Stenosis

A. Congenital-developmental stenosis of the spinal canal
   1. Achondroplastic stenosis
   2. Normal patient with narrowed spinal canal
B. Acquired stenosis of the spinal canal
   1. Stenosis due to degenerative changes
   2. Stenosis due to degenerative spondylolisthesis
   3. Iatrogenic—postfusion stenosis
   4. Post-traumatic
   5. Miscellaneous skeletal diseases; e.g., Paget's disease
C. Combined A and B

From Arnoldi CC, Brodsky AE, Cauchoix J, et al. Lumbar spinal stenosis and nerve root entrapment syndromes: definitions and classification. *Clin Orthop.* 1976;115:4–5 with permission.

conditions, such as a narrowed or abnormally shaped spinal canal. Purely congenital or developmental spinal stenosis is uncommon and receives but brief mention in this chapter.

No better description of the lateral recess zone has been given than in Macnab's well-read and often quoted article on "Negative Disc Exploration" (21), in which he introduced the term "hidden zone" (Fig. 12-1). Since that time, spinal surgeons have struggled to decompress that zone without removing the inferior facet to cause spinal instability. All too often, in the orthopaedic community, the facet has been saved to the detriment of an adequate decompression of the foramen, whereas in the neurosurgical community, an adequate decompression has been completed at the expense of the facet joint, which has possibly led to subsequent instability.

This chapter concerns itself with the three most common forms of SCS.

1. SCS with degenerative spondylolisthesis, the most common stenotic condition, occurs most often in women (female-to-male ratio = 6:1) (9,10,20) (Fig. 12-2) and predominantly in the first story of each anatomic segment.

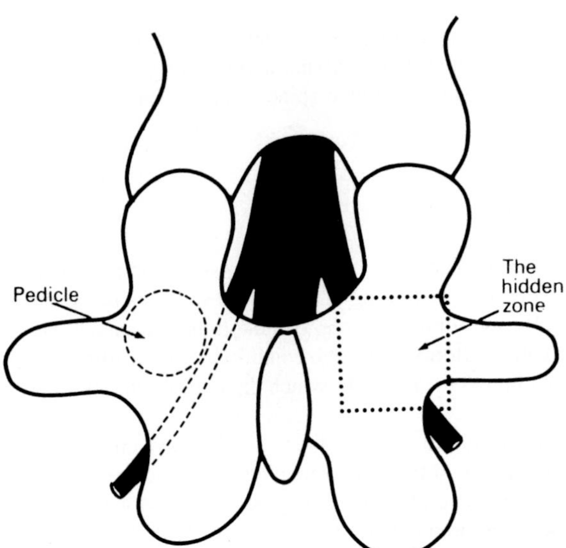

FIGURE 12-1 ● The hidden zone.

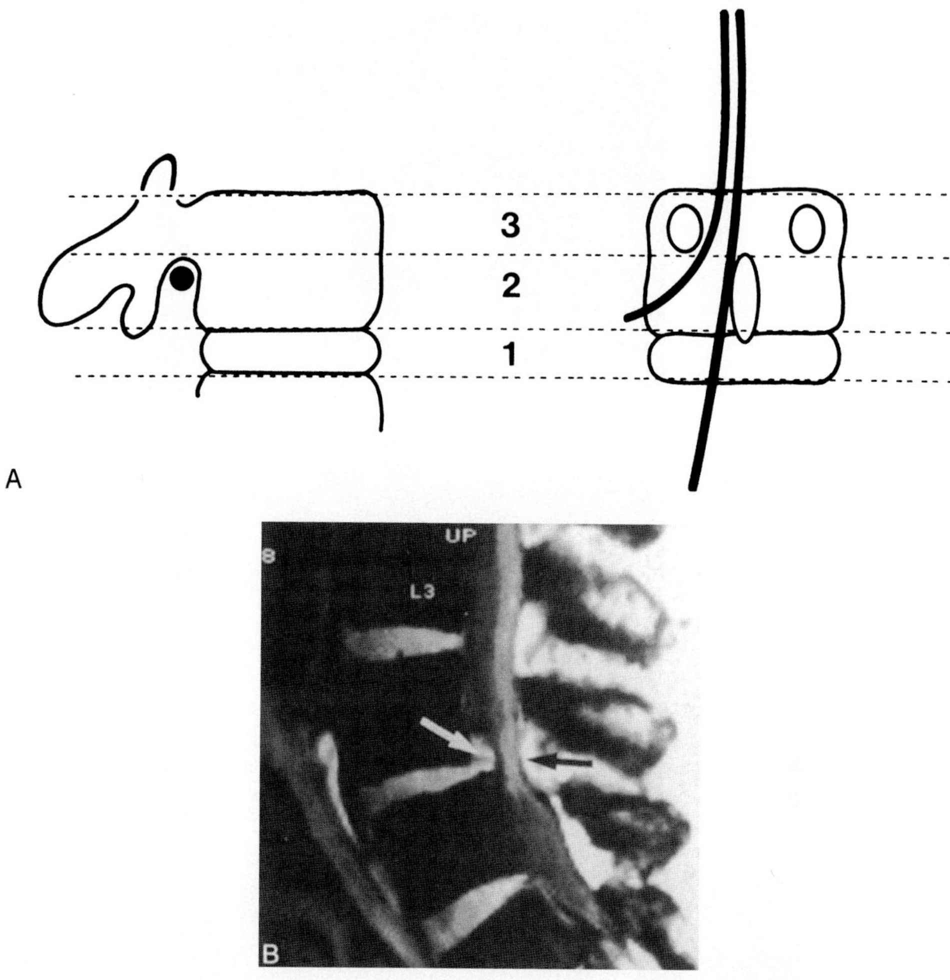

FIGURE 12-2 ● **A:** The three stories of each anatomic segment. (How many times have you seen this schematic!) **B:** Sagittal MRI of degenerative spondylolisthesis and spinal stenosis showing annular bulging *(white arrow)* and ligamentum flavum hypertrophy *(black arrow)* causing stenosis in first story and upper portion of adjacent third story. **C:** Axial MRI in same patient showing ligamentum flavum hypertrophy, or folding, also contributing to stenosis.

2. SCS without vertebral body translation is a condition equally distributed among men and women. (Fig. 12-3).
3. SCS may be due to a combination of a congenitally (developmentally) small spinal canal, superimposed on which are degenerative changes, further narrowing the spinal canal. This condition most commonly occurs in men of large stature and often before age 50 years (Fig. 12-4).

PATHOANATOMY: A SUMMARY

To understand the pathoanatomy of SCS, the reader is referred back to Chapter 1 on anatomy, paying specific attention to the first story of the anatomic segment (Fig. 12-2), which is usually the greatest point of acquired stenosis (Fig. 12-5). Aside from the less frequent congenital narrowing of the spinal canal, the three structures that contribute to the canal stenosis are the ligamentum flavum, the facet joints, and the disc space. Notice in Figures 12-2 to 12-5 how this maximum effect is largely confined to the first story and upper reaches of the third story of the level below. This intrasegmental degenerative "napkin-ring" concept is the key to understanding the message of this chapter.

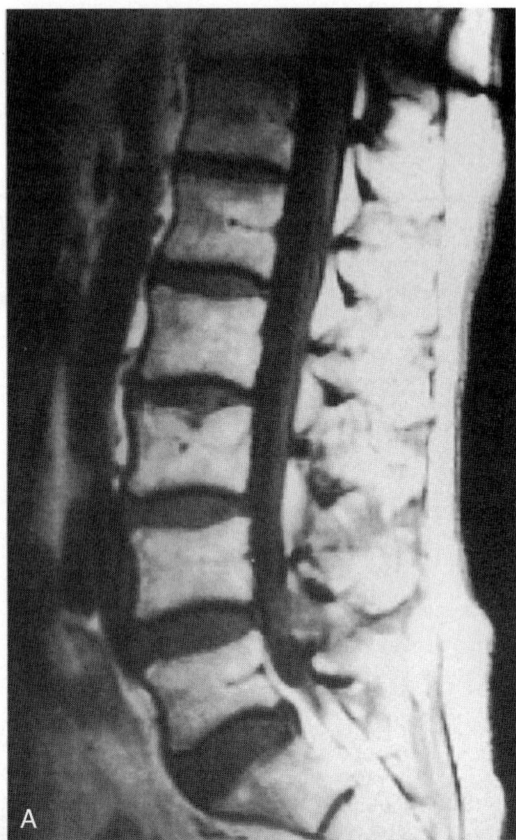

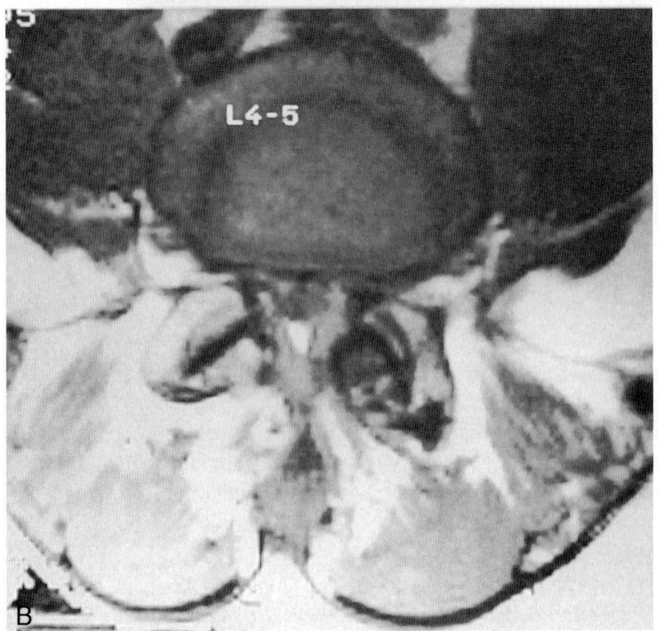

FIGURE 12-3 ● Spinal canal stenosis without a slipped vertebrae: **A:** T1 sagittal—the stenosis does not appear that severe. **B:** T1 axial shows the true extent of the stenosis at L4-L5.

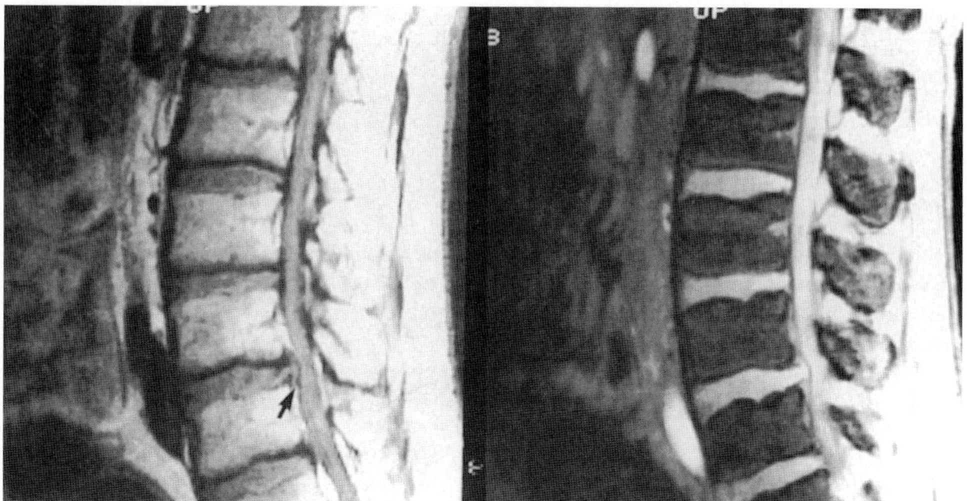

FIGURE 12-4 ● Spinal canal stenosis without a slip but with a significant congenital narrowing of the spinal canal. Note the "global" nature of the pencil thin canal. This was a young patient tipped into symptoms by a disc herniation at L4-L5 *(arrow).*

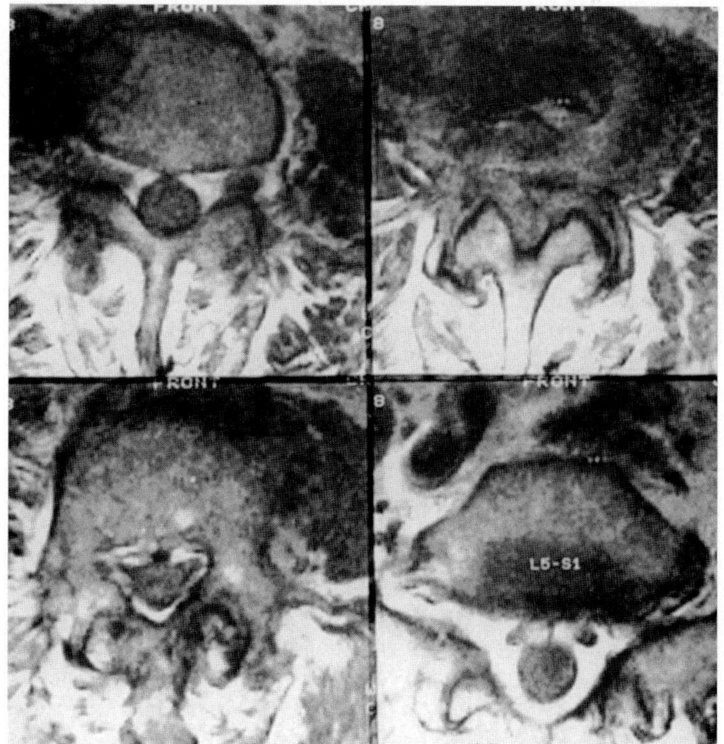

FIGURE 12-5 ● Adjacent MRI T1 axial slices to show first story spinal canal stenosis **(top right)**. Top left is second story of the fourth anatomic segment; bottom left is third story of fifth anatomic segment; and bottom right is first story of fifth anatomic segment (L5-S1 disc space).

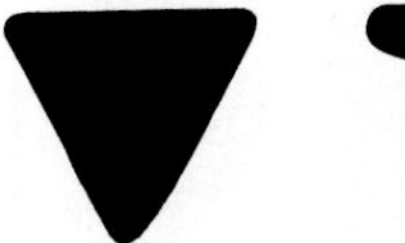
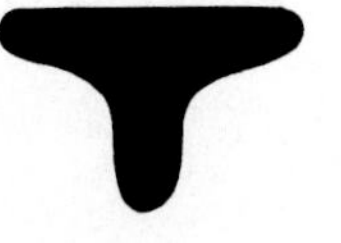
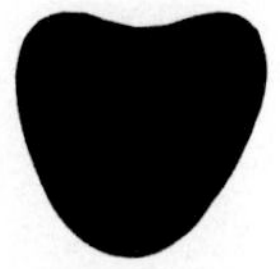

FIGURE 12-6 ● The three shapes of the spinal canal as seen on CT scan or MRI: round (really triangular), trefoil, oval.

SHAPE OF THE CANAL

Figure 12-6 illustrates the three basic shapes of the lumbar spinal canal. The most common shapes are round and ovoid. Perhaps 15% of humans have a trefoil canal, and canals of trefoil shape are most vulnerable to the degenerative changes that decrease the space occupied by the neurologic structures.

DEGENERATIVE CHANGES

Degenerative changes can affect the disc, the soft tissue supports, and the facet joints. (7,15,19,24) Annular bulging, ligamentum flavum infolding or hypertrophy, and osteophyte formation encroach on the spinal canal to decrease the space available to the cauda equina (Fig. 12-7).

The hypertrophied ligamentum flavum enfolds to encroach posteriorly and is the major lesion in stenosis of the first story. Further first story canal encroachment occurs when the facet subluxation of a degenerative spondylolisthesis contributes inferior and superior facet bony masses to narrow the space available to the cauda equina (Fig. 12-8). Finally, annular bulging, with or without retrospondylolisthesis, contributes to anterior narrowing of the canal.

In the second story, the anterior canal wall is formed by the inferior half of the vertebral body, which does not contribute to spinal stenosis. The one place in the second story where stenosis is said to occur is the very midline and posterior common meeting point of the superior edges of the lamina and spinous process (Fig. 12-9). This cortical edge can be likened to the wishbone of a chicken and is said to encroach on the midline of the dura at the junction of the second and third stories. But look at Figure 12-9B, this is the second story of Figure 12-7B and there is no stenosis.

The lateral portion of the second story is the foramen. As mentioned previously, superior capsular hypertrophy, especially in degenerative spondylolisthesis, can protrude into this lateral recess/foraminal interval, producing radicular symptoms due to root encroachment in the lateral zone (Fig. 12-10).

Within the third story, there is virtually nothing that can cause acquired spinal stenosis. At the top end of the pedicle (third story) lies the bottom end of the superior facet. If it is hypertrophied, then lateral zone stenosis (subarticular form) can occur, but virtually nothing in the lower portion of the third story of an anatomic segment can contribute to central canal stenosis.

TRANSLATION

When one anatomic segment translates on the next, a guillotining effect of the spinal canal occurs. The most common type of translation is degenerative spondylolisthesis, a forward or lateral slip of one anatomic segment on the next. Because of the intact neural arch, it has often been stated that the posterior elements of the cephalad segment impinge on the contents of the spinal canal (Fig. 12-11), when, in fact, the major lesion is still the ligamentum flavum and the facet joints. Lateral spondylolisthesis (Fig. 12-12) has the same effect on the space occupied by the cauda equina. Retrospondylolisthesis or posterior translation impinges least on the space occupied by the cauda equina except that it is usually part of the degenerative changes previously listed (Fig. 12-13).

CONGENITAL/DEVELOPMENTAL NARROWING OF THE SPINAL CANAL

The vertebral canal reaches its maximum size by 4 years of age. Thereafter, pedicles/vertebral bodies increase in size and the canal may change its shape, but the overall size of the canal changes little. Intrauterine factors such as drugs, alcohol, and smoking and environmental factors such as

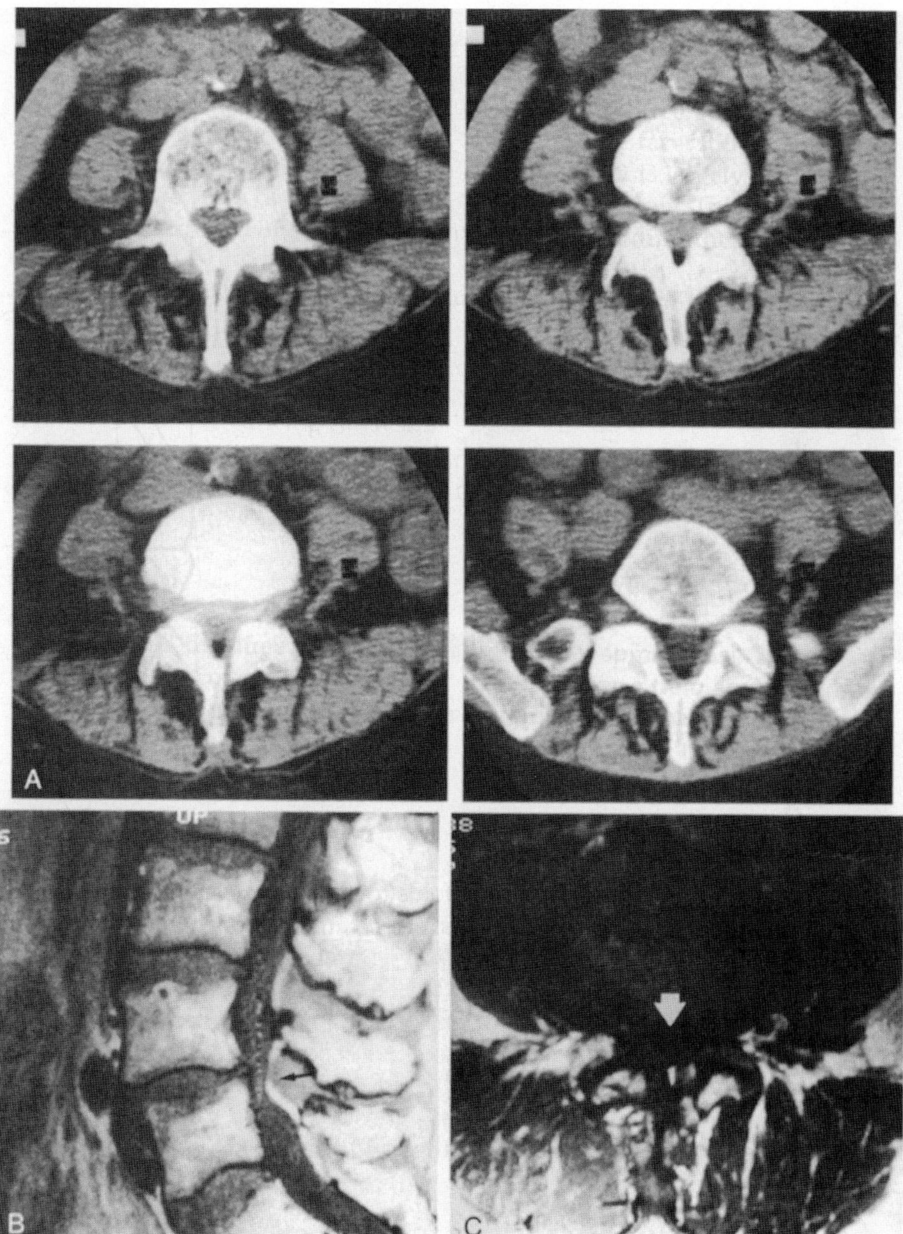

FIGURE 12-7 ● **A:** CT of spinal canal stenosis. The stenotic lesion is greatest in first story of L4 *(bottom left).* The third and second story of L4 **(top)** and the second story of L5 **(bottom, right)** are relatively free of stenosis. **B:** Sagittal MRI showing a similar picture. Spinal canal stenosis is a lesion in the first and upper reaches of the adjacent third story, produced largely by the buckling of the ligamentum flavum from behind *(arrow).* **C:** Axial T1 MRI showing encroachment on space available for cauda equina *(arrow)* by hypertrophied ligamentum flavum and facet joints.

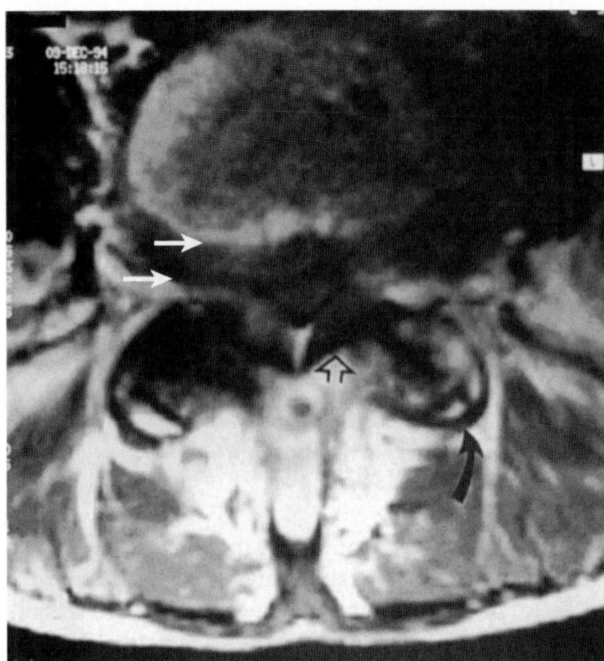

FIGURE 12-8 ● Another example of spinal canal stenosis on T1 axial showing the two margins of the posterior vertebral body *(arrows)* of the "slip" and the ligamentum flavum hypertrophy *(open arrow)* and facet joint hypertrophy *(curved arrow).*

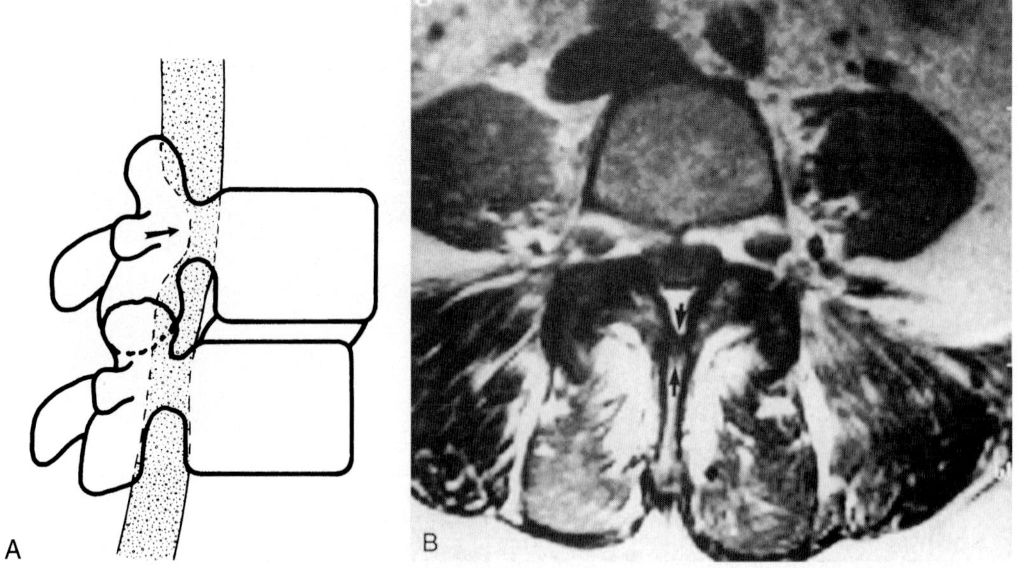

FIGURE 12-9 ● **A:** The wishbone effect. It seems to be present at surgery, yet so rarely seen on CT or MRI. **B:** An axial T1 MRI to show the wishbone *(arrows)*; the junction of the spinous process and two lamina. This is an example of a degenerative spondylolisthesis (Figs. 12-2 and 12-3), with no stenosis at the "wishbone."

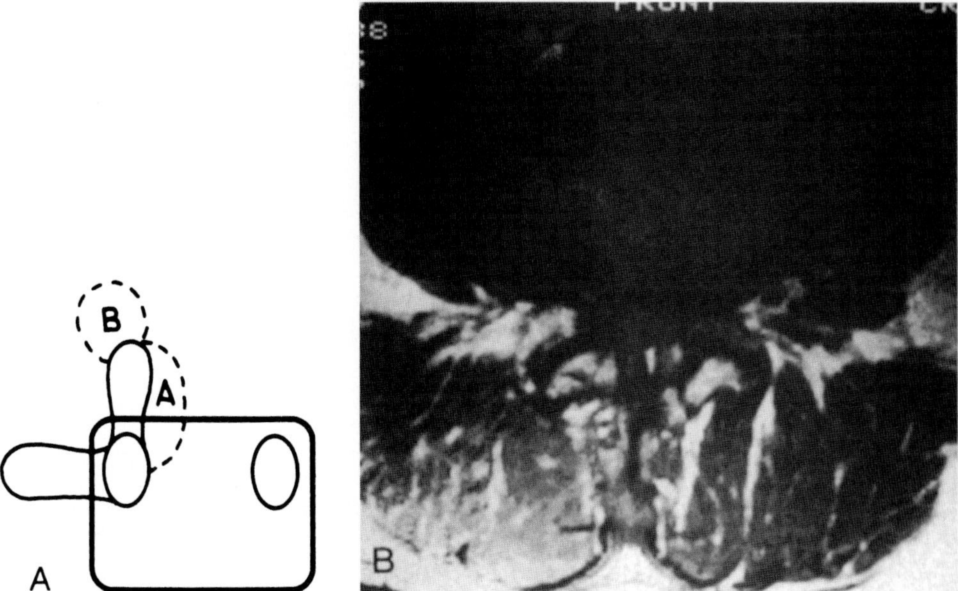

FIGURE 12-10 ● **A:** Schematic showing effect of capsular encroachment on foraminal zone *(B),* and medial edge facet hypertrophy on the subarticular zone *(A).* **B:** MRI showing actual lesion.

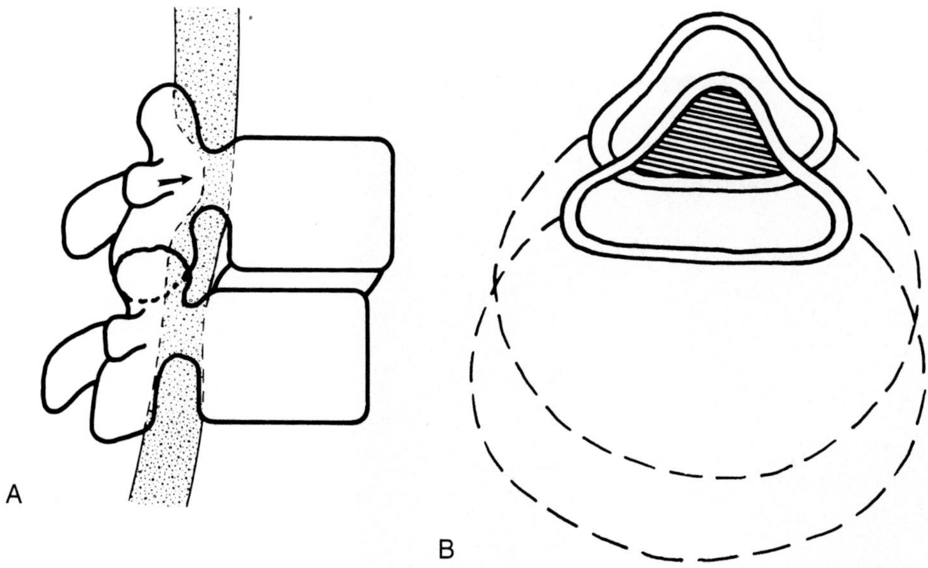

FIGURE 12-11 ● **A:** The wishbone effect. It seems to be present at surgery, yet so rarely seen on CT or MRI. **B:** The so-called guillotining effect on the cauda equina of one posterior arch sliding over its mate. Hatched area is space left for cauda equina.

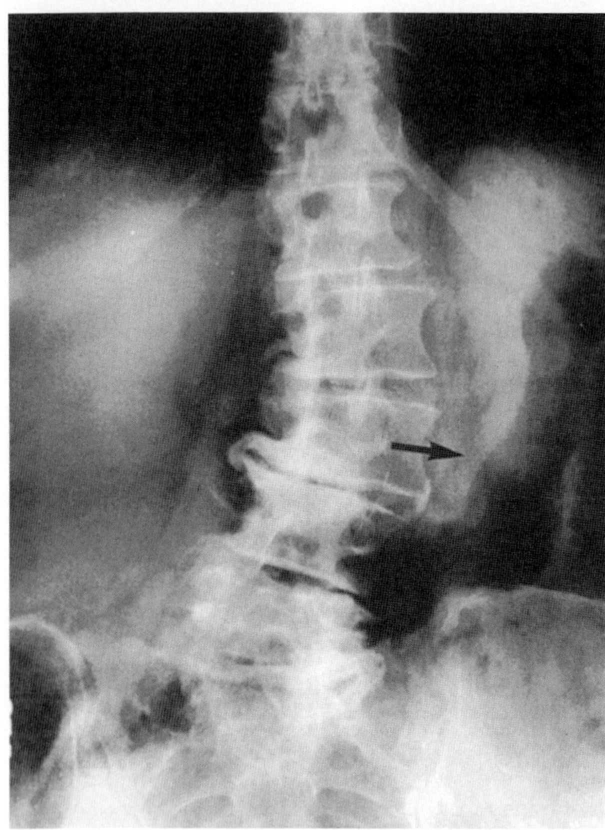

FIGURE 12-12 ● Radiograph of a lateral spondylolisthesis *(arrow)* at the apex of a degenerative scoliosis.

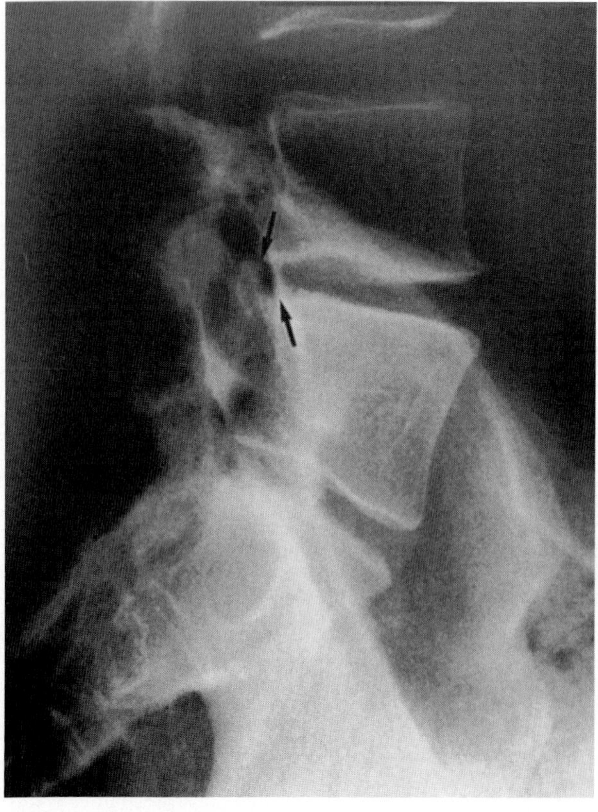

FIGURE 12-13 ● A retro-spondylolisthesis on plain radiograph at L4-L5 (arrows point to the respective corners of the vertebral bodies). Note how L4 is posterior to L5.

infectious diseases and malnutrition may potentially reduce canal size and result in a congenitally narrow canal. Because congenital/developmental stenosis is so prevalent among men of large stature (e.g., the front line of football players), one has to wonder if spurts in vertical height before the age of four somehow reduce the cross-sectional area of the spinal canal. The analogy is a sausage tube held up by one hand maintains its maximal diameter, but when stretched fully by two hands (Fig. 12-14) quickly narrows in diameter. Whatever the insult, the spinal canal can be left in a narrowed state, vulnerable to isolated traumatic events or cumulative trauma causing degenerative changes, which leads to symptomatic SCS (Fig. 12-15).

DIMENSION OF THE NORMAL SPINAL CANAL

Porter (24) has done considerable work in measuring the normal lumbar spinal canal. The bony dimensions are fairly constant from L1 to L5 and are listed in Table 12-2.

MEASUREMENTS IN SPINAL CANAL STENOSIS

Verbiest (31) made a major contribution to our knowledge of how much the canal narrows in patients with spinal stenosis. Careful intraoperative measurements (at the level of the disc space, i.e., first story) led him to identify three degrees of canal stenosis: no stenosis, relative stenosis, and absolute canal stenosis. Absolute SCS occurs when a sagittal diameter of less than 10 mm is noted. In a normal canal, the sagittal diameter is greater than 12 mm and may range up to 20 to 25 mm at L5-S1, normally the largest section of the spinal canal. The normal large diameters at L5-S1 contribute to the fact that SCS is rare at L5-S1 and is the reason why surgical decompression of the L5-S1 segment is so rarely indicated. Relative spinal stenosis occurs when the sagittal diameter is

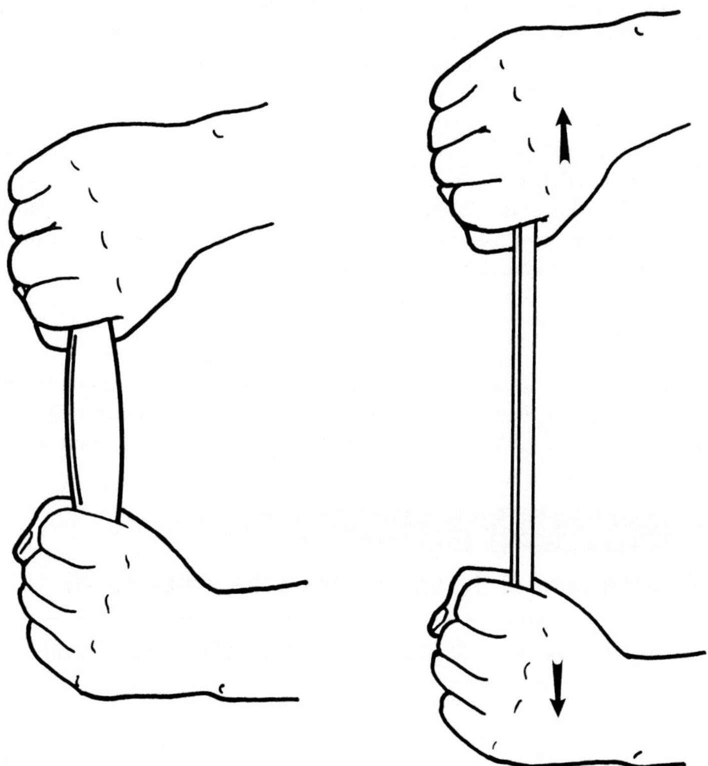

FIGURE 12-14 ● In trying to understand congenital stenosis, think of the unstretched sausage tube **(left)** being stretched through sudden growth **(right)**.

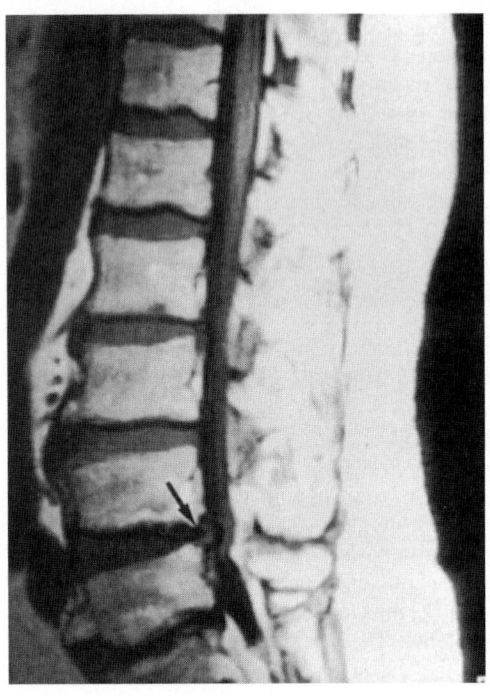

FIGURE 12-15 ● An example of congenital (global) spinal canal stenosis and an HNP *(arrow)* that precipitated the patient into a symptomatic state.

between 10 and 12 mm. Many attempts have been made to relate Verbiest's intraoperative measurements to plain radiographic films, all with limited success. Measurements applied to anteroposterior (AP) and lateral myelograms, axial computed tomography (CT) scans, and magnetic resonance imaging (MRI) are a better indication of the extent of stenosis (22). Spengler's group (27), (in a CT scan study), took into account soft tissue encroachment on the spinal canal, to conclude that the space available for the cauda equina should be measured as an area rather than a diameter. An area less than 100 mm^2 is considered to be indicative of relative spinal stenosis and a cross-sectional area of less than 65 to 70 mm^2 is indicative of absolute stenosis. As more MRIs are studied, further understanding of the anthropometric aspects of SCS will follow. The use of CT and MRI to reveal both bony and soft tissue encroachment on the space available for the cauda equina have largely made spinal canal measurements obsolete (30).

NEUROPATHOLOGY

Obviously, narrowing of the spinal canal constricts the dura and cauda equina within. The nerve roots themselves are constricted and often become adherent due to arachnoid changes. In a histologic examination of the roots, Watanabe and Parke (32) found a reduction in the number of

TABLE 12-2

Dimensions of the Spinal Canal (Midpedicle Level)

Midpedicle Level	Sagittal (mm)	Corona (interpedicle) (mm)
L1	16	22
L2	15	22
L3	14	23
L4	13	23
L5	14	24

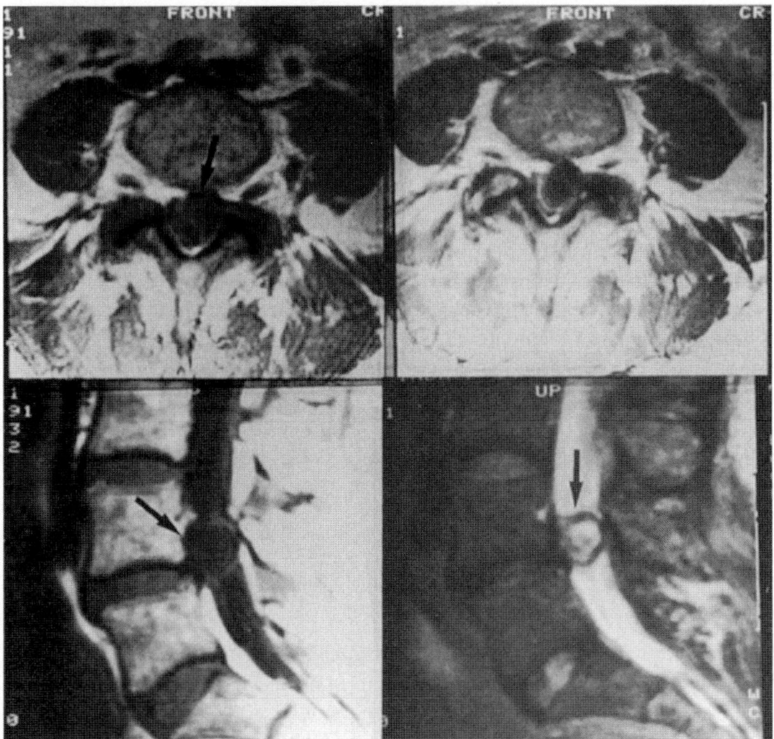

FIGURE 12-16 • A synovial cyst *(arrow)* at a very low grade "slip" L4-L5 contributing to some spinal canal stenosis. Gadolinium enhancement clearly outlines the cyst on axial T1 **(top right)**. The bottom right is a T2 sagittal highlighting the "water" in the cyst.

neurons, especially affecting large-caliber fibers. There were varying degrees of degeneration and demyelination with regeneration of nerve tissue. Morphologic assessment of the vessels revealed that the arterioles were absent at the level of the constriction and more coiled on either side of the constriction. Venules were collapsed at the level of the lesion and engorged proximally, and there appeared to be more arterial venous shunts proximal to the stenotic lesion.

Synovial cysts are reasonably common in SCS (Fig. 12-16). They arise as outpouchings from the degenerative (synarthrodial) facet joint, and if they enlarge into the canal they may further compress a nerve root. They often become very adherent to the dura and can be difficult to excise because of this.

PATHOPHYSIOLOGY

SCS is a chronic rather than an acute compression of the nerve roots in the cauda equina. Although the cauda equina is often considered a peripheral nerve structure, its coverings and vascular anatomy are more like those of a central nervous system structure than those of a peripheral nerve, which makes them more susceptible to compression.

Compression of the cauda equina affects nerve conduction, resulting in the leg symptoms, with it likely that aging nerves are more susceptible to this compressive phenomenon. It is well known that the symptoms of spinal stenosis are exacerbated by activity, specifically involving extension of the back. Thus, any theory to explain the symptoms of spinal stenosis must account for this mechanical component. It is likely that symptoms are caused by a combination of mechanical and ischemic nutritional factors (8,24,25).

The pathophysiology of spinal stenosis can be summarized as follows: The canal constriction or encroachment mechanically affects the cauda equina nerve bundle and the free flow of cerebrospinal fluid around this bundle. In turn, the nerve fiber is constricted and changes occur in the pia-arachnoid. When increased demands are placed on the cauda equina, such as when the patient walks, the body cannot satisfy the nutritional needs of the nerve roots because of the mechanical constriction and the associated ischemia. As well, the noxious by-products of metabolism build up in the constricted area and are not removed because of venous engorgement. Because of the mechanical compression shutting off the arterial blood flow to the constricted area of the cauda equina, arteriovenous shunts open on either side of the nerve root constriction, which in turn upset normal neurophysiologic function. The result is ectopic nerve impulses that produce some of the painful paresthetic and cramping symptoms of spinal stenosis. It is obvious from clinical facts that this neurophysiologic malfunctioning is more sensory than motor, which suggests that the large fiber sensory nerves are more susceptible to the compression than the motor fibers.

If the compression persists long enough, intraneural edema and fibrosis ensues. It is important to intervene surgically before symptoms progress to this stage, which is clinically evident as measurable weakness in the distal extremities.

Do not forget that the patient also experiences the mechanical symptoms of skeletal disease. These symptoms arise from degeneration within the disc spaces and the facet joints, resulting in varying degrees of skeletal instability (backache).

CLINICAL PRESENTATION

SYMPTOMS

Patients symptomatic with SCS may be categorized as (a) patients with only canal stenosis and (b) patients with both canal stenosis and lateral zone stenosis. The various combinations of canal and lateral zone stenosis are the reason for the rather confusing clinical picture presented by patients with SCS. For now, we have agreed to split and discuss the clinical presentation of canal stenosis.

Back Symptoms

Although back pain has been present for some years, almost all patients with spinal stenosis will present because leg symptoms have become disabling. They have put up with and adjusted to the back pain over the years, but the increasing limitation to walking due to leg "symptoms" is the "straw that broke the camel's back" and brought them to the doctor.

Leg Symptoms

The patient with canal stenosis commonly has bilateral radicular symptoms. The bilateral leg symptoms are very diffusely localized and often described as a heaviness, general soreness, or weakness that occurs in both lower extremities, especially with walking. The reason for the diffuse vague leg symptoms rather than discrete radicular pain is due to compression of multiple roots rather than a single root and an ischemic rather than an acute inflammatory origin of the radiculopathy. The distribution of the pain is most frequently to the buttocks, thighs, and calves because most stenotic lesions occur at L4-L5. If there is a higher level symptomatic stenotic lesion, anterior thigh discomfort will present. In addition, mild sensory symptoms in the form of paresthetic tingling or actual numbness are common. The patient may also describe night symptoms of restlessness in the legs or muscle cramps. The classic revelation by the patient is to volunteer that the symptoms are less aggravating in the grocery store, unbeknown to him or her because he or she is leaning on the shopping cart in the flexed position (Fig. 12-17).

These symptoms are almost always of insidious onset, with the patient seldom presenting before 55 years of age. A sudden worsening of these symptoms is equated with a sudden increase in vertebral body translation or the occurrence of an HNP within the stenotic segment, an infrequent event. This latter condition usually occurs at a slip level and is usually accompanied by a dramatic increase in the radicular component of the symptoms.

Within the diffuse cauda equina syndrome may be a sharper radicular component. If it involves a single nerve root in the lateral zone, the patient will describe a better defined radicular distribution to the extremity pain, affecting one leg more than its mate. The radicular symptom of lateral zone stenosis described by the patient is more specific than the diffuse bilateral leg symptoms

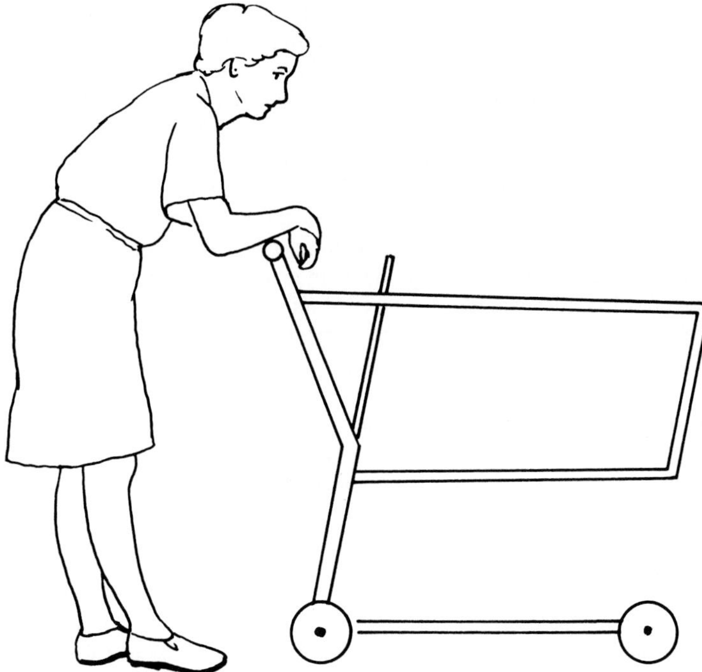

FIGURE 12-17 ● The shopping cart sign: Most patients with spinal canal stenosis have noticed that they are able to walk further when leaning on a shopping cart [because they are flexing their stenotic canal and tensing (unfolding) the ligamentum flavum], which increases the space available for the cauda equina. It is such a common description in spinal canal stenosis that it is worth making it a specific question in your history.

described by patients with SCS. However, the radicular component does not dominate the history, as with a disc herniation. Both sets of symptoms are usually aggravated by walking and relieved by rest or standing in the forward flexed position.

Clinical symptoms of bladder and bowel upset are unusual in patients with SCS. However, many patients with SCS have a subclinical upset in their bladder control and other local causes of impaired bladder control.

At least 50% of stenotic patients will report an upset in balance or an unsteadiness of gait. On the rare occasion, a patient will present with symptoms of collapsing legs due to their weakness and will come to the spinal surgeon only after negative cardiac investigation.

Both the backache and the leg symptoms of SCS are mechanical in nature. That is, they are aggravated by activity and often relieved significantly by rest. They are distinguished from vascular claudication in that the rest required for relief of neurogenic claudication is usually many minutes rather than a brief interruption in activities.

SIGNS

It is necessary to state clearly that often there is virtually nothing to find on physical examination (8,10,11,26), a fact that often relegates these patients to the scrap heap of a "functional illness." The diagnosis of SCS is made on history and verified on investigation. The main reason for doing a physical examination is to note that other conditions, such as vascular disorders, hip disease, or neurologic conditions, such as amyotrophic lateral sclerosis, are not present.

Examination of the back of a patient with SCS can show a loss of lumbar lordosis, sometimes associated with a degenerate scoliosis. Stiffness is often present and a step in the posterior spinous processes may be present if there is an associated degenerate spondylolisthesis.

Neurologic examination of the extremities is often fruitless unless the stenotic condition has been present for a long time and is well advanced. In these infrequent cases, one sees a significant amount of weakness and sensory upset along with an absence of reflexes. However, patients with SCS are more usually seen early in the progression of symptoms, and one records little in the way of reduced straight leg raising. Although paresthetic discomfort is a common symptom in SCS, it is unusual to find a loss of sensation to pinprick testing, temperature, or light touch. Because of the age of patients, loss of distal vibratory sensation is frequent. Although many patients complain of weakness in their legs, a specific weakness is rarely noted unless the stenosis has been present for a considerable time. It is usual to note that the ankle reflexes are much diminished over the knee reflexes (symmetric or asymmetric). However, that observation is frequent in many older patients without spinal stenosis. The observation of a discrepancy in reflexes gives us one useful rule: If a patient has brisk ankle reflexes he or she usually does not have SCS. (The patient may still have neurogenic claudication on the basis of bilateral subarticular stenosis of the fifth lumbar roots.) A femoral stretch test, if positive, suggests fourth root involvement either in the lateral zone or the cauda equina. There is a tendency for all signs to be more obvious immediately after the patient has been active.

The biggest problem with the history and physical examination of spinal stenotic patients is the fact they are in an age group in which a host of other conditions may be in tandem with their spinal stenosis.

TANDEM STENOSIS

This is a term introduced by Epstein et al. (10) and Dagi et al. (5) to describe a patient with both a lumbar canal stenotic lesion and cervical SCS. It is reasonable to assume that the ravages of degenerative disc disease that narrow the lumbar spinal canal can also do the same thing to the cervical spinal canal. The cervical stenotic lesion causes cord compression or myelopathy [upper motor neuron lesion (UMNL)], whereas the lumbar stenosis causes nerve root compression [lower motor neuron lesion (LMNL)]. This causes a mixed picture in the lower extremities. Patients will have hyper-reflexic knee jerks (UMNL), absent ankle jerks (LMNL), and equivocal or upgoing toes. The examiner focused on the lumbar canal stenosis will miss the cervical lesion, and an examiner similarly focused on the neck will miss the tandem lumbar stenosis.

DIFFERENTIAL DIAGNOSIS

The differential diagnosis of SCS (neurogenic claudication) versus vascular claudication is presented in Table 12-3. Although this table makes good script, and may even help you pass an examination, it is important to remember that spinal stenosis has many faces of presentation, some not clearly defined until the end of complete vascular and spinal investigation. Obviously, vascular claudication is the number one differential diagnosis. But other conditions that cause upset in walking also have to be included in the differential diagnosis. The "big four" in the differential diagnosis of SCS are osteoarthritis of the hips, referred leg pain, peripheral neuropathy (PN), and vascular claudication.

Bilateral Hip Joint Disease

It is surprising the number of times this diagnosis is missed and patients are labeled as having SCS. Noting the groin pain along with the thigh pain (both aggravated by walking) will alert you to the possibility of hip joint disease. Inability to rotate the hip for daily tasks (e.g., putting on one's socks and shoes) associated with a loss of hip range of motion on examination are the clues to radiograph the hips (Fig. 12-18).

Referred Leg Pain

Referred pain is a diffuse discomfort in the legs not unlike that of SCS. It differs from the leg symptoms in SCS in that:

1. Although it may occur with walking, it does not limit walking distance.
2. It rarely goes below the knees.
3. It is not associated with neurologic symptoms (numbness, paresthesia).
4. The associated backache dominates the history.

TABLE 12-3

Differential Diagnosis of Claudicant Leg Pain[a]

Findings	Vascular Claudication	Neurogenic Claudication (SCS)
Back Pain	Rare	Always in the past or present history
Leg Pain		
Type	Sharp, cramping	Vague and variously described as radicular, heaviness, cramping
Location	Exercised muscles (often calf, but may be buttock and thigh). May be one leg	Either typical radicular or extremely diffuse and almost always buttock, thigh, and calf in location. Always both legs in canal stenosis
Radiation	Rare after onset, but may be distal to proximal	Common after onset, usually proximal to distal
Aggravation	Walking, not standing	Usually aggravated by walking, but can be aggravated by standing
Walking uphill	Worse	Better (because back is flexed)
Walking downhill	Better (less muscular energy needed)	Worse (because back is extended)
Relief	Stopping muscular activity even in the standing position	Walking in forward, flexed position more comfortable; once pain occurs, relief comes only with lying down or sitting down
Time to relief	Quick (minutes)	Slow (many minutes)
Neurologic symptoms	Not present	Commonly present
Straight leg raising tests	Negative	Mildly positive or negative
Neurologic examination	Negative	Mildly positive or negative
Vascular examination	Absent pulses	Pulses present
Skin appearance	Atrophic changes	No changes

SCS, spinal cord stenosis.
[a]Note that both vascular and neurogenic claudication can coexist.

Peripheral Neuropathy

PN is the toughest differential diagnosis of all, and missing it has to be the most common reason for a failed outcome following spinal stenosis surgery. The two conditions (SCS and PN) may co-exist in the stenosis age group. The clinical presentation of PN is dominated with neurologic symptoms more so than pain and produces a more uniform distal stocking pattern of neurologic deficits. These patients do not necessarily become aggravated by walking but they do experience unsteadiness that interferes with walking. Often, electrophysiologic testing is required to differentiate these conditions. Of course the absence of a stenotic lesion on MRI is a good reason to step back and consider the diagnosis of PN.

A Word about Trochanteric Bursitis

All too often spinal stenotic patients are given the diagnosis of trochanteric bursitis. This is followed by an injection of local anesthetic and steroid into the trochanteric area giving relief of symptoms due to a placebo effect. The relief is short-lived because the real condition is spinal stenotic alteration of the pelvic mechanics to accommodate changes in the lumbar spine (Fig. 12-18).

INVESTIGATION

Investigation of a patient with SCS is often difficult to sort out. Because of the age group affected, it is important to rule out other conditions, such as infection, tumors, and other nonmechanical causes of back pain. A high percentage of these patients may also have vascular disease, and it is important

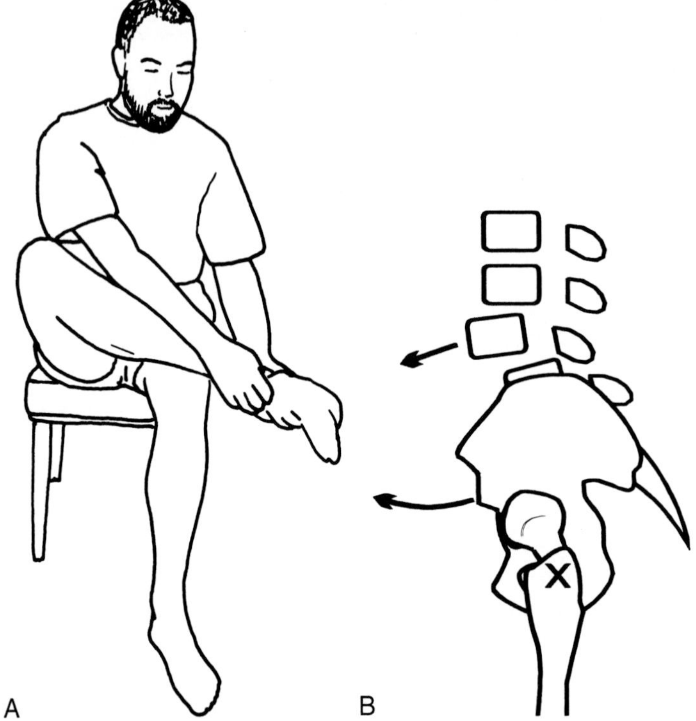

FIGURE 12-18 ● **A:** A patient with an osteoarthritic hip has trouble externally rotating the hip to get a sock on: not a problem in spinal canal stenosis. **B:** The development of pain over the greater trochanter (X) is from a pelvic tilt *(lower curved arrow)* to compensate for the forward slip of the body (at L4-L5). The tensor fascia lata comes into play in an attempt to rotate (compensate) the pelvic balance. This causes pain over the greater trochanteric region. Another form of compensation is backward subluxation (retrospondylolisthesis) above, as shown in this schematic.

to rule out symptomatic aortoiliac or femoral arterial insufficiency. Neurologic symptoms require consideration of all possible causes, including generalized disorders unrelated to the spine.

RADIOLOGIC INVESTIGATION

Plain radiographic films of most patients with low back pain are routinely ordered but yield little information about a patient with SCS except to show vertebral subluxations. Their greatest use is to rule out other conditions, such as tumors or infection. Radiographic films do reveal the degenerative changes within the disc space and the facet joints along with osteophytic formation. Subluxations are also obvious on plain radiographic films and bear on the surgical decision. In the presence of a spondylolisthesis, flexion and extension films give information on the degree of instability.

CT myelography is a useful investigation in the patient suspected of having spinal stenosis. Water-soluble, nonionic compounds are best used for myelographic examination. They are much better than older oil-based myelographic compounds because they offer superior demonstration of the nerve roots. Another advantage of low-viscosity compound is its ability to slide by the block to show levels below the stenotic obstruction. This is most evident on CT myelography (Fig. 12-19). CT myelography allows detailed analysis of the first, second, and third stories of each segment (Fig. 12-19). In addition, myelography allows for screening of the higher lumbar levels to exclude unusual pathologic conditions. Redundant nerve roots are more readily demonstrated by water-soluble contrast material (28) and the incidence of contrast-induced arachnoiditis is much less.

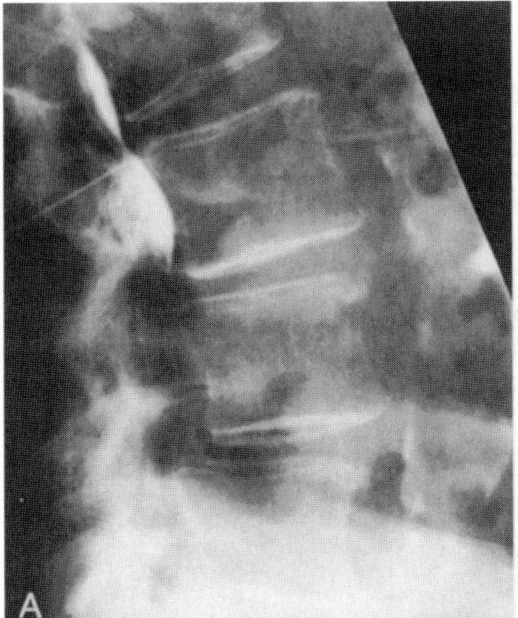

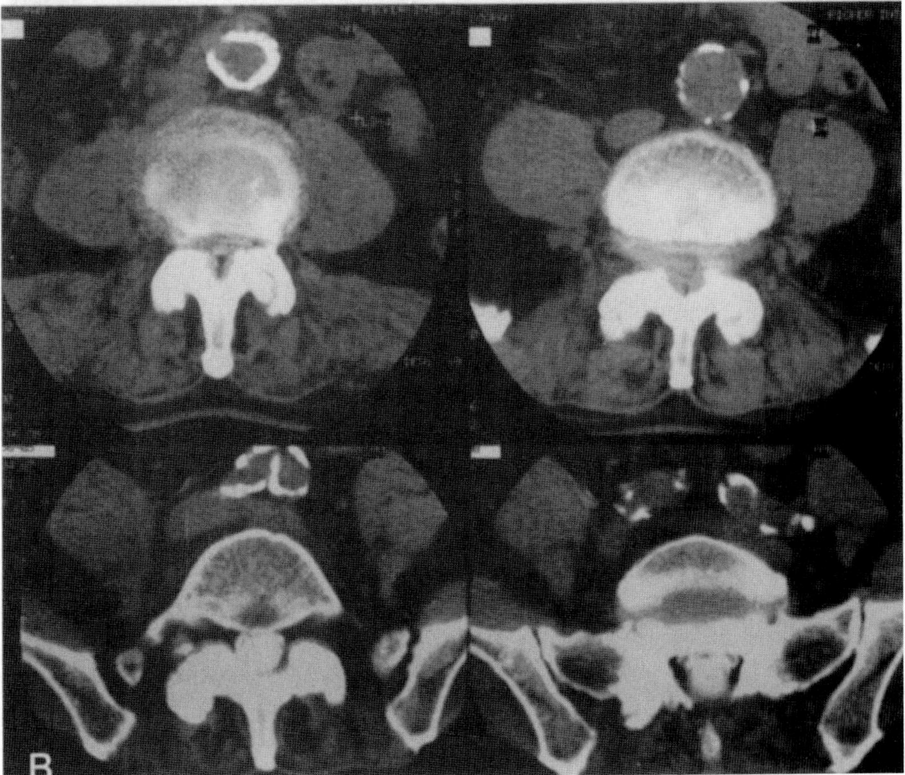

FIGURE 12-19 ● **A:** Myelogram showing apparent complete block at stenotic site, L3, with no contrast at lower segments. **B:** Subsequent CT myelogram showing flow of contrast past the obstruction at L4-L5 to L5-S1.

The myelographic block of SCS is typical and described as either single level or multiple level. An incomplete obstruction is described as having an apple-core appearance (Fig. 12-20) and a complete obstruction as having a paintbrush appearance (Fig. 12-21). These two changes are to be distinguished from the meniscal-like change that occurs with tumors of the spinal canal (Fig. 12-22). Functional myelography including flexion and extension views can be used to bring out subtle encroachments influenced by positioning.

MAGNETIC RESONANCE IMAGING

MRI is used increasingly for imaging in SCS (3). In most situations, except for a scoliotic patient with stenosis, it is superior to any other form of investigation (Figs. 12-2, 12-3, 12-4, 12-8). It is noninvasive, involves no radiation exposure, and provides two views at right angles to each other

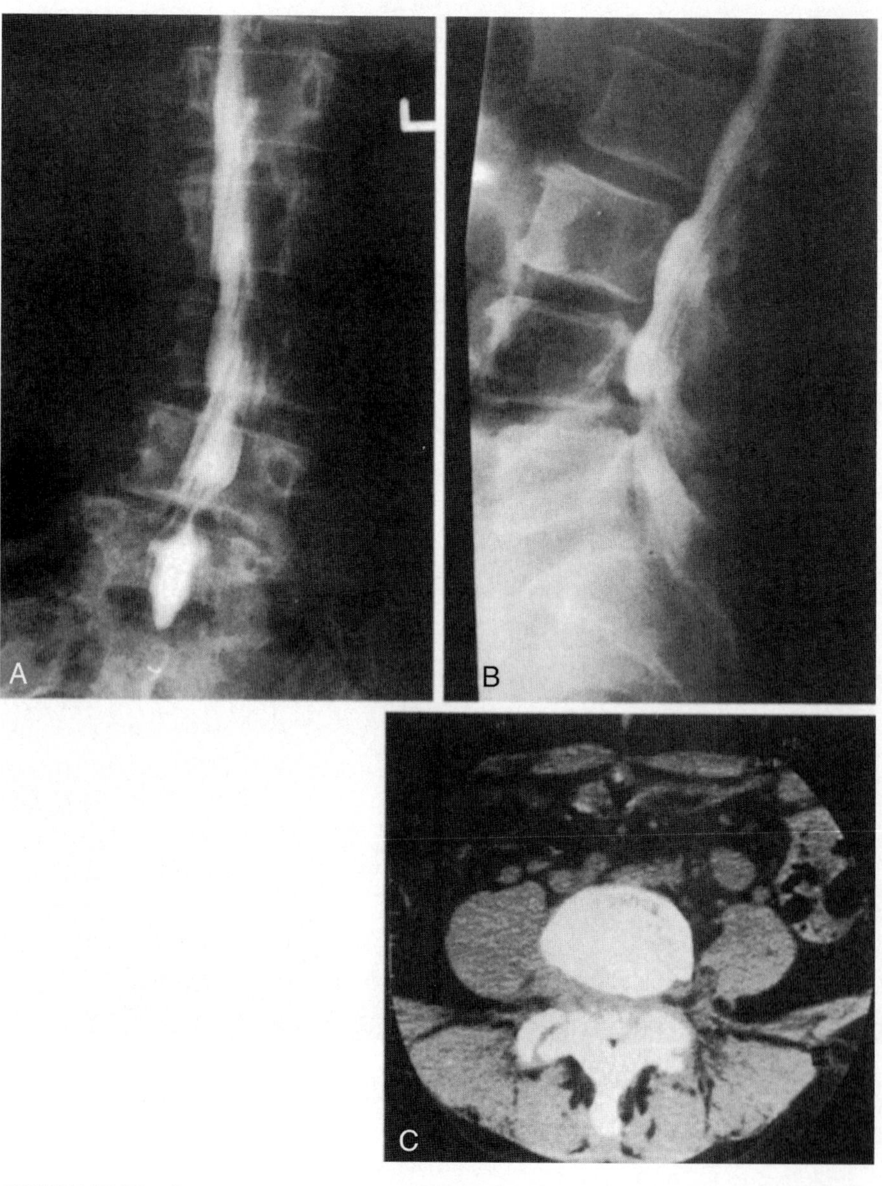

FIGURE 12-20 ● **A:** AP myelogram showing lateral spondylolisthesis. **B:** Lateral myelogram, same patient, showing forward spondylolisthesis. **C:** CT myelogram, axial slice, showing resulting stenosis.

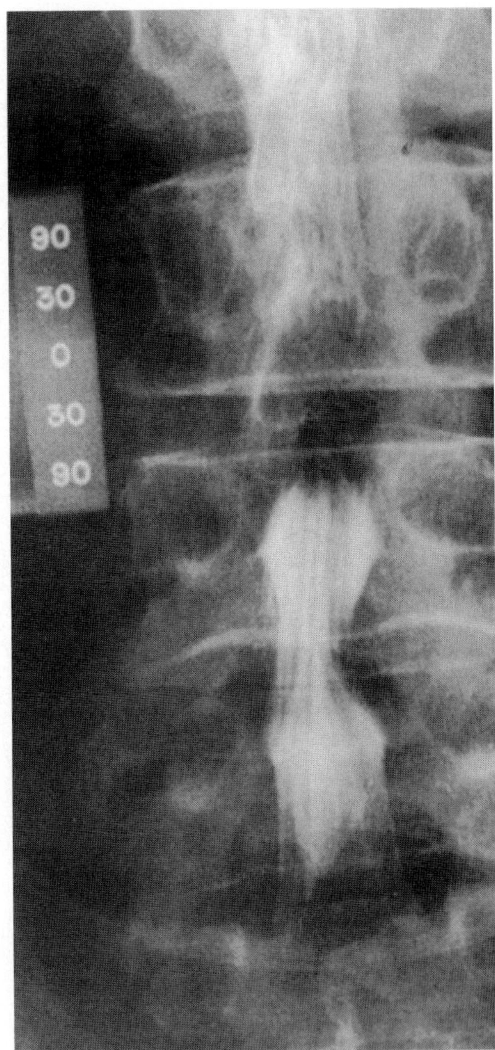

FIGURE 12-21 • Complete obstruction producing paint-brush effect. Note the redundant nerve roots above the block.

(sagittal and axial). Most important, the sagittal images are of all areas of the lumbar spine from the conus to S1. However, MRI is notorious for underestimating the degree of canal stenosis.

Miscellaneous Tests

Electromyograms and nerve conduction studies have not been useful in the assessment of a patient with SCS except to rule out other neurologic disorders. Much work is presently proceeding on the use of somatosensory-evoked potentials to decide on the level of involvement in spinal stenosis (6). To date, this work is not clinically applicable.

TREATMENT

CONSERVATIVE CARE

There is nothing fancy about conservative care in SCS (14). Rest in the form of corset support, weight loss, and the use of a cane can be prescribed. Obviously, anti-inflammatory medication is useful but be mindful of the side effects that are very prone to occur in this older age group.

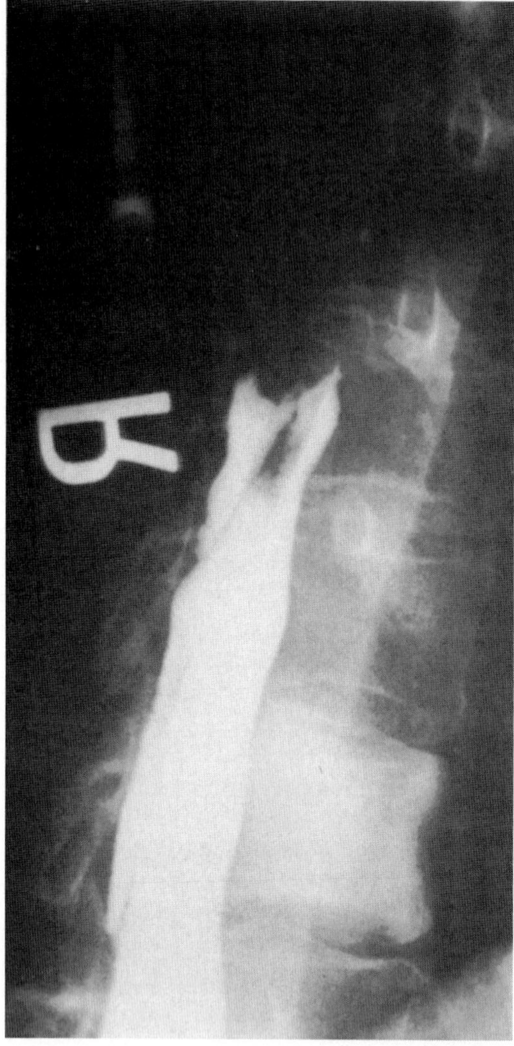

FIGURE 12-22 ● Meniscal-like lesion of tumor obstruction to contrast flow.

Narcotic pain medication and muscle relaxants should be avoided because you are dealing with a chronic condition. A Williams exercise program to reduce lumbar lordosis is very beneficial. Hyperextension exercises are to be avoided. Heat and/or ice and modalities such as ultrasound are of limited benefit. It is unusual that manipulation affects leg symptoms, although it may be very beneficial for back pain.

Epidural cortisone is often prescribed for the treatment of SCS, but the literature contains conflicting evidence of efficacy (23). In addition, successful installation of materials in the extradural space in older patients with the degenerative changes associated with stenosis can be very difficult.

NATURAL HISTORY OF SPINAL STENOSIS

Although some patients with SCS experience temporary relief with conservative care (15,16), any patient with significant narrowing of the spinal canal and the disabling symptoms of SCS will ultimately need surgical intervention because of the progressive, relentless nature of SCS. Patients with a minimal to moderate lesion on MRI and moderate symptoms can often be helped by conservative care. Approximately 50% will not progress and may be managed conservatively, but 50% will experience increasing symptoms despite conservative care and eventually require surgery.

The following are indications for surgical intervention:

1. Failure of a patient with SCS to respond to standard conservative treatment measures.
2. Significant pain and disability in walking regardless of neurologic findings and duration of symptoms.
3. Established weakness that is clinically measurable, regardless of duration of symptoms and conservative treatment.

TIMING OF SURGERY

Patients may become aware of a progression of symptoms despite bracing, therapy, and medication and are discouraged by the prospect of further conservative care. They are counting the years and often want to stay active. All degenerative spinal conditions deserve a trial of conservative care, but, in particular, SCS deserves a good dose of common sense in making treatment decisions. Surgery is obviously elective and can be done when the patient is medically fit. Surgery should not be delayed many months or years, during which the patient may develop signs of weakness.

GENERAL MEDICAL CONSIDERATIONS

Spinal stenosis usually occurs in older patients, who often have associated medical problems. Often patients are wrongly denied surgery because of such conditions. Monitoring and fine-tuning of anesthetic agents in today's world are so good that only patients with severe general medical problems, for example, unstable angina, severe hypertension, or severe respiratory insufficiency, should be denied surgery. As long as the patient is aware of the risks, benefits, and alternatives, indicated surgery should proceed.

Many of our older patients are highly motivated and want to be active, and it is unfair to withhold surgery. Probably the most significant indicator of a good outcome of surgery is this high degree of motivation: "I would rather die than live the rest of my life immobile and restricted to the house."

One important point: Older patients with SCS often have associated (symptomatic) vascular disease and osteoarthritis of the hip(s). It is best to deal with those conditions first, including surgery if indicated. In a significant number of these patients, symptoms thought to be due to spinal stenosis disappear when the vascular disease or hip disease is fixed. The opposite can happen as well. After the vascular disease or hip is fixed and the patients attempt to increase their activity, they may find limitations from the neurogenic claudication due to the spinal canal.

SURGERY

Although the primary goal is to relieve the patient's leg symptoms, one must not lose sight of the mechanical back pain that is present. It is important to explain to patients before surgical intervention that although relief of leg pain often occurs, it may not be complete and some back pain will almost certainly remain. But the residual symptoms should not restrict activities nearly to the extent of the preoperative symptoms.

Two surgical procedures, alone or in combination, are necessary to deal with SCS: (a) decompression of neurologic structures and (b) stabilization of vertebral elements. Let us deal with each one of the three clinical presentations of SCS.

SPINAL CANAL STENOSIS WITHOUT VERTEBRAL BODY TRANSLATION

Usually these patients have very little back pain and a fusion is not part of the game plan. If there is a reasonable component of back pain, it is usually due to multiple level degenerative changes and fusion is not a reasonable option. This latter situation is fortunately not common and the surgical decision centers around the nature and extent of the decompression.

DECOMPRESSION

Length of Decompression

A number of general statements apply to decompression. Is it necessary to decompress every stenotic level seen on radiograph? Some decompress only those levels causing symptoms; others prefer to decompress every stenotic segment seen on radiograph. The tendency today is to do more levels, but limit the extent of the decompression at each level, an approach that is commented on later. Fortunately, in 50% of the SCS cases, the decompression can be confined to a single level, usually L4-L5, and usually the first story of L4 (Fig. 12-23). Decompression is usually not required in the first and second stories of L5, and thus stability of the lumbosacral junction can be maintained.

It is often stated that one should decompress to the level of a pulsating dura or to the level of epidural fat. Although this is a good goal, many times it is not achievable (10,18). The clinical presentation and the structural defects as seen on investigation should guide the surgeon in assessing how far decompression should extend proximally and distally.

Suggested Guidelines for Length and Width of Decompression

1. Decompress all contiguous levels of canal stenosis (Fig. 12-24).
2. Ignore skip lesions (e.g., L1-L2 when doing an L4-L5 decompression) unless the stenosis is severe and/or is producing specific symptoms.
3. Decompress both subarticular regions in each anatomic segment being decompressed (Fig. 12-25).
4. Read the foramen on MRI (Fig. 12-26) and decompress only those that are narrowed.

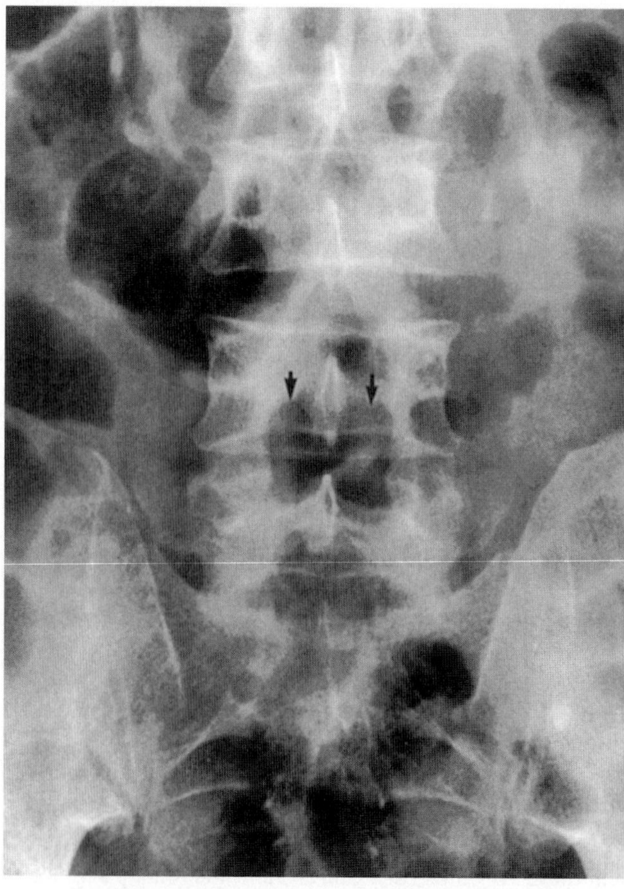

FIGURE 12-23 ● AP radiograph of a single-level spinal canal stenosis decompression (laminoplasty) at L4-L5 (arrows at upper margin of laminar decompression).

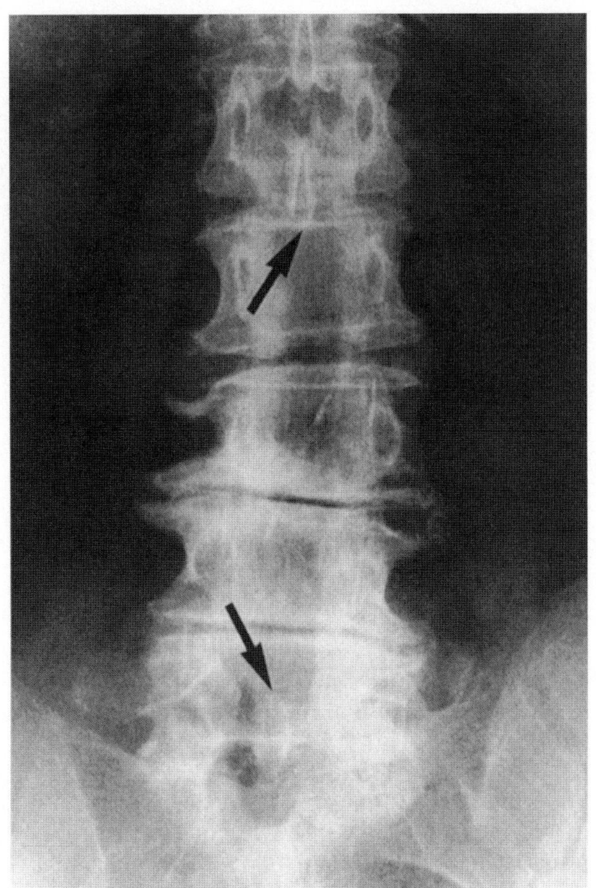

FIGURE 12-24 ● A multilevel decompression for spinal canal stenosis extending from L1-L2 *(top arrow)* to L4-L5 *(bottom arrow).*

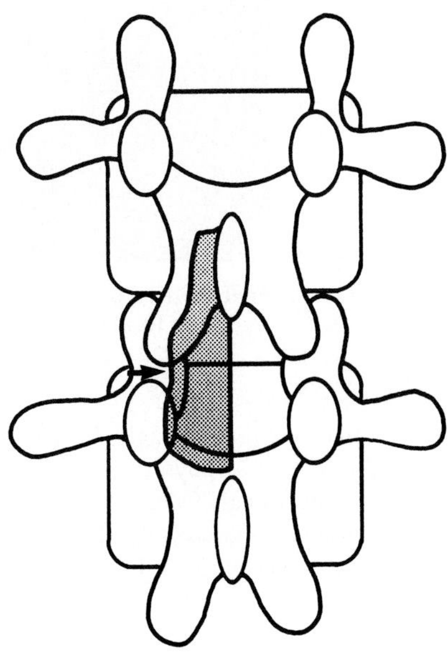

FIGURE 12-25 ● The method of subarticular decompression by taking off the medial edge of the facet joint *(arrow).*

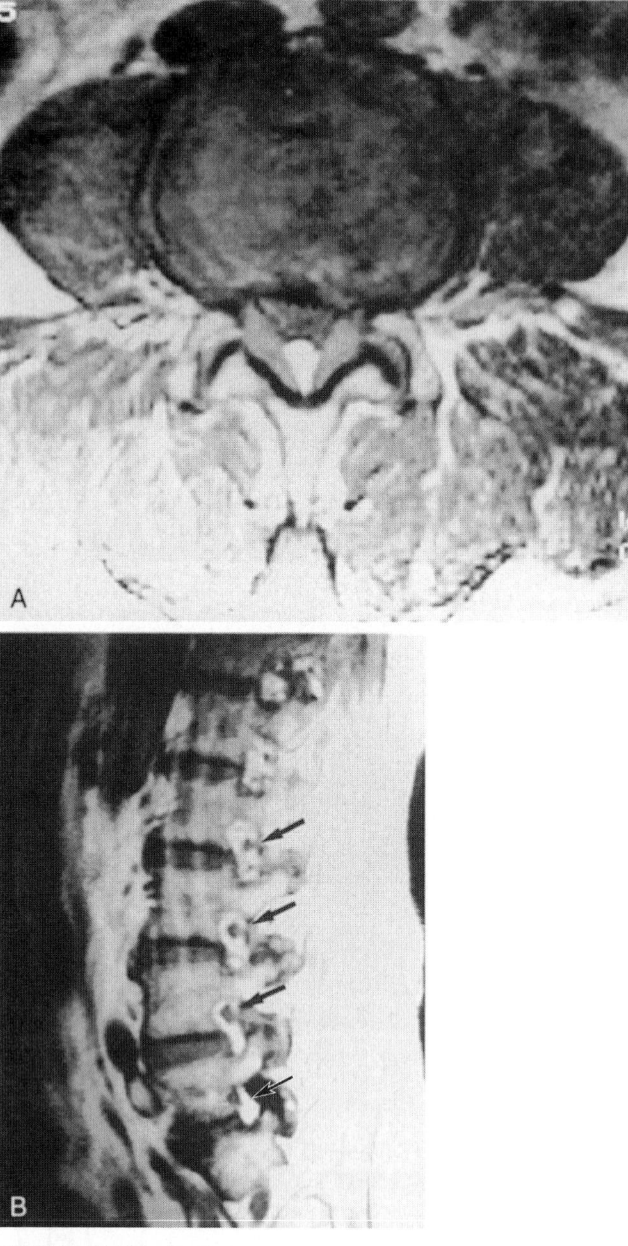

FIGURE 12-26 ● **A:** T1 axial MRI showing spinal canal stenosis. **B:** The foramina on T1 sagittal MRI are all wide open *(arrows).*

5. You may sacrifice a single facet joint in a patient with a narrowed disc space that has been stabilized by osteophytes.
6. Sacrificing a single facet joint in a younger patient with a wide disc space is likely to lead to future problems. Fortunately, this is a rare surgical problem because narrowed foramina tend not to occur at a nonslip level with a wide disc space.

ADHESIONS

It is often reported that adhesions are present between the dura and surrounding tissues, which make dissection difficult. In fact, adhesions de novo are rare; they do occur in the presence of a synovial cyst and can also be associated with a calcified ligamentum flavum. In addition, adhesions can be seen in the concavity of a longstanding degenerative scoliosis.

THE FACET JOINT

If no vertebral body translation is present, it is recommended that stability be preserved by saving each facet joint.

DISC

It is rare for discopathology to be a significant component of spinal stenosis (21) and thus, disc surgery is rarely needed at the time of a spinal stenosis decompression. It is prudent to avoid interfering with discal integrity because this increases postoperative instability. Be aware of the stenotic patient with dominant leg pain, especially of sudden onset. They likely have a disc herniation hidden in their stenotic canal that will be impossible to see on MRI, but easy enough to find at surgery only if you go looking for it!

POSTOPERATIVE CARE

Aside from the medical problems attendant in most of these patients, postoperative care for the decompression and fusion is very limited. The patients are ambulated as soon as possible (the day of surgery) in a light canvas corset. Discharge is usually 2 to 4 days after surgery with the activity level prescribed being a renewed commitment to walk.

SPINAL CANAL STENOSIS WITH VERTEBRAL BODY TRANSLATION

Degenerative spondylolisthesis (Fig. 12-7B) was first described by Macnab (20) as spondylolisthesis with an intact neural arch: the so-called pseudospondylolisthesis. It is the second most common form of spondylolisthesis in adults and affects the L4-L5 level most frequently. It may affect multiple levels (Fig. 12-27) and is at least five times more common in women. It is also more common when the last formed level is fixed to the pelvis (Fig. 12-28).

It is thought to be more common at L4-L5 because of the sagittal orientation of the facet joints at this level compared with the more coronally oriented facet joints at L5-S1. As well, L5-S1 is a more stable level because it is set down in the pelvis and anchored by the iliolumbar ligaments (Fig. 12-29).

The condition is aptly designated "degenerative" because it is thought to occur after long term instability (backache) due to degenerative changes in the posterior ligamentous structures, the disc space, and especially the facet joints. All these changes allow for the forward slip of the cephalad vertebral body on its mate—not the reverse (Fig. 12-30).

When degenerative spondylolisthesis is associated with SCS, the patients can be divided into three groups.

GROUP ONE (AGE OLDER THAN 70 YEARS, NARROW DISC SPACE, NO FLEXION-EXTENSION INSTABILITY, MINOR BACK PAIN)

This group has reached the stabilization phase of Kirkaldy-Willis et al. (19). The body, as natural defenses, through fibrosis of the disc and facet joint capsules and osteophyte formation, has stabilized the segment. These patients can be managed just like the spinal stenosis without slip group—that is, decompression of the symptomatic segments without fusion (Fig. 12-31).

GROUP TWO (AGE YOUNGER THAN 60 YEARS, WIDE DISC SPACE, INSTABILITY ON FLEXION-EXTENSION, BACK PAIN)

Obviously, patients in this group have unstable motion segments and require a fusion at the time of decompression (12,17). The addition of the fusion stabilizes the slip segment and prevents further postoperative increase in the slip, which may lead to a poor surgical outcome. (17). Having to remove a facet joint to decompress a foramen in this group makes a fusion a necessity (Fig. 12-32).

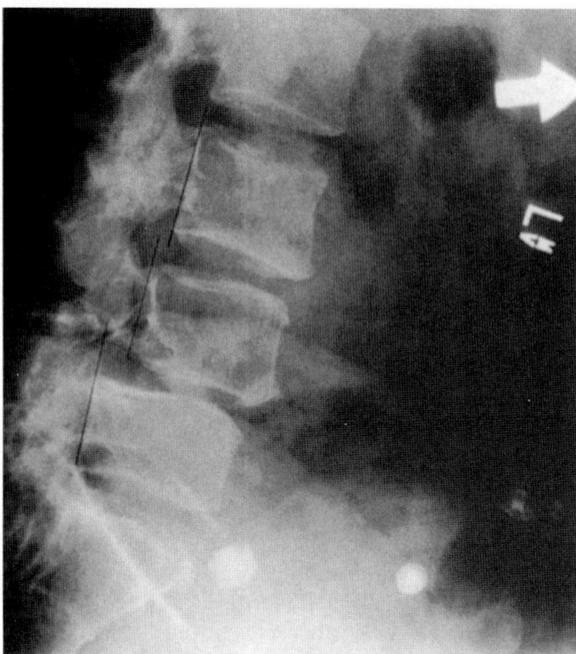

FIGURE 12-27 ● A stair-step degenerative spondylolisthesis on flexion: L3 is slipped forward on L4, and L4 is slipped forward on L5.

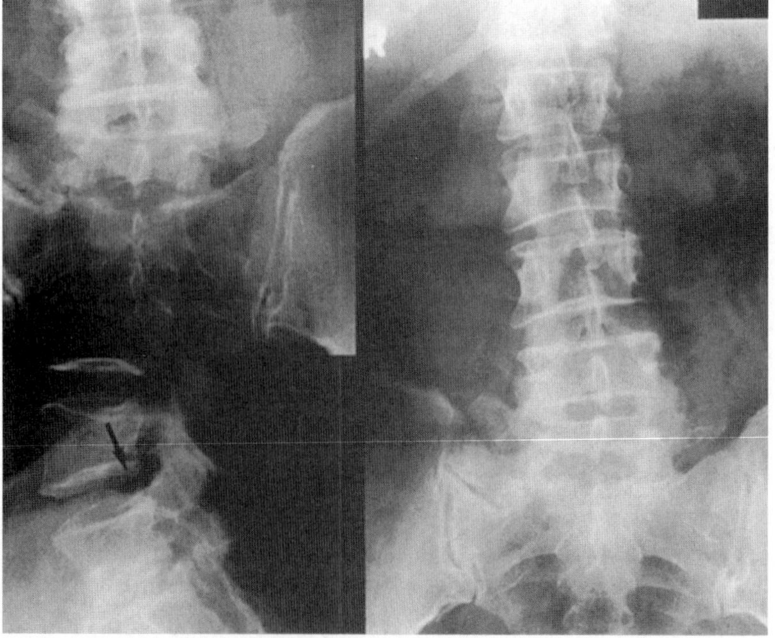

FIGURE 12-28 ● Degenerative spondylolisthesis is more common when the last formed level is fixed to the pelvis. If you look closely at the bottom left lateral radiograph, you can see that the last mobile level (LML) is slightly forward on the last formed level (LFL) *(arrow).*

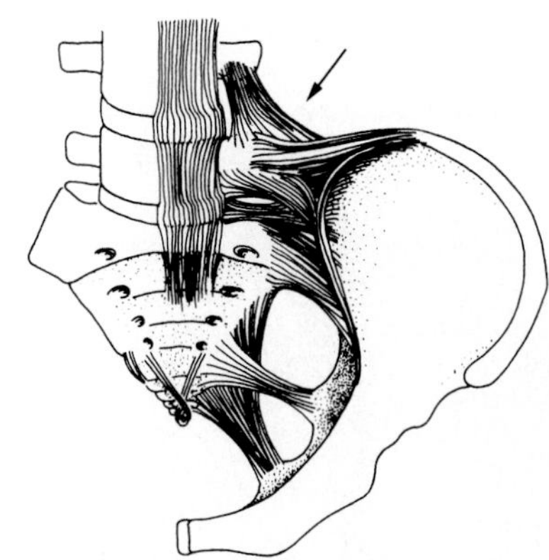

FIGURE 12-29 ● The iliolumbar ligaments.

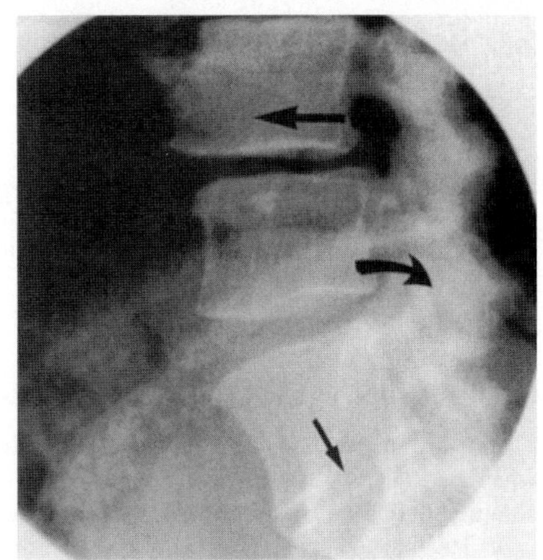

FIGURE 12-30 ● A degenerative spondylolisthesis *(top arrow)* is shown and compared with a retrospondylolisthesis *(curved arrow).* The bottom arrow points to a fixed last formed level.

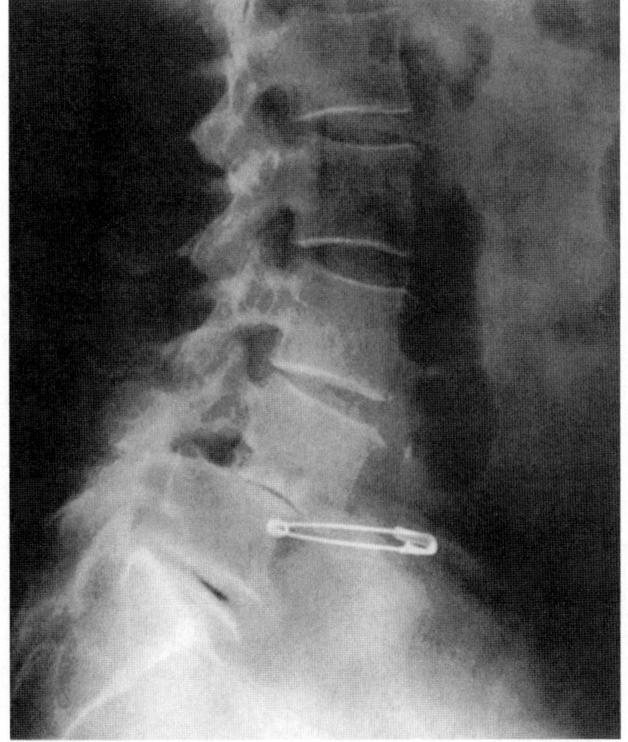

FIGURE 12-31 ● The lateral plain film shows a degenerative spondylolisthesis with a narrowed disc space at the level of the slip: a fairly stable situation.

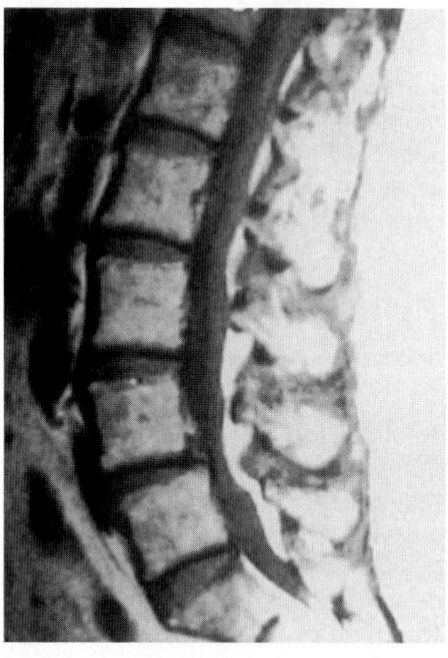

FIGURE 12-32 ● The sagittal (T1) MRI shows a wide disc space (L4-L5) at the slip level: a relatively unstable situation.

GROUP THREE (ASSOCIATED DEGENERATE SCOLIOSIS/LATERAL LISTHESIS)

There is no more vexing problem in a degenerative spine than a degenerative scoliosis, particularly when associated with a lateral slip (lateral listhesis) that contributes to a spinal curve. Despite decompressions and fusions with or without instrumentation in this group, the results are universally poor. The management of this problem calls for a very sophisticated level of surgical expertise that is beyond the scope of this text.

FACET JOINTS

In the presence of a complete spinal canal obstruction with degenerative spondylolisthesis, there is a reasonable possibility of significant foraminal encroachment (Fig. 12-26). This feature serves as the basis for those proposing an interbody fusion with instrumentation (Fig. 12-33). There are three ways to deal with a tight foramen.

1. Directly open the foramen, which may mean removing the inferior facet (Fig. 12-34).
2. Restore disc space height with an interbody fusion (Fig. 12-33).
3. Immobilize the segment (Fig. 12-35).

The last of the three options is not often considered but is a viable consideration based on the fact that no matter how small the nerve root canal, if there is no movement, the nerve will not be a source of pain. The necessity for decompression of the foramen (second story) in slip levels comes from the fact that capsular hypertrophy is often present, impinging on the nerve root in the foramen (Fig. 12-36). Failure to decompress the foramen in this patient, by removing the inferior facet and the capsule of the facet joint will leave the patient with residual leg symptoms (13). In the case of an L4-L5 slip level, this would leave encroachment on the L4 roots, resulting in persisting postoperative anterior thigh discomfort.

FUSION

Stabilization of Vertebral Elements

The controversy about stabilization or fusion of slip levels in spondylolisthesis has been resolved by long-term results (12,13,15,17). If a slip level is not fused at the time of decompression, there is

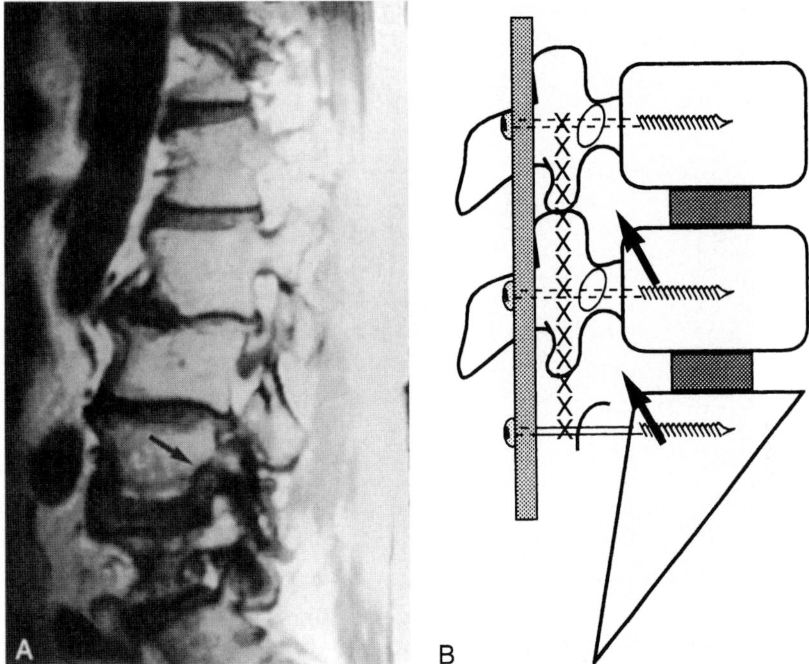

FIGURE 12-33 • **A:** A degenerative spondylolisthesis with foraminal encroachment at one level *(arrow)*. **B:** The 360-degree fusion: interbody and posterolateral; the interbody fusion restores disc space height and reestablishes the patency of the foramen *(arrows)*.

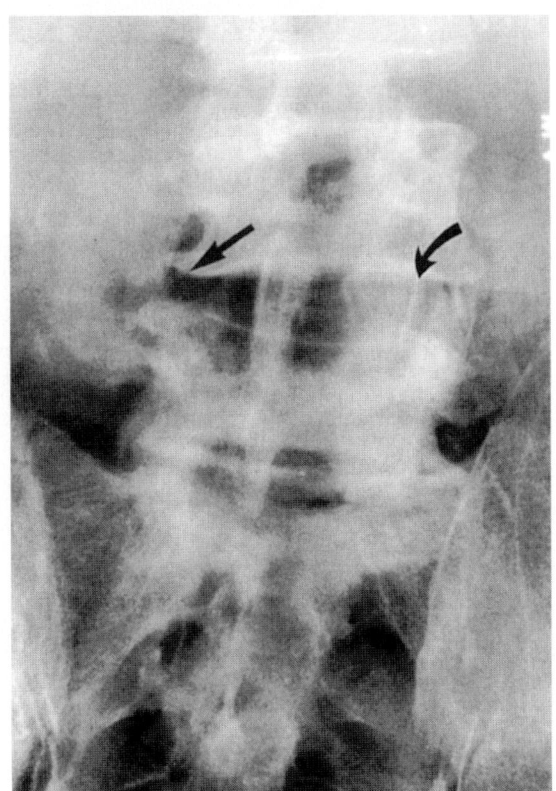

FIGURE 12-34 • To open the foramen on the left, the facet joint had to be removed *(straight arrow)*, and on the right the facet joint was left intact but fused after removing the cartilaginous surfaces *(curved arrow)*.

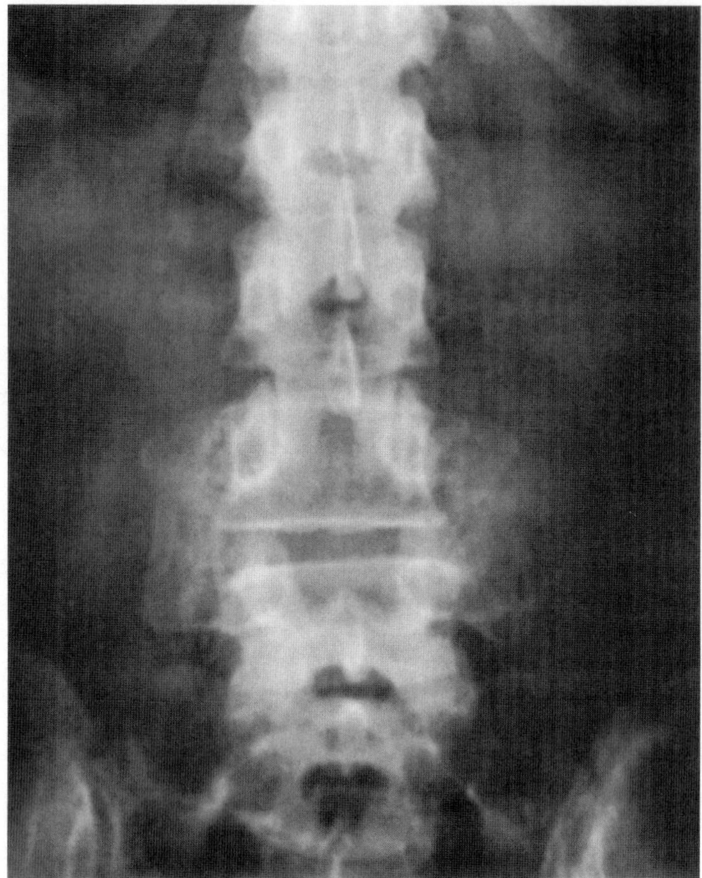

FIGURE 12-35 ● Spinal canal stenosis. Another example of a single level decompression (L4) and a floating fusion, leaving L5-S1 untouched. (A fixed, formed level is below "L5-S1.")

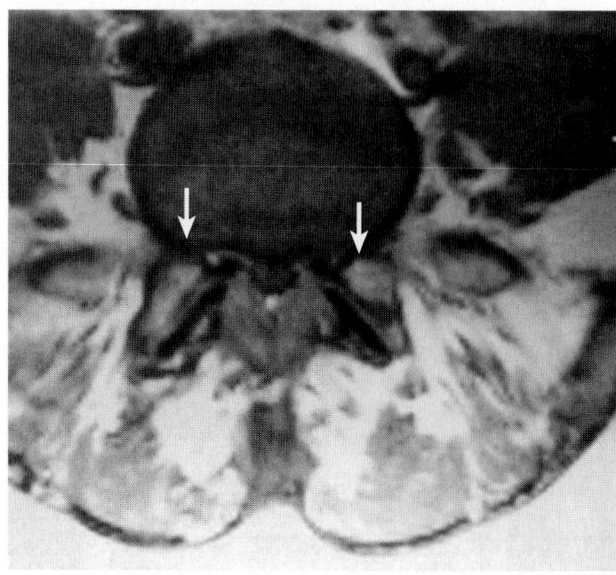

FIGURE 12-36 ● An axial T1 MRI showing congenital stenosis with degenerative changes in the ligamentum flavum and capsule that increase the canal stenosis, and contribute to bilateral foraminal narrowing *(arrows).*

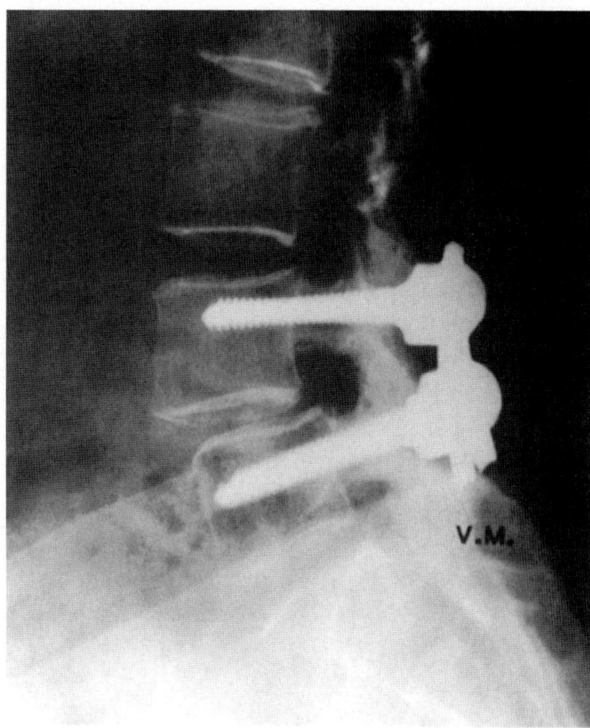

FIGURE 12-37 • Lateral view of an instrumented decompression and fusion for a degenerative spondylolisthesis.

a tendency toward a postoperative increase in the slip and a higher incidence of disabling back pain (17). It is recommended that all slip levels, forward and lateral, be fused at the time of decompression, regardless of whether or not facet joints have been removed during the decompression. The recommended fusion is intertransverse (Fig. 12-37; Fig. 12-35). Up for grabs is whether or not the fusion should be augmented with instrumentation (4).

CONGENITAL/DEVELOPMENTAL SPINAL CANAL STENOSIS

This condition is not at all uncommon, although it does not occur with the frequency of acquired SCS with and without degenerative spondylolisthesis. The mistake in this condition is to miss the global (congenital) stenosis (Fig. 12-36) and see this as a simple degenerative SCS meriting a laminoplasty type of decompression.

There are some basic rules to follow in understanding congenital SCS.

1. The condition usually occurs in men of large stature (male-female ratio = 10:1).
2. The patients present at a younger age and may present the classic picture of a disc herniation. It is only after an imaging study that the SCS is noted.
3. The stenosis affects all three stories of each anatomic segment (Fig. 12-38) (i.e., global nonsegmental) and is not intrasegmental as in degenerative SCS (Fig. 12-7B).
4. It is unusual for a degenerative spondylolisthesis to be present. Therefore most operative decisions center around a decompression only (Figure 12-38 is the exception, not the rule!).
5. It is unusual for foraminal stenosis to be present.
6. If neurologic changes are present (e.g., with an HNP), the neurologic tissues are very sensitive to surgical retraction, and it is easy to increase a neurologic deficit.
7. Most important, all three stories of each stenosed anatomic segment need to be decompressed. This usually means a multilevel decompression that most often extends from L2-L3 to L5-S1. Rarely is a fusion needed provided you save the facet joints.
8. Excessive retraction of nerve roots at the time of decompression, and especially if a disc herniation is present, will result in an increased neurologic deficit postoperatively.

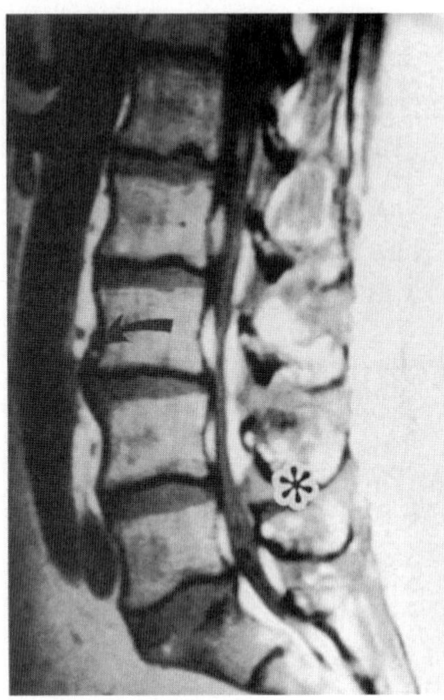

FIGURE 12-38 ● A combined congenital and acquired spinal canal stenosis. Note the "pencil-thin" common dural sac from L1-L2 to L5-S1. This is a congenital "global" stenosis rather than an intrasegmental (first story) stenosis. In addition, there is ligamentum flavum hypertrophy at L4-L5 (*), a slight forward slip (degenerative spondylolisthesis) at L4-L5, and an obvious forward slip at L3-L4 *(arrow).*

OUTCOMES OF SURGERY

Surgery for SCS makes patients better not normal (2,29). Relief of leg pain is a reasonable expectation although chronic neurologic changes (e.g., weakness) will not be improved. Hopefully their progression will be arrested. Relief of back pain, even with a fusion, is a little more tenuous, with most patients ending up with some degree of residual backache. Fortunately, most patients are in an age group in which they do not wish to dig ditches and move furniture on a regular basis, and this lessened demand usually spares the back.

A poor initial result will not improve over time. If the patient's clinical improvement is less than expected within 3 to 6 months, re-evaluation may be prudent. Possible explanations include a missed diagnosis of associated conditions such as a PN, hip arthritis, and vascular claudication. Other causes of a poor result comprise decompression at the wrong level, an inadequate decompression at the right level, or irreversible neurologic changes.

Overall, two thirds of patients can anticipate a good, but not excellent, long-term result.

CONCLUSION

SCS is a relentlessly progressive narrowing of the lumbar spinal canal that insidiously decreases the space available for neurologic structures. The resulting symptoms are quite disabling yet present little clinical evidence of nerve root involvement. The diagnosis is often elusive until the patient undergoes myelographic and/or CT investigation and/or MRI.

Surgery is the fate of at least 50% of patients with SCS. Symptoms can be temporarily relieved by conservative measures, but the degenerative changes of aging are relentless. The spinal canal may continue to narrow, and surgery may eventually be required.

The surgical procedures that are useful are a simple midline canal decompression, a wider decompression with removal of the facet joints, and stabilization procedures for slip levels. These three approaches have met with good results. Fortunately, because patients with SCS are older, they do not make great demands on the back postoperatively. If these patients required the ability to do heavy lifting, then backache postoperatively would be a limiting factor. In general, the results of surgical intervention for these patients are very gratifying.

REFERENCES

1. Arnoldi CC, Brodsky AE, Cauchoix J, et al. Lumbar spinal stenosis and nerve root entrapment syndromes: definitions and classification. *Clin Orthop.* 1976;115:4–5.
2. Atlas SJ, Keller RB, Robson D, et al. Surgical and non surgical management of lumbar spinal stenosis: four-year outcomes from the Maine lumbar spine study. *Spine.* 2000;25:556–562.
3. Boden SD, Davis DO, Dina TS, et al. Abnormal magnetic resonance scans of the lumbar spine in asymptomatic subjects. A positive investigation. *J Bone Joint Surg Am.* 1990;72:403–408.
4. Bridwell KH, Sedgewick TA, O'Brien MF, et al. The role of fusion and instrumentation in the treatment of degenerative spondylolisthesis with spinal stenosis. *J Spinal Disord.* 1993;6:461–472.
5. Dagi TF, Tarkington MA, Leech JJ. Tandem lumbar and cervical spinal stenosis. *J Neurosurg.* 1987;66:842–849.
6. Dvonch V, Scarff T, Bunch W. Dermatomal somatosensory-evoked potentials: their use in lumbar radiculopathy. *Spine.* 1984;9:291–293.
7. Ehni G. Significance of the small lumbar spinal canal: cauda equina compression syndromes due to spondylolysis. *J Neurosurg.* 1969;31:490–494.
8. Epstein JA, Epstein BS, Lavine LS. Nerve root compression associated with narrowing of the lumbar spinal canal. *J Neurol Neurosurg Psychiatry.* 1962;25:165–176.
9. Epstein JA, Epstein BS, Lavine LS, et al. Degenerative lumbar spondylolisthesis with an intact neural arch (pseudospondylolisthesis). *J Neurosurg.* 1976;44:139–147.
10. Epstein NE, Epstein JA, Carras R, Lavine LS. Degenerative spondylolisthesis with an intact neural arch: a review of 60 cases with an analysis of clinical findings and the development of surgical management. *Neurosurgery.* 1983;13:555–561.
11. Getty CJM. Lumbar spinal stenosis: the clinical spectrum and the results of operation. *J Bone Joint Surg Br.* 1980;62:481–485.
12. Herkowitz HN, Kurz LT. Degenerative lumbar spondylolisthesis with spinal stenosis. A prospective study comparing decompression and intertransverse process arthrodesis. *J Bone Joint Surg.* 1991;73:802–808.
13. Herno A, Airaksinen O, Saari T. Long-term results of surgical treatment of lumbar spinal stenosis. *Spine.* 1993;18:1471–1474.
14. Hilibrand AS, Rand N. Degenerative lumbar stenosis: diagnosis and management. *J Am Acad Orthop Surg.* 1999;7:239–249.
15. Johnsson K. *Lumbar Spinal Stenosis: A Clinical, Radiological and Neurophysiological Investigation.* Malmo, Sweden: Special publication of Department of Orthopaedics, Malmo General Hospital, Lund University; 1987.
16. Johnsson K, Rosen I, Uden A. The natural course of lumbar spinal stenosis. *Acta Orthop Scand.* 1993;64(suppl 251):67–68.
17. Johnsson KE, Willner S, Johnsson K. Postoperative instability after decompression for lumbar spinal stenosis. *Spine.* 1986;11:107–110.
18. Katz JN, Lispon SJ, Larson MG, et al. The outcome of decompressive laminectomy for degenerative lumbar spinal stenosis. *J Bone Joint Surg Am.* 1991;73:809–816.
19. Kirkaldy-Willis WH, Wedge JH, Yonk-Hing K, Reilly J. Pathology and pathogenesis of lumbar spondylosis and stenosis. *Spine.* 1978;3:319–328.
20. Macnab I. Spondylolisthesis with an intact neural arch—the so-called pseudospondylolisthesis. *J Bone Joint Surg Br.* 1950;32:325–333.
21. Macnab I. Negative disc exploration. *J Bone Joint Surg Am.* 1971;53:891–903.
22. Porter RW. Management of Back Pain. Edinburgh, Scotland: Churchhill Livingstone; 1993:59–72.
23. McLain RF, Kapural L, Mekhail NA. Epidural steroid therapy for back and leg pain: mechanisms of action and efficacy. *Spine J.* 2005;5:191–201.
24. Porter RW. Central spinal stenosis: classification and pathogenesis. *Acta Orthop Scand.* 1993;251(suppl):64–66.
25. Rydevik B. Neurophysiology of cauda equina compression. *Acta Orthop Scand.* 1993;251(suppl):52–55.
26. Schatzker J, Pennal GEF. Spinal stenosis, a cause of cauda equina compression. *J Bone Joint Surg Br.* 1968;50:606–618.
27. Schonstrom HSR, Bolender NF, Spengler DM. The pathomorphology of spinal stenosis as seen on CT scans of the lumbar spines. *Spine.* 1985;10:806–811.
28. Tsuji H, Tamake T, Itoh T, et al. Redundant nerve roots in patients with degenerative lumbar spinal stenosis. *Spine.* 1985;10:72–82.
29. Turner JA, Ersek M, Herron L, Deyo R. Surgery for lumbar spinal stenosis: an attempted meta-analysis of the literature. *Spine.* 1992;17:1–8.
30. Ullrich CG, Binet EF, Sanecki MG, Kieffer SA. Quantitative assessment of the lumbar spinal canal by computed tomography. *Radiology.* 1980;134:137–143.
31. Verbiest H. Pathomorphologic aspects of developmental lumbar stenosis. *Orthop Clin North Am.* 1975; 6:177–196.
32. Watanabe R, Parke W. Vascular and neural pathology of lumbosacral spinal stenosis. *J Neurosurg.* 1986; 64:64–70.

CHAPTER 13

The Investigation

"Seek, and ye shall find..."

—Matthew 7:7

When you are seeing patients with low back pain (and other spinal pain) day in and day out, you quickly realize how easy it is to miss or err in diagnosis (Tables 13-1 and 13-2). As a clinician, you start to "build a better mousetrap" so you do not make these errors. Various investigations will aid in the evaluation and ultimate diagnosis.

BLOOD WORK

The following laboratory tests are useful as a screening mechanism:

- Hemoglobin, hematocrit, white blood cell count, differential, microscopic, erythrocyte sedimentation rate, and sometimes C-reactive protein.
- Serum chemistries, especially calcium, acid and alkaline phosphatase, and serum protein electrophoresis.
- HLA-B27 antigen.

It is a good routine to agree to do the hematologic tests and serum chemistries in the following individuals: patients who have a significant nonmechanical component to their pain, patients with systemic symptoms such as fevers, any patient with an atypical pain pattern or distribution, and all patients who do not respond to standard conservative treatment directed at the mechanical causes of low back pain. Be particularly vigilant in older patients (older than age 55 years).

BONE SCANNING (SCINTIGRAPHY)

Since the first edition of this book in 1977, bone scanning has come a long way. From whole body scanning for metastases with strontium, a tracer element that is difficult to work with and results in a high radiation dose to the patient, we are now to a stage of selective regional imaging using the workhorse radionuclide of nuclear medicine, technetium-99m-labeled phosphorus (^{99m}Tc).

INDICATIONS FOR BONE SCAN

The location of metastatic bone lesions remains the most common indication for bone scanning, and this technology has virtually displaced the radiographic skeletal survey in the adult (except for

TABLE 13-1

Differential Diagnosis of Nonmechanical Low Back Pain

Causes of nonmechanical low back pain
Referred pain (e.g., from the abdomen or retroperitoneal space)
Infection
Bone
Disc
Epidural space
Neoplasm
Primary (multiple myeloma, osteoid osteoma, and so on)
Secondary
Inflammation: arthritides such as ankylosing spondylitis
Miscellaneous metabolic and vascular disorders such as osteopenia and Paget's disease

multiple myeloma). The second most common reason for considering the use of bone scintigraphy is for early detection of bone infection, days before regular radiographic changes occur. Bone scanning is also being used in detection of osteonecrosis, the study of failed joint prostheses, the investigation of unexplained bone pain (especially in the high-powered athlete who may suffer a stress fracture), and the dating of fracture age (1,2).

TECHNETIUM-99M-LABELED PHOSPHORUS

^{99m}Tc is currently the most frequently used radionuclide in nuclear medicine (5). This predominance exists because the radionuclide is readily available and cheap and has an ideal biologic behavior

TABLE 13-2

Differential Diagnosis of Sciatica

Intraspinal causes
Proximal to disc: conus and cauda equina lesions (e.g., neurofibroma, ependymoma)
Disc level
Herniated nucleus pulposus
Stenosis (canal or recess)
Infection: osteomyelitis or discitis (with nerve root pressure)
Inflammation arachnoiditis
Neoplasm: benign or malignant with nerve root pressure
Extraspinal causes
Pelvis
Cardiovascular conditions (e.g., peripheral vascular disease)
Gynecologic conditions causing sacral plexus pressure
Orthopaedic conditions (e.g., osteoarthritis of hip)
Sacroiliac joint disease
Neoplasms (invading or compressing lumbosacral plexus)
Peripheral nerve lesions
Neuropathy (diabetic, tumor, alcohol)
Local sciatic nerve conditions (trauma, tumor)
Inflammation (herpes zoster)

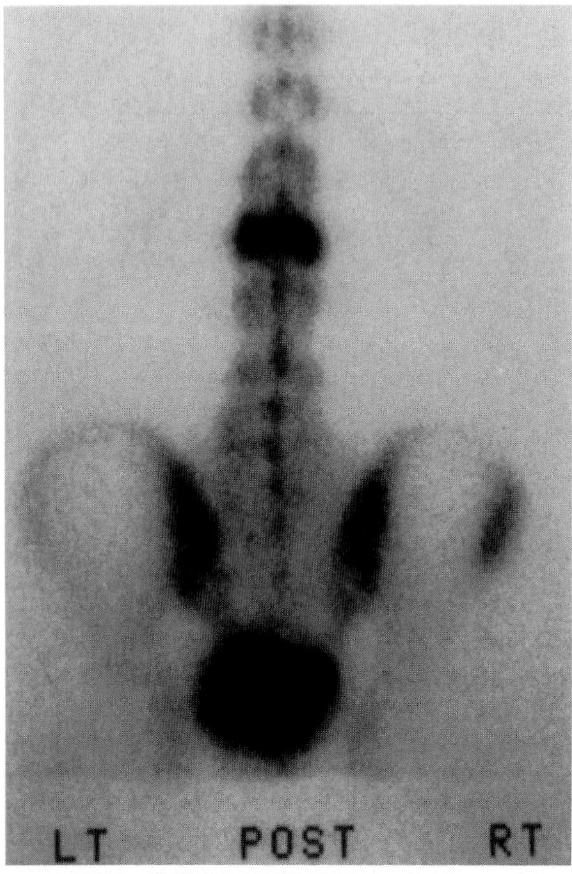

FIGURE 13-1 ● Bone scan (Tc-99m) showing a hot spot in L2—a metastatic tumor.

pattern. This includes easy incorporation in bone, timing of incorporation that suits hospital procedures, and a low radiation dose to the patient.

This is the basis of the "hot spot" (Fig. 13-1).

GALLIUM SCANNING

^{99m}Tc-labeled phosphorus scanning identifies areas of increased bone turnover and is nonspecific for infection. This led to the search for compounds that would specifically bind to sites of infection, the most popular (until recently) being gallium 67 citrate (^{67}Ga). This tracer binds to transferrin and other proteins associated with inflammation and infection. Unfortunately, it emits four gamma rays (photons) ranging from low to high energy, which cause more patient exposure to radiation while making the scan less clear.

More recently, a number of reports on the limited accuracy of gallium scanning, especially in low-grade infections, are appearing in the literature (3,4).

INDIUM-111-LABELED LEUKOCYTES

Because of the limited accuracy of ^{67}Ga scanning, further research has led to the proposal that indium-111-labeled leukocytes have a greater specificity for musculoskeletal (and other) infective foci.

SINGLE PHOTON EMISSION COMPUTED TOMOGRAPHY (SPECT)

Normal nuclear imaging is recorded on only two planes [anteroposterior (AP) and posteroanterior and/or lateral] of the three-dimensional skeleton. The significant overlapping of anatomic structures can blur the localization of radionucleotides in the posterior elements of the lumbar spine. With more sophisticated camera systems and the principle of rotating the gamma camera 360 degrees, multiplanar images of the spine, similar to computed tomography (CT), can be obtained. The rotation of the more sensitive cameras minimizes the superimposed activity from over- or underlying structures that occurs in planar imaging. The principles of "slicing" tissue planes into thin wafers that is discussed later in the CT sections applies to SPECT scanning.

CONCLUSION

Although bone scintigraphy is commonly used today, major changes in nuclear imaging are occurring and will change the indications for use of bone scintigraphy. An example is SPECT, a newer imaging technique just discussed.

PLAIN RADIOGRAPHS

In the assessment of routine mechanical low back pain, the question always arises, "Should a radiograph be taken?" A radiograph is not harmful, but it is about as illogical to take a radiograph of every patient who has a backache as it is to order a barium study on every patient who has a touch of indigestion. A radiograph on the first attendance of a patient with back pain is, however, indicated under the following circumstances:

- Severe back pain after significant trauma.
- Incapacitating back pain.
- A history suggestive of vertebral crush due to osteoporosis or malignancy. These patients, usually older than 50 years, report a history of pain coming on without provocative injury, punctuated by sudden cramps of pain in the back.
- The excessively anxious patient. In such people, a radiograph is an essential part of treatment. These patients cannot be reassured by clinical examination alone.
- Patients in whom the history and examination are suggestive of ankylosing spondylitis. A specific request should be made for views of the sacroiliac joint.
- Patients with a clinically apparent spinal deformity.
- Patients with significant root tension and those presenting evidence of impairment of root conduction. In these patients, a radiograph is of importance to exclude the possibility of malignancy.
- If severe pain persists despite treatment for more than 2 weeks, a radiograph is indicated, not only to exclude the possibility of some obscure spinal abnormality but also to reassure the patient that he/she is not suffering from a serious progressive disease.

Radiographs have limited function in diagnosis and treatment. In diagnosis, the main function of a radiograph is to exclude serious disease, such as infections, ankylosing spondylitis, and neoplasms. If radiographs of the spine show disc degeneration, this radiologic change merely demonstrates a segment that is vulnerable to trauma. Such a demonstration, however, does not necessarily indict this segment as the cause of the presenting symptoms. Treatment is determined by clinical assessment not by the radiologic findings.

The term "degeneration" implies to the average patient a type of "rotting away," like bad cheese. A patient should never be presented with the bald statement, "the radiographs of your spine show arthritis." First, this is rarely true. The presence of osteophytes or, more correctly, "spondylophytes" on the vertebral bodies does not denote arthritis. Second, the term "arthritis" carries with it an evil connotation for the patient. Given this diagnosis, the patients frequently foresee a progressive restriction in their way of life leading eventually to a wheelchair existence.

Detailed assessment of radiologic findings indicative of mechanical insufficiency of the spine is only of value in the preoperative assessment of a patient. At this time, a thorough analysis of the radiographic findings is of importance in determining whether surgical intervention is feasible and, if so, the type of operative correction required.

In reading plain radiographs (Fig. 13-2), look at the nonskeletal areas first. Review the retroperitoneal area with specific regard to the kidneys and ureters and the abdominal aorta. Be sure that the psoas shadows are intact. After reviewing the nonskeletal part of a lumbar spine radiograph, consider the skeleton. Look at the sacroiliac joints, survey the pedicles and vertebral bodies for erosions, and finally consider the structural defects that may have a potential for causing the patient's syndrome. Such observations as narrowing of the disc space and translation of vertebral bodies should

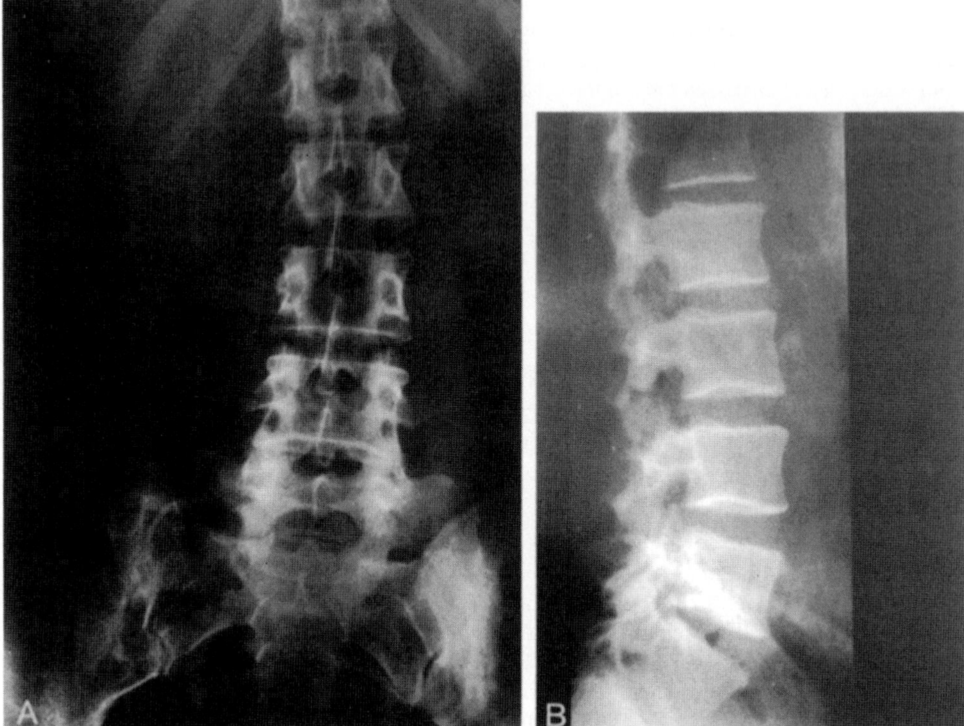

FIGURE 13-2 ● **A:** Standard AP with psoas shadows evident, no abnormal kidney shadows, no calcification in aorta, and normal joints. Note the congenital lumbosacral anomaly. **B:** Lateral showing good disc space integrity and no vertebral body translations ("slips").

be noted, and may turn out to be important. Various measurements on plain radiographs are not helpful in assessment of canal or recess narrowing.

MYELOGRAPHY, COMPUTERIZED AXIAL TOMOGRAPHY, AND MAGNETIC RESONANCE IMAGING

The demands of lumbar spine surgery require a precise definition of not only the nature of the lesion but also the location of the offending pathology. This can be provided only by CT scanning or magnetic resonance imaging (MRI). It is getting more difficult to meet the requirements of precise surgical technique with myelography alone, which results in an increased use of CT scanning and MRI. At the time of this writing, MRI is assuming a primary role in patient assessment because it has the potential to deliver all of the necessary information on which to base a surgical game plan. In this milieu of change in imaging technique, myelography is assuming a less important place in investigation.

PHILOSOPHY OF INVESTIGATING A PATIENT WITH LUMBAR DISC DISEASE

The cornerstone of diagnosis of lumbar disc disease is the history and physical examination—not the investigation.

CT and MRI are ordered for two reasons: (a) almost always to verify the clinical diagnosis as correct and at the same time to plan a surgical approach to the problem and (b) infrequently to solve a differential diagnosis problem.

Investigative procedures used to resolve a differential diagnostic problem may fall short of helping to plan surgery. An example is the water-soluble myelogram, which was the "gold standard" for diagnosis of lumbar disc disease. It is valuable in differential diagnosis, such as ruling out a conus tumor, but it fails to provide all of the necessary information to plan a surgical procedure, especially one with limited exposure.

When viewing the investigation, do so in light of the clinical information. You are seeking to identify the anatomic level and the structural lesion. If there is not a perfect marriage among the clinical presentation, anatomic level, and the investigation, something is wrong. To proceed with surgery at this stage sets the stage for a poor outcome.

Consider the following clinical information and respective implications:

- A patient with an acute radicular syndrome with significant straight leg raising (SLR) reduction and S1 neurologic symptoms and signs should have an unequivocal lesion involving the S1 nerve root on CT scan or MRI.
- A patient with anterior thigh pain and a positive femoral stretch with a decreased knee reflex should not be accepted as having a herniated nucleus pulposus (HNP) at L4-L5 unless it extends into the foramen to involve the fourth root.
- A patient with a long history of back pain and claudicant leg pain should have a clear-cut stenotic lesion on investigation before making the diagnosis of spinal stenosis.

The potential for false-negative and false-positive investigative findings is great (17). CT scans and MRIs are so sensitive that it is possible to show pathology in almost every patient. CT scans show only what is scanned. If a conus tumor is present, and the scan is confined to L3 to the sacrum, the lesion will be missed. MRI covers this CT deficiency but at the same time introduces many false-positive results because of overinterpretation. Beware of the clinical diagnosis lacking substance and borderline investigative findings.

A poor quality investigative test is no good to anyone. An extradural myelogram cannot be interpreted, a poorly done electromyograph is misleading, a blurred CT scan is useless, and a patient rushed through an MRI machine will result in a bad MRI scan. It is essential for clinicians to keep the pressure on our radiologic colleagues to deliver the best quality images possible to reduce the risk of operative misadventure.

There is a tendency in the United States to order major spine investigative procedures too early in the progress of disc disease. Tests such as myelography, CT scanning, and MRI are part of an operative procedure; they are not routine radiographs to be ordered without hesitation. If a clinician is in trouble with spine differential diagnosis to the point where frequent myelograms or myelogram/CT scans and MRI are part of the practice routine, then a careful clinical examination is missing. If a significant number of tests ordered by a clinician are negative, the indications for ordering such radiologic tests are too broad and need to be reassessed. Almost every myelogram, CT scan, or MRI examination of the lumbar spine should be positive and followed by an operation. If this is not the case, indiscriminate early ordering of these tests is occurring.

HISTORY

"Myelography" was introduced in 1922 by Sicard (15), using iodized poppy seed oil (Lipiodol) injected into the epidural space. Steinhausen et al. (16) at the University of Rochester introduced iophendylate in 1940, and Pantopaque remained the medium of choice for years. The difficulty in using large needles necessary to introduce the viscous fluid, the necessity of poststudy removal of the contrast material sometimes injuring nerve roots, late arachnoiditis, and other complications (7) led to the incongruous situation of many surgeons ordering the test, yet few themselves prepared to submit to the procedure. Obviously, Pantopaque was not a great medium for myelography, which stimulated the search for better agents. By the mid-1970s, water-soluble contrast agents had virtually eliminated Pantopaque for lumbar myelography, and since the late 1980s we have had available relatively nontoxic, cheap, water-soluble agents; these newer myelographic agents have been developed all in time to see myelography being surpassed as the procedure of choice by better CT scanning and newer MRI (7,9,11).

DYNAMIC EXAMINATION

Some radiologists use flexion/extension films to accentuate midline stenotic lesions. Patients with spinal stenosis aggravate their symptoms in extension and are likely to show more of a myelographic defect in this position.

ADVERSE REACTIONS TO MYELOGRAPHY

Severe adverse reactions to the instillation of contrast material occur in approximately 1:35,000 procedures. They can be divided into adverse neurologic reactions (13), anaphylactoid reactions, and renal toxicity.

Anaphylactoid reactions are rare, especially with the newer water-soluble contrast materials. Screening of patients historically, corticosteroid and antihistamine pretreatment when indicated, and in some cases refusing to do myelography in a sensitive patient have reduced the incidence of anaphylactoid reactions to a minimum.

Renal toxicity from the doses of contrast material used for lumbar myelography are much rarer compared with the use of the higher doses of these agents that are used for vascular studies. There is a possibility that a patient with pre-existing renal disease can have a toxic reaction from intrathecal water-soluble contrast agents (8).

Adverse neurologic reactions (7,9,11,14) are the reactions that concern myelographers. They include, most frequently, headache, nausea, and vomiting; less frequently, the following reactions occur: increased pain, seizures, myoclonic spasms, psychomotor disturbances, fever, vertigo, and urinary retention.

Patients prone to adverse effects are the older patient, the patient with a previous reaction, and the long-term psychoactive drug user; extra precautions are needed with these patients. Most important, it is necessary to identify these patients with a careful preinjection history.

MYELOGRAM CHANGES

Figure 13-3 demonstrates a normal myelogram. Abnormalities in myelography indicative of an HNP are as follows:

1. Defects in the sac alone. The most difficult defects to interpret involve the dural sac alone. A double density (Fig. 13-4) is usually indicative of a disc herniation toward the midline, but

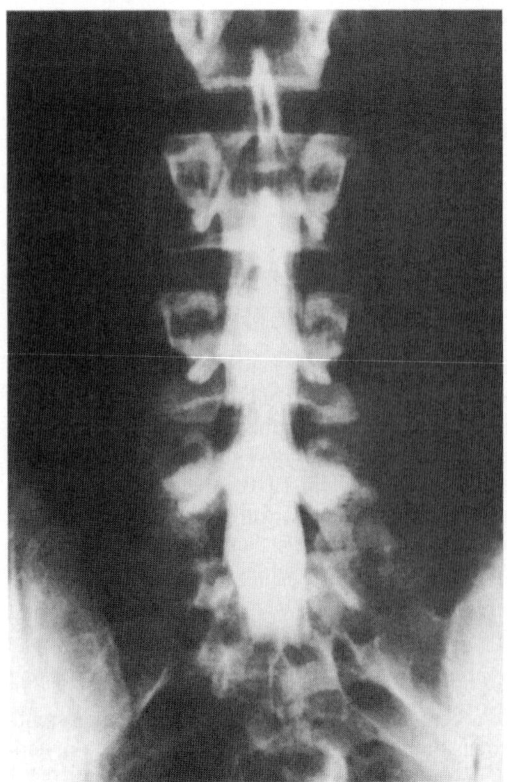

FIGURE 13-3 ● A normal AP myelogram.

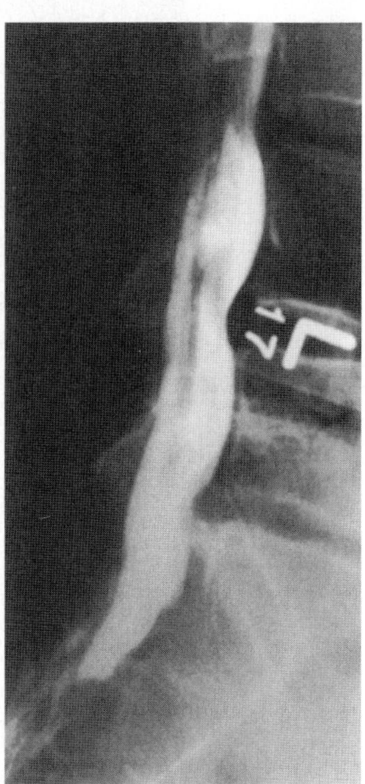

FIGURE 13-4 • A lateral myelogram with a double density at L5-S1 and annular bulging deforming the sac at L4-5.

still eccentric enough to produce the typical defect. On occasion, an HNP fragment will migrate up or down from a disc space and produce a defect on the sac alone (Fig. 13-5). Simple, smooth midline defects are not to be interpreted as HNP (Fig. 13-6). These defects are known as "sucker discs" and are caused by annular bulging as part of the phenomenon of degenerative disc disease. Often, they will be accompanied by degenerative changes, especially retrospondylolisthesis.

2. Defects affecting the root sleeve. The low viscosity of water-soluble contrast materials makes it possible to readily fill the root sleeves (radiculogram). The defects demonstrated can be an absent root sleeve (Fig. 13-7).
3. A root sleeve shortening or cut-off (Fig. 13-8), a root sleeve deformity (Fig. 13-9), and a swollen root sleeve (Fig. 13-10).
4. Defects affecting sac and root. These are the most obvious defects and are depicted in Figure 13-11.

SENSITIVITY AND SPECIFICITY OF MYELOGRAPHY

Although there are numerous reports in the literature on false-positive and false-negative myelograms (9,10), most reports are poor in that they do not follow up on patients to completion of treatment. False-negative myelograms can still occur with water-soluble agents in the following situations:

- Foraminal HNP (Fig. 13-12).
- Unscanned area (high lumbar disc not scanned).
- Insensitive space at L5-S1 (Fig. 13-13).
- Short or narrow dural sac at L5-S1 (Fig. 13-14).
- Conjoint nerve roots distorting the contrast column.

OUTPATIENT MYELOGRAPHY

With the North American desire to ration health care (contain costs), more patients are undergoing outpatient myelography (6). In the second edition of this book we did not support outpatient

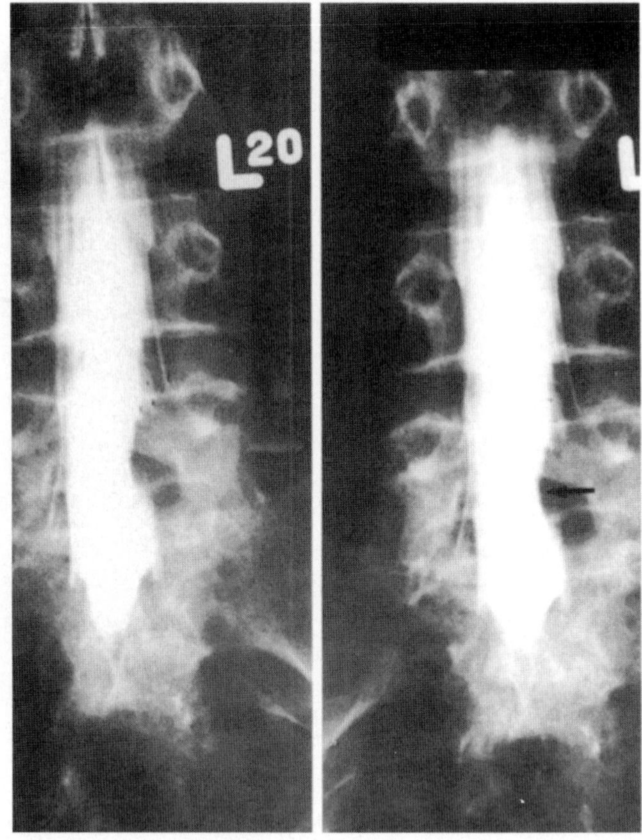

FIGURE 13-5 ● AP myelogram showing a large herniated nucleus pulposus (HNP) behind the vertebral body of L5 distorting the sac (the S1 root is also obliterated) *(arrow).*

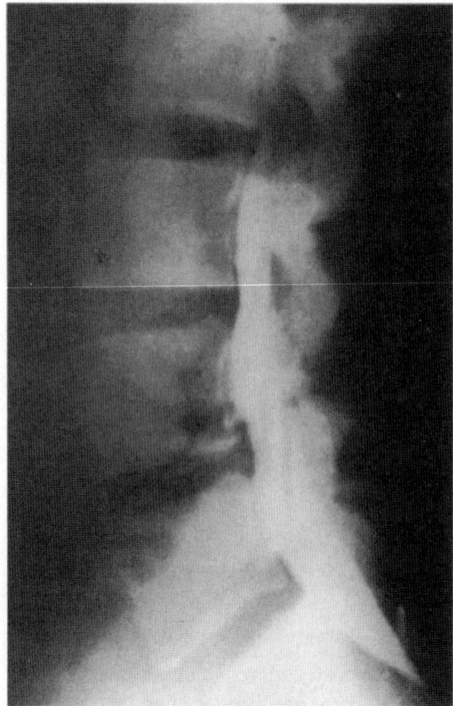

FIGURE 13-6 ● Lateral myelogram showing annular bulging at L4-L5. This is the lateral of Fig. 13-3, the so-called sucker disc.

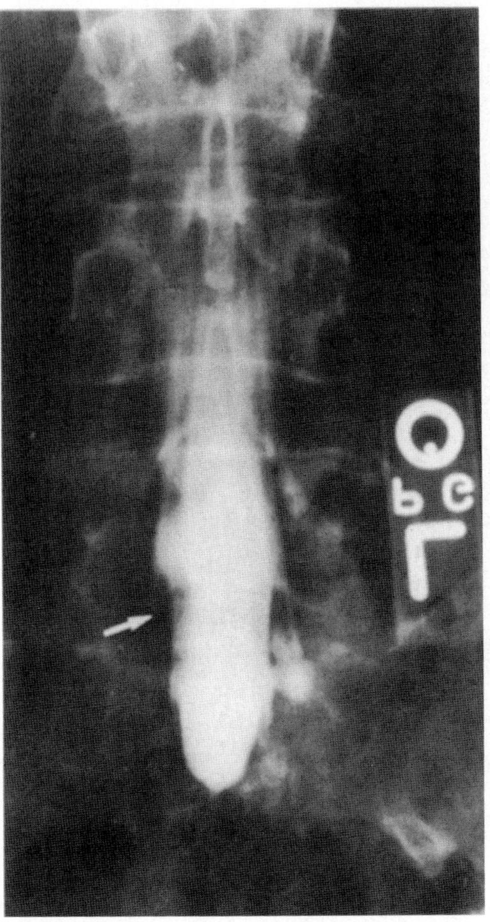

FIGURE 13-7 ● AP myelogram showing S1 root sleeve absent on right (herniated nucleus pulposus, L5-S1, right) *(arrow).*

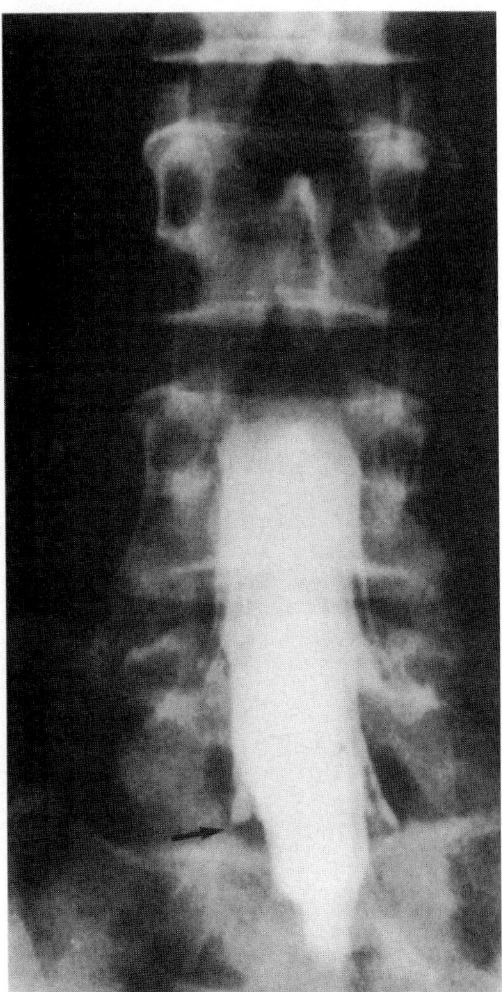

FIGURE 13-8 ● Root sleeve shortening on AP myelogram *(arrow).* Compare the length of S1 root filling on the right (shorter) with the left S1 root. Now, compare the shortening of this S1 root with the absence of the S1 root in Fig. 13-7.

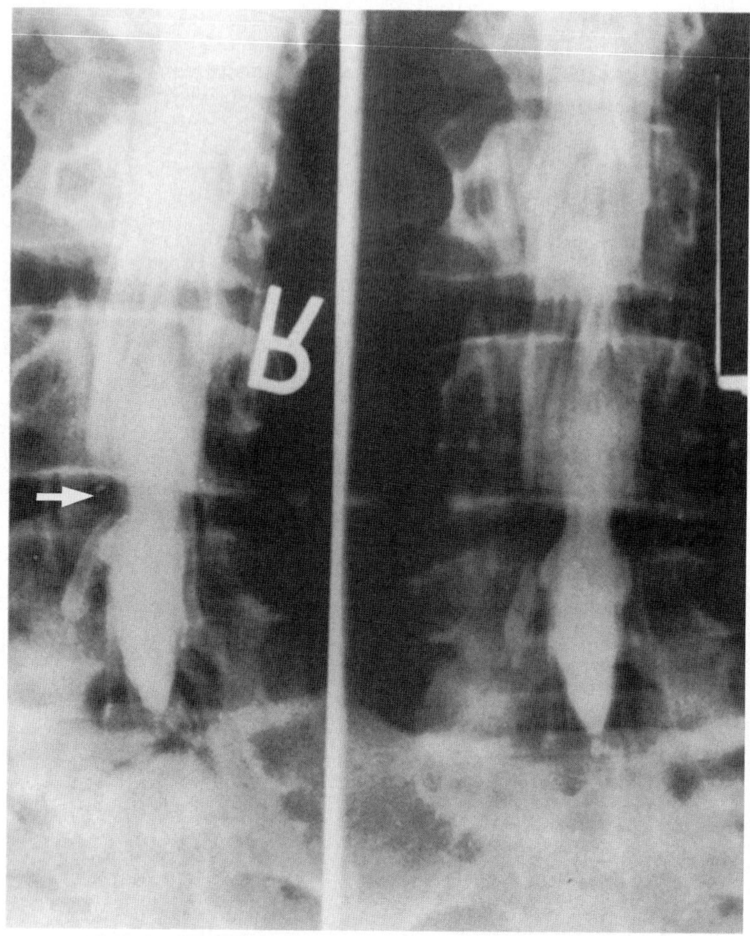

FIGURE 13-9 ● AP and oblique myelogram showing herniated nucleus pulposus (HNP) L4-L5 distorting the LS root sleeve *(arrow).*

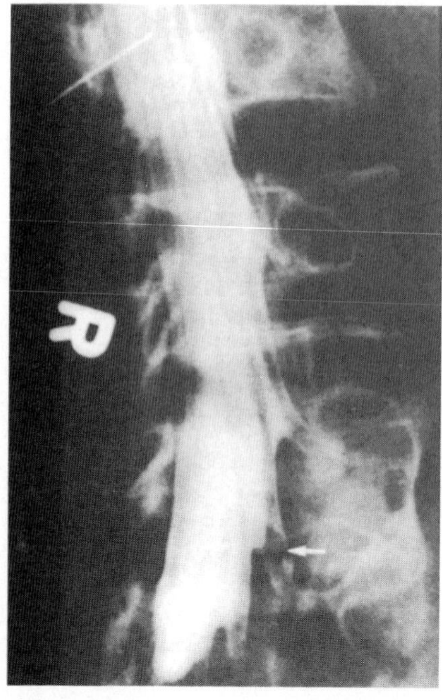

FIGURE 13-10 ● The S1 root, left, is swollen *(arrow).* (Compare with the L5 root at the level above.)

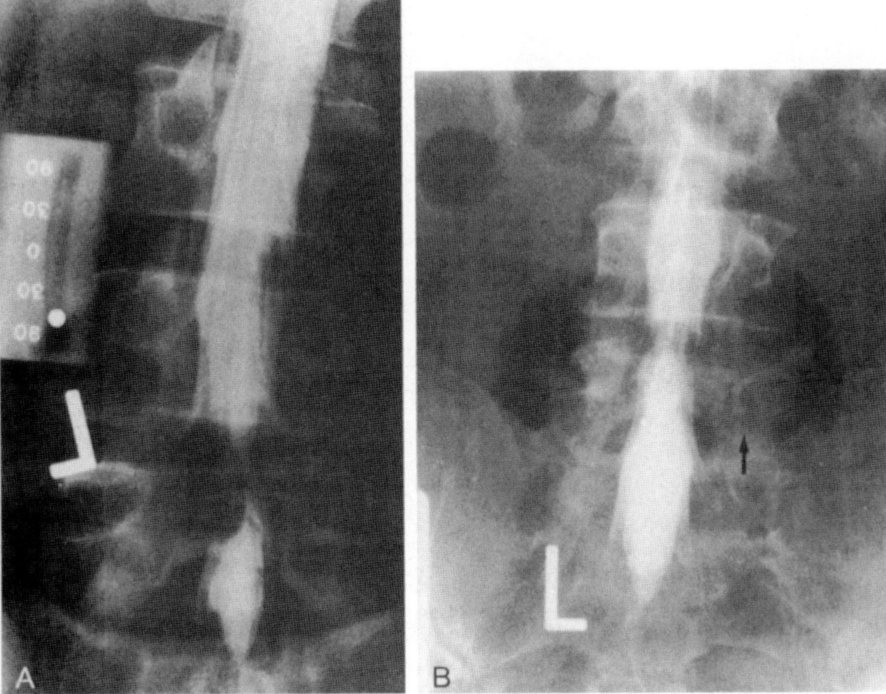

FIGURE 13-11 • **A:** AP myelogram showing herniated nucleus pulposus (HNP) L4-L5, left, with significant distortion of sac and root. This is a large HNP that has trapped down behind the vertebral body of L5. **B:** Apparent defect of sac and root, L4-L5, right. Did you notice the absent pedicle, L5, right *(arrow)*? This was a secondary carcinoma from a lung malignancy.

myelography. With the increasing use of low-osmolality contrast agents, outpatient myelography is most often completed without adverse patient events.

CONCLUSION

Virtually no one is doing myelography alone these days; almost all myelograms are followed by a CT examination. The issue today is whether to continue to use CT myelography or switch to MRI as the primary investigative step before surgery. We prefer the MRI, but there are still situations where a myelogram, followed by CT, is indicated:

1. An equivocal CT or MRI in a patient who the surgeon feels has a surgical lesion.
2. An obese patient who cannot fit into the CT or MR gantries.
3. Multilevel spinal stenosis, especially with scoliosis (scoliosis interferes with proper CT or MRI "slicing" of each segment).
4. Patients in whom metal implants (e.g., pedicle screws) will distort the CT scan or MRI.
5. Less-than-optimal MRI scanning machines (which are not that uncommon).

HIGH-RESOLUTION COMPUTED TOMOGRAPHY

It is becoming more difficult to plan a surgical procedure on the spine without investigation that shows not only the level but also the precise location and nature of the pathology. Myelography is often capable of showing the level at which the pathology lies (20) but fails to show the nature of the lesion or its precise location in the anatomic segment (18,25) (see Chapter 1). This limits the value of water-soluble myelography in surgery for lumbar disc disease, a void that is fortunately filled by CT scanning and, more recently, MRI.

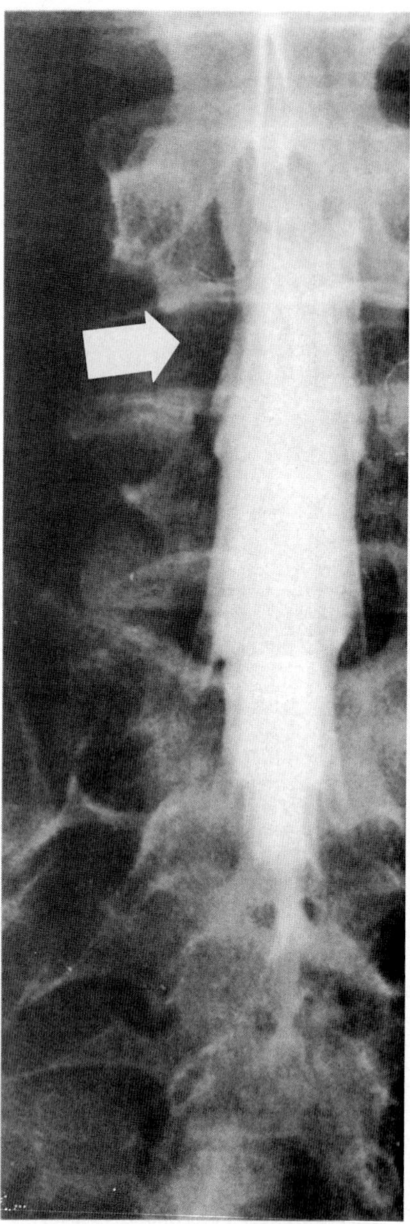

FIGURE 13-12 ● Foraminal herniated nucleus pulposus (HNP), L4-L5, right. Arrow points to slight distortion of contrast column, a change easily missed.

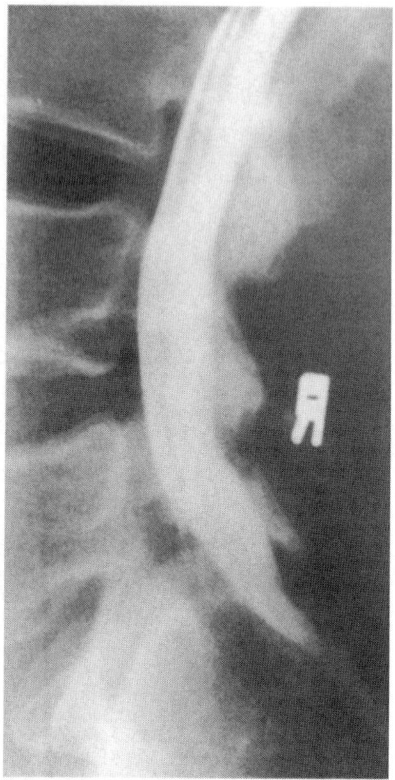

FIGURE 13-13 ● Lateral myelogram showing wide "insensitive space" between back of L5-S1 disc space and front of "dye" column where pathology, such as a herniated nucleus pulposus (HNP), could reside and not be detected on myelography.

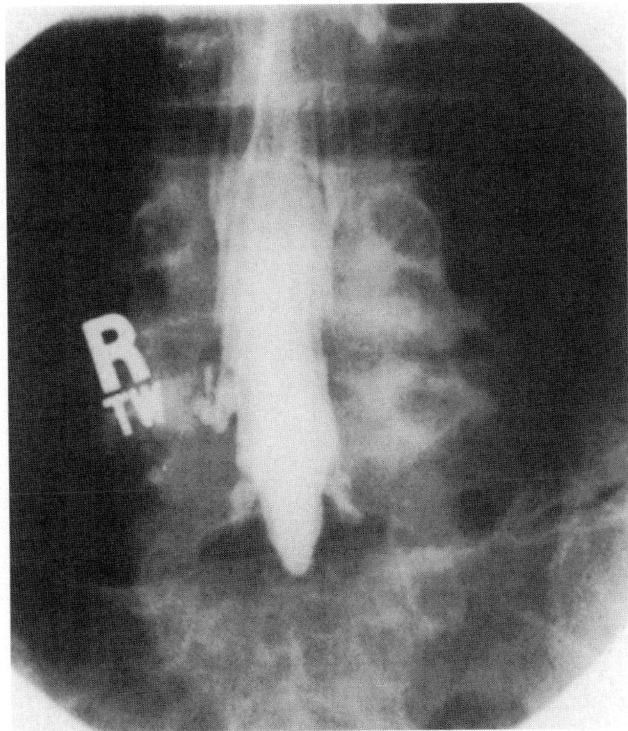

FIGURE 13-14 ● AP myelogram showing a short dural sac, ending before it reaches the level of L5-S1. There is no hope that this myelogram would reveal a herniated nucleus pulposus (HNP) of L5-S1. Fortunately, the HNP was at L4-L5, left, demonstrated by an absent root.

ADVANTAGES AND DISADVANTAGES

Table 13-3 lists the advantages and disadvantages of CT scanning. The most serious problem with routine CT scanning is the ease with which the procedure can be done. With no requirement for hospitalization or injection into the body, the CT scan becomes too simple a step to take, and this procedure is capable of delivering erroneous data (30) that can lead to ill-advised surgical intervention.

TABLE 13-3

Advantages and Disadvantages of Computed Tomography (vs. Myelography)

Advantages	Disadvantages
1. Noninvasive, outpatient procedure	1. Poor detail in obese patient
2. Clear picture of nature and location of pathology	2. Only see what you scan (higher conus pathology obviously will not be seen)
3. Can see canal detail below the level of a myelographic block	3. Too sensitive (high false-positive rate)
4. Lower false-negative rate than myelography at L5-S1	4. Intradural changes (arachnoiditis and tumors) not well seen
5. Shows bone and soft tissue detail better than myelography	5. Radiation exposure compared with MRI (no radiation)
6. Shows paraspinal soft tissues	
7. Reduced tissue radiation compared with myelography	

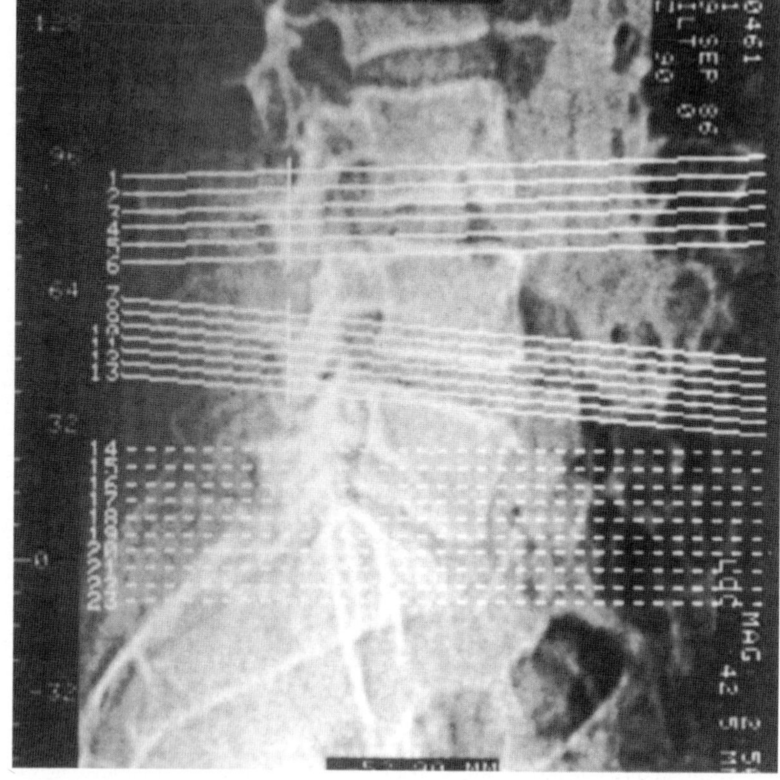

FIGURE 13-15 ● Gantry angulation on lateral scout view. Successful at L4-L5 but not possible at L5-S1.

Originally, most scanning protocols called for angled gantry cuts parallel to the disc space (perpendicular to the spinal canal) (Fig. 13-15). The following limitations of this approach have become evident:

1. Increased patient through-put time while the gantry angle is changed.
2. Difficulty, especially at L5-S1, to get the gantry angled parallel to the disc space.
3. Inability to do sagittal reconstructions.

The most important limitation of gantry angulation is demonstrated in Figure 13-16. It is essential to view the entire spinal canal so as not to miss portions of the third story that can harbor migrated disc fragments, spondylolysis, and the most inferior portion of the subarticular recess. For this reason, a number of departments have adopted the protocol as depicted in Figure 13-17. If a patient is scanned for an HNP, and the radiologist cannot unequivocally see the HNP on the standard scanning protocol, the gantry is angled for cuts parallel to the disc space. This latter requirement rarely occurs in our center.

RADIATION DOSE

Although the total dose of radiation emitted during a CT scan can be equivalent or greater than a myelogram, the collimation of the radiographic beam limits surface radiation dose to 1.6 to 2.5 rad/slice. This results in a radiation dose to the bone marrow in the order of 0.2 to 0.4 rad, which is approximately the same marrow dose received during myelography. A full series of plain lumbar spine radiographs (AP, lateral, both obliques, and spot lateral of the lumbosacral junction) delivers approximately the same surface radiation dose as a CT scan slice (21).

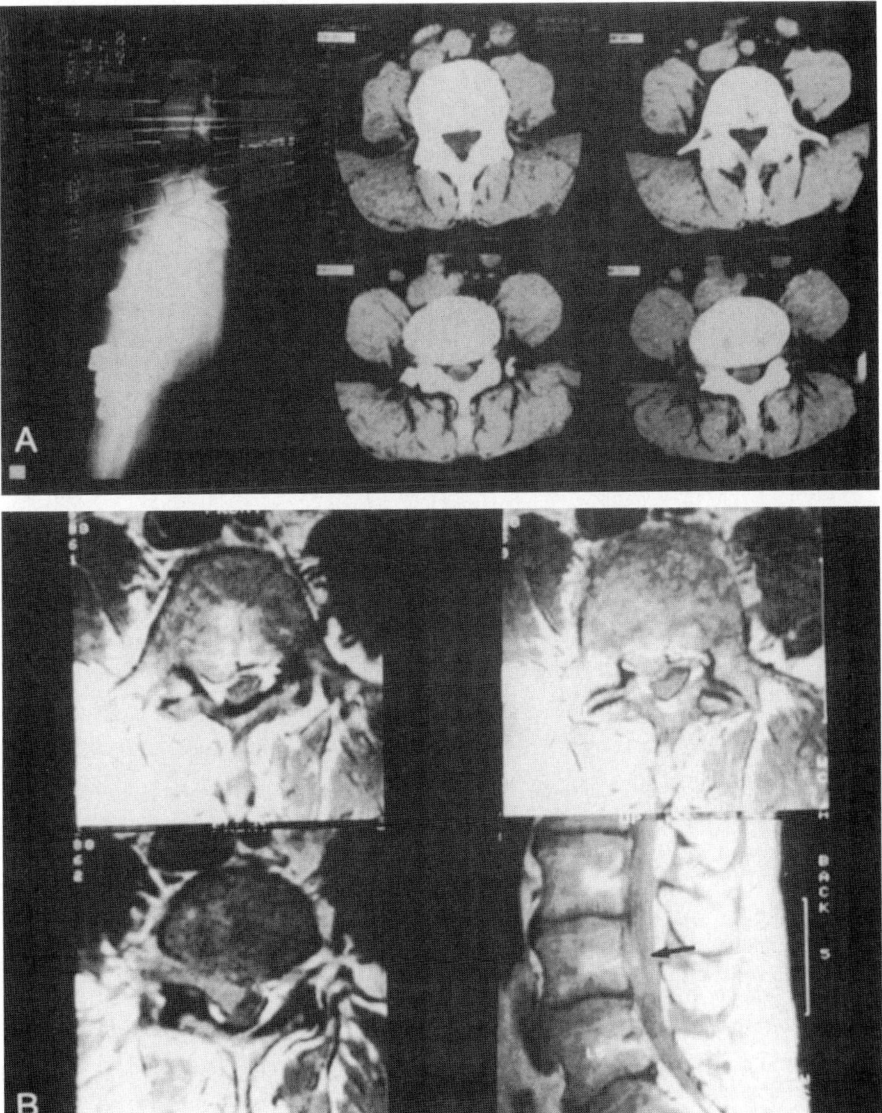

FIGURE 13-16 ● **A:** CT showing gantry angulation and sample of axial slices. No disc herniation is to be found in this patient with significant right leg pain. **B:** Now, look at the MRI and see the large herniated nucleus pulposus (HNP) from the L3-L4 space, trapping down behind the vertebral body of L4 *(arrow).* Look back at the scout view of the CT scan in **A** and see that the gantry angulation missed the upper two thirds of the spinal canal behind the body of L4 where the disc herniation lay. Unless the scout views show all of the canal (compare Fig. 13-17), the scan is not complete.

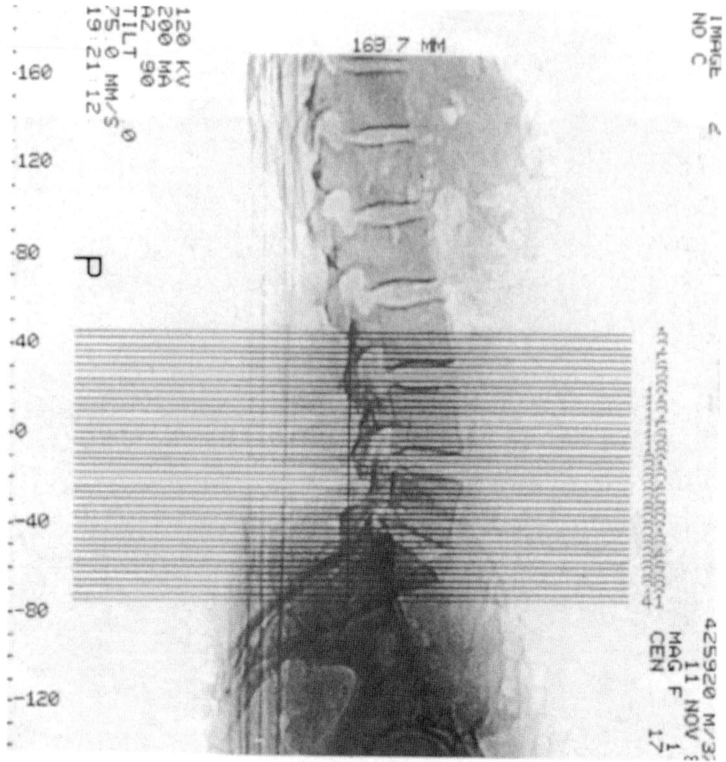

FIGURE 13-17 ● A standard CT protocol as depicted on a lateral scout film.

MIDLINE HERNIATED NUCLEUS PULPOSUS

There is no more CT scan diagnosis fraught with a higher rate of false-positive readings than the diagnosis of a midline HNP (23). MRI will rescue us from this dilemma, but today's technology dictates that we address the issue of the midline HNP on CT scan.

Computed Tomography Scan Diagnosis of a Midline Herniated Nucleus Pulposus

The foundation of all CT diagnosis of an HNP is "focally dominant" extension of disc material beyond the normal peripheral limits of an intervertebral disc (into the epidural space). The "midline disc herniation" is no exception. Figure 13-18 is an example of a midline HNP. An important clue to the diagnosis is the patient's statement to the effect that although both legs are symptomatic, one leg dominates in its affliction over the other. If the midline HNP can be shown to be eccentric to that dominant side on CT scan, this is support for the diagnosis.

The final support for the diagnosis of a bilateral radicular syndrome due to a midline HNP lies in the successful relief of symptoms with removal of the HNP, a criterion often not met or even discussed in this syndrome.

LATERAL ZONE

The lateral zone of the spinal canal is outlined in detail in Chapters 1 and 12. In summary, the zone is defined (Fig. 13-19) as subarticular, foraminal, and extraforaminal.

CENTRAL CANAL

Aside from an HNP, central canal neurologic territory can be encroached on by degenerative or congenital changes (21,29). Spinal canal stenosis due to degenerative changes is by far the most common and is depicted in Figure 13-20.

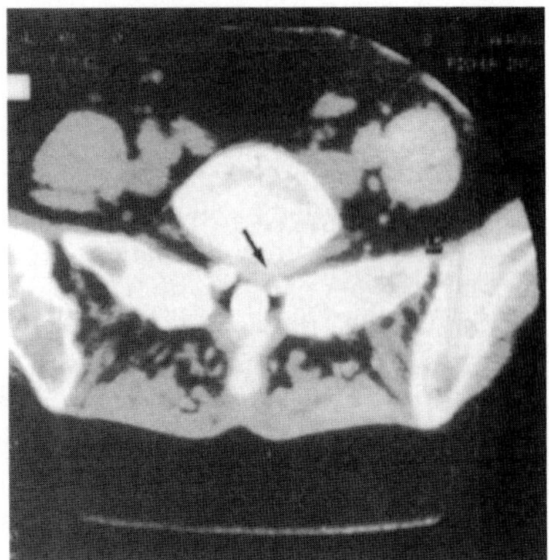

FIGURE 13-18 ● An axial CT showing a midline herniated nucleus pulposus (HNP) at L5-S1; the disc herniation and symptoms were eccentric left *(arrow)*.

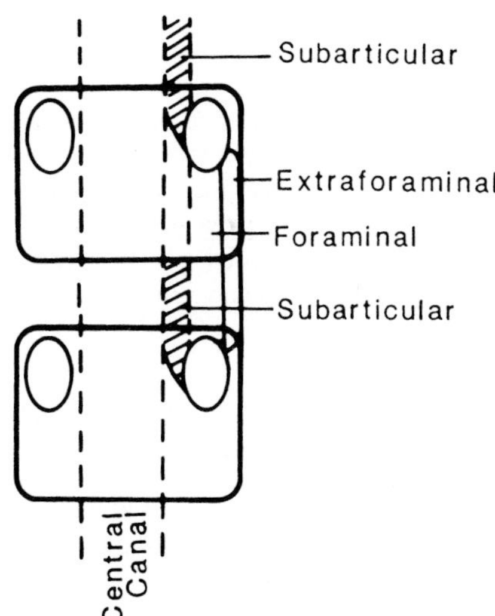

FIGURE 13-19 ● Schematic depicting the three regions of the lateral zone.

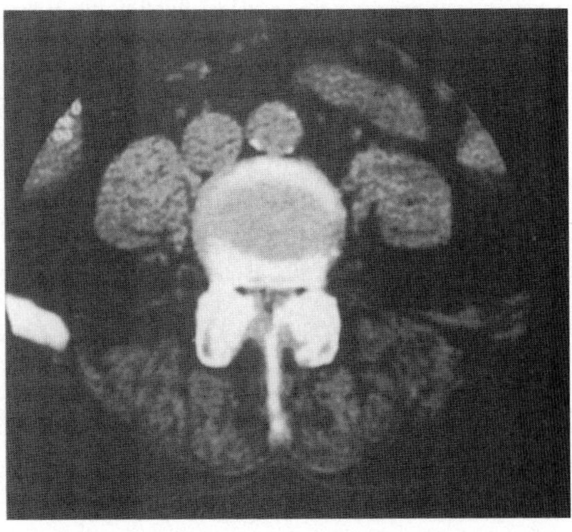

FIGURE 13-20 ● Axial CT showing significant canal stenosis.

FACET JOINTS

Degenerative facet joint changes are akin to degenerative disc changes: Their presence does not necessarily mean the patient is having symptoms. The changes are common and are shown in Figure 13-21.

SPONDYLOLISTHESIS

In an adult spinal surgical practice, lytic and degenerative spondylolisthesis is the common CT scan change seen. This condition's appearances were shown in Chapter 6.

CT SCAN APPEARANCE OF CONJOINT ROOTS

Figure 13-22 shows conjoined nerve roots (19,28). The nerve root tissue is isodense, with the cauda equina compared with an HNP that is denser (whiter) than nerve tissue. Reviewing scan slices from proximal to distal will reveal that the conjoint roots are closely related to the dural sac proximally, and separate distally, in preparation for their exit through the neural foramen.

The bony canal changes that usually accompany conjoined nerve roots have been well described by Helms et al. (19) and are shown in Figure 13-22.

CONCLUSION

The conjoined nerve root is easily observed on myelography (Fig. 13-23), which makes the diagnostic exercise easy. But with more surgery being based on MRI or CT scanning without myelography, conjoined nerve roots are important to recognize preoperatively.

A good test of the value to neuroradiology, CT scanning, and surgical intervention occurs in the patient who has sciatica due to an HNP and at the same level has a conjoined nerve root and lateral zone stenosis. Fortunately, the occurrence is rare because the diagnosis is difficult, and the surgery is tedious.

SAGITTAL RECONSTRUCTIONS/THREE-DIMENSIONAL RECONSTRUCTION AND HELICAL (SPIRAL) COMPUTED TOMOGRAPHY

Most CT scanning machines sold today are capable of spiral scanning (Fig. 13-24). Although the technique has many advantages in other parts of the body (lung, brain), it is of limited use in the spine. To date, the only known advantage is faster scanning of the cervical spine in polytrauma patients. Its use in the lumbar spine is limited because the time (and number of spirals) to scan from

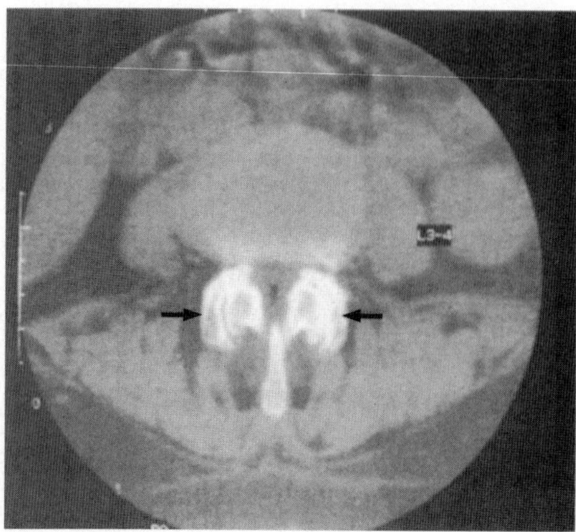

FIGURE 13-21 ● Axial CT showing degenerative facet joints *(arrows)* and significant canal stenosis.

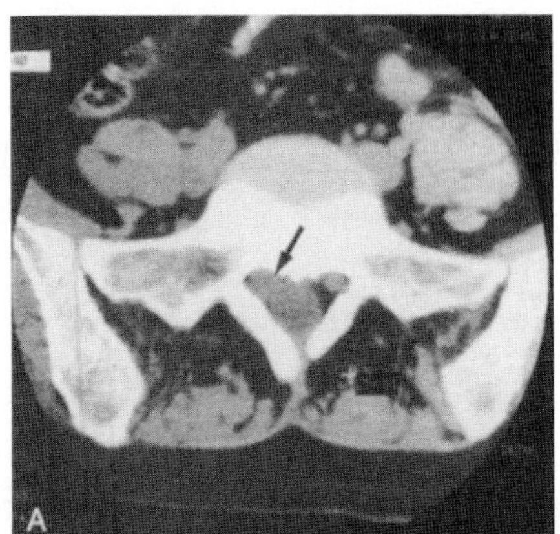

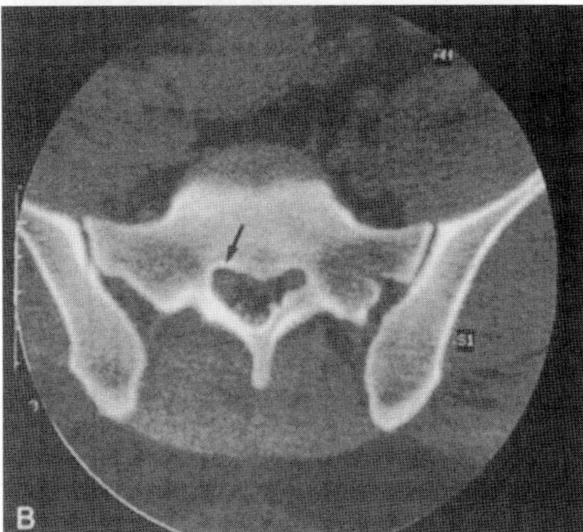

FIGURE 13-22 • **A:** Axial CT showing conjoined nerve root (S1, right) *(arrow).* Note the difference in the shape of the "root canal"—it is larger on the right. **B:** Axial CT (bone window) showing congenitally larger bony subarticular zone on right *(arrow)* to accommodate larger sized conjoined root.

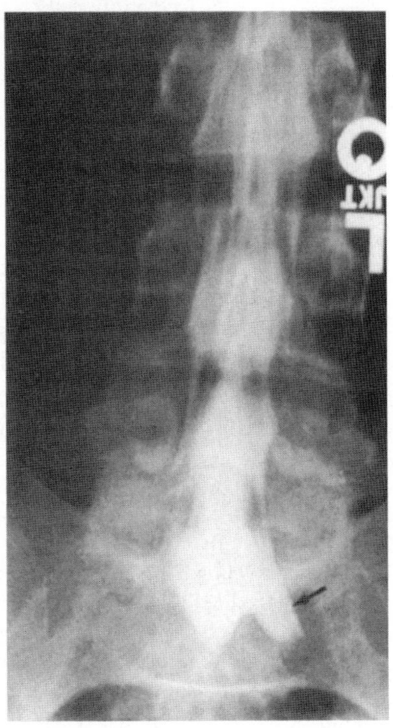

FIGURE 13-23 • An AP myelogram showing obvious conjoined root at S1 level on left *(arrow).*

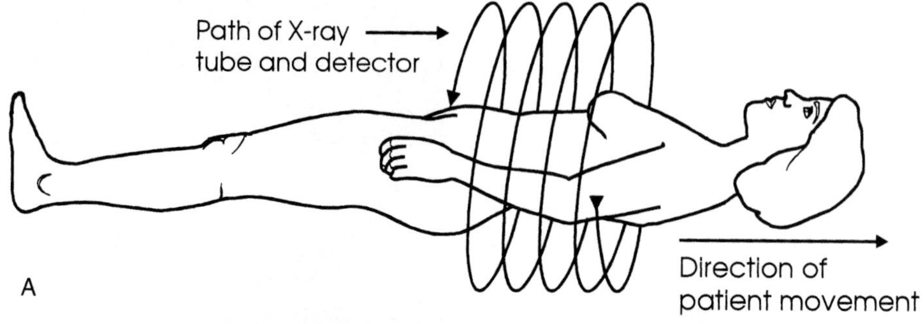

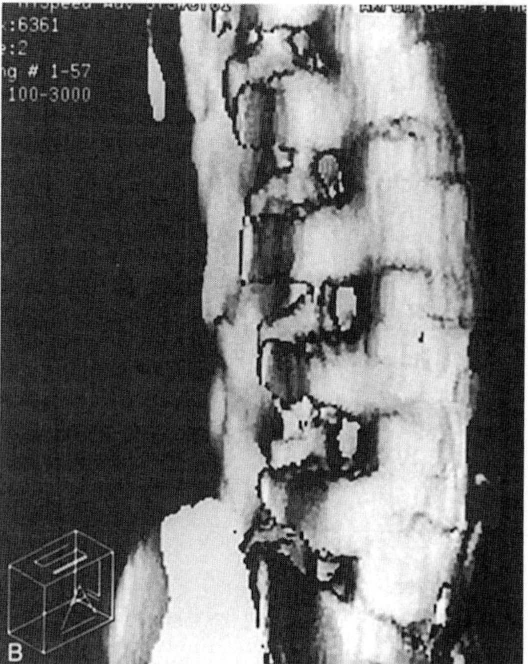

FIGURE 13-24 ● **A:** The spiral scan technique. **B:** A spiral scan technique was used to obtain this three-dimensional image of the foraminal zone.

L3-S1 is so long that the radiograph tube overheats. The only proposed use of the spiral CT scan in the lumbar spine has been for sagittal reconstruction and three-dimensional reconstruction of the lumbar spine in difficult cases such as failed back surgery (31) (Fig. 13-24). The strength of CT over MRI has always been the superior depiction of bony detail. Add to this the even more superior resolution of helical CT with three-dimensional reconstruction, and you are better able to see residual bony encroachment, especially in the foramen.

CT MYELOGRAMS

There was an initial reluctance on the part of the surgeon to give up the gold standard of myelography while traveling the learning curve of CT scanning. This led to the use of a relatively low dose, pre-CT subarachnoid-injected, water-soluble contrast material: the CT myelogram. (22) (Fig. 13-25).

With improved CT scanning hardware and software resulting in clearer images, the necessity for subarachnoid instillation of contrast material has waned. The final step in relegating myelography to an infrequent procedure has been the increasing use of MRI as the primary diagnostic test in lumbar disc disease.

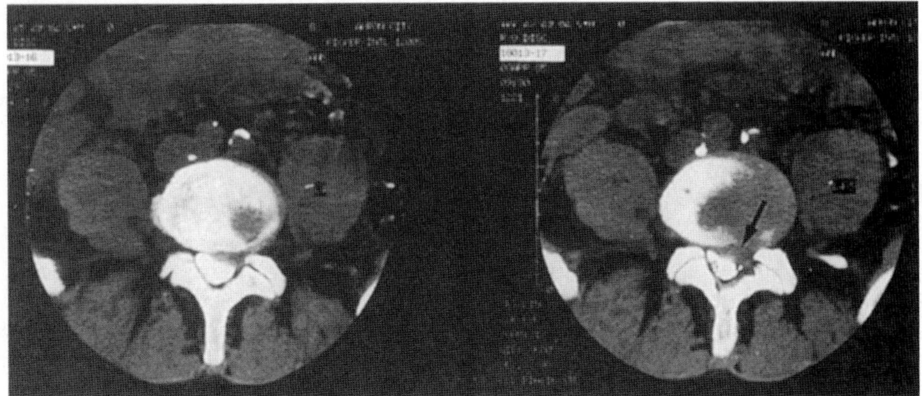

FIGURE 13-25 • A CT myelogram showing a herniated nucleus pulposus (HNP), L4-L5, left *(arrow)*. With increasing familiarity by clinicians for the increasing imaging capabilities of CT and MRI, the myelogram and CT myelogram will largely disappear.

At present, CT myelography is not routine in our center, but this procedure is useful for:

1. An obese patient, in which case scanning images are anticipated to be of poor quality.
2. Anticipation of a difficult differential diagnosis that might include higher lumbar lesions.
3. The older patient with spinal stenosis symptoms and the following:
   - Proximal leg symptoms suggesting a high lumbar lesion.
   - Scoliosis on plain radiograph.
   - A questionable diagnosis (e.g., high erythrocyte sedimentation rate, positive bone scan). (A patient with classic spinal stenosis symptoms and no associated abnormal tests can be investigated adequately with MRI scanning alone.)
4. A young patient with a suspected midline HNP used to be an indication for CT myelography, but MRI has supplanted this need.
5. A confusing CT scan due to a perineural cyst (27), conjoined nerve roots, and so on.

The decreasing use of CT myelography in the face of improved CT and MRI is a trend supported in the literature.

DISCOGRAPHY AND CT DISCOGRAPHY

A number of articles (24,26) have appeared in the literature describing CT discography (Fig. 13-26) as a method of assessing patients with lumbar symptoms. The authors of the first editions

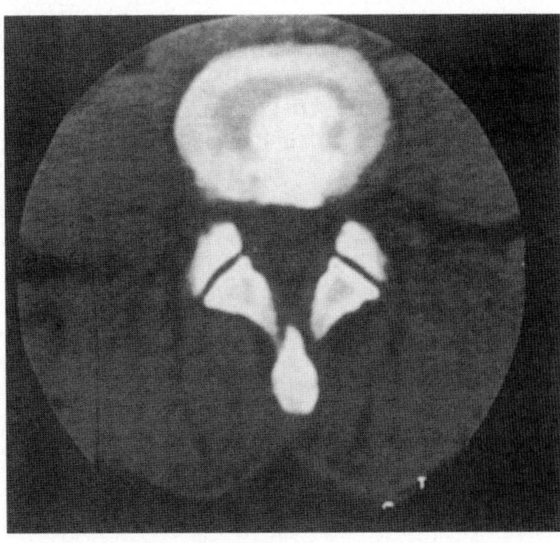

FIGURE 13-26 • A CT/discogram.

(Macnab and McCulloch) have performed more than 10,000 discograms and remained unimpressed with the value of discography as a basis for surgical decision making. To extend this technique to CT examination of instilled contrast material increases the risk of false-positive findings and improper surgery. Until further studies on the scientific validity of CT discography appear in the literature, their routine use for surgical decision making is to be discouraged.

CONCLUSION

There is no question that spine surgical practice has been immensely enhanced by CT scanning technology. Understanding the strengths and weaknesses of any investigation or technique will only help the procedure grow and become even more useful. The final missing link in this growth potential for CT is an increased joint effort for neuroradiologists to deliver quality images and clear diagnoses and for clinicians to relate the clinical material to this effort. This should result in more collaborative studies on surgical outcomes appearing in the radiologic literature. The difficulty in obtaining an unbiased intraoperative determination of normal, bulging, or herniated disc can be balanced only by independent surgical follow-up: The radiologist made a diagnosis. The surgeon operated. Did the patient get better?

A satisfactory patient outcome is the only way to verify that the radiologic diagnosis was firm. Simple observation at surgery is no longer good enough.

MAGNETIC RESONANCE IMAGING

MRI is the major medical imaging development of the century. Its effect on the practice of medicine will be even more profound than Roentgen's original proposal for the use of radiographs to view internal structures. We said in the second edition of this book that MRI developments are coming so quickly that by the time the chapter was published, it would likely be out of date. Things have not changed in MRI; there is still rapid change. The rate of advancement is bewildering, and it is important that the clinician grasp the basics now and hang on for the ride.

For years (32,41), molecular biologists and chemists used magnetic resonance spectroscopy for the laboratory study of molecular and pharmacologic structures. It was not until 1971 (33) that MRI was proposed for human use, and it was in 1981 (34) (only 25 years ago!) that the first high-quality image of the brain was generated at Hammersmith Hospital in London, England. Today, clinicians are getting high-quality images of spinal structures, yet the radiologic scientists have only scratched the surface. MRI has become the imaging modality of choice for investigation of degenerative conditions of the spine, with CT scan and myelography assuming a secondary role.

PHYSICS

A clinician's chance of understanding the physics of MRI is remote. However, a grasp of the basic physics is helpful in appreciating the potential for growth in MRI. There are two magnets essential to MRI:

1. The external magnet (32). That is, the magnet that is part of the imaging machine. Its strength is described in tesla (T) units, and the most common sizes are 0.5, 1.0, and 1.5 T. Work is ongoing with 4 T units as experimental magnets [not Food and Drug Administration (FDA) approved]. As of this writing, the strongest commercially available magnet is 3T.
2. The internal magnets (zillions); that is, the miniature magnet of the hydrogen atom contained in the body.

Resonance

A resonating system is a system "in sync," that is, all the violins are on the same wavelength to produce a nice sound for the audience. Resonance in MRI-talk is the matching of the frequency of the radiowaves (the violins) used for excitation with the frequency of the spinning hydrogen atoms (the audience) in the magnet field. Like an audience that leaves a concert with renewed vigor, the hydrogen atoms absorb energy from the radiowaves, which changes the magnetic vector. Some audience members fail to get excited during a concert (some even fall asleep!) because the resonating sound from the stage simply did not excite them. Similarly, hydrogen atoms have to be resonated with the correct frequency, or they will not respond (fortunately, the hydrogen atoms are much more predictable than a symphony audience!).

The atom used for MRI is the hydrogen (H) atom because it is abundant in the body and capable of giving off a strong signal when excited. Hydrogen is a simple element with one proton in the nucleus, no neutrons, and no orbiting electrons. This atom is everywhere in the body: water, lipids, proteins, and nucleic acids. It is the hydrogen ion in water that is available for excitation. To a lesser extent, the hydrogen ion of lipids will contribute to the MRI signal, with protein and nucleic acid hydrogen ions offering nothing to the signal.

The predetermined frequency is called the "resonant frequency." Some of the hydrogen magnets will absorb some of the energy from the series of radiowave energy and tilt over. The "excited" hydrogen atoms have absorbed the energy from the radiofrequency (RF), and in their tilted position are said to be at a higher energy level, which results in an overall change in direction of the net magnetic vector. The series of the RF pulse is repeated in cycles of finite time known as "repetition time" (TR). During a gap in the pulsatile RF wave, the hydrogen magnets (atoms) will try and reorient themselves in the magnetic field, returning the net magnetic vector to its original position. In doing so, the hydrogen atoms will release energy by rebroadcasting the RF signal they absorbed on deflection. This rebroadcasted RF wave can be picked up with an antenna just as a car radio picks up a broadcast signal. By "tuning in" to a particular frequency, the echo of the RF signal can be picked up. The time in the gap in the RF wave when "tuning in" is done is known as the echo time (TE). The TE can be altered by altering the time when the detection antenna is turned on.

As the net magnetic vector returns to its original position, the rebroadcasted signal is detected by an antenna in the form of a surface coil applied to the patient's spine. (The patient is actually lying on the coil.) As explained later, the use of surface coils in spinal imaging has resulted in much improved images. Different RF signals from different regions of the sample are recorded as digital data by the computer.

IMAGES AVAILABLE IN MRI

The varying shades of gray produced in CT depend on the varying densities of the tissues absorbing the radiation. Thus, only one parameter, electron density of different tissues, determines the image in CT.

Images can be formed in axial, sagittal, and coronal planes by varying the direction of the magnetic gradients across the patient. The type of image formed depends on the computer detection of the parameters as listed previously, that is, signal strength; relaxation time (T1); relaxation time (T2); and state of motion of protons (blood flow, because of its motion, gives no signal, i.e., black, unless the computer converts it to white).

The signal received, like a light bulb, is either bright (white) or dim (black), with many shades of gray (brightness) in between. The exact shade of gray is determined by the H ion concentration of the various tissues scanned and the T1 and T2 characteristics of the tissues imaged.

Each study represents a set of characteristics predetermined by the computer software and ordered up by the radiographic technician. Most scanners reproduce three separate studies: sagittal T1-weighted, sagittal T2-weighted, and axial (T1>) images.

Field Strength

MRI machines are built with varying magnet sizes measured in tesla. The strength of the magnet is many times the earth's gravitational pull and is capable of twisting aneurysm clips, pulling hair pins out of the head, moving wheelchairs, and decoding credit cards. Magnet sizes commonly used in medicine today are 0.5, 1, and 1.5 T. It is not necessarily true that the bigger magnet is better, but imaging of difficult areas, such as the posterior fossa and base of the brain, is better with the higher field strengths. Although the manufacturers state that it is possible to get good spinal images from the lower field strength machines, the authors' early and continuing experiences would suggest that the most consistently good spinal images come from the machines with the highest field strength (38).

Pulse Sequence

In reading about MRI, clinicians will see the term "pulse sequence" mentioned often. There are three types of pulse sequences commonly used today: One (spin echo) was used exclusively for clinical imaging of the spine in the original protocols; a second (gradient echo) acquisition of a new pulse

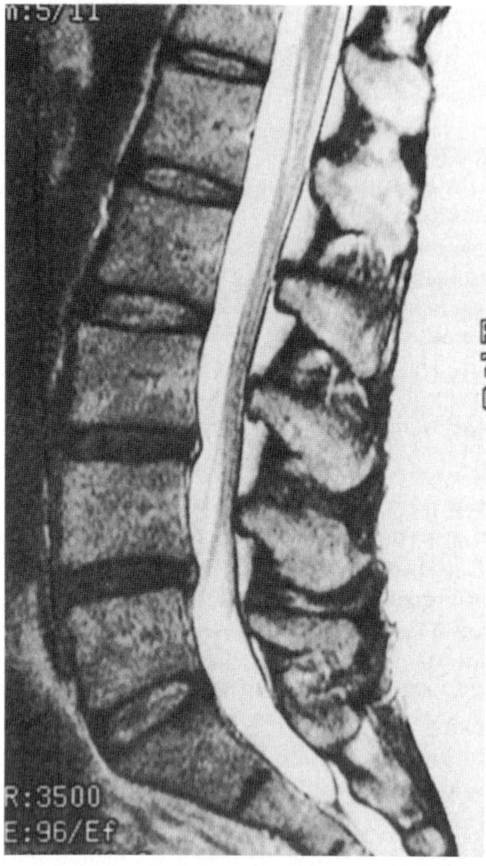

FIGURE 13-27 ● A fast spin ECHO sagittal showing high signal intensity (white) cerebrospinal fluid (CSF), gray marrow of vertebral bodies, and blackened (degenerative) discs, especially at L3-L4 and L4-L5.

sequence has recently been introduced to speed up image acquisition time and give more contrast between cerebrospinal fluid (CSF) and its surrounding tissues. The latest pulse sequence to come along is "fast spin-echo," which simply reduces image acquisition times without significant loss of image quality, a particularly useful tool in the acquisition of T2 spin-echo images (Fig. 13-27).

OTHER TERMS

Echo Time

TE is the time between the initial pulse, which deflects the hydrogen atom 90 degrees, and the middle of the spin echo production when the antenna "listens in" to detect the amount of signal.

Repetition Time

TR represents the period of time between one RF pulse and the next. By varying TE and TR, various tissue relaxation times are produced, and different tissue contrasts can be produced. The differences in the strengths of the primary magnetic field (0.5 to 1.5 T) also change tissue relaxation times, a factor to be aware of when reviewing scans from different centers.

Relaxation Times

This is the intrinsic property of tissue, after being magnetized and struck with RF waves. It is determined by the behavior of atoms in a magnetic field and can be used to produce images of varying tissue contrast. By varying TR and TE, two basic types of tissue contrast are produced. The two types of relaxation mechanisms are as follows:

- T1 relaxation time (T1-weighted images) (spin lattice or longitudinal relaxation time). Produced by using a short TR/TE, it is the time required for spinning atoms to realign themselves with the externally applied magnetic fields after displacement with RF waves.

A good analogy would be the length of time it takes a regiment of soldiers, briefly at ease and talking to one another, to "present arms."

- T2 relaxation time (T2-weighted images) (spin-spin or transverse relaxation time). Produced by longer TR/TE times, it represents the time required for the loss of signal caused by interaction of adjacent nuclei.

The analogy here would be giving the regimental soldiers a little more time to intermingle and then let them go home, their disappearance being the signal.

Each tissue, be it normal or abnormal, has characteristic T1 and T2 relaxation times, dependent on chemical composition. This composition determines the signal intensity and thus the ultimate image produced.

Signal intensity. The ranges of signal intensity are low (a black image) to high (a white image) (Table 13-4).

Those tissues that give off a high intensity signal (high hydrogen ion concentration that can be affected by the magnet and the RF wave) are water, fat, marrow, and nerve tissue. Intermediate signal intensity comes from muscle and articular cartilage. Low signal intensity (black) structures are cortical bone, ligaments, tendons, and menisci. Because of the flow of blood (i.e., the hydrogen ions will not stand still long enough to be counted), no signal intensity is produced by blood vessels that appear black.

THE MAGNETIC RESONANCE IMAGING GRAY SCALE

The varying shades of gray produced in CT and other radiographic studies are determined by one factor: the different densities of the tissues (to be exact, the density of the orbiting electrons of each atom). The varying shades of gray produced on MRI are based on four independent components of tissue, one physical (proton density) and three biochemical (relaxation time T1, relaxation time T2, and motion or flow of materials).

T1, T2, and the Gray Scale

It should be noted that:

- Substances with the shortest T1 relaxation time give off the brightest signal (fat, lipid-containing molecules, or proteinaceous fluid).
- Substances with the longest T1 relaxation time [edema, CSF, pure fluid, tumors (benign and malignant)] give off a low signal and appear grayer (Fig. 13-28 and Table 13-4).

By selecting a scanning protocol with a short TR and TE, the image is weighted to emphasize these T1 characteristics, but weighting too heavily will ruin the image by invoking other physics equations that affect signal-to-noise ratios, scan time, and so on, a subject far beyond this chapter. Just the correct amount of TR and TE is needed to produce a useful T1 image.

A protocol that lengthens both TR and TE (Table 13-4) is called a T2-weighted image, in which the reverse signal characteristics occur: that is, the longer the T2 relaxation time, the brighter the signal (remember, the longer the T1 relaxation time, the grayer the picture) (Fig. 13-29).

Substances with a short T2 relaxation time include muscle and tendons. Substances with a long T2 (brighter image) include water and CSF and edematous and inflamed tissue. Thus, many common disease processes become conspicuous on T2-weighted images because the increased free water of edema and inflammation gives a brighter (whiter) signal.

The T1- and T2-weighted images are summarized in Tables 13-4 and 13-5.

TABLE 13-4

The Gray Scale

Brightest Image	=	Short T1 and long T2 relaxation time in tissues
Darkest Image	=	Long T1 and short T2 relaxation time in tissues

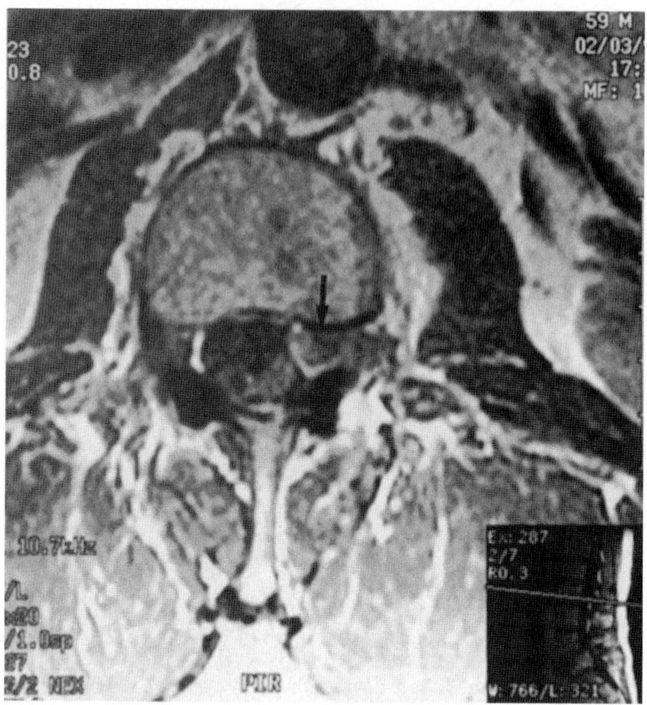

FIGURE 13-28 ● An axial T1-weighted MRI to show gray scale: note signal intensity from water [cerebrospinal fluid (CSF)], muscle, fat. An arrow points to a disc herniation.

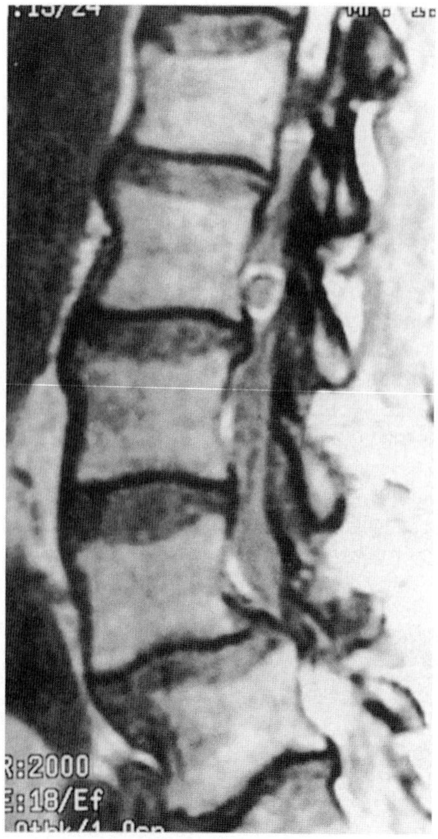

FIGURE 13-29 ● A sagittal proton density showing the same disc herniation behind the vertebral body of L2.

TABLE 13-5

The Gray Scale in Various Tissues

Tissue	T1-Weighted	T2-Weighted
CSF	Black	White
Gray matter	Gray	White
White matter	White	Gray
Marrow	Gray	Whiter
Disc nucleus	Gray	White
Disc annulus	Less gray	Black
Fat	Bright	Gray
Subacute hemorrhage	Bright	Gray
Gadolinium-enhanced tissues	Very white	Gray
Muscle	Gray	Gray

CSF, cerebrospinal fluid.

IMAGES PRODUCED BY MAGNETIC RESONANCE IMAGING

Most protocols for the spine produce one axial and two sagittal images. Advantages of each image are as follows:

Sagittal T1 (Fig. 13-30) depicts the following:

Root canals (foramina).
Facet joints.
Vertebral bodies.
Spinal cord.

Sagittal T2 (Fig. 13-31) brightens (whitens) fluid (H_2O)-containing structures, and thus boundaries:

CSF.
Internal structure of disc.
Osseous structures are poorly seen on T2-weighted image.

Axial T1 (Fig. 13-32) depicts:

Facet joints.
Ligamentous flavum.
Foramina.

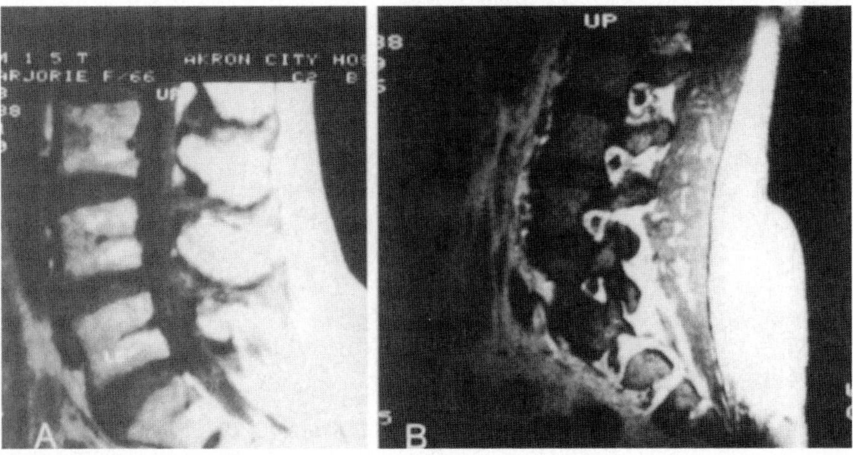

FIGURE 13-30 • Sagittal T1 MRI. **A:** Midline. **B:** Lateral, showing neural foramina.

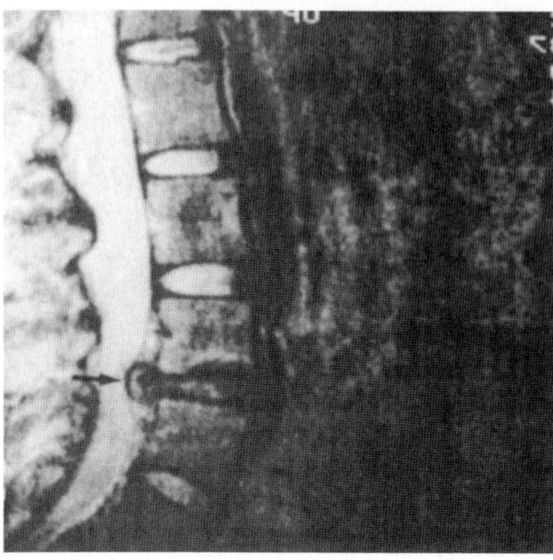

FIGURE 13-31 ● Sagittal T2 MRI. Note the large midline herniated nucleus pulposus (HNP) at L4-L5 *(arrow)* and the whiteness of the cerebrospinal fluid (CSF) and nucleus.

ADVANTAGES OF MAGNETIC RESONANCE IMAGING OVER COMPUTED TOMOGRAPHY

1. MRI does not require the use of ionizing radiation (which also means that the quality of the MR images is not affected by patient size).
2. MRI produces excellent sagittal sections, that is, images at 90 degrees to axials.
3. MRI produces excellent soft tissue detail. In fact, clinicians trying to travel the MRI learning curve are struggling to contend with the superior (exaggerated) detail as they try to avoid a high incidence of false-positive MRIs.
4. MRI will detail intradural lesions such as tumors, syrinx, and arachnoiditis.
5. MRI signal is not impeded by bone, which results in better images in the posterior fossa and the base of the brain.
6. MRI does not produce artifact from nonferromagnetic metals in surgical clips and prostheses.

DISADVANTAGES OF MRI

1. The gantry for MRI is smaller and longer than the CT gantry and is more prone to producing a claustrophobic feeling for the patient.

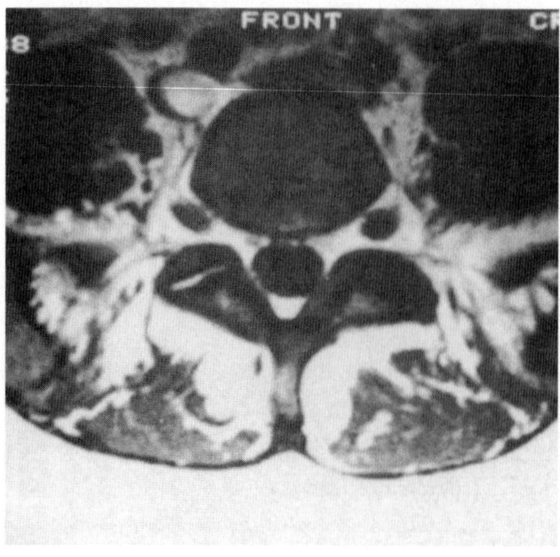

FIGURE 13-32 ● Axial (T1) MRI. Note facet joint and foramina/detail.

2. The scan time is longer for MRI, and a patient in pain may find it difficult, if not impossible, to be still for the time required.
3. Patients with ferromagnetic materials in their body cannot be scanned if the following conditions apply:
   - Cerebral aneurysm clips will be torqued by the magnet.
   - Pacemakers will be converted to a fixed rate.
   - Transcutaneous electrical nerve stimulation units will be drawn into the magnet.
   - Ocular metallic foreign bodies may be moved and result in damage to vision.
   - Metallic cardiac valves are at risk.
   - Life support devices are at risk.

Fortunately, most orthopaedic implants are not ferromagnetic and thus do not affect image quality, unless directly in the field, for example, pedicle instrumentation.

4. The MRI machine is more costly to purchase and install in a specially shielded room. This high initial capital cost transfers into the necessity for a higher fee for MRI compared with CT. In the future, both hardware and software changes will hopefully lead to reduced costs.
5. MRI does not image bone as well as CT, resulting in somewhat poorer delineation of calcified discs or osteophytes. Changes in the MRI protocol are likely to result in improved bone images.
6. MRI is very operator dependent: If the radiologist does not keep on top of the changing technology, or if the technologist does not operate the equipment properly, poor images will result.

TODAY'S INDICATIONS FOR MAGNETIC RESONANCE IMAGING (FOR DEGENERATIVE SPINE CONDITIONS)

The title of this section is "Today's Indications" because tomorrow's will be different. There is reasonable expectation today in many leading centers that MRI will be the imaging modality of choice for all spinal problems.

Today's indications are as follows:

- The only necessary investigation of a patient with a disc rupture who has failed conservative care and is being considered for surgery.
- Young patient with a suspected midline HNP!
- Young patient with a suspected HNP!
- Any patient with an HNP (38)!
- A patient with single level degenerative disc disease and no radicular symptoms who is being considered for a single level fusion. An MRI will verify (a) there is no root encroachment within the canal or lateral zone and (b) the discs above or below are normal.
- A patient with a classic story of spinal stenosis, with no unusual neurologic presentation and no scoliosis.
- A patient suspected of having arachnoiditis.
- Recurrent HNP.

In addition, MRI has been very useful for other spinal problems, such as tumors, trauma, and infection, and it has been extremely useful for assessment of a host of intraspinal lesions, such as multiple sclerosis and syrinx.

PATIENT PREPARATION

Most imaging centers will give patients preparatory instructions that include such things as follows:

- Do not wear metal items to the examination (e.g., belts, hairpins, metal arched high-heeled shoes, jewelry, zippers).
- Do not wear eye makeup, some of which contains iron or cobalt.
- Do not bring credit cards; they all contain a magnetized code.
- Do not wear a dial-type wrist watch.

It is unnecessary for a patient to fast before an MRI.

WEIGHT RESTRICTIONS

There is a patient weight restriction of approximately 300 lb. This has as much to do with the size of the gantry (tunnel) as with the ability of the table to carry a heavy patient. Taller patients a little heavier than 300 lb may fit into the tunnel and shorter patients weighing less than 300 lb may not fit into the tunnel. Open, low field strength permanent magnet units are available to accommodate the very large patient.

ABNORMAL MAGNETIC RESONANCE IMAGING

Figures 13-33 to 13-42 show examples of degenerative spine problems.

NEWER TECHNIQUES

Contrast-Enhanced Magnetic Resonance Imaging

The word "contrast" in radiograph (e.g., myelography) implies a direct effect of a compound on the image produced. Contrast enhancement in MRI is purely an indirect effect of a pharmaceutical on signal intensity (40). These pharmaceuticals are in the form of three paramagnetic compounds known as gadolinium chelates: Magnevist, ProHance, and Omniscan. When administered intravenously, they are deposited in tissues with high water content, provided there is a good blood supply. These compounds will not deposit in tissues with poor blood supply (e.g., disc material). Within edematous tissues, these paramagnetic compounds lower T1 relaxation values and increase their signal intensity. Thus, scar in the lumbar spine enhances, whereas recurrent disc ruptures do not enhance (Fig. 13-43). The enhancement of scar tissue is more pronounced on high field strength magnets.

Fat-Suppression Techniques

The spine is surrounded by a lot of fat: the marrow spaces, the epidural space, and the neural foramina. This is useful on T1 images because it improves contrast between the normal fatty marrow and the pathologic tumor or infection that is replacing the marrow (Fig. 13-44). On infusion of contrast material (gadolinium), the fat has a tendency to obscure the enhancement of the tumor or edema. By suppressing the high intensity of the fat signal on T1-weighted images, the contrast enhancement of pathology is more evident (Fig. 13-44). For inflammatory and neoplastic diseases of the spine, fat suppression plus gadolinium contrast material helps to demonstrate early lesions of the posterior elements and disease extension into the epidural space. In failed

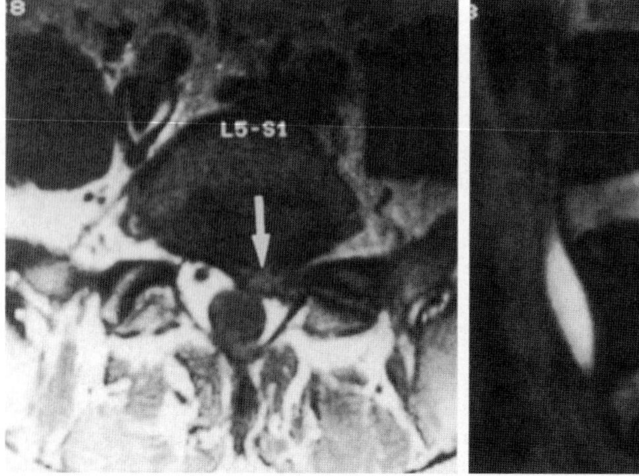

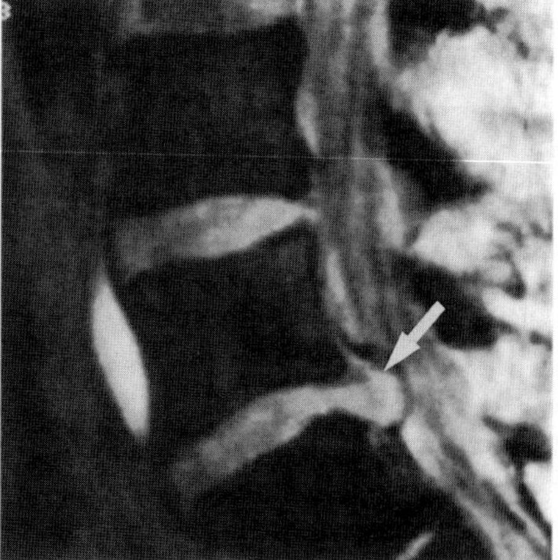

FIGURE 13-33 ● Axial T1 weighted showing herniated nucleus pulposus (HNP), L5-S1, left *(arrow)*. Sagittal gradient echo showing same HNP *(arrow)*.

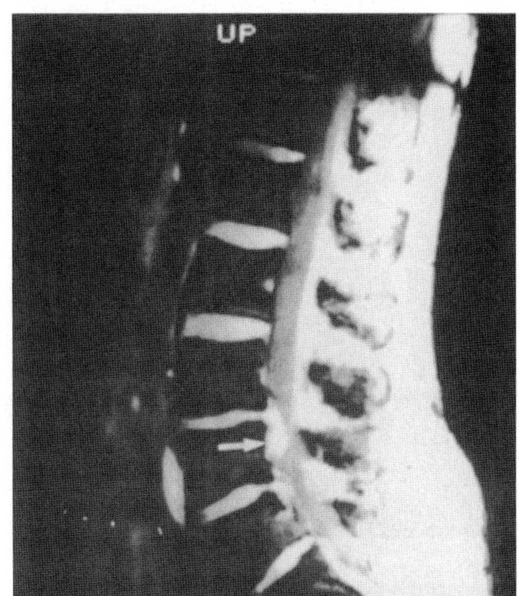

FIGURE 13-34 ● Sagittal gradient echo image showing herniated nucleus pulposus (HNP), L3-L4, trapping down into third story of L4 *(arrow).*

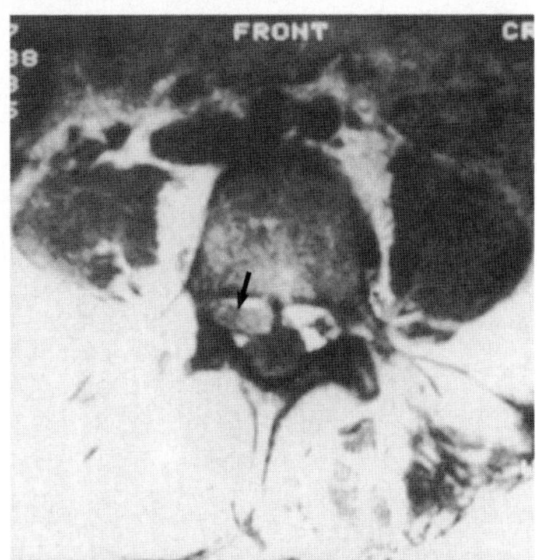

FIGURE 13-35 ● Free fragment of disc material well down into third story of L4, right (T1 axial) *(arrow).*

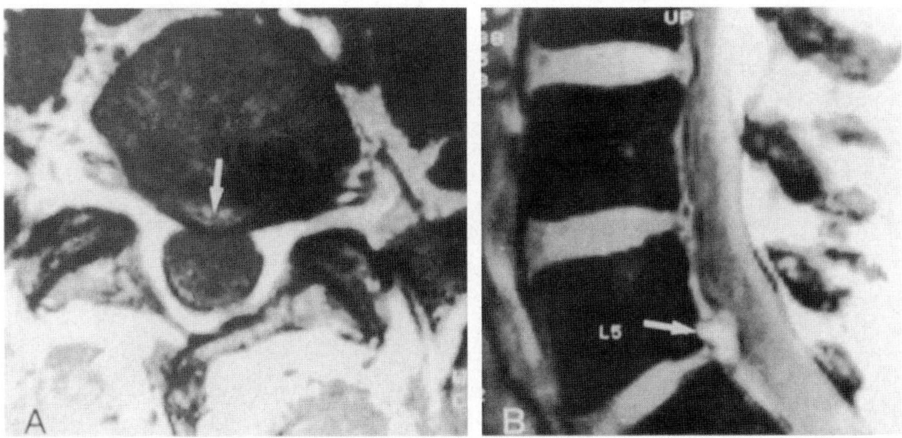

FIGURE 13-36 ● Midline herniated nucleus pulposus (HNP) (L5-S1). **A:** Axial T1 *(arrow).* **B:** Sagittal gradient echo *(arrow).*

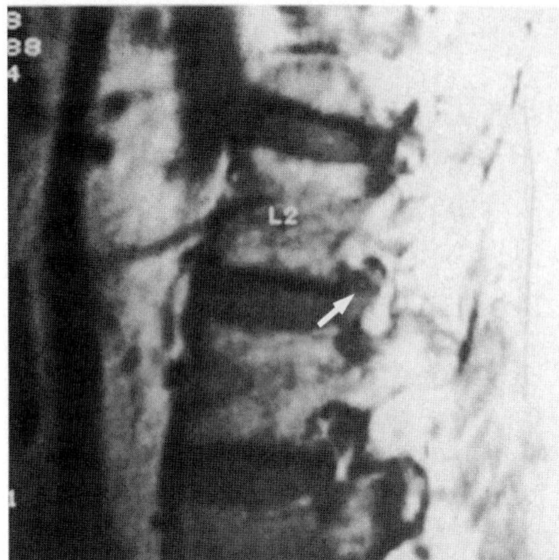

FIGURE 13-37 ● Sagittal T1—foraminal herniated nucleus pulposus (HNP), L2 *(arrow).*

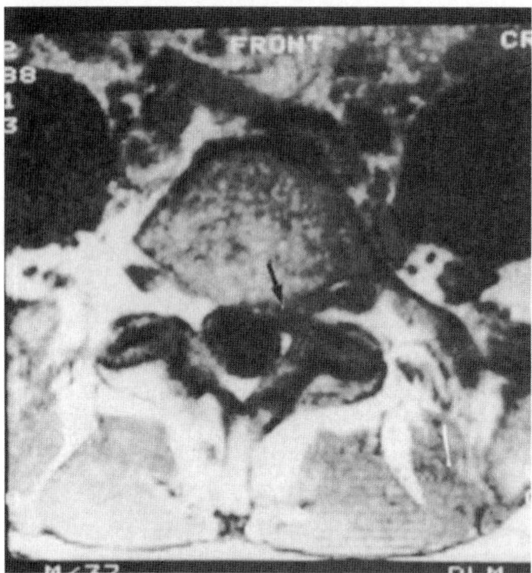

FIGURE 13-38 ● Herniated nucleus pulposus (HNP), L5, left, second story, on T1 axial *(arrow).*

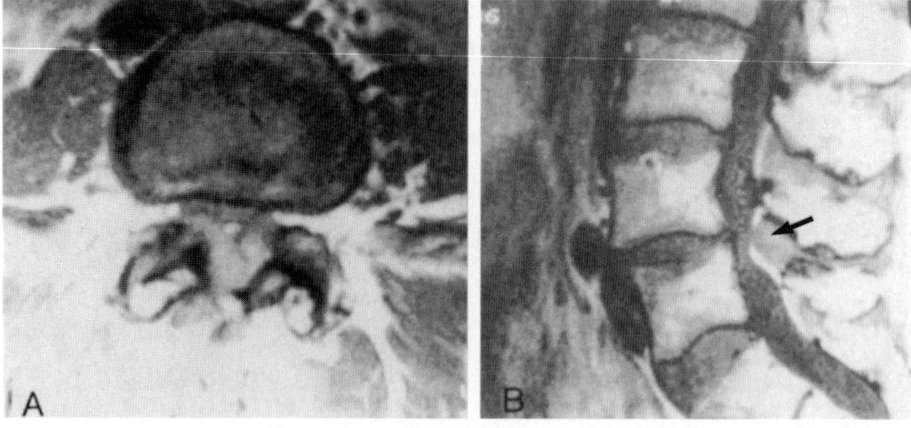

FIGURE 13-39 ● Spinal canal stenosis at degenerative spondylolisthesis level, L4-L5. **A:** Axial T1. **B:** Sagittal T1 *(arrow).*

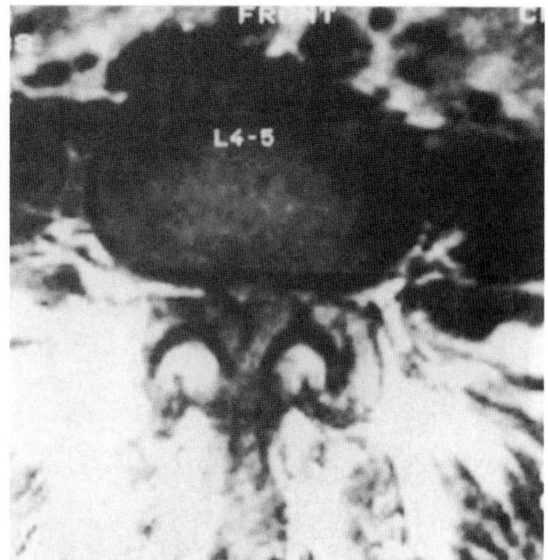

FIGURE 13-40 ● Spinal canal stenosis (L4-L5)—axial T1.

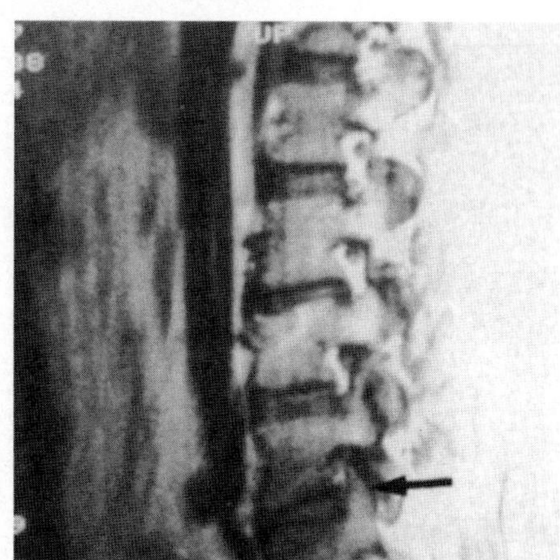

FIGURE 13-41 ● Spinal stenosis, lateral zone, L5 foramen on axial T1. Note the subluxed superior facet of S1 filling the L5 foramen *(arrow).*

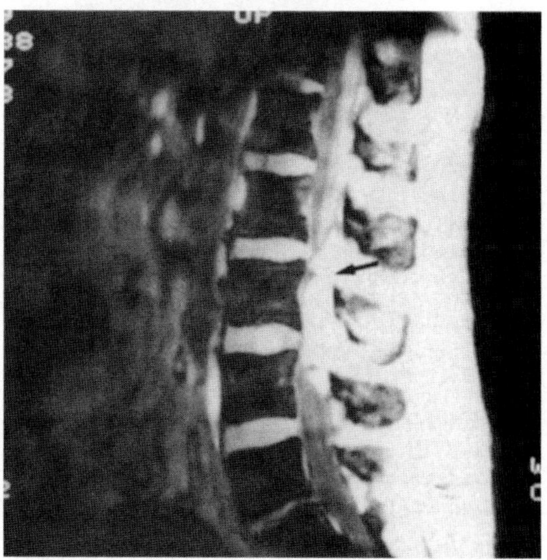

FIGURE 13-42 ● Extradural tumor (lymphoma), L2 to L4 *(arrow),* on gradient echo image, sagittal slice in midline.

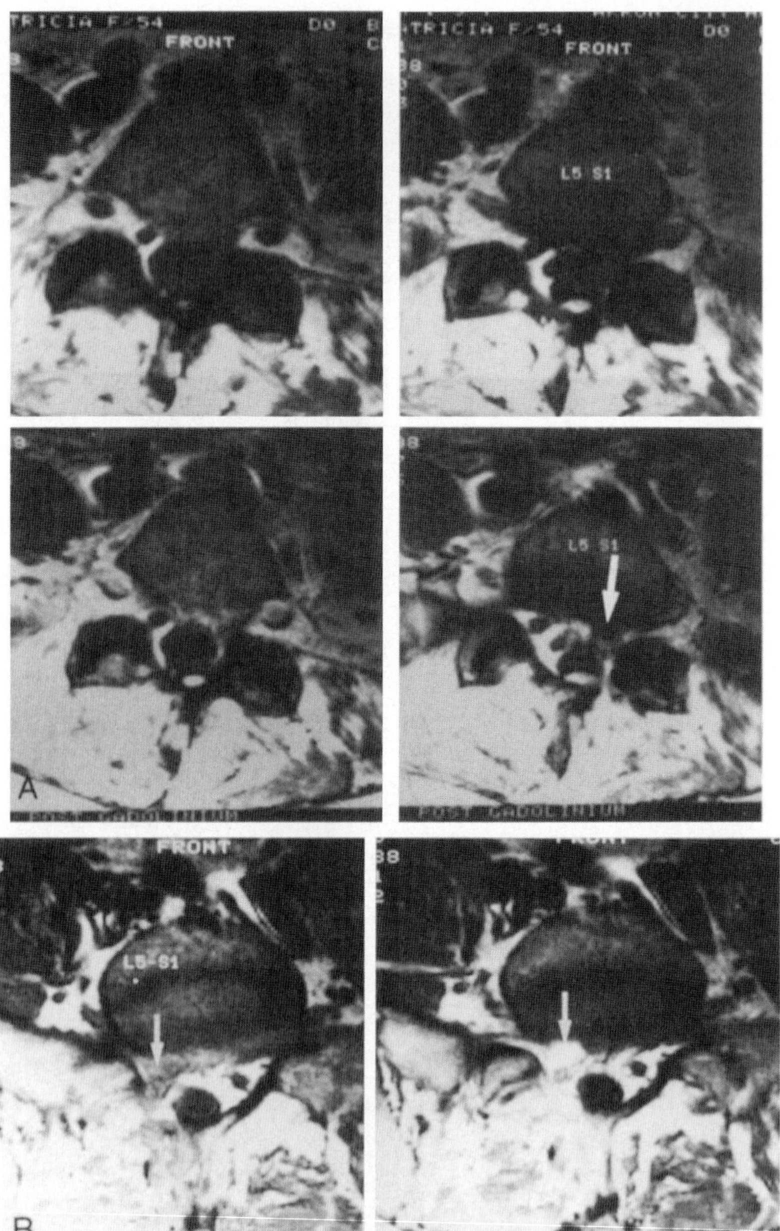

FIGURE 13-43 ● **A: Top row:** axial MRI (T1) of patient with recurrent leg pain 15 years after L5-S1 discectomy, left. **Bottom row:** axial MRI (T1) after injection of gadolinium-DTPA. Scar, lit up by the gadolinium-DTPA, is evident on the left; a nonenhanced recurrent disc herniation is evident in the lower right cut (L5-S1, left) *(arrow).* **B:** A young doctor, 6 weeks after operation, had continuing right leg pain. An enhanced MRI shows bright scar tissue and no recurrent herniated nucleus pulposus (HNP) *(arrows).*

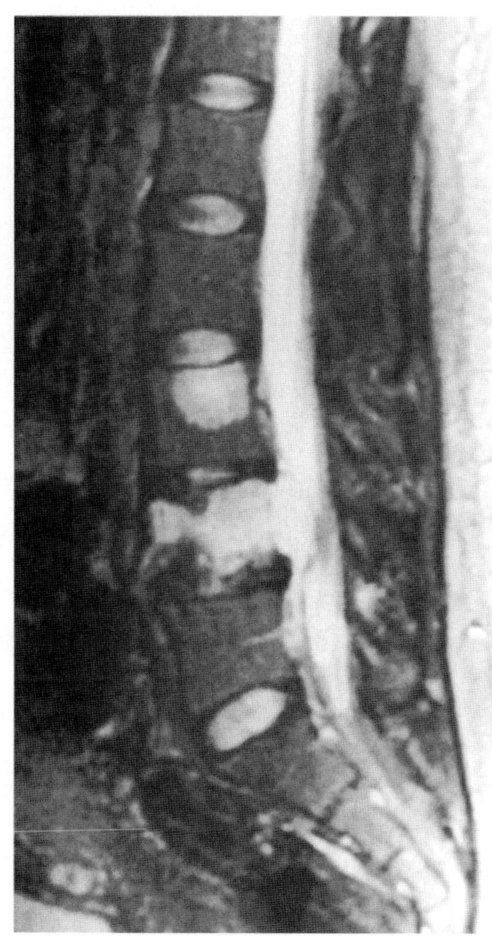

FIGURE 13-44 • The fat suppression technique has obliterated the marrow fat to reveal metastatic carcinoma of lumbar vertebral bodies 3 and 4.

spine surgery, the technique also increases conspicuousness of epidural fibrosis and nerve roots individually and within the common dural sac (e.g., demonstration of arachnoiditis) (Fig. 13-45) and helps distinguish ganglia from disc fragments.

Nothing in life is free. Fat-suppression techniques decrease spatial resolution because of a decreased signal-to-noise ratio, that is, the images just are not as sharp (36). The images take longer to acquire, and sometimes the fat suppression is uneven. Despite these drawbacks, fat suppression of T1 gadolinium-enhanced MRI images is a useful sequence to have available when looking for tumors and infections and when trying to assess scar tissue in the postoperative lumbar spine.

CONCLUSION

To date, the MRI has been used to substitute for CT, but Haughton (37) believes that the future use of MRI will expand to include the study of the following pathologic and chemical changes:

- Disc bulge versus disc herniations.
- Water content and disc degeneration (39).
- Annular tears.
- Intervertebral disc pH measurements relative to degenerative disc disease.
- Scars and adhesions.
- Pulsations and movement of the CSF in such conditions as spinal stenosis (35).

From the first brain images in 1982 to the excellent spine images today, MRI has made dramatic advances. Even more rapid changes are in store for the clinician, making it essential to stay close to the science. Failure to do so may result in MRI technology running away from clinical.

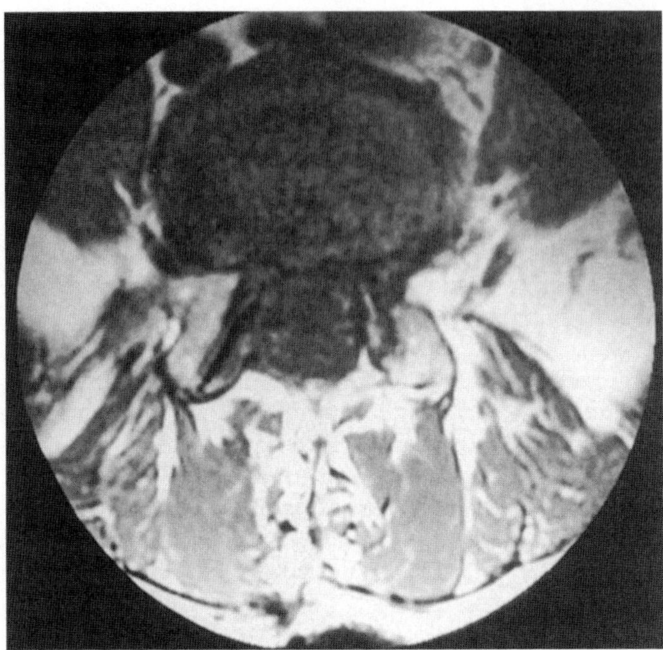

FIGURE 13-45 ● Arachnoiditis without the fat suppression technique: note the clumping of the nerve roots around the periphery of the common dural sac in this postoperative patient.

THERMOGRAPHY

Thermography, once a promising diagnostic test, has largely been dropped from clinical use because of the lack of scientific support.

ELECTROMYOGRAPHY/NERVE CONDUCTION TESTS

The neuromuscular system is an electrical circuit board, and its activity can be measured with appropriate equipment. The electrophysiologic tests used are electromyography and nerve conduction tests (NCTs). Other electrical testing methods that are being used in spine problems include somatosensory-evoked potentials and motor-evoked potentials. These are beyond the interests of this book, and readers are referred to other texts.

Electrical physiologic testing is used to study two basic groups of problems:

1. Orthopaedic—nerve root lesions.
   Overuse and entrapment syndromes.
   Plexus injuries.
2. Neurologic—neuropathies.
   Myopathies.
   Spinal cord [upper motor neuron lesion (UMNL)] mixed with lower motor neuronal lesions such as amyotrophic lateral sclerosis, multiple sclerosis, and Friedreich's ataxia.

The two basic ways of studying these problems are as follows:

1. Nerve conduction test (NCT).
2. Electromyography (EMG).

NERVE CONDUCTION TESTS

NCTs are used to evaluate nerve entrapment syndromes. As such they are not particularly valuable in assessment of low back problems unless you have a differential diagnostic problem such as an L5 nerve lesion that could be due to a root lesion (disc rupture) or entrapment neuropathy in the

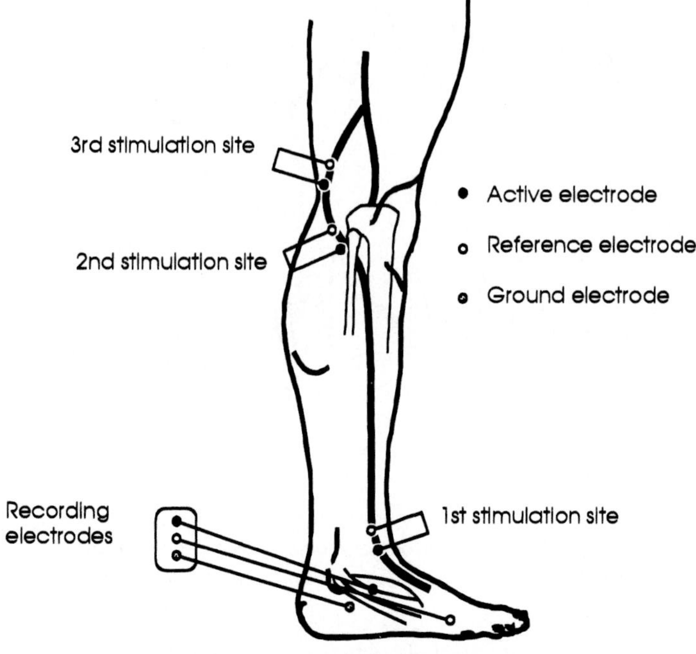

FIGURE 13-46 • A nerve conduction test of the peroneal nerve showing the various locations for stimulation and the sight of recording in the extensor digitorum brevis.

pelvis or around the knee. NCTs are very valuable in cervical disc/upper extremity entrapment neuropathies, in which differential diagnosis can be very confusing.

An NCT is shown in Figure 13-46. After stimulating proximally and measuring the action potential distally (usually no more than 8 to 10 cm away from stimulation), the duration to travel the distance can be calculated as follows.

The NCT can then be compared to the standard tables (e.g., normal limit for conduction along peroneal nerve around fibular head is 41.65 msec). If the NCT is longer than what the tables say it should be, there is a delay in nerve conduction time, that is, an entrapment between the stimulation site and the recording site. By moving proximally and distally along the nerve, sites of entrapment can be localized.

ELECTROMYOGRAPHY

EMG is a method of studying the intrinsic electrical activity of individual motor units of muscle. After inserting a needle electrode into muscle (Fig. 13-47), both spontaneous and volitional electrical impulses can be recorded on an oscilloscope. EMG is largely a study of lower motor neuron phenomena and is useful for diagnosing neuropathies and myopathies.

Five parameters of electrical activity are studied (Fig. 13-48):

1. Voltage: the amplitude of the wave from peak to peak (normal is up to 4,000 or 5,000 microvolts).
2. Duration: how long the wave lasts (normal is 8–12 msec).
3. Waveforms: how many dips in waveform (normal is a bi- or triphasic wave).
4. Frequency: number of waves/second (normal is 1–60/sec).
5. Sound: the actual sound the waves make on the oscilloscope.

These normal values change from muscle to muscle (e.g., flexors vs. extensors) and from young to old. Electrical potentials are examined on insertion of the needle electrode, with the muscle at rest and with the patient providing maximum contraction of the muscle being examined.

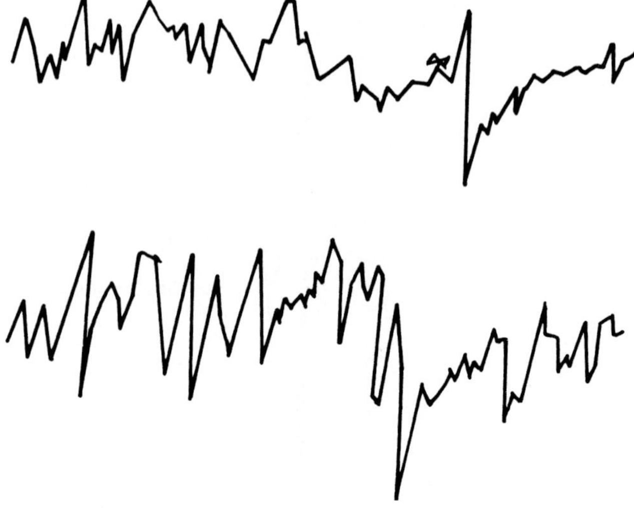

FIGURE 13-47 ● Electromyography (EMG) volitional motor unit activity.

EMG can be used to localize the level of lumbar nerve root involvement. Healthy, normally innervated muscle is electrically "silent" at rest, and the insertion of an electromyographic needle does not produce sustained electrical discharges. However, in the presence of a nerve root lesion, a series of involuntary electrical discharges can be recorded. These are characterized by a shortened potential and reduced amplitude (fibrillation potentials) or by altered waveforms (positive waves). The positive waveforms are produced only on needle insertion, but the fibrillation potentials can be recorded all of the time (Fig. 13-48).

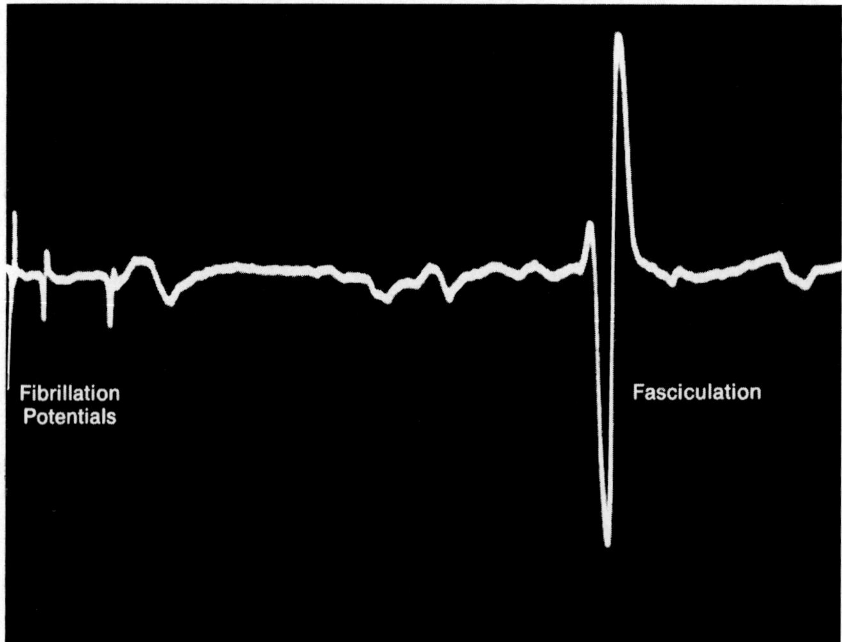

FIGURE 13-48 ● A drawing of normal and abnormal electromyography (EMG) changes.

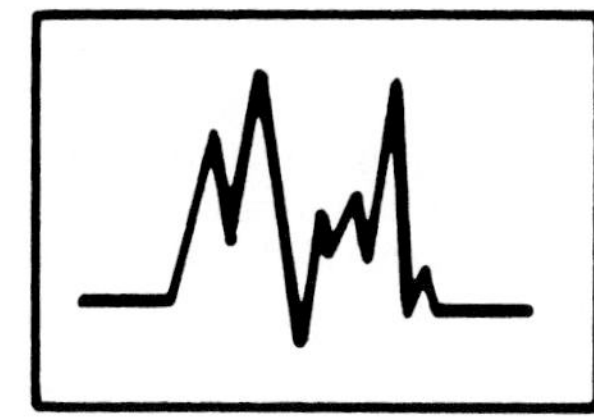

FIGURE 13-49 • Abnormal polyphasic potentials.

On voluntary contraction of a normal muscle, the motor unit action potentials evoked are biphasic or triphasic in form. With partial denervation, the quantity of motor units recording is decreased, and polyphasic waves are seen (Fig. 13-49).

The paraspinal muscles are supplied by the posterior primary rami of the emerging lumbar nerve roots. In the electromyographic examination of a patient suffering from nerve root compression, the electrical activity of the paraspinal muscles at rest and on voluntary activity is observed. Lesions producing interference of root conduction will demonstrate the electromyographic changes described.

Hoffmann's reflex, sometimes referred to as the H-reflex, is seen with S1 root involvement. The time between the sensory stimulus and the motor response will be prolonged, and the pattern of the evoked potential may be abnormal. Despite the apparent science of EMG, it takes great skill and a lot of subjective input on the part of the electromyographer to arrive at a suitable conclusion. This explains why some electromyographic reports are more useful than others.

With the availability of MRI and CT to accurately demonstrate anatomic levels of nerve root involvement, the use of EMG in the evaluation of obvious nerve root lesions is not needed. However, if you have a differential diagnostic problem, for example, a diabetic patient presenting with an acute radicular syndrome who may have diabetic neuropathy and not a disc herniation, EMG is very valuable; diabetic mononeuropathy will spare the paraspinals, and despite its label, will show signs of denervation in more than one nerve root distribution.

SUMMARY

After 25 years of practice, the authors are awed by the sophistication of investigation available to evaluate a patient with low back pain. After a careful history and physical examination, it is possible with the appropriate choice of investigation to be fairly certain of the diagnosis. When planning a surgical procedure for degenerative disc disease problems (e.g., a ruptured disc), an MRI will so precisely localize the nature of the problem and the anatomic level that very limited surgical procedures can be planned. These investigations have become the "eyes" of the surgeon, allowing for precise surgery, only when a problem is clearly identified on testing.

REFERENCES

BONE SCANNING (SCINTIGRAPHY)

1. Holder LE. Radionuclide bone imaging in the evaluation of bone pain. *J Bone Joint Surg Am.* 1982;64:1391–1396.
2. Kirchner PT, Simon MA. Current concepts review, radioisotopic evaluation of skeletal disease. *J Bone Joint Surg Am.* 1981;63:673–681.
3. Magnusson JE, Brown ML, Hauser MF, et al. In-111-labeled5 leukocyte scintigraphy in suspected orthopedic prosthesis infection: comparison with other imaging modalities. *Radiology.* 1988;168:236–239.
4. Merkel KD, Brown ML, Dewanjee MK, Fitzgerald RH. Comparison of indium-labeled leukocyte imaging with sequential technetium-gallium scanning in the diagnosis of low-grade musculoskeletal sepsis. *J Bone Joint Surg Am.* 1985;67:465–476.
5. Subramanian G, McAfee JG. A new complex of 99mTc for skeletal imaging. *Radiology.* 1971;99:192–196.

PLAIN RADIOGRAPHS AND MYELOGRAPHY

6. Badami JP, Baker RA, Scholz FJ, McLaughlin M. Outpatient metrizamide myelography: prospective evaluations of safety and cost effectiveness. *Radiology.* 1985;158:175–177.
7. Neurotoxicity of metrizamide (editorial). *Arch Neurol.* 1985;42:24–25.
8. Eldevik OP, Nakken KO, Haughton VM. The effect of dehydration on the side effects of metrizamide myelography. *Radiology.* 1978;129:715–716.

9. Eldevik OP, Nakstad P, Kendall B, Hindmarsh T. Iohexol in lumbar myelography: preliminary results from an open noncomparative multicentered clinical study. *AJNR.* 1983;4:299–301.
10. Hindmarsh T, Ekholm SE, Kido DK, et al. Lumbar myelography with iohexol and metrizamide. A double blind clinical trial. *Acta Radiol Diagn.* 1984;25:365–368.
11. Kuuliala IK, Goransson HJ. Adverse reactions after iohexol lumbar myelography: influence of post-procedural positioning. *AJR.* 1952;149:389–390.
12. Mason MS, Raaf J. Complication of pantopaque myelography: case report and review. *J Neurosurg* 1952;19: 302–305.
13. Meador KI, Hamilton WJ, El Gammal TAM, et al. Irreversible neurologic complications of metrizamide myelography. *Neurology.* 1984;34:817–821.
14. Nakstad P, Helgetveit A, Aaserud O, et al. Iohexol compared to metrizamide in cervical and thoracic myelography. *Neuroradiology.* 1984;26:479–484.
15. Sicard JL. Roentgenologic exploration of the central nervous system with iodized oil (Lipiodol). *Arch Neurol Psychiatry.* 1926;16:420–426.
16. Steinhausen TB, Ramsey G, French JD, et al. Iodinated organic compounds as contrast media for radiographic diagnoses. *Radiology.* 1944;43:230–235.
17. Wiesel SW, Tsourmas N, Feffer HL, et al. A study of computer-assisted tomography: I. The incidence of positive CAT scans in an asymptomatic group of patients. *Spine.* 1984;9:549–551.

CT SCANNING

18. Haughton VM, Eldevik OP, Magnaes B, Amundsen P. A prospective comparison of computed tomography and myelography in the diagnosis of herniated lumbar discs. *Radiology.* 1982;142:103–110.
19. Helms CA, Dorwart RH, Gray M. The CT appearance of conjoined nerve roots and differentiation from a herniated nucleus pulposus. *Radiology.* 1982;144:803–807.
20. Hitselberger WE, Witten RM. Abnormal myelogram in asymptomatic patients. *J Neurosurg.* 1968;28:204–207.
21. John V, Ewen K. Vergleichende Untersuchungen zur Strahlenexposition des Patienten bei des spinalen Dunnschicht. *Computertomographie Strahlentherapie.* 1983;159:180–183.
22. Ketonen L, Gyldensted C. Lumbar disc disease evaluated by myelography and postmyelography spinal computed tomography. *Neuroradiology.* 1986;28:144–149.
23. Macnab I. Negative disc exploration—an analysis of the cause of nerve root involvement in sixty-eight patients. *J Bone Joint Surg Am.* 1971;53:891–903.
24. McCutcheon ME, Thompson WC. CT scanning of lumbar discography. *Spine.* 1986;11:257–259.
25. Modic MT, Masaryk T, Boumphrey F, et al. Lumbar herniated disc disease and canal stenosis: prospective evaluation by surface coil MR, CT and myelography. *AJNR.* 1986;7:709–717.
26. Sachs BL, Vanharanta H, Spivey MA, et al. Dallas discogram description: a new classification of CT/discography in low-back disorders. *Spine.* 1987;12:287–294.
27. Tarlov IM. Spinal perineural and meningeal cysts. *J Neurol Neurosurg Psychiatry.* 1970;33:833–843.
28. Torricelli P, Spina V, Martinelli C. CT diagnosis of lumbosacral conjoined nerve roots. *Neuroradiology.* 1987;29:374–379.
29. Verbiest H. The significance and principles of computerized axial tomography in idiopathic development stenosis of the bony lumbar vertebral canal. *Spine.* 1979;4:369–378.
30. Wiesel SW, Tsourmas N, Feffer HL, et al. A study of computer-assisted tomography. I: the incidence of positive CT scans in an asymptomatic group of patients. *Spine.* 1984;9:549–551.
31. Zinreich SJ, Long DM, Davis R, et al. Three-dimensional CT imaging in post-surgical "failed back" syndrome. *J Comput Assist Tomogr.* 1990;14:574–580.

MAGNETIC RESONANCE IMAGING (MRI)

32. Bloch F, Hansen WW, Packard ME. Nuclear induction. *Phys Rev.* 1946;69:127–135.
33. Damadian R. Tumor detection by nuclear magnetic resonance. *Science (Washington, DC).* 1971;171:1151–1153.
34. Doyle FE, Gore JC, Pennock, et al. Imaging of the brain by nuclear magnetic resonance. *Lancet.* 1981;2:53–57.
35. Enzmann DR, Rubin JB, De La Paz R, Wright A. Cerebrospinal fluid pulsation: benefits and pitfalls in MR imaging. *Radiology.* 1986;161:773–778.
36. Georgy BA, Hesselink JR. MR Imaging of the spine: recent advances in pulse sequences and special techniques. *AJR.* 1994;162:923–934.
37. Haughton VM. MR imaging of the spine. *Radiology.* 1988;166:297–301.
38. Jenkins JPR, Hickey DS, Zhu XP, et al. MR imaging of the intervertebral disc: a quantitative study. *Br J Radiol.* 1985;58:705–709.
39. Panagiotacopulos ND, Pope MH, Krag MH, Bloch R. Water content in human intervertebral discs: part 1. Measurement by magnetic resonance imaging. *Spine.* 1987;12:912–917.
40. Peterfy CG, Linares R, Steinbach LS. Recent advances in magnetic resonance imaging of the musculoskeletal system. *Radiol Clin North Am.* 1994;32:291–311.
41. Purcell EM, Taurry HC, Pound RV. Resonance absorption by nuclear magnetic moments in a solid. *Phys Rev.* 1946;69:37–46.

CHAPTER 14

Differential Diagnosis of Low Back Pain

"Physicians think they do a lot for a patient when they give his disease a name."

—Immanuel Kant (1800)

This question is frequently asked by doctors at various stages of training and practice experience: "How can I assess and treat a patient with back pain when the diagnosis is so elusive?" It is hard on the ego to assess a patient and fail to arrive at a concrete diagnosis on which to base a treatment program. The result often is a treatment program based more on hope than science. This should not be so. In today's medical world, our clinical skills and our investigative tools are such that we should be able to arrive at the correct diagnosis for most patients with "lumbago or sciatica." This chapter outlines the simple steps needed to assess a patient who presents with a complaint of low back pain.

ASSESSMENT METHOD

Do not initiate your assessment with a long list of time-consuming differential diagnoses on your menu. In family practice, this presents an overwhelming burden to the multitude of chief complaints heard during a day. Instead, adopt a simple, methodical approach. Your goal is to sort those patients who have mechanical or structural problems in the low back from those who have not. In a family practice setting, perhaps 20% to 25% of patients presenting with low back pain will have a source outside of the back as the cause of their symptoms. This fact presents many pitfalls for the unwary. For this reason, accurate evaluation requires a logical, step-by-step method. The foundation of this method is the clinical assessment/the good old-fashioned history and physical examination. Investigations such as computed tomography (CT) scanning and magnetic resonance imaging (MRI) should play a secondary role to clinical assessment. Today, our investigative tools are so sophisticated that one can find pathology on investigation in almost every patient whether or not the patient is sick (1,2). Moreover, minor insignificant pathology can become the red herring that causes you to miss the symptom producing lesion.

THE CLINICAL APPROACH

In assessing a patient with a low back complaint, ask yourself five questions:

1. Is this a true physical disability or is there a setting and a pattern on history and physical examination to suggest a nonphysical or nonorganic problem?
2. Is this clinical presentation a diagnostic trap?
3. Is this a mechanical low back pain condition, and if so, what is the syndrome?
4. Are there clues to an anatomic level on history and physical examination?
5. After reviewing the results of investigation, what is the structural lesion and does it fit with the clinical syndrome?

Although these questions may not be answered sequentially during the history and physical examination, they ultimately must be answered sequentially before arriving at a diagnosis and prescribing a treatment program. That is to say, do not answer Question 5 and plan a treatment program until you have satisfactory answers to each preceding question. Probably the biggest pitfall is to answer Question 3 before you have satisfactorily answered Questions 1 and 2. The answers to Questions 1 and 2 should routinely be made outside the hospital, and before CT, myelography, MRI, and other sophisticated investigative modalities are used. The classic trap is to ignore Questions 1 and 2 and admit a patient with a complaint of low back pain to the hospital, with sophisticated investigative tools, and then prescribe a treatment plan based on false-positive findings.

QUESTION 1

Is this a true physical disability, or is there a setting and a pattern on history and physical examination to suggest a nonphysical or nonorganic problem? That medicine should concern itself with the whole person is often stated but frequently ignored. The hallmark of a good clinician is the ability not only to diagnose disease but also to assess the "whole patient." No test of the art of medicine is more demanding than the identification of the patient with a nonorganic or emotional component to a back disability.

Remember the disability equation:

$$\text{Disability} = A + B + C$$

where:

A = the physical component (disease).
B = the patient's emotional reaction.
C = the situation the patient is in at the time of disability (e.g., compensation claim, motor vehicle accident).

Each patient presenting with a back disability may have some component of each of these entities entwined in their disability. For example, a patient presenting a collection of symptoms, with no physical disability evident on examination, should lead one to think of the other aspects of the equation and look for emotional disability or situational reactions.

A classification of nonorganic spinal pain is presented again in Table 14-1. The term nonorganic has been chosen over other terms such as nonphysical, functional, emotional, and psychogenic. The conditions classified in Table 14-1 are such a common part of practice you cannot remind yourself enough to consider them in your differential diagnosis.

Commit Table 14-2 to memory. If you are puzzled by a patient with a complaint of low back pain, revisit Question 1: Is this a true physical disability? Specifically look for some or all of these symptoms and/or signs. If they are present, stop! Do not order expensive tests and treatment but rather seek help from someone more skilled in the evaluation of these nonorganic syndromes.

It is important to stress that one swallow does not make a spring! The fact that a patient has one of these findings does not mean the patient should be classified as a exaggerator or litigant reactor. It is important to stress that a collection of symptoms and signs should be present with

TABLE 14-1

Classification of Nonorganic Spinal Pain

Psychosomatic spinal pain
  Tension syndrome (fibrositis)
Pure psychogenic spinal pain
  Psychogenic spinal pain
  Psychogenic modification of organic spinal pain
Situational spinal pain
  Litigation reaction
  Exaggeration reaction

TABLE 14-2

Symptoms and Signs Suggesting a Nonorganic Component to Disability

Symptoms
- Pain is multifocal in distribution and nonmechanical (present at rest)
- Entire extremity is painful, numb, and/or weak
- Extremity gives way (as a result, the patient carries a cane)
- Treatment response:
  - A. No response
  - B. "Allergic" to treatment
  - C. Not receiving treatment
- Multiple crises, multiple hospital admissions/investigations, and multiple visits to doctors

Signs
- Tenderness is superficial (skin) or nonanatomic (e.g., over body of sacrum)
- Simulated movement tests positive
- Distraction tests positive
- Whole leg weak or numb
- Academy Award performance

the appropriate clinical setting to make the diagnosis of exaggeration behavior. Waddell et al. (3) have documented the significant symptoms and signs that, when collected together, suggest that a nonorganic component to a disability is present. These symptoms and signs have been scientifically documented as valid and reproducible. As a screening mechanism they are an excellent substitute for pain drawings and psychological testing.

Every human attends the school of survival. Sometimes the lessons lead patients to modify or magnify a physical disability at a conscious or unconscious level. Another word of caution: The presence of one of these nonorganic reactions does not preclude an organic condition such as a herniated nucleus pulposus. The art of medicine is truly tested by a patient with a physical low back pain who modifies the disability with a nonorganic reaction of tension, hysteria, depression, or emotional factors.

QUESTION 2

Is this clinical presentation a diagnostic trap? It is too easy, when trying to arrive at a mechanical diagnosis, to fall into the many traps in the differential diagnosis of low back pain. An example is the young man in the early stages of ankylosing spondylitis who presents with vague sacroiliac joint pain and mild buttock and thigh discomfort who is thought to have a disc herniation. The patient with a retroperitoneal tumor invading the sacrum or sacral plexus may present with classic sciatica and also be diagnosed as having a disc herniation. It is not uncommon that patients with pathology within the peritoneal cavity will refer pain to the back. To avoid missing these various diagnostic pitfalls, always ask yourself the second question: Is this clinical presentation a trap?

Two broad categories of disease are included in this question:

1. Back pain referred from outside the spine may come from within the peritoneal cavity (e.g., gastrointestinal tumors or ulcers) or from the retroperitoneal space (genitourinary conditions, abdominal aortic conditions, or primary or secondary tumors of the retroperitoneal space). These patients can be recognized clinically on the basis of two historic points. First, the pain is often nonmechanical in nature and troubles the patient just as much at rest as it does with activity. Second, the pain in the back often has the characteristics of the pain associated with the primary pathology, that is, if the primary pain is colicky, the back pain will be colicky.
2. Painful, nondegenerative conditions arising from within the spinal column, including its neurologic content. This group is subdivided into the following:
   a. The differential diagnosis of low back pain or lumbago (Table 14-3).
   b. The differential diagnosis of radicular pain or sciatica (Table 14-4).

TABLE 14-3

Differential Diagnosis of Nonmechanical Low Back Pain

Referred pain (e.g., from the abdomen or retroperitoneal space)
Infection: bone, disc, epidural space
Neoplasm
- Primary (multiple myeloma, osteoid osteoma, etc.)
- Secondary

Inflammation
Miscellaneous metabolic and vascular disorders such as osteopenias and Paget's disease

These patients have nonmechanical back pain or a pain characteristic for the primary pathology. Radiating extremity pain is not common unless neurologic territory has been invaded by the disease process, which usually occurs late in the disease. Unfortunately, many of these conditions are not obvious on history and physical examination and are often missed on reviewing plain radiographs. The following diagnostic tests are useful as a screening mechanism:

1. Hemoglobin, hematocrit, white blood cell count, differential, and erythrocyte sedimentation rate (ESR).
2. Serum chemistries, especially calcium, acid and alkaline phosphatase, and serum protein electrophoresis.
3. Bone scan. These three screening tests can be completed outside of the hospital and almost routinely identify these conditions. MRI will start to play a bigger role in the diagnosis of these various nonmechanical conditions.

TABLE 14-4

Differential Diagnosis of Sciatica

- Intraspinal causes
  - Proximal to disc: conus and cauda equina lesions (e.g., neurofibroma, ependymoma)
  - Disc level
    - Herniated nucleus pulposus
    - Stenosis (canal or recess)
  - Infection: osteomyelitis or discitis (with nerve root pressure)
  - Inflammation: arachnoiditis
  - Neoplasm: benign or malignant with nerve root pressure
- Extraspinal causes
  - Pelvis
    - Cardiovascular conditions (e.g., peripheral vascular disease)
    - Gynecologic conditions
    - Orthopaedic conditions (e.g., osteoarthritis of hip)
    - Sacroiliac joint disease
    - Neoplasms
  - Peripheral nerve lesions
    - Neuropathy (diabetic, tumor, alcohol)
    - Local sciatic nerve conditions (trauma, tumor)
    - Inflammation (herpes zoster)

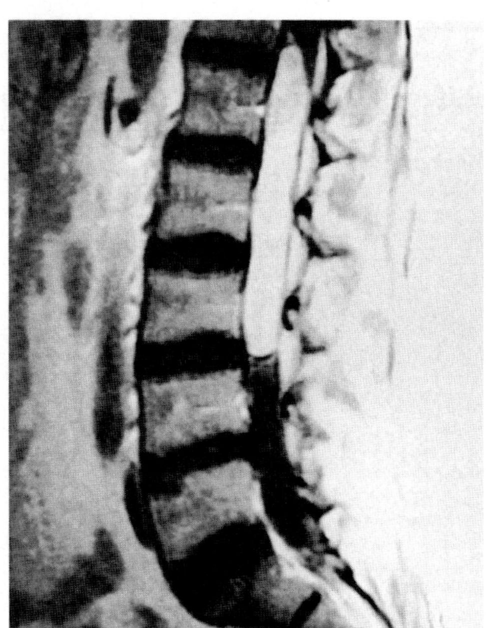

FIGURE 14-1 • Gadolinium-enhanced sagittal MRI of high lumbar schwannoma that was not seen on initial unenhanced MRI.

Although the most common cause of leg pain in a radicular distribution is a structural lesion in the lumbosacral region, there are many other causes of radiating leg discomfort that must be considered. Missing these conditions is probably the most common error made in a spine surgical practice. For example, the high sensitivity of today's investigative modalities is capable of showing a minor and insignificant herniated nucleus pulposus when, in fact, the patient has a conus tumor higher in the spinal canal (Fig. 14-1). This situation is being abetted by the tendency to perform a CT scan and skip myelography in an attempt to arrive at a structural diagnosis for mechanical low back pain. This may seem a good idea to avoid the complications of myelography, but it will present problems unless you adhere to the following rule: An equivocal CT scan requires completion of myelography. As more MRI is done, the issue is going to be resolved. Soon, all patients with low back pain who do not respond to usual conservative treatment measures will be mandated by government or an insurance clerk to have an outpatient hematologic and serum screen, a bone scan, a CT scan, or MRI. (Is it far down the road that one day robots will deal with the structural lesion?)

Etiology of Radiating Leg Pain

Space does not permit discussion of all the differential diagnoses of radiating leg pain, but three common conditions must be recognized:

1. Cardiovascular conditions (peripheral vascular disease).
2. Hip pathology.
3. Neuropathies.

Cardiovascular conditions. Cardiovascular disorders in the form of peripheral vascular disease can cause leg discomfort that is easily confused with nerve root compression. Because these conditions tend to occur in the older patient population, they may coexist. Table 14-5 separates vascular claudication from neurogenic claudication.

Hip pathology. Usually, it is easy to diagnose conditions of the hip because they so commonly cause pain around the hip and specifically pain in the groin. An early clue to hip pathology is the patient's statement that he/she cannot comfortably put on his/her socks (external rotation) (Fig. 14-2). In addition, walking causes a limp, and physical examination reveals a loss of internal rotation early

TABLE 14-5

Differential Diagnosis of Claudicant Leg Pain[a]

Findings	Vascular Claudication	Neurogenic Claudication
Pain		
Type	Sharp, cramping	Vague and variously described as radicular, heaviness, cramping
Location	Exercised muscles (usually calf and rarely includes buttock, almost always excludes thigh)	Either typical radicular or extremely diffuse (usually including buttock)
Radiation	Rare after onset	Common after onset, usually proximal to distal
Aggravation	Walking, especially uphill	Not only aggravated by walking, but also by standing
Relief	Stopping muscular activity even in the standing position	Walking in the forward flexed position more comfortable; once pain occurs, relief comes only with lying or sitting down
Time to relief	Quick (seconds to minutes)	Slow (many minutes)
Neurologic symptoms (Paresthesia)	Usually not present	Commonly present
Straight leg raising tests	Negative	Mildly positive or negative
Neurologic examination	Negative	Mildly positive or negative
Vascular examination	Absent pulses	Pulses present

[a]Be wary of the patient in whom both conditions coexist.

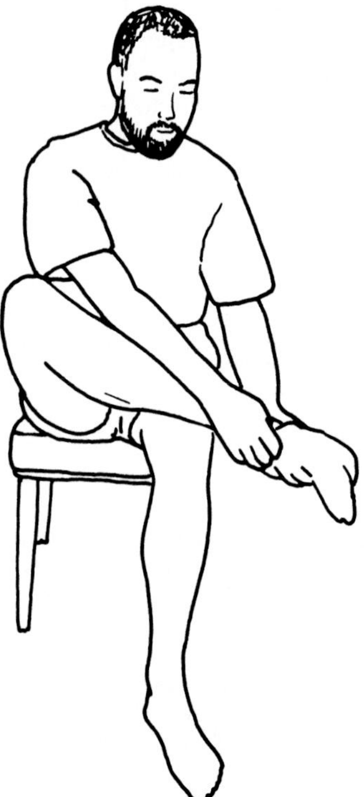

FIGURE 14-2 ● A patient with hip disease has trouble getting his or her leg into position (hip externally rotated) to put on socks. A patient with an acute disc herniation cannot get socks on because he or she cannot even sit to try and get the leg into this position!

in the disease. Occasionally, however, a patient with hip pathology will have no pain around the hip and will have only referred pain in the distal thigh. In these patients, it is easy to miss hip pathology unless one specifically examines the hip for loss of internal rotation. If there is any doubt, an radiograph of the hips must be taken, and if still in doubt a bone scan will be required.

Neurologic disorders. Someone who sees a lot of patients with low back pain will quickly realize that they must be a good neurologist. This is a major advantage of a neurosurgically trained spine surgeon over an orthopaedically trained spine surgeon. But all is not lost if one takes a simple step by step approach to the patient who presents with weakness, sensory upset, pain, and instability in the lower extremities. If pain is the predominant lower extremity symptom and follows a typical radicular distribution, there is a reasonable chance you are dealing with nerve root encroachment from a disc or osteophyte. But if weakness, sensory upset and/or instability is/are the dominant symptom(s), watch out: There is a good chance you are dealing with a primary neurologic disorder. How do you approach such a patient?

Weakness as a Symptom

Weakness comes in many forms. For the poor historian it is one of the first words they reach for to describe almost any problem with the legs. It is used to describe generalized fatigue regardless of cause, for example, anemia. A true motor weakness will affect one or both limbs or a muscle group and will originate in the motor unit or the proximal motor pathways in the spinal cord, brainstem, and cortex. Table 14-6 outlines the clinical aspects of weakness to help distinguish central from peripheral lesions. The next step in evaluating weakness is to separate the myopathies form the neuropathies. A good general rule is that the more proximal and symmetric the weakness, the more likely you are dealing with a myopathy. The more distal lesions, symmetric or asymmetric, are more likely polyneuropathies.

Table 14-7 classifies extremity weakness and sensory upset. Look back at Table 14-4 and recognize it as a table outlining the differential diagnosis of radiating leg pain. When you look at Table 14-7 you are looking at a different set of symptoms—that is, weakness and sensory deficit.

As depicted in Table 14-7, these neurologic disorders can be classified according to etiology, anatomic level, and symptoms. Because the nerve fiber tracts involved lie so close to each other in the spinal cord and brainstem, it is often the case that the symptom complex for these deficits will be mixed.

Table 14-8 shows the working classification used in this section. Lesions are discussed according to their anatomic level, that is, spinal cord, anterior horn, peripheral nerve, myoneural junction, and muscle. This is a simple classification but is not always correct in that some of the disorders discussed will affect more than one anatomic location. Also, etiologic factors are considered in a simplistic fashion and sometimes are not clear-cut etiologic factors. Even the subclassification of neurologic presentation is simplistic in its concept but complicated in its

TABLE 14-6

Symptoms and Signs of Central Versus Peripheral Weakness

	Central	Peripheral
Symptom	Diffuse weakness, associated stiffness	Localized to specific muscle group
Distribution	Proximal > distal	Proximal or distal
Tone	Increased (spastic)	Decreased (flaccid)
Reflexes	Increased	Decreased or absent
Path reflexes	Upgoing toes	None
Rapid alternating movement	Poor	Slight impairment unless gross weakness
Atrophy	Limited	Limited to significant
Fasciculation	Absent	Present

TABLE 14-7

Classification of Extremity Weakness/Sensory Deficit

Etiologic classification	Anatomic level	Symptoms
Congenital	Spinal cord	Weakness
Acquired	Anterior horn	Sensory
Trauma	Dorsal root ganglion	Combined motor/sensory
Infection	Peripheral nerve	Associated symptoms (e.g., pain)
Neoplasm	Myoneural junction	
Degeneration	Muscle	
Metabolic		

application. If this were not the case, there would be no need for the specialty of neurology! Finally, many of these conditions bear little resemblance to differential diagnostic factors in sciatica. They are mentioned for completeness.

Anatomic Level: Anterior Horn Level (Table 14-9)

Motor neuron disease. This is a general term used to designate a progressive disorder of motor neurons resulting from degeneration in the spinal cord, brain stem, and motor cortex. It occurs most commonly in middle-aged men and is manifest clinically by muscular weakness, atrophy and corticospinal tract signs in varying combinations. It usually ends in death in 2 to 6 years.

Amyotrophic Lateral Sclerosis. This is the most common motor system disorder with amyotrophy and hyperreflexia combined. It most often starts in the hand, with awkwardness of fine movements and stiffness in the fingers. It may also start in the neck and trunk, and on the rare occasion its initial manifestations will be in the lower extremities. Eventually, the trait of atrophic weakness of hands and forearms, slight spasticity of the legs, and generalized hyperreflexia is present in the absence of any sensory or sphincter upset. Later, the disease spreads to involves the neck, tongue, pharynx, and laryngeal muscles. The confusion for the spinal surgeon comes about when the initial symptom of this disorder is a dropped foot, but on careful examination, the patient will be noted to have a diffuse lower extremity weakness and spasticity with hyperreflexia.

Progressive Muscle Atrophy. This is a symmetrical wasting and weakness of the intrinsic hand muscles. It slowly progresses to involve the rest of the arm. It is a variant of amyotrophic lateral sclerosis and is usually symmetrical.

Progressive Bulbar Palsy. The first manifestation of bulbar palsy is an affliction of the muscles of the jaw, face, tongue, and pharynx. Its earliest manifestation is difficulty in articulating. It eventually spreads to respiratory muscles. It is not usually a differential diagnostic problem for the spinal surgeon.

TABLE 14-8

Workable Classification

Anatomic level
Etiologic classification
  Neurologic presentation

TABLE 14-9

Anterior Horn Disorders

Motor neuron disease
Amyotrophic lateral sclerosis
Progressive muscular atrophy
Primary bulbar palsy
Spinal muscular atrophy
Poliomyelitis
Tetanus

Heredofamilial Forms of Progressive Muscular Atrophy (Spinal Muscular Atrophy). This condition is represented by the floppy baby syndrome, which is the infantile form of spinal muscular atrophy known as Werdnig-Hoffmann atrophy. It can have a later onset between the ages of 3 and 18, and this proximal spinal muscle atrophy results in a significant scoliosis.

Poliomyelitis. Poliomyelitis is a familiar condition of an acute febrile systemic illness that results in a lower motor neuron lesion of muscles. It is due to a viral invasion of the anterior horn cells. It can affect higher centers in the form of a bulbar palsy, but the most common form is an affliction of the extremities.

Tetanus. Three bacterial toxins affect humans. Tetanus affects the motor neuron; diphtheria affects the peripheral nerve; botulism affects the neuromuscular junction. Tetanus toxin attaches to the motor neuron cell and causes tetanic spasms, which first affect the jaw, face, and swallowing, and subsequently spread to involve the entire body. Tetanus is never a differential diagnostic problem to the spinal surgeon.

Dorsal root ganglion. Herpes zoster is the viral infection that affects the dorsal root ganglion. The virus migrates up the peripheral nerve to the dorsal root, a migratory pattern that may occur early in life, leaving the virus dormant for years. It is then excited as an etiologic agent and causes acute inflammatory reaction in the dorsal root ganglion. The initial manifestation is pain in a nerve root distribution followed by a skin rash in the same distribution. It can also spread to the anterior horn and cause a poliolike illness.

Clinically, usually only one root is affected. Although it is primarily in the lower thoracic region, it can occur in the lumbar region and present confusion to the spinal surgeon because of the radicular distribution of the pain. Eventually, a chickenpoxlike rash appears in the same radicular distribution to establish the diagnosis. The pain may be present prior to the appearance of the rash by a few days, but eventually the rash will appear and disappear in 1 to 4 weeks. There are occasions, especially in the debilitated patient, in whom the syndrome persists as a painful rash.

Peripheral Nerve Polyneuropathies

Table 14-10 classifies the polyneuropathies. Polyneuropathies are slowly developing afflictions of multiple peripheral nerves. They may start primarily in one nerve (mononeuritis) and spread to involve multiple nerves (polyneuritis), a spread that is usually slow. Some may remain as mononeuropathies. Polyneuropathies are most often sensory in their onset, distal in their location, and lower extremity in their affliction. They are most characteristically asymmetrical. Subsequently, they will include weakness as part of their presentation. On physical examination, there is loss of reflexes. [Electromyogram (EMG) assessment will demonstrate loss of innervation in the form of fibrillation potentials, the pathology in neuropathies, and other degenerative neuropathies.] In the hereditary and toxic neuropathies, the pathologic lesion is in the axon.

TABLE 14-10

Polyneuropathies

Genetically determined	Nutritional (undernourished)
Hereditary motor and sensory neuropathies	Infectious diseases
Peroneal muscular atrophy (Charcot-Marie-Tooth)	Guillain-Barré syndrome
Neuronal type of peroneal muscular atrophy	Leprosy
Hypertrophic neuropathy (Dejerine-Sottas)	Collagenoses
Polyneuropathy or porphyria	Periarteritis nodosa
Metabolic	Toxic
Diabetic	Lead and alcohol
Symmetrical distal diabetic neuropathy	Miscellaneous
Asymmetrical proximal diabetic neuropathy	Neoplastic
Amyotrophy or myelopathy in diabetes	Ischemic
Hypothyroidism	

Genetically determined polyneuropathies

Peroneal Muscular Atrophy (Charcot-Marie-Tooth). There is a relationship between Charcot-Marie-Tooth atrophy and Friedreich's ataxia. A pure Charcot-Marie-Tooth disorder is considered an inherited peripheral neuropathy affecting particularly the distal reaches of the peroneal nerve, manifested by pes cavus in childhood. It is associated with absence of ankle jerks. It can occur in this pure form, but often there are additional degenerative changes in the pyramidal tracts and the posterior columns, putting it into the same family as Friedreich's ataxia.

The neurologic manifestations are weakness and wasting in the distal peroneal nerve distribution. This may be manifest as a drop foot with overpull of the gastrocnemius and posterior tibial muscle to give an equinovarus deformity with a caval foot and claw toes. In the more severe forms, there is an affliction of the upper extremities. These is rarely a sensory component to this neurologic disorder, although there may be impairment of vibration sense distally.

Neuronal Type of Charcot-Marie-Tooth Atrophy. This is a neurologic disorder that appears later in life and affects predominantly the peripheral nerves of the lower extremities. The lesion is actually in the anterior horn cell, and this condition should be classified as an anterior horn cell disorder.

Hypertrophic Neuritis (Dejerine-Sottas disease). This is a polyneuropathy not unlike Charcot-Marie-Tooth atrophy. It begins early in childhood and is manifest by a motor involvement much more severe than Charcot-Marie-Tooth atrophy.

Porphyria. Porphyria usually presents with acute abdominal symptoms in the form of colic, constipation, and vomiting. In addition, there is a generalized polyneuropathy that can be severe to the point of flaccid tetraplegia.

Metabolic peripheral neuropathies. The most common peripheral neuropathy that a spinal surgeon will face as a differential diagnostic problem is diabetic neuropathy. This is a disease of the Schwann cell. The Schwann cell needs insulin to make myelin; when this cell is deprived of insulin, there will be myelin degeneration. Ischemia also plays a role in these disorders. There are various forms of diabetic peripheral neuropathy listed in Table 14-11.

Symmetrical Distal Diabetic Neuropathy. This is predominantly a sensory neuropathy that occurs in the elderly mild diabetics. They complain of restlessness, pain, and inability to sleep at night because of the distal lower extremity symptoms. They can have extraordinary complaints, yet they have virtually nothing in the way of physical finding. If present long enough as a pathologic entity, the patients will display a stocking and glove type of sensory loss. By the time the polyneuropathy extends up to the level of the thighs, there will be a similar phenomenon occurring in the hands.

There is a motor form of symmetrical distal diabetic neuropathy that occurs in upper extremities in men. It is a rare phenomenon, occurring in 1 of 200 sensory neuropathies seen.

TABLE 14-11

Diabetic Peripheral Neuropathy

Symmetrical distal
Asymmetrical proximal mononeuropathies and cranial neuropathies
Diabetic amyotrophy

Asymmetrical Proximal Mononeuropathy [Single Root or Local Involvement of Two or More Nerves (Multiplex)]. This condition results from a stroke of the vasa nervorum of the peripheral nerve. It is manifest by radicular pain of sudden onset, almost identical to a herniated nucleus pulposus. However, the pain is more commonly in the femoral nerve distribution, most common in the older patient; the pain is nonmechanical in nature in that it bothers the patient day and night. The vital point on historical examination is the absence of back pain. The vital observation on physical examination is the unusual absence of root tension signs such as straight leg raising (SLR) reduction. Although the sensory symptoms predominate, mononeuropathy affecting the formal of the lumbosacral roots had a more significant motor and reflex component on examination. The diagnosis is supported by abnormal blood sugars and electrical studies showing slowed nerve conduction velocities and the presence of fibrillation potentials, positive waves at rest, and a decrease in the number of motor unit potentials on EMG. As time passes, this condition tends to improve. Symptoms of asymmetrical proximal diabetic neuropathy can be precipitated by a minor disc herniation that may point the treating surgeon to operative intervention, only to result in a poor outcome because of the undetected diabetic neuropathy.

Diabetic Amyotrophy. This is a particular problem of the adult-onset, obese, mild diabetic. It is a generalized condition of rapid onset manifested by weight loss and proximal weakness, especially in the psoas, gluteal, and quadriceps muscles. There is often a mild associated prodromal state. Over the course of a few weeks, the patient is unable to walk because of the severe weakness. These patients may have had a preexisting symmetrical distal sensory neuropathy and then experienced the onset of their proximal pain and severe weakness with wasting. Bladder and bowel function are always spared. From a differential diagnoses aspect, there is no back pain in diabetic amyotrophy and the neurologic manifestations are of significant proximal weakness and less in the way of pain. In addition, the severe neurologic involvement, symmetrical in nature, in the absence of bladder and bowel involvement, is a clue to the diagnosis.

Infectious Diseases

Guillain-Barré Syndrome. The Guillain-Barré syndrome occurs following viral infection and is predominantly motor (and minimally sensory) in its manifestations. It occurs in young or middle-aged adults, more commonly men than women. It begins as a paresthetic sensation in the hands and/or the feet. It is at this moment that it can be seen by a spinal surgeon. Quickly, it spreads to become severe weakness of the extremities, especially in the proximal girdle muscles. This weakness may be accompanied by a general feeling of soreness. Cranial nerves can be involved. Again, bladder and bowel functions are spared, and there are minimal sensory findings. The patient is areflexic.

The concern with Guillain-Barré syndrome is the severe respiratory problems that can ensue.

Collagen Disorder

Polyarteritis Nodosa with Mononeuropathy Multiplex. This is another peripheral neuropathy in which there is an upset in the vascular supply to a nerve. It has a presentation typical to a disc herniation, with radicular pain and paresthesia. Very quickly, a significant paralysis ensues and spreads to multiple nerves. Usually, the patient will experience the systemic manifestations of the collagen disorder, such as painful joints. Hypertrophic superficial cutaneous nerves, secondary to collagen deposition, may be palpated.

Disease of the Neuromuscular Junction

Myasthenia gravis. This is an acquired autoimmune disease in which antibodies are formed that bind to the acetylcholine receptors at the myoneural junction, resulting in interference with the transmission of nerve impulses. The condition occurs in young adults, more commonly in women than men (3:1). In the generalized form, there are varying degrees of severity. It often starts in the bulbar nerves, especially those nerves controlling the eyes. It then spreads to the neck, arms, and legs, and is ultimately manifest by significant weakness. Symptoms fluctuate during the day's activities, with the patient usually better in the morning and worse by the end of the day.

Muscular Lesions

Polymyositis. This is an inflammatory myopathy in the category of autoimmune disease. It is frequently of insidious onset and occasionally of acute onset. Symptoms are progressive weakness of the limb girdle, trunk, and neck flexor muscles. Muscle pain may be associated with the condition, and if the changes are more pronounced around the neck and shoulders, the condition is easily confused with cervical disc disease having bilateral referred shoulder pain. Some patients have the typical skin changes of dermatomyositis.

Clinically detectable weakness distinguishes this condition from polymyalgia rheumatica. The diagnosis can be confirmed by muscle biopsy (showing muscle necrosis and repair), increased serum levels of muscle enzymes, and EMG changes (increased insertional activity and fibrillation potentials).

Polymyalgia rheumatica. This disease of elderly patients who have symptoms of malaise, weight loss, and an increased ESR as part of a myalgic picture. The pain may be confined to the shoulder girdle region, but is more often diffuse.

The absence of weakness, with normal creatine phosphokinase enzymes and normal EMG examination, distinguishes this problem from polymyositis.

Conclusion

Although there are many other causes of extremity symptoms not listed in this Table 14-10, it is important to recognize that the table includes most causes of lower extremity pain. Extremity symptoms such as numbness and weakness, in the absence of pain, should suggest very strongly that a primary neurologic disorder is possible rather than a mechanical low back condition.

QUESTION 3

Is this a mechanical low back pain condition, and if so, what is the syndrome? The two important words are "mechanical" and "syndrome." Mechanical pain is pain aggravated by activity such as bending and lifting, and relieved by rest. There may be specific complaints relative to household chores or specific work efforts. These mechanical pains are usually relieved by rest. Although these statements seem straightforward, clinical assessment is not always easy. A poor historian may not be able to relate a history of mechanical aggravation or relief. In addition, if significant leg pain is present, implying a significant inflammatory response around the nerve root, then much rest will be needed before the patient describes a relief of leg pain. Significant mechanical back pain may sometimes be aggravated by simply rolling over in bed. To the unsophisticated historian, this may have the appearance of nonmechanical back pain. However, if one takes a careful history, and if a patient is a good historian it is possible to determine that mechanical back pain is pain aggravated by activity and relieved by rest.

The second important word is "syndrome." It is much safer to make a syndrome diagnosis for mechanical low back pain and then, after investigation, try matching a structural lesion with the clinical syndrome. There are two reasons for taking this approach:

Today's investigative techniques are so sophisticated that it is possible to find abnormalities whether a patient has symptoms or not. A patient may have an obvious structural lesion such as spondylolisthesis, yet may have an acute radicular syndrome due to a disc herniation at a level other than that of the spondylolisthesis. In fact, a patient with spondylolisthesis may have any one of the

TABLE 14-12

Syndromes in Mechanical Low Back Pain

Lumbago: mechanical instability
Sciatica: radicular pain
 Unilateral acute radicular syndrome
 Bilateral acute radicular syndrome
 Unilateral chronic radicular syndrome
 Bilateral chronic radicular syndrome

potential diagnoses discussed in this chapter. To focus on the structural lesion of spondylolisthesis shown on radiograph and ignore the history and physical examination will lead to errors in diagnosis and treatment.

There are basically two syndromes in mechanical low back pain (Table 14-12): (a) lumbago (back pain) and (b) sciatica (radicular leg pain syndrome). Before enlarging on these syndromes, it is well to take a moment to reflect on the concept of "referred pain." Many experts state that leg pain that does not go below the knee and is associated with good SLR ability is likely referred leg pain. This idea is further entrenched if there is an absence of neurologic symptoms or signs. The gate control theory of pain is one of the theories used to explain referred pain. The phenomenon is thought to occur when painful stimuli are reflexively shifted around at the cord level. This shunting results in pain being felt in a myotomal or dermatomal distribution (e.g., legs) away from the origin of the pain. The concept is altogether too simplistic and needs to be reworked in light of new investigative techniques such as CT scanning and MRI. We predict that referred leg pain will be a lot less common than originally thought. It is more likely that patients labeled as having referred pain for their leg radiations have various degrees of radicular pain due to nerve root encroachment by either bone or chronic disc herniations.

The diagnosis of referred leg pain should be reserved for the patient who has the following clinical presentation:

1. There is significant mechanical back pain present as the source of referral.
2. The leg pain affects both legs, is vague in its distribution, and has no radicular component.
3. The degree of referred leg discomfort varies directly with the back pain. When the back pain increases in severity, the referred leg pain occurs or increases in severity. Conversely, a decrease in back pain results in a decrease in the referral of pain. Referred pain is less likely to radiate below the knee.
4. There are no neurologic symptoms or signs in concert with the complaint of referred leg pain.

It is safer to assume that any patient with radiating leg pain, especially unilateral leg pain, has a radicular syndrome until proven otherwise.

Lumbago–Mechanical Instability

The lumbago–mechanical instability syndrome is easy to recognize. These patients present exclusively with lumbosacral backache aggravated by activities such as bending, lifting, and sitting. The pain may radiate toward either iliac crest, but does not radiate down into the buttocks or legs. The pain is almost always relieved by various forms of rest, for example, reduced activity, weight reduction, corset support, or bed rest. Most patients have no trouble describing these relieving efforts.

Most importantly, there are no associated leg symptoms or signs. (See Chapter 5 for a complete discussion of these patients.)

Radicular Syndromes

The radicular syndromes have been described in Chapters 11 and 12. If you have time, go back and browse!

TABLE 14-13

Criteria for the Diagnosis of Acute Radicular Syndrome[a]

Leg pain (including buttock) is the dominant complaint when compared with back pain
Neurologic symptoms that are specific (e.g., paresthesia in a typical dermatomal distribution)
Significant SLR changes (any one or a combination of these)
A. SLR less than 50% of normal
B. Bowstring discomfort
C. Crossover pain
D. Neurologic sign (see section on anatomic level)

SLR, straight leg raising.
[a]Three or four of these criteria must be present, the only exception being young patients who are very resistant to the effects of nerve root compression and thus may not have neurologic symptoms (Criterion 2) or signs (Criterion 4).

Summary

Tables 14-13, 14-14, and 14-15 summarize some of the important historic and physical features on which to build the diagnosis of an acute radicular syndrome.

(The cauda equina syndrome) bilateral acute radicular syndrome. Fortunately, the bilateral acute radicular syndrome is rare. Unfortunately, there is frequent delay in diagnosis, jeopardizing long-term function of the bladder and bowel. Although we have covered this topic in Chapter 11, let us review it again because it is such an important clinical setting. To start, recognize that the chronic cauda equina encroachment of spinal canal stenosis does not cause bladder and bowel impairment, even in the face of significant physical compression of the cauda equina roots. On the other hand, a large sequestered disc rupture (acute) at L3-L4, L4-L5, or L5-S1 can seriously impair cauda equina function. Patients usually have a problem of back symptoms that suddenly worsen. The syndrome includes back pain, bilateral leg pain, saddle anesthesia, bilateral lower extremity weakness, bladder (urinary) retention, and lax rectal tone. This presentation requires urgent medical attention almost always including a CT myelogram or MRI and surgical decompression within hours of first seeing the patient. It is usually due to a massive midline sequestered disc. The syndrome is manifest by the sudden onset of bilateral leg pain usually accompanied by bladder and bowel impairment. It is obviously an emergency and is a diagnosis that is rarely missed.

TABLE 14-14

The Difference in Presentation of the Acute Radicular Syndrome in Various Ages

	Young (<30 y)	Adult (35–55 y)	Older (60+ y)
Symptoms			
Leg pain	Usually the only symptom	Some BP, but LP dominates	Usually BP, but LP still dominates
Paresthesia	Often absent	Usually present	Almost always present
Signs			
SLR	Very positive (often 10–20% of normal)	Less than 50% of normal	Occasionally good ability
Neurologic signs	Absent in at least 50% of patients	Sometimes absent	Almost always present

BP, buttock pain; LP, leg pain; SLR, straight leg raising.

TABLE 14-15

Common Neurologic Changes in Acute Radicular Syndrome

Change	L4	L5	S1
Motor weakness	Knee extension	Ankle dorsiflexion	Ankle plantar flexion
Sensory loss	Medial shin to knee	Dorsum of foot and lateral calf	Lateral border of foot and posterior calf
Reflex depression	Knee	Tibialis posterior	Ankle
Wasting	Thigh (no calf)	Calf (minimal thigh)	Calf (minimal thigh)

Unilateral chronic radicular syndrome. The difference between acuteness and chronicity in a radicular syndrome is often difficult to measure. The severity and the duration of the syndrome usually combine to distinguish acute from chronic radicular pain. Chronic unilateral radicular pain is usually a complaint for many months or more. It follows a typical radicular distribution, including pain below the knee, and is usually associated with much in the way of mechanical back pain. Both pains are usually aggravated by walking. Neurologic symptoms are less prevalent than in the acute radicular syndrome, and are sometimes extremely diffuse and nonlocalizing. SLR ability is usually much better than 50% of normal, and bowstring discomfort and crossover pain are not seen in this syndrome. Neurologic findings are very few and usually not helpful in localizing the degree of nerve root involvement. For a complete discussion of this syndrome, see Chapter 11.

Bilateral chronic radicular syndrome. The bilateral chronic radicular syndrome is known as neurogenic claudication and is discussed in Chapter 12. However, bilateral leg symptoms specifically aggravated by walking are present in only 50% of patients with chronic bilateral radicular syndrome. For this reason, the term chronic bilateral radicular syndrome is preferred. This syndrome differs from the unilateral radicular syndrome in two ways:

1. Both legs are affected rather than one leg.
2. The pain of the bilateral radicular syndrome may not be a typical radicular-type pain. Some patients describe typical claudicant leg pain in a radicular distribution. Other patients describe a diffuse type of claudicant leg discomfort that cannot be localized to a radicular distribution.

Many other symptoms are present in this syndrome, including weakness, "heaviness," and "rubberiness" in the legs. Numbness is also prevalent in this syndrome and is often of no value in localizing which nerve roots are compromised. There is a typical march phenomenon with the chronic bilateral radicular syndrome. Symptoms get much worse with prolonged walking, radiate further down the leg, and ultimately interfere with the ability of the patient to ambulate. Some patients may report noticing that if they attach themselves to a shopping cart and walk in the flexed position, they can get more distance before their leg symptoms appear. Characteristically, physical examination in chronic bilateral radicular syndrome reveals little. SLR is usually very good, and if the syndrome is due entirely to canal narrowing rather than lateral recess narrowing, there are limited neurologic findings except for mild weakness in the roots distal to the lesion and bilateral ankle reflex suppression. Rarely does the syndrome progress to the point where the patient has significant weakness requiring a wheelchair.

QUESTION 4

Are there clues to an anatomic level on history and physical examination? Is there an anatomic level clinically? This is an important intermediate question to consider between a syndrome diagnosis and a structural diagnosis. If it is possible to determine an anatomic level clinically, then any structural lesion has to be at the appropriate level. Otherwise, it cannot be considered a significant defect. A patient who has an anatomic level of S1 root involvement rarely should have a structural diagnosis localized to the L3-L4 interspace!

There are three ways to determine an anatomic level: distribution of leg pain, neurologic symptoms, and neurologic signs.

Distribution of Leg Pain

Pain in the posterior thigh and posterior calf distribution incriminates the fifth lumbar root or the first sacral root. Whether this pain is posterior or posterolateral in the thigh and calf is of little use in separating fifth lumbar root lesions from 1st sacral root lesions. However, pain down the anterior thigh almost certainly incriminates the 4th lumbar nerve root or higher lumbar nerve roots, and excludes involvement of the fifth lumbar or first sacral roots.

Neurologic Symptoms

A paresthetic discomfort with a dermatomal distribution is the most helpful historic feature in localizing an anatomic level. Paresthetic discomfort along the lateral edge of the foot incriminates the first sacral nerve root, paresthetic discomfort over the dorsum of the foot and the lateral calf incriminates the fifth lumbar nerve root, and paresthetic discomfort down the medial shin incriminates the fourth lumbar nerve root.

Neurologic Signs

The diagnosis of acute radicular syndrome is in totally dependent on the demonstration of root impairment as reflected by signs of motor weakness or changes in sensory appreciation or reflex activity. However, the presence of such changes reinforces the diagnosis. The common neurologic changes are summarized in Table 14-15.

QUESTION 5

After reviewing the results of investigation, what is the structural lesion and does it fit with the clinical syndrome? The potential structural lesion diagnoses are listed in Table 14-16. This table covers only degenerative conditions of the spine; it omits postoperative scarring of arachnoid or nerve roots and fractures and dislocations. It is important to stress here that it is possible to have multiple syndromes related to a single structural lesion. For example, a degenerative spondylolisthesis can cause both mechanical instability (back pain) and bilateral claudicant leg pain as a result of encroachment on the spinal canal. Table 14-17 links syndromes with structural lesions.

Conclusion

It is important to make a clear-cut syndrome diagnosis on the basis of a history and physical examination, and match it to a clear-cut bona fide structural lesion on investigation. Failure to do this leads to wrong diagnoses and futile treatment interventions.

METHODS USED TO DOCUMENT THE STRUCTURAL LESION

Steps to document the presence of a structural lesion in mechanical low back pain should be taken only after a satisfactory answer has been obtained for Questions 1, 2, and 3. Seeking a structural lesion in a patient with an unrecognized nonorganic problem is usually a waste of time and money and is a danger to the patient.

TABLE 14-16

Structural Lesions in Mechanical Low Back Pain

Instability	Soft tissue lesions—muscle spasm; ligamentous strain
Intrinsic to disc—degenerative disc disease	Herniated nucleus pulposus (HNP)
Extrinsic to disc	Narrowing of spinal canal
Facet joint disease	Spinal canal stenosis (SCS)
Spondylolisthesis	Lateral zone stenosis (LZS)

TABLE 14-17

Relationship of Syndromes and Structural Lesions

Lumbago	DDD
	FJD
	Spondylolysis/spondylolisthesis
	Soft tissue
Unilateral acute radicular	HNP
	HNP +LRS
Unilateral chronic radicular	LRS
	HNP
Bilateral acute radicular	Central HNP
Bilateral chronic radicular	SCS

DDD, degenerative disk disease; FJD, facet joint disease; HNP, herniated nucleus pulposus; LRS, lateral recess stenosis; SCS, spinal canal stenosis.

False-positive investigative findings are easy to come by with today's sophisticated techniques (2). Before entertaining each of these possible investigative procedures, it is assumed that a thorough history, physical examination, and other necessary investigations have satisfactorily answered Questions 1 and 2. For a runthrough of the investigative procedures useful and useless, you are referred back to Chapter 13.

CONCLUSION

The assessment of a patient with a low back disability does not need to be difficult. By keeping a simple system in mind, it is possible to arrive at a good clinical impression by asking yourself the following five questions and committing yourself, eventually, to sequential answers.

1. Is this a true physical disability, or is there a setting and a pattern in the history and physical examination to suggest a nonphysical or nonorganic problem?
2. Is this clinical presentation a diagnostic trap?
3. Is this a mechanical low back pain condition, and if so, what is the syndrome?
4. Are there clues to an anatomic level on history and physical examination?
5. After reviewing the results of investigation, what is the structural lesion, and does it fit with the clinical syndrome?

Do not commit yourself to any major investigative step until Questions 1 and 2 have been adequately answered. Then, if you are satisfied that you have a mechanical low back pain problem, dissect it into a syndrome first, an anatomic level second, and a structural lesion third. The structural lesion diagnosis should fully support the clinical syndrome and the anatomic level. If not, take one step back and repeat the history and physical examination. Listening to the patient's story, doing a thorough physical examination, and supporting your diagnosis with investigation is the best way to avoid erroneous diagnoses and ill-fated surgery.

REFERENCES

1. Bell GR, et al. A study of computer-assisted tomography. *Spine*. 1984;9:552–556.
2. Boden SD, Davis DO, Dina TS, et al. Abnormal magnetic resonance scans of the lumbar spine in asymptomatic subjects. *J Bone Joint Surg*. 1990;72:403–408.
3. Waddell G, McCulloch JA, Kummel EG, et al. Non-organic physical signs in low back pain. *Spine*. 1980;5: 117–125.

CHAPTER 15

Injections

"Necessity's sharp pinch!"

—W. Shakespeare, *King Lear*

Injection procedures, both diagnostic and therapeutic, have become an established tool in the evaluation and treatment of spinal pathology.

DISCOGRAPHY

The most controversial diagnostic injection is the discogram (Fig. 15-1). Since first introduced by Lindblom (18) in the late 1940s the discogram has been a constant source of debate. Touted as an indicator of discogenic back pain, the procedure has been dogged with questions about its specificity and reliability. Attitudes toward discography have swung back and forth over the years. Dye injection can fairly definitively outline annular defects, leaks, and disc herniations. However, uncertainty has persisted on the ability of intradiscal injection to activate concordant pain reproduction. Physician perspectives have been influenced on the one hand by papers suggesting a relatively high incidence of positive discography in normal subjects (15) or those with minor back pain (6) versus more positive articles indicating refined methodology and improved specificity (8,9). Technique modifications have included routine monitoring for pain hypersensitivity by including a control level injection, differential intradiscal pressure manometry, gauging a postinjection anesthetic effect on pain, use of minimal sedation, and alternating levels of injection all may help better scrutinize a patient's pain response. Psychologic factors may invalidate the discogram as a reliable test (7). Serious complications such as postinjection discitis have been described (11). The "two needle" technique has been used to reduce the incidence of infection by avoiding having a skin plug from the initial puncture of the dermis carried into the injection site.

A 2003 Contemporary Concepts Review from the North American Spine Society (14) suggested that the use of discography was reasonable for the following situations:

1. Further evaluation of demonstrably abnormal discs to help assess the extent of abnormality or correlation of the abnormality with the clinical symptoms. Such may include recurrent pain from a previously operated disc and lateral disc herniation.
2. Patients with persistent, severe symptoms in whom other diagnostic tests have failed to reveal clear confirmation of a suspected disc as the source of pain.
3. Assessment of patients who have failed to respond to surgical procedures to determine if there is painful pseudarthrosis or a symptomatic disc in a posteriorly fused segment, or to evaluate possible recurrent disc herniation.
4. Assessment of discs before fusion to determine if the discs within the proposed fusion segment are symptomatic and to determine if discs adjacent to this segment are normal.
5. Assessment of minimally invasive surgical candidates to confirm a contained disc herniation or to investigate dye distribution pattern before chemonucleolysis or other intradiscal procedures.

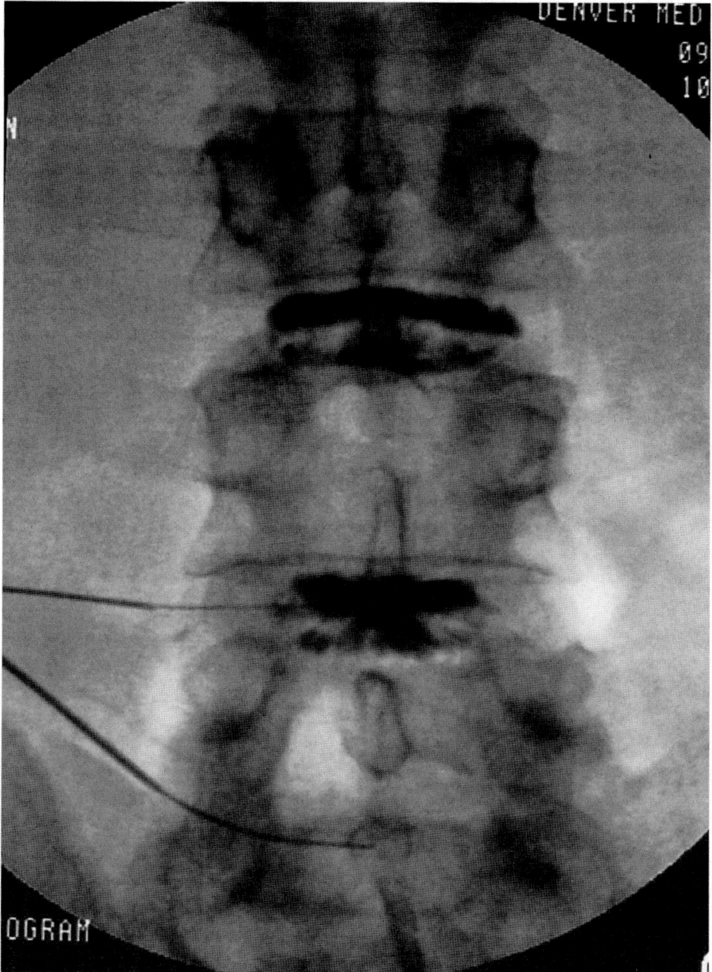

FIGURE 15-1 • AP x-ray of a three-level lumbar discogram. Normal "cookie" appearance at L3-L4. Mild fissuring of the annulus at L4-L5. Note the double-needle technique.

FACET BLOCKS/MEDIAL BRANCH BLOCKS

Facet blocks serve a diagnostic and therapeutic purpose but do not appear completely reliable in diagnostic accuracy. The diagnostic aspect of facet injections can be accomplished using intra-articular injection of anesthetic agents (Fig. 15-2) or medial branch blocks (3). However, false-positive rates as high as 38% are reported (24). In an effort to be more reliable, complimentary procedures have evolved. Differential blocks have been touted as a method to improve dependability. In this approach, a positive response depends not only on the amount of pain relief (generally more than 50%), but must also correlate with the expected time frame for anesthetic effect from a short- versus long-acting analgesic injection. This has been termed the double-block technique (2,24). A triple-block method has also been described (2). In this application, an initial injection of short-acting anesthetic serves as a preliminary screening examination. Only those patients having a positive response proceed to have two additional injections as confirmatory procedures. An accurate pain response to both a placebo extra-articular saline injection and introduction of an intra-articular anesthetic agent (both performed in a blinded fashion) validates the facet as a pain generator. Reliability of medial branch blocks can be confirmed with appropriate response to injection with anesthetic agents and placebo.

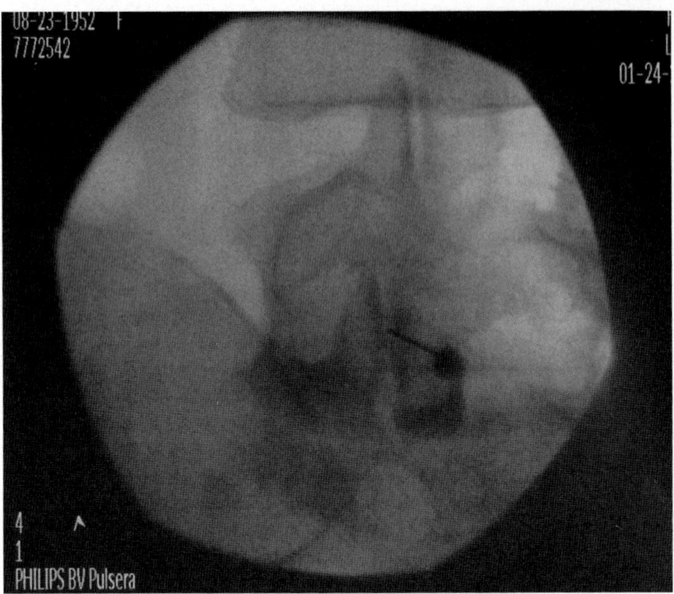

FIGURE 15-2 ● Intra-articular facet injection. Oblique fluoroscopic view of needle placement. The anatomic "Scotty dog" is visible. Snout is the L5 transverse process, ear is the superior facet, front leg the inferior spinous process, face is the pedicle of L5, and the body is the lamina.

FACET RHIZOTOMY

There has been a recent resurgence in the interest and use of this procedure. Initial use of radiofrequency ablation of the medial branches providing pain fibers to the facets dates back more than 30 years (4,20). Although these early studies were encouraging in terms of initial relief of low back pain originating from the facet, improvement tended to recede with time. Subsequent investigations have advanced our knowledge of facet innervation and have led to refinements in technique. A two-point lesion has been employed (7). However, a more intimate knowledge of anatomy has led to use of a more extensive, broad based lesion extending as much as a centimeter along the route of the nerve (10). Therapeutic temperatures are considered to be in the 80°C to 85°C range with an ablation time of 60 to 90 seconds (25). Three prospective randomized trials have shown facet rhizotomy to be effective at follow up intervals varying between 3 and 12 months (13,17,26). Studies showing longer term improvement are lacking.

EPIDURAL STEROID INJECTIONS

The most commonly employed therapeutic injection is the epidural steroid injection (ESI) (Fig. 15-3). Indications include radicular pain from both herniated discs and spinal stenosis. Pathways for injection include the standard translaminar approach, caudal (via the sacral hiatus), and transforaminal routes. Steroids serve as an anti-inflammatory agent against an irritated nerve root. A number of inflammatory mediators including phospholipase A2 (PLA 2) (21), substance P, and vasoactive intestinal peptide (1) are influenced by corticosteroids. Efficacy rates vary according to a number of variables. In a randomized trial of patients with lumbar disc herniations, Butterman (5) found that although discectomy gave faster and more long-lasting relief of sciatica, almost half of the patients who had been randomized to ESI still noted an improvement in symptoms nearly 3 years out from injection. The most bothersome complication is the spinal headache, which usually comes after a wet tap. Aggressive fluid intake, especially with caffeinated beverages, rest, and occasionally an epidural blood patch can be necessary to overcome the effects. There has been a

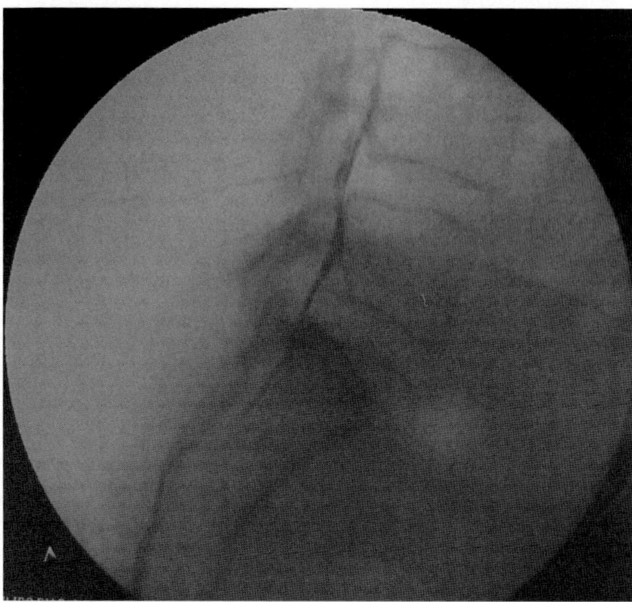

FIGURE 15-3 ● Lateral view of an epidural steroid injection. Needles placed under fluoroscopic control have helped reduce the incidence of a "wet tap." Dye can be seen coursing around the dura with an excellent spread pattern.

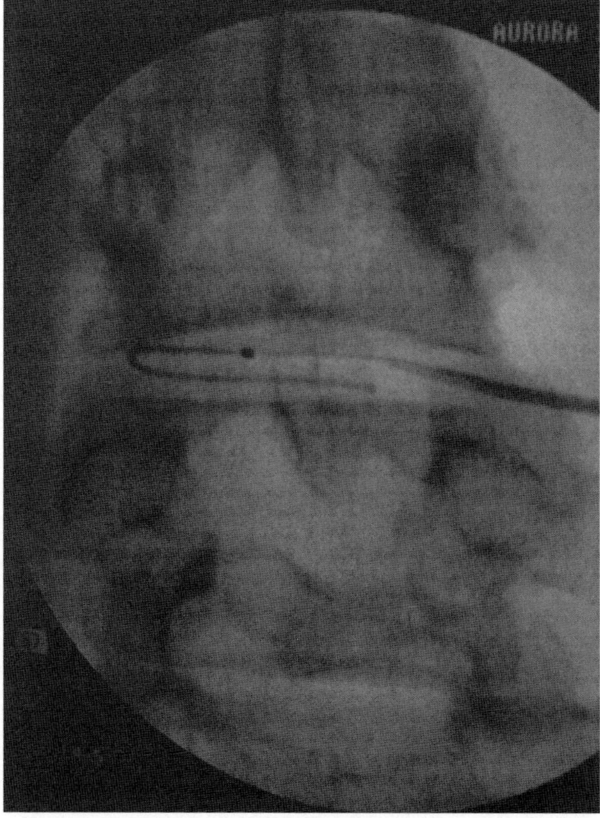

FIGURE 15-4 ● Intradiscal electrothermal treatment (IDET). AP x-ray with intradiscal catheter positioned around the periphery of the annulus.

movement to carry out epidurals with image intensifier control to try to reduce the incidence of dural breech and associated spinal fluid leakage.

Major complications such as epidural abscess and cauda equina syndrome have been reported in rare instances (16).

Selective nerve root blocks serve the purpose of helping confirm a specific nerve root as a pain generator. This function is particularly helpful in circumstances of multiple levels of mild to moderate pathology on imaging studies of the spinal canal associated with a mixed clinical picture on physical examination. The injection may also be therapeutic.

Facet injections are definitely best performed with guidance from an image intensifier to ensure proper needle positioning and a remedial injection.

INTRADISCAL ELECTROTHERMAL TREATMENT

There has been movement in recent years toward converting techniques which cannulate the disc from essentially diagnostic into a route of therapeutic intervention. Probably the most frequently used therapeutic cannulation procedure has been the intradiscal electrothermal treatment (IDET) (22,23) (Fig. 15-4 on page 359). There have been two published randomized clinical trials of IDET (12,19). These studies have not given a definitive answer to the question of clinical effectiveness of IDET. One series showed a minor statistical improvement in the IDET cohort versus placebo and the other showed no significant difference. There have been reports of complications including dysesthetic lower extremity pain and back spasms (23).

REFERENCES

1. Ashton IK, Roberts S, Jaffray DC, et al. Neuropeptides in the human intervertebral disc. *J Orthop Res.* 1994;12:186–192.
2. Boas RA. Diagnostic neural blockade. In: Cousins MJ, ed. *Neural Blockade in Clinical Anesthesia and Management of Pain,* 2nd ed. Philadelphia: J.B. Lippincott; 1988:885–898.
3. Bogduk N. International Spinal Injection Society guidelines for the performance of spinal injection procedures. Part I: zygapophysial joint blocks. *Clin J Pain.* 1997;13:285–302.
4. Burton CB. Percutaneous radiofrequency facet denervation. *Appl Neurophysiol.* 1976–1977;39:80–86.
5. Buttermann G. Treatment of lumbar disc herniation: Epidural steroid injection compared with discectomy. *J Bone Joint Surg Am.* 2004;86:760–679.
6. Carragee E, Alamin T, Miller J. Discographic, MRI and psychosocial determinants of low back pain disability and remission: a prospective study in subjects with benign persistent back pain. *Spine J.* 2005;5:24–35.
7. Carragee E, Alamin T, Miller J, Grafe M. Provocative discography in volunteer subjects with mild persistent back low pain. *Spine J.* 2002;2:25–34.
8. Colhoun E, McCall IW, Williams L, Pullicino VNC. Provocative discography as a guide to planning operations on the spine. *J Bone Joint Surg Br.* 1988;70:267–271.
9. Derby R, Howard MW, Grant JM, et al. The ability of pressure-controlled discography to predict surgical and nonsurgical outcomes. *Spine.* 1999;24:364–371.
10. Dreyfuss P, Halbrook B, Pauza K, et al. Efficacy and validity of radiofrequency neurotomy for chronic lumbar zygapophysial joint pain. *Spine.* 2000;25:1270–1277.
11. Fraser R, Osti OL, Vernon-Roberts B. Discitis after discography. *J Bone Joint Surg Br.* 1987;69:26–35.
12. Freeman B, Fraser R, Cain C, Hall D. *A randomized, double-blind controlled efficacy study: intradiscal electrothermal therapy (IDET) versus placebo.* Paper presented at International Society for the Study of the Lumbar Spine, 30th annual meeting; May 13–17, 2003; Vancouver, Canada.
13. Gallagher J, Petriccione di Vadi PL, Wedley JR, et al. Radiofrequency facet joint denervation in the treatment of low back pain: a prospective controlled double-blind study to assess its efficacy. *Pain Clin.* 1994;7:193–198.
14. Guyer R, Ohnmeiss D. Lumbar discography. *Spine J.* 2003;3:11S–27S.
15. Holt EP. The question of discography. *J Bone Joint Surg Am.* 1968;50:720–726.
16. Houten J, Errico T. Paraplegia after lumbosacral nerve root block: report of three cases. *Spine J.* 2002;2:70–75.
17. Leclaire R, Fortin L, Lambert R, et al. Radiofrequency facet joint denervation in the treatment of low back pain: a placebo-controlled clinical trial to assess efficacy. *Spine.* 2001;26:1411–1417.
18. Lindblom K. Diagnostic puncture of the intervertebral discs in sciatica. *Acta Orthop Scand.* 1948;17:213–239.
19. Pauza K, Howell S, Dreyfus P, et al. A randomized, placebo-controlled trial of intradiscal electrothermal therapy for the treatment of discogenic low back pain. *Spine J.* 2004;4:27–35.
20. Rashbaum RF. Radiofrequency facet denervation. A treatment alternative in refractory low back pain with or without leg pain. *Orthop Clin North Am.* 1983;14:569–575.
21. Saal JS, Franson RC, Dobrow R, et al. High levels of inflammatory phospholipase A2 activity in lumbar disc herniations. *Spine.* 1990;15:674–678.
22. Saal JA, Saal JS. Intradiscal electrothermal treatment for chronic discogenic low back pain. Prospective outcome study with a minimum 2-year follow-up. *Spine.* 2002;27:966–974.

23. Saal J, Saal J, Wetzel T, et al. *IDET related complications: a multicenter study of 1675 treated patients with a review of the FDA MDR Data Base.* Paper presented at: 16th annual meeting of the North American Spine Society; October 31–November 3, 2001; Seattle, WA.
24. Schwarzer AC, Aprill CN, Derby R, et al. The false positive rate of uncontrolled diagnostic blocks of the lumbar zygapophysial joints. *Pain.* 1994;58:95–100.
25. Slipman CW, Bhat AL, Gilchrist RV, et al. A critical review of the evidence for the use of zygapophysial injections and radiofrequency denervation in the treatment of low back pain. *Spine J.* 2003;4:310–316.
26. van Kleef M, Barendse GAM, Kessels A, et al. Randomized trial of radiofrequency lumbar facet denervation for chronic low back pain. *Spine.* 1999;24:1937–1942.

CHAPTER 16

Pain

"It is as important to know as much about the man who has the pain as it is to know about the pain the man has."

—Numerous great physicians and surgeons

That medicine should concern itself with the whole person is often stated but frequently ignored. The hallmark of a good clinician is the ability not only to diagnose disease but also to assess the "whole patient." No test of the art of medicine is more demanding than the identification of the patient with a nonorganic or emotional component to a back disability.

To start, recall the disability equation:

$$\text{Disability} = A + B + C$$

where A = the physical component (disease); B = the patient's emotional reaction; C = the situation the patient is in at the time of disability (i.e., compensation claim, motor vehicle accident).

Each patient presenting with a back disability may have some component of each of these entities entwined in their disability. For example, the presentation of a collection of symptoms with no physical disability evident on examination should lead the clinician to think of the other aspects of the equation and look for emotional disability or situational reactions.

PAIN

Back pain has been around for as long as history has been recorded. With the advent of compensation legislation in the 19th century, the concept of pain was attached to the inability to function and initiated the rising tide of "spine disability."

In an attempt to clarify the issues, this chapter is divided into the following sections:

1. Pain.
2. Nonorganic syndromes.
3. Psychological assessment.

As musculoskeletal physicians and surgeons, we spend the majority of our time dealing with pain. Each of us has our own view of pain, based on training, experience, and, ultimately, biases. As time goes by, we lose contact with general theories on pain and develop a narrow tubular view of the patient with pain. The purpose of this chapter is to review the various pathophysiologic theories that affect a patient's pain appreciation.

DEFINITION OF PAIN

The International Association for the Study of Pain (6) defines pain as "an unpleasant sensory and emotional experience, associated with actual or potential tissue damage, or described in terms of such damage."

As such, pain is a perception rather than a sensation. Like vision, hearing, and other senses, there are well-documented pain pathways through the nervous system. Unlike those other senses, pain is a complex set of actions and reactions, modified by intellect, emotion, and many other factors. Pain is unpleasant to the point that the body is motivated to do something to stop the sensation; this situation is very different from the positive motivation of pleasant sounds and sights.

TYPES OF PAIN

Pain can be divided into acute or chronic pain. Acute pain is of short duration, arises from specific trauma or disease, and has associated pain behavior and closely reflects and parallels the stimulus; that is, a small painful stimulus is associated with a small amount of acute pain. Acute pain usually responds to traditional treatment methods such as analgesia, immobilization, and surgery.

Chronic pain occurs once the initial causes of pain have faded. Other non-nociceptive phenomenon have then interceded, such as culture, family, emotion, situation, and drug use. Chronic pain is associated with many subjective symptoms. It fails to respond to the usual treatment measures, especially those for acute pain as just mentioned.

The following discussion is predominantly centered around the concepts of acute pain; set chronic pain aside for now.

CATEGORIZATION OF PAIN

There are four main categories of pain. (8)

Category 1: Pain Due to External Events

- Involves skin receptors.
- Is precise in location.
- Usually precipitates withdrawal.

Category 2: Pain Due to Internal Events

- Organ pain that does not involve skin.
- Is less specific in its identification.
- Cannot be handled by withdrawal.

Category 3: Pain Associated with Lesions of the Nervous System (e.g., Herniated Nucleus Pulposus)

- Prolonged pain that does not directly involve skin but may refer to skin.
- Cannot be handled by withdrawal; the identification of this kind of pain is usually more specific than the pain due to internal events.

Category 4: Pain Associated with Psychological, Environmental, and Other Factors

Research usually centers around pain due to external events. Unfortunately, it is easy to move concepts from this category in an attempt to explain the pain of Category 3.

MORPHOLOGIC ANATOMY OF PAIN RECEPTORS AND PATHWAYS

End Organs

End organs for pain are know as nociceptors—that is, receptors sensitive to a noxious (tissue damaging) or potentially noxious stimulus.

General discussion. The body contains many different sensory receptors that register changes around, adjacent to, and within the body. The specialized sensory organs, to a certain extent, are stimulus specific and are the end organs of the different nerve fibers. After end-organ stimulation, the information is transmitted as an impulse along the sensory nerve.

A classification of end organs (2)

Teleceptors. These end organs record stimuli from a distance. Examples are the receptors in the eyes and in the ears.

Enteroceptors, visceroceptors, and proprioceptors. These end organs provide information about the position and movement of joints and also provide information regarding other phenomena, such as tension within a muscle or tendon. Other receptors that record sensations from within the body are chemoreceptors and baroreceptors.

Exteroceptors. These record stimuli from the skin. They can be subdivided into mechanoreceptors (which record touch and pressure sensation), thermoceptors (which record cold and heat changes), and nociceptors (which record painful stimuli).

Pain receptors can be further classified into (a) free nerve endings and (b) encapsulated end organs.

Free nerve endings cover the entire body and transmit pain and temperature impulses.

Encapsulated end organs are of many morphologic types:

1. Meissner's corpuscles (touch).
2. Pacini's lamellar corpuscles (pressure).
3. Krause's corpuscles (cold).
4. Ruffini's corpuscles (warmth).

Currently, the specificity of stimulation on these nerve endings is in doubt. However, they do exist, and perhaps excessive stretch or pressure activates them; massage, manipulation, acupuncture, and transcutaneous electrical nerve stimulation (TENS) have been used in an effort to modify pain, through stimulation of these end organs. Wall and Melzack (12) have postulated that damage to tissue may directly excite nerve endings by the following:

1. Mechanical effect.
2. Thermal effect.
3. Chemical effect (effects on nerve membrane).

Chemical Mediators of Pain

Chemists have identified non-neurogenic mediators of pain (prostaglandin, bradykinin, and so on) and neurogenic mediators of pain (substance P, vasoactive intestinal peptide, etc.). The neurogenic mediators are thought to originate in the dorsal root ganglion (15). The proteolytic enzymes are produced in response to injury or degeneration and are capable of acting in many ways to introduce pain into what should be a quiet (painless) motion segment. It is thought that the large non-myelinated C nerve fibers are constantly "tasting" the metabolic state of tissues and that, by way of impulses and transfer of the chemicals just mentioned, the C fibers assist in modulating pain.

TRACTS

Peripheral Nerves

A peripheral nerve contains thousands of nerve fibers (axons) that are myelinated or nonmyelinated. Myelin acts as fiber insulation and, along with interspersed nodes of Ranvier, facilitates fast conduction. Modalities such as TENS are partially founded on the basis of manipulation of C-fiber impulses (12).

Proximal Nerve Tracts

The proximal peripheral nerve fiber tracts, to and from the lumbar spine and extremities, are four in number.

The types of nerve fibers and distribution of the tracts are as follows:

1. Anterior (ventral) ramus.
   a. Types of fibers.
      i. Motor and sensory (afferent).

ii. Sympathetic: are present only above L2; below L2, there are no sympathetic fibers in the ventral ramus (Fig. 16-1).

b. Distribution.
   i. Limbs.
   ii. Lateral annulus fibrosus.

2. Posterior (dorsal) ramus.
   a. Types of fibers.
      i. Motor and sensory (afferent).
      ii. Sympathetic.
   b. Distribution to the skin and to the muscles of the back (medial and lateral branches): medial branch goes to the facet joints; lateral branch supplies the paraspinal muscles and skin.
3. Sinuvertebral nerve (recurrent nerve of Luschka or meningeal ramus).
   a. Types of fibers.
      i. Sensory (afferent) branch from the ventral ramus.
      ii. Sympathetic fibers.
   b. Distribution.
      i. Posterior longitudinal ligament.
      ii. Ventral aspect of dural sac (the dorsal aspect of the dural sac does not have nerve supply).
      iii. Blood vessels of the spinal canal.
4. Gray rami communicans (sympathetic fibers).
   a. Types of fibers.
      i. Unmyelinated postganglionic.
   b. Distribution.
      i. Lateral and anterior annulus.
      ii. Anterior longitudinal ligament.

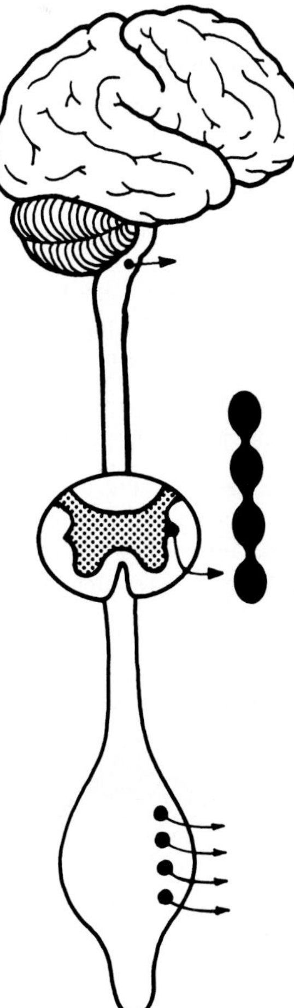

FIGURE 16-1 ● The sympathetic system is considered the thoracolumbar outflow system, and the parasympathetic system is considered the cervical-sacral outflow system *(arrows)*.

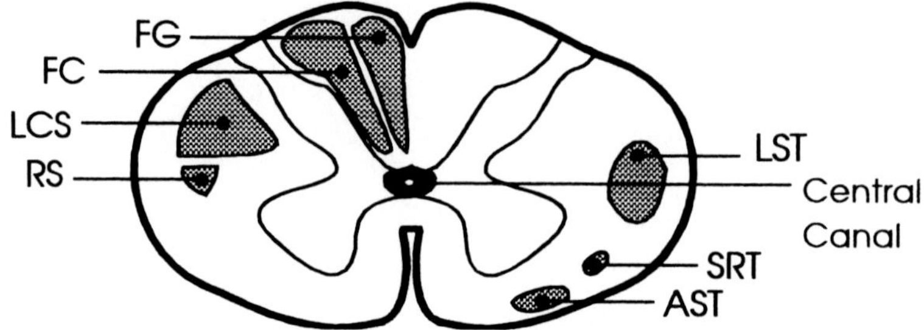

FIGURE 16-2 ● Tracts in the spinal cord: the two important tracts are the lateral spinothalamic (LST) and the lateral cortical spinal (LCS). The dorsal columns are labeled FC and FG. RS, rubrospinal tract; SRT, spinal reticular tract; AST, anterior spinothalamic tract.

The role of the sympathetics in pain is poorly understood. It is thought that they have some modulating effect on the pain receptors. It is known that blocking the sympathetic ganglion, such as a stellate ganglion block, will alter pain appreciation.

SPINAL CORD TRANSMISSION PATHWAYS

Within the human spinal cord, there are approximately five ascending pathways (Fig. 16-2) for the pain impulses:

1. Spinothalamic tract (the most significant).
2. Spinoreticular tract.
3. Spinomesencephalic tract.
4. Spinocervical tract.
5. Second-order dorsal column tract.

The Dorsal Horn

With their gate control theory of pain, Wall and Melzack (12) have called much attention to the dorsal horn.

The concepts and diagrams of the gate control theory of pain are attacked on all sides by the purists, but to the pragmatists they represent the groundwork on which to seek new understanding of pain mechanisms.

- The dorsal sensory afferents travel in the dorsal root entry zone for one or two segments before entering the dorsal horn (Fig. 16-3).

Like a computer, the laminae of the dorsal root entry zone simulate the information delivered, pass it back and forth, and receive descending modulating impulses. It is after this computerized analysis of the information that the pain impulses are ready for collection and discharge up the spinal cord pathways. This section of the dorsal horn is the gate center for pain modulation (Fig. 16-4).

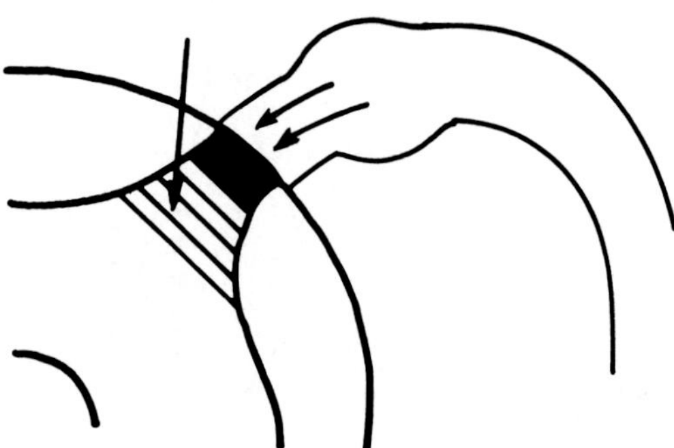

FIGURE 16-3 ● The dorsal root entry zone: striped area.

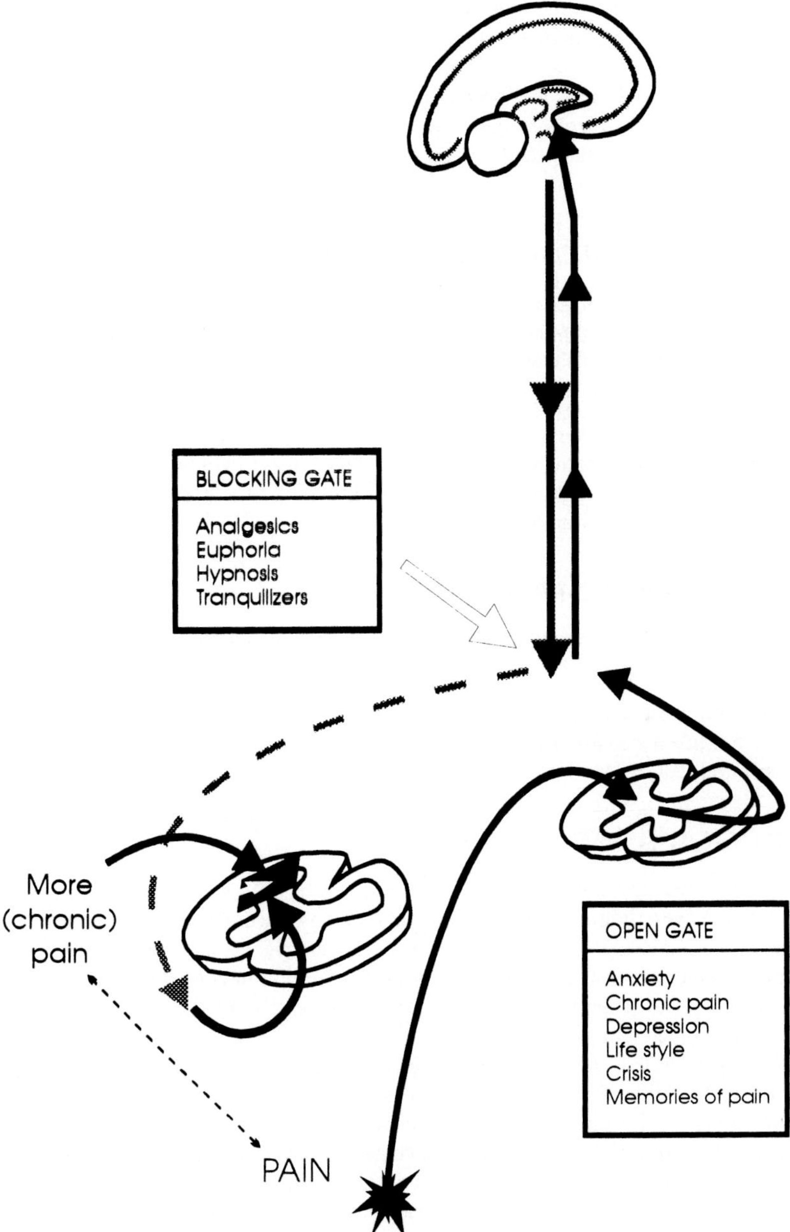

FIGURE 16-4 • The gate control mechanism: the blocking agents close the gate *(white arrow)* to decrease painful impulses.

GATE CONTROL THEORY

As mentioned earlier, this is the theory advanced by Wall and Melzack (12), who are today's most widely read pain researchers. Their theory postulates the presence of a sorting-out center in the dorsal horns of the spinal cord. These sorting-out centers act as a gate, controlling the pain impulses. The gate can act to increase or decrease the flow of nerve impulses from the peripheral fibers to the central nervous system (CNS). How the gate behaves is determined by a complex interaction of distal afferent stimulation and descending influences from the brain. There is a critical level of pain information that arrives in the dorsal horn and that will stimulate and open the gate and allow for higher transmission (Fig. 16-4).

It is thought that activity in the nonmyelinated C fibers tends to inhibit transmission and thus closes the gate; conversely, small myelinated A-delta-fiber activity facilitates transmission and opens the gate.

From a clinical point of view, it is postulated that trigger zones in the skin and muscle keep the gate open. Local anesthetic/steroid trigger injectors are used to ablate this phenomenon. Likewise, TENS units are used to stimulate the C fibers and close the gate to transmission of pain impulses to higher centers.

HIGHER CENTERS FOR RECEIPT OF PAIN FIBERS

As one goes higher in the CNS, the discrete sensory tract blends into many other CNS pathways. To say exactly where every pain pathway goes at this higher level is impossible. Only the most basic concepts are mentioned:

1. Fibers from the spinothalamic tract go to the thalamus.
2. Other afferent sensory tracts end in the brain-stem reticular formation.
3. Fibers from the thalamus going on to higher cortical centers travel through the internal capsule.
4. Many of these fibers will end up in the postcentral gyrus of the cortex, which is considered to be the predominant sensory area of the cerebral cortex.

SUMMARY OF CONCEPTS PRESENTED

When trying to understand the nervous system pathways for pain, one is struck by the multidimensional character of pain:

1. There are multiple nociceptors activating multiple neural systems.
2. There are multiple ascending tracts.
3. There are multiple CNS receptors.

PSYCHOLOGICAL ASPECTS OF PAIN

The greatest gray area in trying to understand pain lies in the obvious psychological modulation of pain that occurs in every human being. As clinicians, we are aware of patients in whom the slightest amount of pain seems to cause significant disability, and we are also aware of patients in whom a significant amount of pain is accompanied by little alteration in acts of daily living. The reason for this discrepancy and range of pain response lies in understanding the psychological aspects of pain. This is best depicted in Figure 16-5 (4).

The nociception circle is the actual injury. The pain response is the result of the injury. Without any psychological modification, a patient would suffer with the pain.

The difficult part of this diagram is the pain behavior circle. This is what is manifest by the patient and what the doctors and relatives observe in a patient experiencing pain. It is wrapped up into

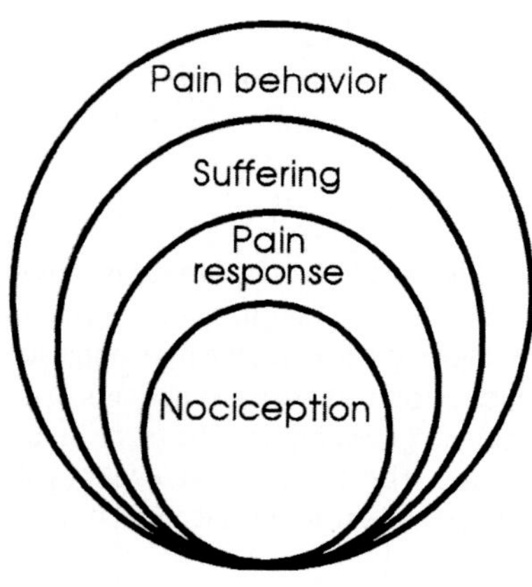

FIGURE 16-5 ● The circles of expanding pain and disability.

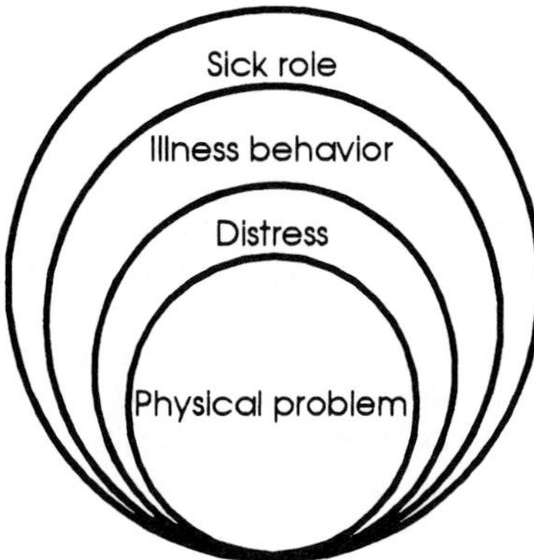

FIGURE 16-6 ● The Glasgow illness model.

the theories of primary and secondary gain and may include moaning, grimacing, limping, excessive talking, excessive silence, refusing to work, seeking health care, and taking medications. One can only conclude that pain is always accompanied by a display of emotions. These emotions are in the form of anxiety, fear, depression, anger, aggression, and so on, and manifest themselves as pain behavior. Waddell et al. (11) has enhanced this concept with his Glasgow illness model (Fig. 16-6), which is more applicable to the back pain sufferer, plied and enticed by such societal phenomena as accidents, lawyers, courts, and financial awards.

The emotional intensity and pain behavior of the patient is significantly related to the genetic makeup, cultural background, and interpretation of past events. It is an extremely complex cognitive process beyond the scope of this book.

REFERRED PAIN

From the original work of Kellgren (3) to the more recent work of Mooney and Robertson (7), the concept of referred pain has enjoyed wide support among spine surgeons.

Many clinicians would accept patients as having referred pain when they present with a very diffuse sensation in their legs, bilateral in nature, not associated with any radicular pattern and not associated with any root tension irritation or compression findings. Provided that those patients do not have spinal stenosis on computed tomography (CT) scan or magnetic resonance imaging (MRI), they probably do have referred pain.

The concept of referred pain is one of two types of discomfort. Either it is a deep discomfort felt in a sclerotomal or myotomal distribution or it may be superficial in nature and felt within the skin dermatomes. The fact that gallbladder pain can be felt in the shoulder obviously supports the fact that referred pain is a phenomenon that does occur.

In theory, somewhere in the nervous system is a convergence and summation of nerve impulses from the primary painful area. This is probably lamina 5 in the dorsal horn. The stimulation of this lamina opens a gate and allows central dispatch of the pain message and distal referral of other sensations, including referred pain.

CONTROL OF ACUTE PAIN

Intrinsic

There are descending analgesic pathways within the CNS that have the potential for modifying acute pain. The midbrain contains areas that, if stimulated, anesthetize an extremity. These areas contain many opiate receptors, and it is postulated that the distal extremity anesthetization comes about because of the release of opiatelike neuropeptides from the midbrain. These are known as endorphins. Somehow, the endorphins affect or travel down the spinal cord to the dorsal horn to modulate the pain impulse.

External

There are external methods to control pain, and these can be summarized as follows:

1. Pain can be controlled by (a) blocking the pathways with local anesthetic, (b) cutting peripheral nerves, and (c) interrupting tracts in the spinal cord.
2. Drugs can be used to (a) block receptors, (b) block the gate center in the dorsal column, (c) block brainstem transmission of pain, or (d) dull the higher-center appreciation of pain.
3. A TENS unit can be used to manipulate the sensory side of the reflex arc. Theoretically, low-level stimulation by the TENS unit selectively activates the large C fibers and closes the gate in the dorsal horn. Acupuncture also works in this fashion. Stimulation of the dorsal columns in the spinal cord provides intense stimulation to the brainstem, which supposedly inhibits the sensory appreciation from below. As fine as the theories appear with regard to the TENS unit, acupuncture, and dorsal column stimulators, in practice these theories appear to work only in those patients with chronic pain who have a significant psychological component to their pain. This raises the spectrum of placebo response, which is a fact of life for spine surgeons evaluating any treatment modality.
4. Obviously, pain can be modified by manipulating psychological factors. This can be accomplished through desensitization, hypnotic training, relaxation training, biofeedback, and behavior modification.

CONCLUSION

A normal motion segment is painless. Even a normal motion segment taken to the extremes of physiologic movement is painless. It is the introduction of pathologic changes (Table 16-1) that brings pain to the motion segment. Pain endings and pain fibers are plentiful in the spinal column, but why do some pathologic changes cause pain, whereas other aging pathologic changes remain asymptomatic? This is an enigma.

NONORGANIC SPINAL PAIN

Now, from pain theory to even more intangible concepts. A classification of nonorganic spinal pain is outlined in Table 16-2.

Before even considering this section, recognize that nonorganic syndromes do not occur in a void. There is always a clinical setting that supports the fact that there is a nonorganic component to the patient's disability, that is, if you make the diagnosis of psychosomatic pain, there will be a tension-producing situation in the patient's life or a patient in anxiety; if you make the diagnosis of psychogenic pain syndrome, you will find a premorbid personality or emotional state that fostered the reaction; if you make the diagnosis of situational spinal pain, a situation such as a motor vehicle

TABLE 16-1

Pathologic Changes That Initiate Pain

1. Within the disc
   Annular tears
   Disc resorption
   Osteophyte formation
2. In facet joints
   Synovitis
   Capsular laxity
   Degeneration of articular cartilage
   Joint subluxation
3. Muscles and ligaments
   Stretch
   Tear and hematoma

TABLE 16-2

Nonorganic Spinal Pain

1. Psychosomatic spinal pain
Tension syndrome (fibrositis)
2. Psychogenic spinal pain
Psychogenic modification of organic spinal pain
3. Situational spinal pain
Litigation reaction
Exaggeration reaction

accident and a lawyer or a compensation claim will exist. *Nonorganic reactions do not occur in a void.*

The following definitions are used:

1. Psychosomatic spinal pain is defined as symptomatic physical change in tissues of the spine, which has anxiety as its cause. The expression of anxiety is mediated as a prolonged and exaggerated state that eventually leads to structural change (spasm) in the muscles of the neck or low back.
2. a. Psychogenic spinal pain is defined as the conversion or somatization of anxiety into pain referred to the neck or back, unaccompanied by physical change in the tissues of these regions. The pain is variously known in the literature as conversion hysteria, psychogenic regional pain, traumatic or accident neurosis, and hypochondriasis.

   The emotional upset brings pains to the back just as it may bring tears to the eyes. The reason for the conversion is found in complex psychodynamic mechanisms beyond the scope of this chapter. The reaction represents a sincere, unconscious emotional illness that offers the patient the primary gain of solving inner conflicts, fears, and anxieties. Inherent in the conversion reaction is the concept of suggestion and hypnosis, the importance of which are apparent later in this chapter.

   b. Psychogenic modification of spinal pain is a sincere emotional reaction that modifies the appreciation of an organic pain. Usually, the organic pain by itself would not be disabling, but with the psychogenic modification, a significant disability ensues. No associated physical change occurs as a result of anxiety, and a conversion reaction may or may not coexist.

   An example is the patient burdened with life situational pressures (mortgage payments, car payments) who, because of the physical illness, feels that he or she cannot sustain the effort necessary to meet these demands. A resulting depression may occur, and the symptoms of fatigue, loss of appetite, insomnia, impotence, constipation, and so on, so dominate the history that the underlying physical condition is missed. Other examples are patients with passive dependent personality, drug or alcohol dependence, or psychosis, who, in the face of a minor physical problem, use their illness as an excuse to step out of the demands of the real world into a lifestyle mode of frequent demand for mood-altering or analgesic medications.

   Some obsessive-compulsive patients cannot adjust to a minor physical problem, and this personality trait leads them to feel that they have a significant disability.
3. Situational spinal pain is a reaction whereby a patient, through a collection of symptoms, maintains a situation (with potential secondary gain) through overconcern or conscious effort.

   a. The litigation or compensation reaction is defined as overconcern by the patient for present and future health, arising out of a litigious or compensable event that initially affected the patient's health. The reaction manifests itself in a patient's complaint of continuing neck or back pain coupled with a concern that, on formal severance from his or her claim to compensation, deterioration in health may occur. The patient with this reaction is neither physically nor emotionally ill.

This reaction is not to be confused with the ambiguous terms "litigation neurosis" or "compensation neurosis." Like "whiplash," the terms "litigation and compensation neurosis" have no medical or legal value and should be dropped from our vocabulary. If a patient has a true neurosis arising out of a litigious or compensable event (accident), then those terms listed under "psychogenic spinal pain (2a or b)" should be used for diagnostic purposes (e.g., traumatic neurosis or accident neurosis). If the patient's disability appears to be based more on an awareness of the commercial value of his or her symptoms, the reaction should not be legitimized by the use of the term neurosis in conjunction with the words litigation or compensation (thus, litigation reaction).

b. Exaggeration reactions are attempts by the patient to appear ill or magnify an existent illness. "Malingering" is a term frequently applied to this reaction and is defined as "the conscious alteration of health for gain."

As described later, it is possible for the physician to detect effort to magnify, but it is not proper to assign motives (gain) to the patient. The lawyer involved is in a reversed role. He or she may raise doubts about the plaintiff's motives (gain) but not be in a position to clinically detect effort to magnify or exaggerate. The choice of the word malingering implies proficiency in two professions, which is an uncommon occurrence. For this reason, the terms malingering and conscious effort are best not used by the physician when discussing nonorganic spinal pain.

Alteration of health to deceive, evade responsibility, or derive gain does occur. Those who would deny its occurrence deny the existence of human nature. The patient who tries to alter or reproduce symptoms or signs of a spinal problem may do so in a number of ways.

PRETENSION

No physical illness exists, and the patient willfully fabricates symptoms and signs. This mode occurs infrequently in the military during wartime and is a rare civilian event.

EXAGGERATION

Symptoms and signs of a spinal disability are magnified to represent more than they really are.

PRESERVATION

Symptoms and signs that were once present have ceased to exist but continue to be described or demonstrated by the patient.

ALLEGATION

Genuine disability is present, but the patient fraudulently ascribes these to some causes associated with gain, knowing that, in fact, his or her condition is of a different origin.

Civilian nonorganic situational spinal pain is usually the exaggeration or preservation type. Pretension and allegation are uncommon forms of gainful alteration of health in civilian practice. Like the patient with the litigation reaction, these patients are neither emotionally ill nor physically ill. However, they differ from the litigation reaction in that they are attempting to demonstrate physical illness through the effort of exaggeration or preservation. The reason for this effort is usually, but not always, found in secondary financial gain.

CLINICAL DESCRIPTION

Before describing each of these entities, it is important to emphasize:

1. This is a simplistic classification that is useful only to the family practitioner or the spinal surgeon. It does not allow for the complex assessments done by psychologists, psychiatrists, and so on, but it does allow for a foundation on which to build clinical recognition of these entities so that the patient can be referred to others more skilled in the field.

2. One cannot rigidly define disability, because there are gray areas. However, there is a tendency for a nonorganic disability to fall largely into one category.
3. It is most important to determine whether the setting exists for one of these nonorganic disabilities.
   a. A patient who has had previous emotional problems is prone to have an emotional component to a disability. Symptoms such as fatigue, sleeplessness, agitation, gastrointestinal upset, and excessive sweating should signal that an emotional component is likely present.
   b. A patient who is in a secondary gain situation such as a motor vehicle accident claim has the potential for these nonorganic reactions. It is important to establish the presence of such circumstances early in the patient encounter. If a patient states that low back pain started suddenly with an incident, it is important to document whether the incident is a claim type of accident and whether insurance and legal factors are involved. Conversely, if there is no secondary gain detected on history, it is unusual for the clinician to arrive at a secondary gain diagnosis such as litigation reaction or magnification exaggeration reaction.
4. A vague and confusing history, a baffling physical examination, and an elusive diagnosis signal a possible nonorganic diagnosis. Reflect on this before taking the expensive step of hospital admission and sophisticated and expensive testing that has the potential to give a false-positive result.
5. A patient who quickly establishes an abnormal doctor/patient relationship has a potential nonorganic component to his disability. These abnormal doctor-patient relationships include patients who are hostile or effusively complimentary, those who have had many other doctors involved in care before your assessment, some who fail to respond to standard (physical) conservative treatment measures, and patients who are critical of other doctors.

PSYCHOSOMATIC BACK PAIN

The psychosomatic phenomenon of muscle spasm arising out of tension states usually affects the neck but may affect the low back. It should be known as the "orthopaedic ulcer" but more often is given the label of fibrositis. Patients with this problem are overtly strained and tense, as evidenced by facial expression. They are fidgety and restless and may sit on the edge of the chairs while they wring their hands. Some of these patients will place their hands on their neck or back during the history and literally wring the area while describing the pain. They have a general feeling of restlessness and a specific feeling of a tightness in their neck with associated sensations of cracking and a constant feeling of the need to stretch out the neck and shoulder muscles. The pain is not specifically mechanical but does tend to accumulate with the day's activity, especially when that activity is carried out in the tension-producing environment (e.g., work).

The pain typically responds to chiropractic or physiotherapeutic intervention, but relief is usually temporary, a fact that makes the patient tend to seek prolonged care.

Physical examination reveals a good range of movement in the back, with a complaint of pain only if movement is done too quickly or carried to extremes. The significant physical finding is the presence of firm, tender muscles when the affected part is examined in a position of rest. The patient may be able to demonstrate the "cracking" to the touch or auditory perception of the examiner.

No evidence of nerve root involvement exists in the lower extremities. Skin tenderness, the significance of which is explained later, is not an unusual finding.

PSYCHOGENIC BACK PAIN

The patient with psychogenic spinal pain is emotionally ill. These patients often have a history of past illnesses replete with emotional problems. It follows that the history of present illness contains a preponderance of emotional symptoms, and the description of the pain will not be typical of any organic condition. The patient is convinced that he or she is ill, and that conviction extends to the frequent demand for consultations with numerous doctors. Considerable financial hardship and aggravation will occur in some cases when these consultations take the patient great distances to and from major clinics or spas throughout the world. Throughout their constant demand for care, these patients notice times when their symptoms do improve. This is due to the institution of some new

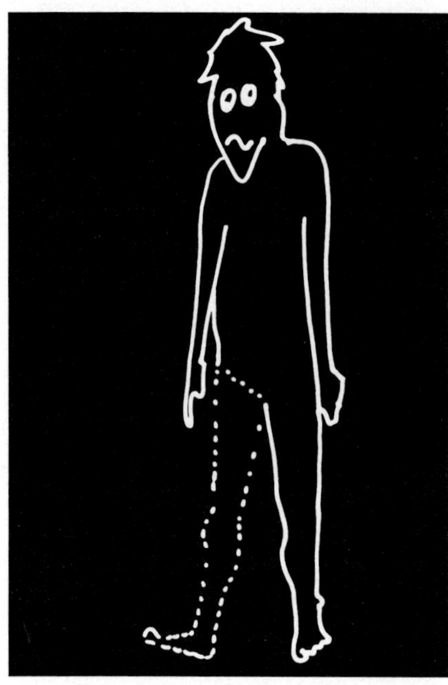

FIGURE 16-7 ● During sensory testing, it is evident that the sensory loss extends over many dermatomes and is, in fact, a loss indifferent to matters of innervation or anatomic relationships. The whole leg appears numb.

form of treatment that affects the patient through suggestion or hypnotism, a fact that makes placebo trial of little value in the evaluation of these problems.

It follows that because these patients are emotionally ill, no causative organic problem will be found on physical examination. The conversion reaction is associated with an upset body image appreciation such that a topographical unit (the back and leg), indifferent to matters of innervation or anatomical relationship, will contain physical findings of skin tenderness and dulled sensory appreciation (11) (Fig. 16-7). The somatization infrequently reaches the stage of weakness, with wasting and depression of all of the reflexes in the contiguous part, for example, an arm or leg.

However, the important observation on physical examination of this patient is the paucity of physical findings, which separates him or her from the magnifier and exaggerator, who by definition has many "physical" findings.

PSYCHOGENIC MODIFICATION OF ORGANIC PAIN

Of all of the nonorganic causes of spinal pain, the patient who psychogenically modifies organic pain presents the most difficult diagnostic and therapeutic challenge. Sometimes, but not always, the organic problem by itself would not be disabling. Thus, the historical and physical component of the disability related to the organicity is not significant. Those findings indicative of a physical illness will be appropriate and a quantitative guide to the extent of physical illness. However, the life situational pressures or the personality of the patient modify the disability to a significant point. As well, the psychogenic reaction interferes with response to treatment and leads to persistence of the disability. In a surgical practice, this failure to respond to conservative treatment is the classic indication for operative intervention. If the surgeon fails to recognize that the failure to respond to physical treatment measures is due in this instance to a psychogenic disability, he or she will gradually build a practice containing a number of spinal surgery failures.

Psychogenic modifications are commonly seen in the patient with an inadequate personality. By definition, this patient's personality may limit advancement up the social, educational, and occupational ladder and confine him or her to the unskilled worker classification. Some of these patients can be found in the workmen's compensation board population, which may be one of the reasons for poorer results of treatment sometimes obtained in the compensation patient.

These patients are seen with a minor physical problem (e.g., back strain), yet they have a total disability. All attempts at treatment fail to return the patient to the workforce. Frequent office visits reinforce the disability for the patient. If the doctor fails to recognize this maladaptive reaction and reinforcement, he or she may initiate treatment that will not help the patient in any way.

Other psychogenic modifications come about through drug addiction and alcohol dependence. Occasionally, psychotic behavior will convert a minor physical problem into a prolonged disability.

Physical examination will reveal the nature and extent of the physical impairment. Usually, the physical impairment by itself would not be significantly disabling. The loss of movement in the back is minor, the limitation of straight leg raising (SLR) is minimal, and the neurologic changes are of questionable significance. In the face of repeated assessments and a continuing statement of disability, the patient's minor physical problem may become magnified in the mind of the clinician who does not assess personality and life situational factors.

SITUATIONAL SPINAL PAIN

Litigation Reactions

This patient is neither physically nor emotionally ill. Thus, few emotional symptoms will be present on historical examination. The patient is in the process of litigation or under the care of the workmen's compensation board. These patients often state that they do not care about the litigious or compensation issue, yet they also state that they are afraid to settle or return to work for fear that further illness will develop. Their continuing complaints are rather vague and would not normally be incapacitating. If they are receiving treatment, they are not improving. Physically, there may be an increased awareness of the body part in question, as manifested by skin tenderness in the affected area, but no organic illness is detectable, and there is no attempt to exaggerate or magnify a disability.

Magnification-Exaggeration Reaction

Some or most of the following historical characteristics will be obtained from this patient. The most obvious historical point is the secondary gain situation that usually has involved the fault of someone else and/or payment of financial compensation. Other secondary gain situations can occur. The initiating event is usually a trivial or minor incident. There may be a latent period of hours or days between the incident and the onset of symptoms, during which time the patient speaks to friends and relatives and learns of the commercial value of the injury.

The patient describes the pain with some degree of indifference, as evidenced by a smile or a laugh when describing the severe disability. He or she is vague in describing and localizing the pain, giving the examiner the impression of someone struggling to remember a dream. Specificity and elaboration require memory for repetition, a quality not present to a significant degree in this type of patient. The individual wishes you to believe this pain is unique and severe. This attempt to have you believe in the pain is often accompanied by a salesmanlike attitude, with many examples of the disability spontaneously listed. Inability to engage in sex is usually at the top of the list.

Despite the trivial initiating event, the disability may have been present for a long time. Three types of treatment patterns occur:

1. The patient follows a "straight line" course of treatment; he or she does not respond to the standard physical treatment or to the inherent suggestion and hypnosis of treatment; that is, he or she does not improve or gets worse.
2. The patient is not receiving treatment because he or she is "allergic" to all medications prescribed, "suffocates" in the neck or back braces, or becomes ill in a physiotherapy setting.
3. The patient is not receiving treatment because he or she has failed to seek treatment.

Certain behavior patterns become apparent after seeing a number of these patients. Some never appear for appointments despite weeks of notification. Others appear late for the appointment and do not apologize or state indifferently that the traffic was heavy. There may be an attempt to manipulate your feelings with a compliment about your reputation or your office. There may be an effort to play one doctor against another by making false statements about another doctor. Finally, hostility may appear during the assessment. A patient truly ill will not be aware or afraid of an exposure and will not be hostile unless provoked. A patient exaggerating a disability is suspicious. He or she may start out hostile, but the usual pattern is one of developing hostility as discrepancies in the history and physical examination are exposed. Examiners are advised, for obvious reasons, not to precipitate this final behavioral pattern.

The patient who is magnifying or exaggerating a disability can be exposed only through an adequate physical examination. Those physicians who do not physically examine patients will not recognize this reaction, which may explain the reluctance of the psychiatric community to accept this clinical entity.

The physical findings of magnification or exaggerated reaction are classified into those that demonstrate acting behavior, those that indicate anticipatory behavior, and those that fail to support the patient's claim to illness.

Acting behavior. Exaggerating a disability requires acting by the patient. This acting may be general in nature such as the Academy Award performances put on by some patients as they moan and groan through the examination, walk around the examining room with their eyes closed, and either reach for objects to support themselves or reach for their painful areas. The incongruity of this acting behavior may be evident when the patient mounts the examining table with considerable ease and/or dresses within minutes of the examination and smiles and waves goodbye as he or she leaves the office.

Specific examples of acting behavior are the rigid back, a condition that disappears on the examining table (Fig. 16-8); the reduction of SLR that disappears in the sitting position (Fig. 16-9); tender skin; and the paralyzed, insensitive extremity. That these findings are a result of acting can be demonstrated through the use of distraction testing (Table 16-3). Using nonpainful, nonemotional, and nonsurprising examination techniques, it is possible not only to change the acting behavior but also to demonstrate normal physical function. It is the authors' opinion that proper distraction testing that abolishes an acted physical finding and demonstrate normal physical function is a method of demonstrating magnification-exaggeration behavior. The best distraction test is simple observation of the patient as he or she gets undressed and moves about the examining room.

Varying degrees of acting behavior occur in different patients. In general, the more sophisticated the patient, the more sophisticated the acting behavior, and the more sophisticated the examination must be (Fig. 16-10).

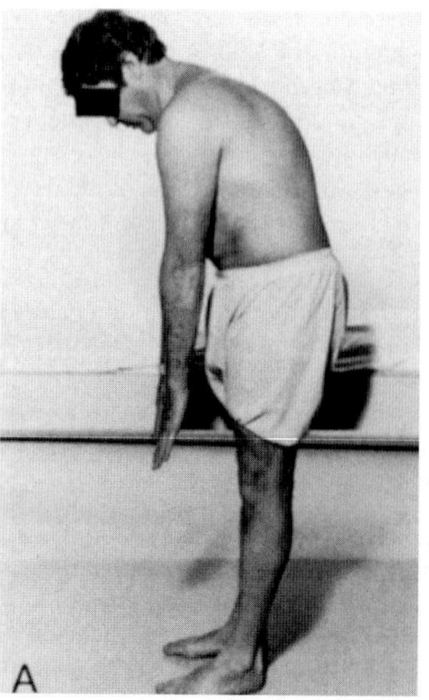

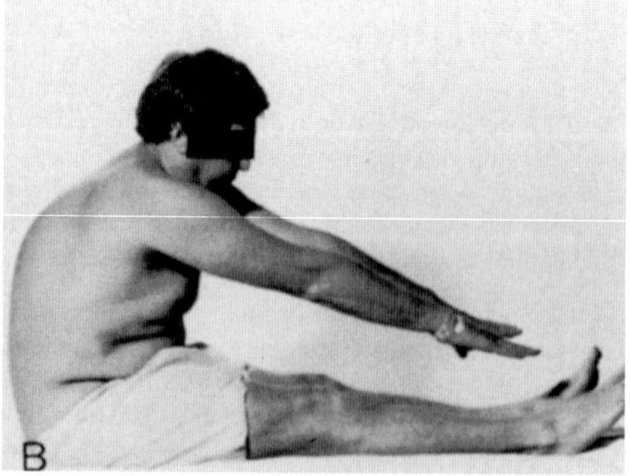

FIGURE 16-8 ● **A:** Acting behavior. During testing of flexion, the patient pretends that very limited flexion is possible. **B:** Acting behavior. Later in the examination, a similar test of flexion is possible by asking the patient to sit as shown. If the patient shows not only good flexion ability but also reverses the lumbar lordosis, no physical stiffness in the lumbar spine is evident.

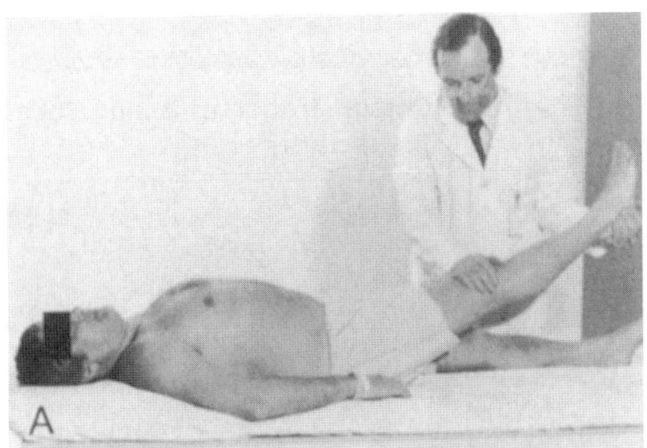

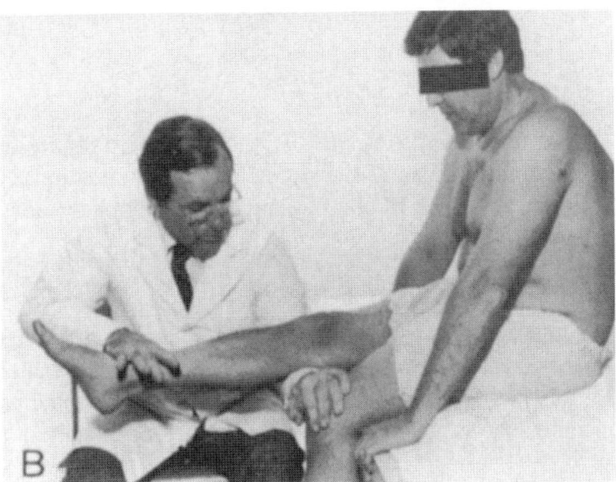

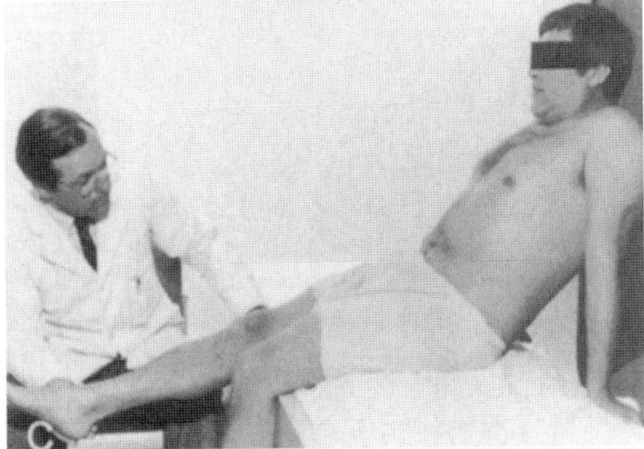

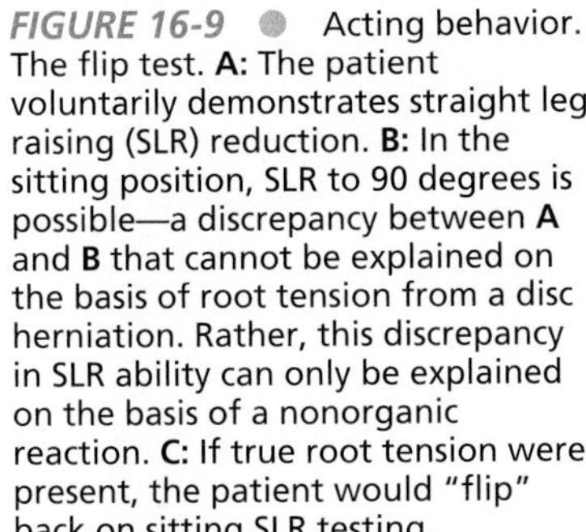
FIGURE 16-9 ● Acting behavior. The flip test. **A:** The patient voluntarily demonstrates straight leg raising (SLR) reduction. **B:** In the sitting position, SLR to 90 degrees is possible—a discrepancy between **A** and **B** that cannot be explained on the basis of root tension from a disc herniation. Rather, this discrepancy in SLR ability can only be explained on the basis of a nonorganic reaction. **C:** If true root tension were present, the patient would "flip" back on sitting SLR testing.

TABLE 16-3

Demonstration of Acting Behavior Through Distraction Testing

Condition	Response
Physical finding (acting behavior)	Reduction in straight leg raising
Distraction test, e.g., flip test	Normal straight leg raising
Nonpainful	
Nonemotional	
Nonsurprising	
Result	Normal physical function

Anticipatory behavior. The second group of physical findings in this reaction represents anticipation on the part of the patient to the test situations. This anticipatory behavior leads to an appropriate response by the patient in an attempt to indicate illness. These tests are illustrated in Figure 16-11.

Contradictory Clinical Evidence

Statements by the patient to the effect that he or she is unable to work may not be supported by clinical observations. Some patients will say that they are unable to drive, yet will have driven by themselves great distances to get to the examination. Some patients will say that they require frequent medication, yet will arrive from great distances without their medication. The patient who claims

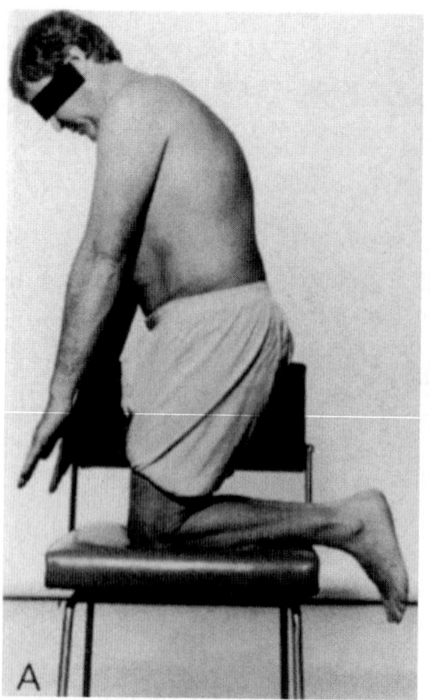

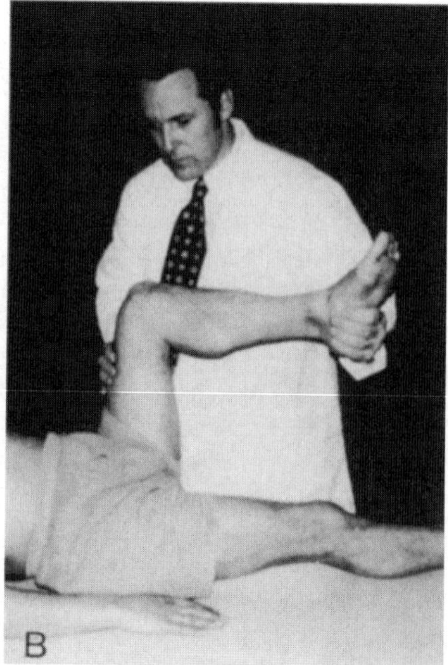

FIGURE 16-10 ● Acting behavior. **A:** In the kneeling position, with the hamstrings relaxed, more lumbar flexion should be available. **B:** With the hip and knee flexed, the patient acts out back pain, which does not occur in organic pain.

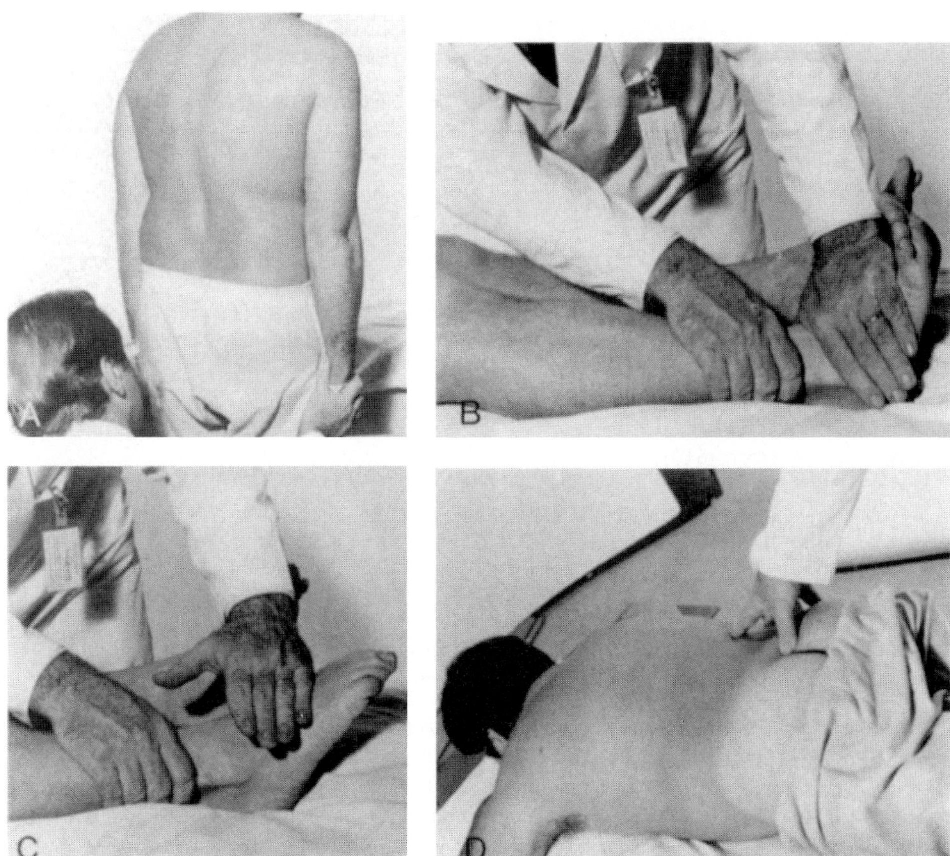

FIGURE 16-11 ● Anticipatory behavior. **A:** Simulated movement: Rotate the patient's trunk through the hip joints. This should not cause pain in organic low back pain because the back is not being moved. **B:** Dorsiflexion testing for strength. The toes will remain extended as pressure is applied to the dorsum of the foot. **C:** The nonorganic patient will give way either in a cogwheel fashion or signal the onset of feigned weakness by giving way voluntarily with the toes and then the foot. **D:** Skin tenderness and/or tenderness over the body of the sacrum is most often nonorganic in nature.

to be continuously wearing a collar or a brace should show signs of this wear on the body and the appliance. If a patient carries the brace to the examination, ask him or her to put it on. It may turn out to be a friend's brace that was borrowed for the doctor visit, and it either does not fit or he or she does not know how to put it on! Patients with calluses on their hands and knees contradict their story of a prolonged inability to work. Other evidence of work may be in the form of paint stains on the skin or a particular distribution of sunburned areas on the skin. Patients with nicotine stains on a grossly paralyzed limb should start to demonstrate similar stains on the opposite hand. Finally, those patients who attempt to demonstrate a prolonged and profound weakness in an extremity should have associated wasting of that extremity.

Just because a patient has one contradictory finding does not mean the patient should be classified as a magnifier-exaggerator or litigant reactor. It is important to stress that a collection of symptoms and signs should be present with the appropriate clinical setting to make the diagnosis of magnification-exaggeration behavior. Waddell et al. (10) have documented the significant symptoms and signs that, when collected together, suggest that a nonorganic component to a disability is present. These symptoms and signs have been scientifically documented as valid and reproducible. As a screening mechanism, they are an excellent substitute for pain drawings and psychological testing (Table 16-4).

TABLE 16-4

Symptoms and Signs Suggesting a Nonorganic Component to Disability

Symptoms	Signs
1. Pain is multifocal in distribution and nonmechanical (present at rest)	1. Tenderness is superficial (skin) or nonanatomic (e.g., over body of sacrum)
2. Entire extremity is painful, numb, and/or weak	2. Simulated movement tests are positive
3. Extremity gives way (as a result, the patient carries a cane)	3. Distraction test is positive
4. Treatment response No response "Allergic" to treatment Not receiving treatment	4. Whole leg is weak or numb
5. Multiple crises, multiple hospital admissions/investigations, multiple doctors	5. "Academy Award" performance

It is one thing to have a fancy classification, and it is another to make that classification work. When interviewing the patient, try to place him or her in one of the following categories:

The everyday, normal patient with low back pain. Fortunately, this group is by far the largest group of patients with which most of us deal. It seems, without great socioeconomic studies, that people tend to associate with kindred spirits. Turkeys prefer to flock with turkeys, and eagles like to soar with eagles. Similarly, the hypochondriacal patient tends to associate with other anxious, tension-ridden people. If, as a practitioner, you are oversympathetic and solicitous to patients with emotional components to their disability, then soon their friends start appearing as your patients, and soon the bulk of your patient load ceases to be the normal, everyday patient with low back pain.

The stoic. This patient is usually in your office at his wife's request. When asked why he is there, the patient may state that there is a little pain present in his leg, but "not to worry, I can walk and play." Do not be misled. This patient may have no more than 5 degrees of SLR ability, no ankle reflex, and no plantar flexion power—that is, he has a significant physical problem due to the ruptured disc at L5-S1. But the patient does not have time in his busy life for illness. We have used the male designation for this example because most (but not all) of these patients are men. They are not always from "management"; many who come from the laboring segment of the economy have yet to succumb to the financial inducements to illness behavior inherent in the various workmen's compensation systems.

The Racehorse Syndrome

The racehorse syndrome applies to the group of tense, hard-driving, hyper-reactive patients. In stressful situations, they tend to hyperextend their backs and assume the "fight" position as a result of their chronic muscle spasm. Throughout their lives, they have responded to tense situations in this manner without pain. However, once they develop disc degeneration, segmental instability, and muscle spasm, this allows the related posterior joints to be pushed beyond the permitted physiologic range when this posture is adopted, and pain results. The pain that they experience interferes with their ability to get on with their normal way of life, and the frustrations that they feel increase the tension in the sacrospinalis muscles, thereby aggravating and perpetuating their discomfort. In the treatment of these patients, the significance of this postural change must be explained. In addition to the routine conservative treatment of discogenic back pain, these patients should be taught voluntary muscle relaxation, and they need mild sedation to take the edge off their normal tensions and anxieties. (Classification: This patient has a variety of psychosomatic pain that aggravates the organic condition of degenerative disc disease.)

The Razor's Edge Syndrome. The razor's edge syndrome refers to patients who precariously trend their way through life on the razor's edge of emotional stability. These patients have hysterical personalities, and like people in show business, play their lives in high C.

Before the recent changes in sartorial habits, these patients could be spotted easily. The women loved outlandish hair styles and heavy eye makeup. They decorated themselves with large earrings and rows of necklaces. Multiple bracelets and bangles adorned their wrists, and they wore huge garish rings on their fingers. The men grew beards, and men and women wore dark glasses even indoors. In today's world, dress and hairstyle can no longer be regarded as being of diagnostic significance, but the dramatization of symptoms is characteristic. Superlatives are thrown around with gay abandon. The pain is "agonizing." "I was paralyzed with pain." "It was as though someone was tearing the muscles out of my leg." ". . . like boiling water poured on my back." "I haven't had a wink of sleep in 2 months."

Examination reveals diverse corporal contortions such as twitching, turning, writhing, and rolling about, and the examiner's discovery of tender points is invariably vocally acknowledged by wails, moans, groans, and sharp intakes of breath or uncontrolled and alarming shouts.

No drug will give these patients a chemical vacation from their exhausting reaction to life. If the underlying cause of their symptoms can be recognized through the emotional smokescreen they have put up, it should be treated along routine lines. When the cause of the pain has been overcome, they will return to a way of life that is normal for them.

Hysterical reactions are common in childhood. When a child grazes the knee, he or she walks with a stiff leg. There is no need to do this; it is a hysterical response to injury: an exaggerated response for the purposes of gain—namely, attention and sympathy. In a child, this is understood and tolerated with a smile. In an adult, the same response generally irritates the physician and indeed may irritate him or her to such a degree that examination tends to be superficial, and treatment becomes perfunctory. At times, it is difficult to remember that these patients cannot control or modify their reactions: it is in their genes; they are built this way. The physician is treating a patient not a spine, and regardless of the bizarre description of the symptoms and the histrionics on examination, the physician must accept the possibility of a physical disorder and investigate its probability, if indicated. (Classification: This patient is a psychogenic modifier: more often than not, with a minor physical problem.)

The Worried-Sick Syndrome. Only a moron is totally unconcerned about the development of inexplicable symptoms. Most patients are concerned not only about the cause of their symptoms but also about their significance. Many have seen relatives in the terminal phases of malignancy whose last symptom was low back pain. Many people associate pain in the back with "arthritis," and this fear maybe reinforced by being told previously that the "radiographs of the spine showed arthritic changes." To most patients, arthritis denotes a relentlessly progressive dread disease that leads eventually to confinement in a wheelchair.

These fears are common, although not commonly expressed. Above all else, the physician must reassure the patient and disabuse him or her of unfounded anxieties. If the patient has disc degeneration, he or she must never be told that the diagnosis is "arthritis of the spine."

Anxiety may be a form of intelligent concern, but in some persons who are born to worry, an almost pathologic unfounded concern about their symptoms may be more disabling than the pain itself. These patients confuse the words "hurting" and "harming." Every time they do something that increases pain, they are terrified that they have done themselves irreparable damage. They treat their backs as though they are made of Dresden china and are fearful of doing anything that may be painful. In the routine management of discogenic back pain, these patients may be told to avoid certain activities such as bending, lifting, playing tennis, or bowling. This is good advice, but they must also be told that these modifications of activity are suggested to decrease discomfort—not to prevent damage. Unless told this, patients may gradually cut themselves out of all activities until eventually they just vegetate.

"This back pain is completely ruining my life: I can't bowl, I can't ski, I can't play golf, I can't do anything," the patient may say. The doctor asks, "Do you get a lot of pain when you do these things?" The patient answers, "I don't know: I haven't done anything for 2 years." The doctor again queries, "Why haven't you tried to play a game of golf again?" The patient's answer is: "My doctor told me I shouldn't."

After weeks or months of inactivity, it will be extremely difficult to get these patients back to the business of normal living. Every increase in activity may be associated with a new twinge of pain that may frighten them back to the security of their beds. Their problems are compounded by apprehension and misapprehension, and the physician must deal firmly with both. (Classification: These patients have a variety of situational spinal pain. Although worried about their symptoms, they have not gone through complex psychodynamic mechanisms resulting in somatization. Rather, these patients simply need encouragement to deal in a more positive way with their symptoms and recognize the significant difference between hurt and harm.)

The Last Straw Factor. The havoc wrought on a patient's life by back pain may destroy the patient's emotional stability; for example, look at the case of a patient who speaks little English and has no special skills, who works as a laborer in a small town, and supports a wife and five children. An insecure job situation, because of industrial recession in the area, keeps him constantly concerned about his ability to keep up payments on his debts. The back pain resulting from an accident stops him from working for a few days. A recurrence without provocative trauma makes both the employer and the patient doubtful about his ability to hold down a job, and the third attack results in his unemployment. Inability to find alternative employment increases this man's debts, and articles of furniture are repossessed by the finance company. To this patient, his backache is the major disaster of his life, and his symptoms and signs may well be exaggerated beyond recognition.

This patient cannot be helped solely by measures directed at his back. His whole problem has to be alleviated, and the help of all social services has to be enlisted. (This patient, not uncommonly seen, can be classified as having psychogenic modification of organic spinal pain.)

The Camouflaged Emotional Breakdown. Depressive states are common between the ages of 45 and 55 years. These patients, commonly very active when younger, find that as their energy level decreases, that is, as they move into second gear, they are increasingly unable to cope with the demands made on them. Despite the term "depression," they do not present a picture of melancholia. They demonstrate concealed or overt hostility. They are more easily provoked to anger and tears. They are increasingly critical of the faults they recognize in people around them. They are constantly tired, and sleep does not refresh them. They do not sleep well and frequently awaken early in the morning. They cannot make decisions. They do not want to go out, but they hate staying in. They lose their sense of fun. They claim that this unsociable state is the result of their wretched spine. Remember, a persistent backache seldom makes people miserable, but miserable people frequently have backache and complain loudly about it.

The back pain from which these patients suffer becomes a scapegoat to explain their inability to cope with life. "I was always a very active woman. I was president of the local parents/teachers association, I was one of the campaign organizers for the last election, and I always went with my husband on trips, but, with this backache, I am useless." These patients have an almost delusional belief in the organicity of their symptoms. They believe, and would like you to believe, that had it not been for the backache they would still be a leader in the community and, characteristically when reporting their history, they will constantly refer to this restriction in activities.

The curtailment of these patients' activities is not solely due to their backaches. If they were in better emotional health, they could cope with their discomforts, mollifying and minimizing their pain with mild analgesics and a slight modification of their daily activities. Simple therapeutic measures directed at the organic basis of these patients' complaints will not preempt them to return to normal activities. Failure of conservative treatment may lead to desperation surgery, which is nearly always attended by poor results and an aggravated deterioration in the patient's emotional health. Treatment must be directed at the patient as a whole, and psychiatric guidance must be sought early. (This mode is simply another variety of psychogenic modification.)

The "What If I Settle" Syndrome. These patients bring a vague set of symptoms and little in the way of physical findings to the doctor-patient encounter. They are simply drifting in the sea of their minor symptoms, the wind in their sails sometimes provided by an unscrupulous lawyer hoping for prolonged symptoms, more investigation, and a larger "green poultice" in the end. If an unscrupulous doctor joins in the cause, the situation may never end for the patient. This unsuspecting and usually sincere patient has become a pawn of the professionals involved in his or her claim and care. A simple explanation to the patient will often bring matters to a satisfactory conclusion. (Classification: Obviously, this patient is in a litigation or compensation reaction.)

The "Head to Toe" Syndrome. Although these patients rarely complain "outright" of pain from the tops of their heads to the tips of their toes, it becomes apparent during their history that there is no part of the body that does not hurt. They may represent psychogenic pain or, if secondary gain is involved, they may be magnifying their disability. As soon as the examiner recognizes that pain is present head to toe, there appears a resignation to our natural training as doctors to "give the patient the benefit of the doubt." This may be accompanied by a rather perfunctory examination, missing the historical and physical feature of magnification behavior. The charade goes on in an attempt to pump up damages to which, in the end, an unscrupulous lawyer makes substantial claim.

Rather, in this setting, the doctor should attempt to separate the patients into those who have emotional disability and are in need of counseling from those whose disability will disappear only when contentious issues are removed from their considerations (i.e., settlement of the lawsuit).

It is apparent that these everyday clinical occurrences can be classified into psychosomatic, psychogenic, or situational spinal pains with or without some organic component. Once classified, treatment by the appropriate explanation and/or therapy can be intuited.

But wait! Is there any further help for assessing these patients?

ASSESSMENT OF NONORGANIC SPINAL PAIN

There are additional methods of assessing these conditions, including the pain drawing (9), psychometric testing, and the pentothal pain study (13). Although the orthopaedic literature is full of descriptions of these various assessment methods, it is probably best that these assessment methods are conducted and interpreted by those skilled in the field. Orthopaedic surgeons, by and large, are not skilled in these fields, and it is somewhat dangerous for them to be using these tests. These tests can be used to suggest the presence of a nonorganic component to the disability that results in referral of the patient to someone more skilled in the assessment of this aspect of disability. We do not use any of these ancillary assessment methods, but rather rely on history and physical examination findings described in the preceding sections. A brief description of these three assessment methods is offered.

PENTOTHAL PAIN STUDY

The introduction of the thiopental sodium pain assessment by Walters (13) has been of value in assessing the significance of emotional states in the production of the disability presented by the patient. The basis of this test lies in the fact that, in the state of light anesthesia, although the patient is unconscious, he or she is still capable of demonstrating primitive reactions to pain. The patient is anesthetized with thiopental in a slow fashion and then allowed to rouse until the corneal reflex returns. At this stage of anesthesia, the patient will withdraw from pinprick and will grimace when a painful stimulus is applied, such as squeezing the tendo Achillis. With the patient maintained at this level of anesthesia, maneuvers that were previously painful on clinical examination are re-evaluated. An example would be a patient who had SLR reduction of 20 degrees before induction of the thiopental sodium anesthesia. Theoretically, two extremes can occur. At one extreme, the 20-degree SLR reduction will persist under the light general anesthesia, a finding that may be taken as irrefutable evidence of significant root tension. If, on the other hand, at the stage of anesthesia when the patient will withdraw from pinprick, SLR, which was only 20 degrees on clinical examination, can now be carried out to 90 degrees without any response from the patient, the clinician may safely conclude that there is no evidence of root tension. It is likely that this patient's disability is due to an emotional reaction rather than to any organic source of pain.

If the patient previously had the diffuse, stocking-type of hypesthesia at this stage of narcosis, he or she will withdraw the limb when it is pricked by a pin. If, however, in addition to the hysterical response, there is a sensory loss due to root compression, then the patient will not show any response on pricking the skin over the dermatome of the root involved.

Thiopental sodium pain assessment is used in the patient with a combined nonorganic/organic disability. Its use is best confined to psychiatrists who have an interest in chronic pain, whereas the spinal surgeon relies on the symptoms and signs outlined in Table 16-4 to detect the potential for a nonorganic component to the disability.

PAIN DRAWING

The pain drawing (Fig. 16-12), popularized by Mooney and Robertson (9), is a simple form of psychometric testing that can be done by the patients while in the waiting room. Patients do not mind doing a pain drawing, because they regard this as cooperating with the physician in keeping an adequate record of their symptoms. But patients have just the reverse reaction to psychometric testing. The pattern used by the patient to fill out the pain drawing weighs the disability toward an organic or a nonorganic basis. The pain drawing is based on the assumption that organic back pain will be distributed along axial (low back) or radicular structures. The reverse is true in nonorganic pain syndromes, leading patients to draw less distinct and more widespread pictures to describe their pain (Fig. 16-12).

This is probably the safest assessment method for a spine surgical practice, but there are enough pitfalls in the use and interpretation of the test that it should be used by the orthopaedic surgeon or neurosurgeon in a screening fashion only. Chan et al. (1) have demonstrated a good correlation between nonorganic pain drawings and a Waddell score (nonorganic historical and physical findings). An abnormal pain drawing should then result in referral of the patient to some other professional more skilled in the assessment of nonorganic disability.

PSYCHOLOGICAL TESTING

Psychometric testing is a simple, rough guide to a patient's emotional health. The use and interpretation of these tests depend greatly on the experience of the user. Wiltse and Rocchio (14) have demonstrated convincingly that patients with a good emotional profile as shown on the Minnesota

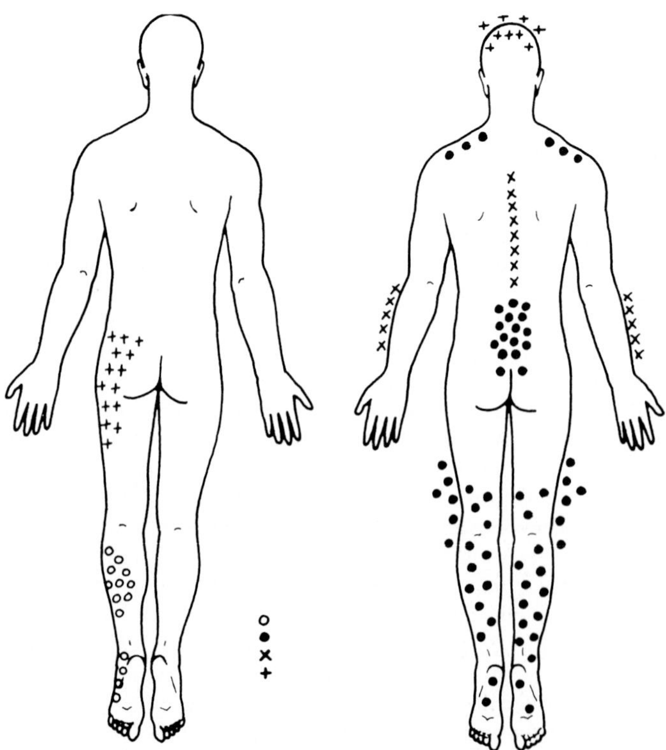

FIGURE 16-12 ● The pain drawing. Each patient is asked to draw with +, o, •, and × (+, stabbing; o, numbness; •, pins and needles; ×, burning) where they feel various pain sensations. The drawing to the left is by a patient with left sciatica. The drawing to the right is typical of a nonorganic pain patient.

Multiphasic Personality Inventory (MMPI) studies could be confidently expected to obtain better results following chemonucleolysis than those patients in whom a psychological profile was abnormal. There are so many psychometric tests with various strengths and weaknesses that it again is suggested that the spinal surgeon who recognized the potential for a nonorganic component to the disability refer the patient to someone skilled in the use of these tests.

It has been frequently mentioned in this text that psychological testing should be conducted by individuals skilled in the field. The suggestion to a patient that you wish to explore psychological or emotional aspects of their disability (step) will often provoke hostile behavior. The basis for this is the patient's perception that this step implies that "there is nothing wrong with my back, it is all in my head." These patient referrals have to be handled with understanding and a clear statement that there is something wrong with their back, but that the step in this direction is an appropriate avenue for them to explore.

TESTS THE PATIENT MAY ENCOUNTER

Minnesota Multiphasic Personality Inventory

This is the most common psychological test used. It contains 550 true-false questions and is scored on 10 clinical scales. Scales 1 and 3, hypochondriasis (Hs) and hysteria (Hy), if high, have been associated with poor treatment outcomes (14). Many studies have questioned the validity of these studies. Along with the fact that this test is long and tedious for patients to take and contains many questions of a psychiatric nature, it is losing favor as a psychological test for low back pain patients.

McGill Pain Questionnaire (5)

This test is used to measure the quality of pain by asking patients to pick adjectives to describe their pain. This is a simpler test for patients and is easily scored.

There are many other tests available for psychological evaluation, and each psychologist has his or her favorites. Fortunately, there are many in the field willing to help in the evaluation of these patients.

CONCLUSION

Every human attends the school of survival. Sometimes, the lessons lead patients to modify or magnify a physical disability at a conscious or unconscious level. One word of caution: The presence of one of these nonorganic reactions does not preclude an organic condition such as an herniated nucleus pulposus (HNP). The art of medicine is truly tested by a patient with physical low back pain who modifies the disability with a nonorganic reaction such as tension, hysteria, depression, or other factors.

Low back pain is only a symptom; it will only become a chronic disease if we poorly diagnose, poorly treat, and carry out injudicious surgery. Then we are dealing with DISABILITY (review the disability equation at the beginning of this chapter and Figures 17-1 and 17-2). The best way to prevent this expensive cascade of events is to understand the physical and nonphysical aspects of back pain and help patients lead as close to normal lives as possible.

REFERENCES

1. Chan CW, Goldman S, Ilstrup DM, et al. The pain drawing and Waddell's nonorganic physical signs in chronic low back pain. *Spine.* 1993;18:1717–1722.
2. Guyton AC. *Textbook of Medical Physiology.* Philadelphia: WB Saunders; 1986.
3. Kellgren JH. On the distribution of pain arising from deep somatic structures with charts of segmental pain areas. *Clin Sci Mod Med.* 1939;4:35–46.
4. Loeser JD. Concepts of pain. In: Stanton-Hicks M, Boas RA, eds. *Chronic Low Back Pain.* New York: Raven Press; 1982;145–148.
5. Melzack R. The McGill Pain Questionnaire: major properties and scoring methods. *Pain.* 1975;1:277–299.
6. Merskey R. Pain terms: a list with definitions and notes on usage. *Pain.* 1979;6:249–252.
7. Mooney V, Robertson J. The facet syndrome. *Clin Orthop.* 1976;115:149–156.
8. Noordenbos W: Prologue. In: Wall PD, Melzack R, eds. *Textbook of Pain.* Edinburgh, Scotland: Churchill Livingstone; 1984.

9. Ransford AO, Cairns D, Mooney V. The pain drawing as an aid to the psychological evaluation of patients with low back pain. *Spine.* 1976;1:127–134.
10. Waddell G, McCulloch JA, Kummel EG, et al. Non-organic physical signs in low back pain. *Spine.* 1980;5:117–125.
11. Waddell G, Morris EW, DiPaola MP, Bircher M, Finlayson D. A concept of illness tested as an improved basis for surgical decisions in low-back disorders. *Spine.* 1986;11:712–719.
12. Wall PD, Melzack R. *Textbook of Pain.* Edinburgh, Scotland: Churchill Livingstone; 1984.
13. Walters A. Regional pain alias hysterical pain. *Brain.* 1961;84:1–18.
14. Wiltse LL, Rocchio PD. Preoperative psychological tests as predictors of success in chemonucleolysis in the treatment of low back syndrome. *J Bone Joint Surg Am.* 1975;57:478–483.
15. Yoshizawa H, O'Brien JP, Smith WT, et al. The neuropathology of intervertebral disc removed for low back pain. *J Pathol.* 1980;132:95–104.

CHAPTER 17

Complications and Failures of Spinal Surgery

"There is not a fiercer hell than the failure in a great object."

—John Keats

Although spine surgery covers a broad range of procedures for trauma, tumors, and degenerative conditions, this chapter limits the discussion to that of failures for degenerative conditions. Failures in spine surgery are a fact of life because of the multifactorial nature of the problem. But should it be that way? There are many factors to consider when dealing with a failure of spine surgery. By reading this chapter perhaps we will all become more discrete in our choice of patients, our diagnosis, and our surgical interventions.

One of the most difficult problems in spinal surgery is the assessment and management of patients still seriously disabled by backache, despite one or more attempts at surgical correction of the underlying lesion (45). Such failures are nearly always compounded by a variable and varying mixture of inadequate preoperative assessments, errors in operative technique, and emotional breakdown of the patient either antedating or following surgery (19). This situation will only become more complex with the recent Food and Drug Administration (FDA) approval of the first artificial lumbar disc (1,42). It is convenient to consider these separately under the headings listed in Table 17-1.

Although surgeons take much of the blame (and somewhat deservedly so) for creating the monstrous problem of the failed back surgery syndrome (FBSS) (45), it is important to remember that some aspects of conservative care are also capable of delivering patients into the failed back syndrome. Nachemson (25) has suggested that nerve root compression beyond 3 months has the potential of permanent sequelae and recommends that nerve root decompression occur before that time has slipped by with prolonged conservative care (32).

PREOPERATIVE FAILURE

SELECTION OF THE WRONG PATIENT FOR SURGERY

It is a constant theme throughout this book that, when contemplating back surgery, one should look at the whole patient. To ignore obvious emotional and situation pressures deflecting the patient toward a larger or longer period of disability will result in failure of the surgical exercise. The reader is reminded that the first question to be asked in the differential diagnosis of any low back disability is:

> "Am I dealing with a true physical disability, or are there features on history or physical examination to suggest there is a nonorganic component to the patient's disability equation?"

TABLE 17-1

Failures of Spine Surgery

Preoperative errors
- Wrong patient
- Wrong diagnosis

Intraoperative errors
- Wrong level
- Wrong operation
  - Wrong syndrome
  - Incomplete surgery
- Complications (immediate/local)

Postoperative failure
- Complications
- Arachnoiditis
- Change of symptoms or recurrence of symptoms

All too often this question is only answered in the affirmative after failed surgery.

It is not infrequent that a surgeon is faced with a patient who has a protracted disability. The patient has been in and out of work, in and out of hospital, in and out of physical therapy departments, and in and out of the offices of drugless practitioners. It is understandably tempting to regard this long period of disability as indicating severe pain. However, if this group of patients, suffering from low back pain only, cannot be retrained to undertake lighter jobs, then a desperation fusion will be unlikely to succeed.

In this regard, it must be emphasized that a patient cannot describe the pain; he or she can only describe the disability. Pain and disability are not synonymous, and the disability complained of is not necessarily indicative of the degree of pain experienced.

In the simplest superficial analysis, disability has three components: the pain, the patient's reaction to the pain, and the situation prevailing at the time of the pain. A certain degree of what might be termed a functional reaction can be regarded as normal. When the functional response is gross, it becomes a major part of the disease process. This concept is best exemplified by describing three hypothetical workmen, three bricklayers who presented with the same degree of disability. They had pain in their backs; although they could walk around, they could not do their work. They could not climb ladders, carry bricks, or stoop to lay the bricks. They were not able to describe the amount of pain they had; they could only describe their disability. They all had degenerative disc disease. The radiographs could not describe how much pain they were experiencing. All that was known was that the disability claimed by all three was the same: They could not work. In one patient (patient A), the disability was largely due to the anatomic basis of his pain. In another patient (patient C), there was little anatomic source of pain, but he was overcome by the functional reaction or the emotional response to his discomforts (Fig. 17-1).

Surgery meticulously performed might overcome 90% of the anatomic basis of the disability. The first patient (A) would be cured and would be able to return to work, but even with 90% of the organic basis of his disability removed, the third patient (C) would still be incapacitated (Fig. 17-2). In such instances, because of failure of treatment, the functional reaction will get worse, and the story of patient C is best exemplified by the letters that were written to the workmen's compensation board about him:

> "Dear Sirs:
> I saw this very pleasant claimant, George Smith, today, and the poor fellow has not responded to conservative therapy at all. He is totally unable to work. His radiographs show marked disc degeneration, and I plan to bring him into the hospital for a local fusion."

> "Dear Sirs:
> I operated on George today, and I am sure he will do well."

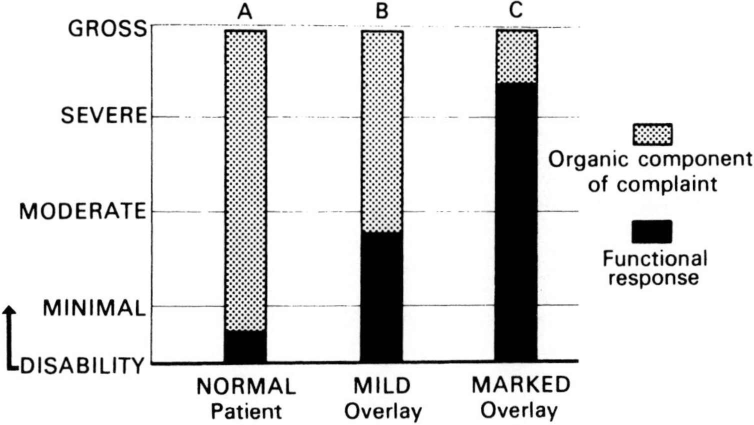

FIGURE 17-1 • Functional overlay. Three patients (A, B, and C) with apparent identical disability.

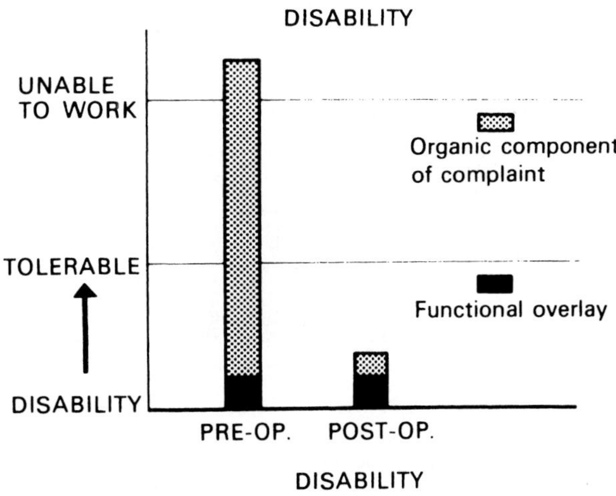

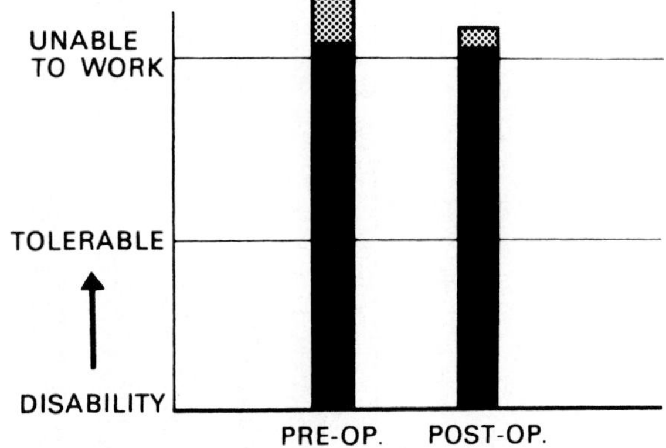

FIGURE 17-2 • Diagram to show that although removal of the organic basis of pain will produce a good result in the emotionally stable patient **(top),** the continuing emotional turmoils in the patient with significant functional overlay **(bottom)** result in perpetuation of the disability after operation.

"Dear Sirs:
I saw George Smith today, and I am a little disappointed with his progress to date."

"Dear Sirs:
Smith's radiographs show a solid fusion, but he shows surprisingly little motivation to return to work."

"Dear Sirs:
This dreadful fellow Smith."

"Dear Sirs:
Smith obviously needs psychiatric help" (Fig. 17-3).

Patients A, B, and C all presented with the same disability. They were bricklayers who could not work. They had the same radiographic changes, but the constitution of their disability varied enormously, and, predictably, the results of operative treatment varied also (Fig. 17-4).

In patient C, the degenerative disc disease was not causing too much pain, and in better emotional health, the discomfort he experienced would not have taken him to a doctor. However, because of factors outside his spine, in fact, outside his soma, he was totally disabled by his discomfort; and this disability was later compounded, perpetuated, and exaggerated by the failure of surgical treatment.

Patients A and C do not really constitute much of a problem because the gross functional overlay of patient C is usually recognizable. These two groups of patients have been discussed in detail throughout this book to emphasize the fact that pain and disability are not synonymous. The middle group, patient B, typifies the most difficult problem. The surgeon who regards a functional overlay as a solid contraindication to operation will not help patient B even though he does have an organic basis of discomfort.

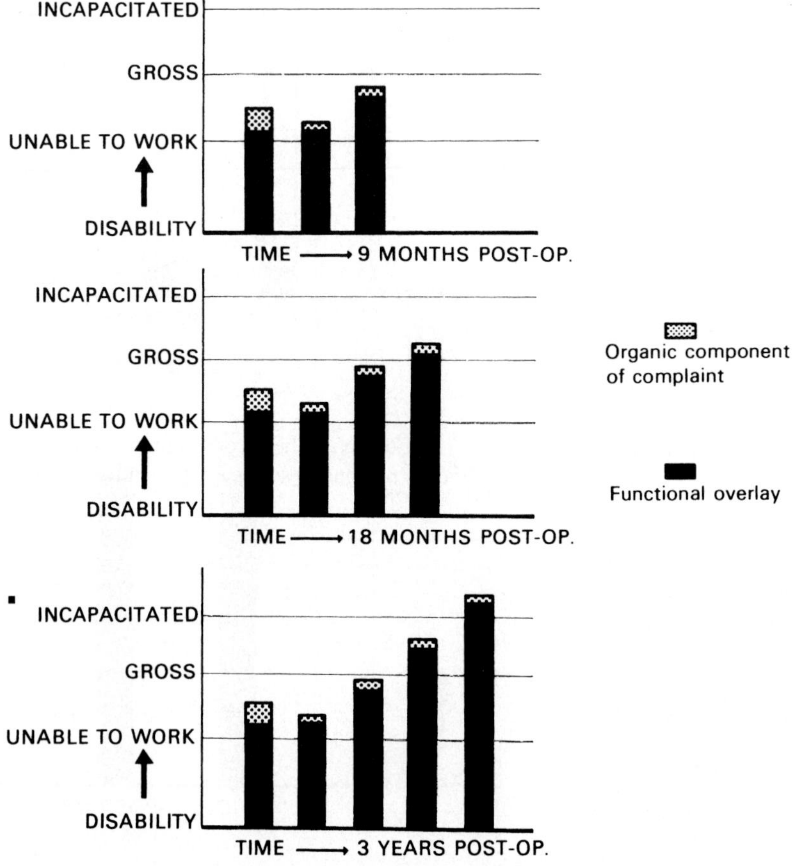

FIGURE 17-3 ● Diagram shows how increasing emotional breakdown will produce increasing disability after surgical intervention.

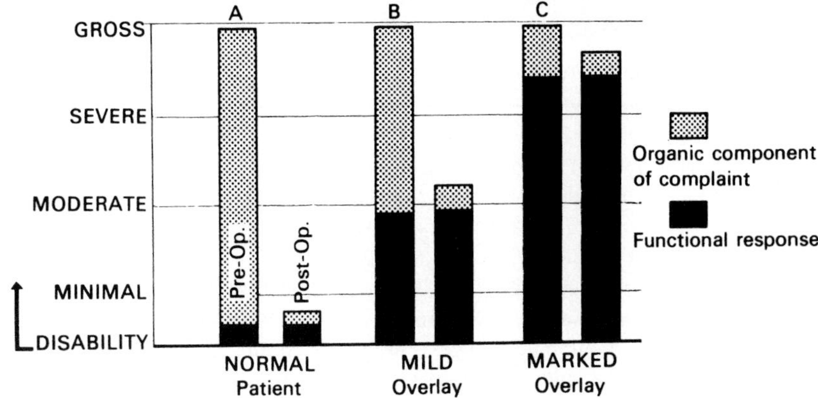

FIGURE 17-4 • Diagram to show the relationship between the functional overlay and the response to treatment in patients A, B, and C.

There are two important aspects in the management of patient B that must always be kept in mind: first, the recognition of the organic basis of pain, despite the clouding of the clinical picture by the functional elements; and second, an analysis of the constitution of the functional component of the disability.

The functional overlay is derived from a combination of many factors. A large part of the emotional overlay is due to the patient's personality; the patient may have no drive, no motivation, and may even be a psychopath. Whatever it is, it probably cannot be altered. It is important to recognize a gross personality defect because these patients will not do well with treatment directed solely at their spines.

Other factors must be considered, such as the patient's affect or mood, the significance of pain to the patient, and the patient's ability to adjust to his or her environment. The importance of financial security and work demands are obvious. Finally, the reaction of the patient to pain must be considered: the individual's pain tolerance and pain threshold. If the patient, because of inheritance or constitution, for example, tends to have an exaggerated reaction to any painful stimulus, it makes it very difficult to recognize the fact that the patient is suffering from an organic lesion.

For example, a patient may react violently at the limit of one phase of clinical examination: straight leg raising (SLR). On experiencing discomfort, the patient may writhe, groan, shout, bang his or her hands, and finally collapse, sobbing and weeping. Such patients react excessively to pain produced by an organic disability. However, when this excessive reaction is of a hysterical nature, it becomes extremely difficult to determine whether the problem is one of a hysterical patient with pain or a patient with hysterical pain. Suffice it to say, if these considerations are made preoperatively, it is less likely that the patient will fail to respond to surgical intervention because of nonorganic factors.

With the heightening criticism directed at spine surgeons for the all too frequent poor outcome, we are looking at the many factors that lead us into failure. It is becoming more apparent that the nutritionally compromised patient does not have the physical foundation for adequate wound healing (11). The authors are becoming more convinced that the heavy smoker and/or drinker has also compromised wound healing, specifically graft incorporation, and is more likely to end up with a pseudarthrosis after attempted fusion (10).

WRONG DIAGNOSIS

There are many pitfalls awaiting the unwary in evaluating and treating low back and leg pain. If an incorrect diagnosis was the basis of the surgical procedure, there is virtually no hope of a successful outcome. The "step back and take a long look" approach is then indicated. The second question to be answered satisfactorily is: Did I fall into a diagnostic trap and make an error in diagnosis (Tables 17-2 and 17-3)?

TABLE 17-2

Differential Diagnosis of Nonmechanical Low Back Pain

Causes of nonmechanical low back pain	
Referred pain (e.g., from the abdomen or retroperitoneal space)	
Infection	bone, disc, epidural space
Neoplasm	primary (multiple myeloma, osteoid osteoma, and so forth) metastatic
Inflammation	arthritides such as ankylosing spondylitis
Miscellaneous metabolic and vascular disorders such as osteopenia and Paget's disease	

INTRAOPERATIVE ERRORS

WRONG LEVEL

It seems rhetorical to state that even though you make the right diagnosis in the right patient, operating at the wrong level will fail to cure the disease. There is more "wrong level" surgery being done than we, as surgeons, have admitted. This occurs in two situations: (a) preoperative selection of the wrong level for surgery (Figs. 17-5 and 17-6) and (b) making the technical error of selecting the wrong level intraoperatively. Systems approaches for consistently arriving at the site of pathology have been proposed. The "Sign, Mark and X-Ray (SMaX)" program from the North American Spine Society is a reasonable methodology (48).

Congenital Lumbosacral Anomalies

The reason congenital anomalies can lead to wrong level exploration is because our radiologic colleagues speak a different language regarding these anomalies. Because of this lack of a common meeting ground, the radiologist reading the film may inadvertently number congenital lumbosacral

TABLE 17-3

Differential Diagnosis of Sciatica

- Intraspinal causes
  - Proximal to disc: conus and cauda equina lesions (e.g., neurofibroma, ependymoma)
  - Disc level
    - Herniated nucleus pulposus
    - Stenosis (canal or recess)
    - Infection: osteomyelitis or discitis (with nerve root pressure)
    - Inflammation: arachnoiditis
    - Neoplasm: benign or malignant, with nerve root pressure
- Extraspinal causes
  - Pelvis
    - Cardiovascular conditions (e.g., peripheral vascular disease)
    - Gynecologic conditions
    - Orthopaedic conditions (e.g., osteoarthritis of hip)
    - Sacroiliac joint disease
    - Neoplasms (invading or compressing lumbosacral plexus)
  - Peripheral nerve lesions
    - Neuropathy (diabetic, tumor, alcohol)
    - Local sciatic nerve conditions (trauma, tumor)
    - Inflammation (herpes zoster)

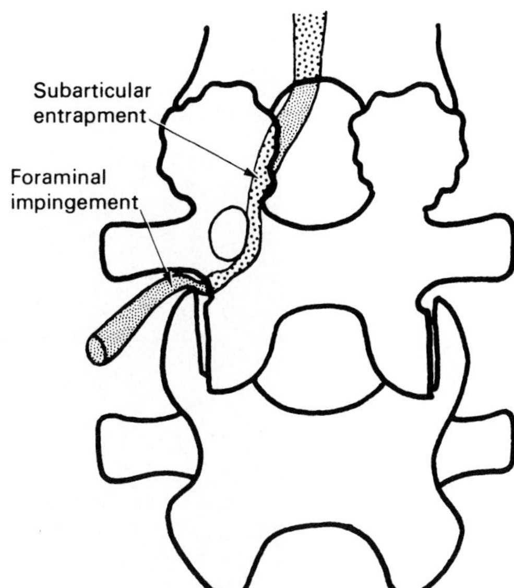

FIGURE 17-5 • The emerging nerve root may be compressed at more than one site. In this diagram, the nerve root is shown to be compressed as it passes through the subarticular gutter. It is also trapped in the foramen by the tip of the superior articular facet. The error in diagnosis occurs when one of the lesions is missed.

anomalies differently than the clinician, which may contribute to a wrong level exploration. The reason for this is that orthopaedic surgeons tend to read lumbar spine radiographs from the bottom up and radiologists tend to read lumbar spine radiographs from the top down (L1 to the sacrum).

Definitions. When faced with congenital lumbosacral anomalies and the potential for numbering errors, the following definitions are offered. A formed lumbar segment is described as any anatomic segment that has an interlaminar space and a formed disc space (Fig. 17-7). A mobile lumbar segment is any lumbar vertebrae free of pelvic or rib attachment (Fig. 17-7). There is a tendency, which makes embryologic sense, that the extent of formation of the disc space parallels the extent of formation of the interlaminar space; that is, the more rudimentary the disc space, the more rudimentary the interlaminar space (Fig. 17-8). Even a rudimentary interlaminar space, exposed in a limited fashion, can appear as a normal interlaminar space. It represents entry into a nonmobile level that rarely harbors pathology, and a wrong level exposure. These congenital anomalies were fully discussed in Chapter 1.

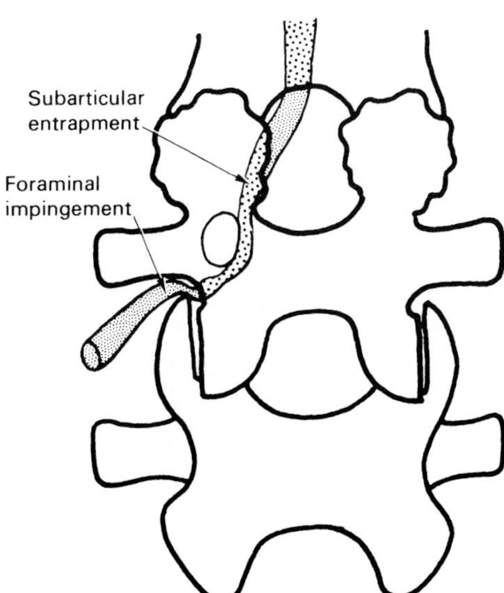

FIGURE 17-6 • Diagram showing apophyseal stenosis that results in the compression of two nerve roots. The diagnostic error occurs when only one root is thought to be causing symptoms.

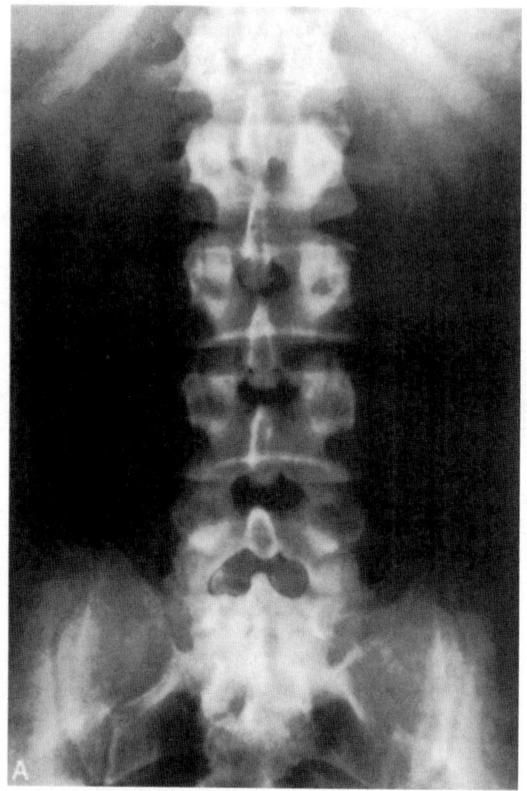

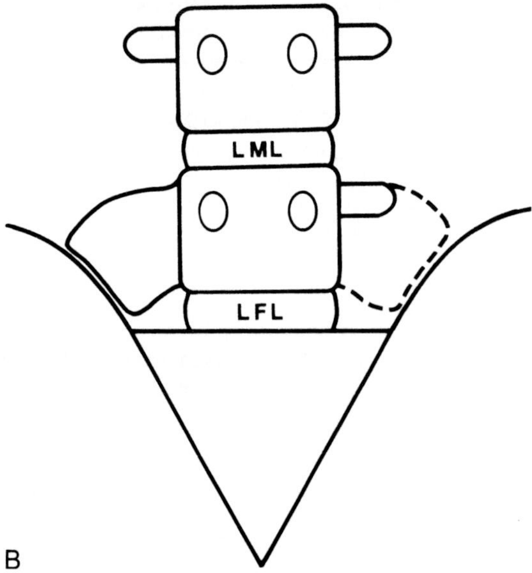

FIGURE 17-7 ● **A:** In a normal lumbar spine, there are five vertebrae, which are free of rib and pelvic bony attachment. The last interlaminar space is outlined. **B:** A schematic depicting the last mobile segment. LML, last mobile level; LFL, last formed level.

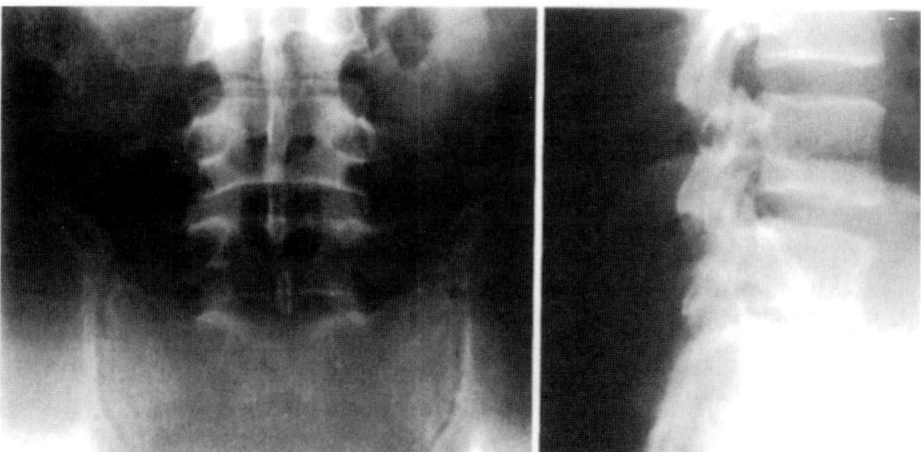

FIGURE 17-8 • A fixed last-formed level with narrow interlaminar space on the AP and corresponding rudimentary disc space on the lateral.

WRONG OPERATION, WRONG SYNDROME

If you are satisfied that no error was made in the differential diagnosis of low back pain or sciatica, and the operation was done at the correct level, then was an error made in the third question? Specifically, is this a mechanical low back pain condition and, if so, what is the syndrome (Table 17-4)?

Surgery for degenerative conditions in the lumbar spine consists of two basic types: (a) decompression surgery for nerve root compromise and (b) stabilization/fusion surgery for a painful motion segment.

There are many occasions when both surgeries (decompression and fusion) are indicated. However, if one type of surgery was carried out and the patient fails to improve, was the wrong operation performed on the basis of an incorrect preoperative diagnosis? Was encroachment surgery done when stabilization surgery was indicated (20)? This is a common error and is most often due to referred leg pain being confused for radicular leg pain; removal of a "sucker disc" (Fig. 17-9) with the result being even more instability and more back pain.

WRONG OPERATION, INCOMPLETE SURGERY

An example might be failure after laminectomy for spinal stenosis due to incomplete apophyseal decompression. Incomplete decompression of the involved nerve roots is seen in the following circumstances: missed fragment of ruptured disc material. A reasonable criticism of microdiscectomy is the potential, because of a limited surgical field, to leave behind fragments of ruptured disc.

TABLE 17-4

Syndromes in Mechanical Low Back Disorders

Lumbago–back pain (mechanical instability)
Sciatica–radicular pain
- Unilateral acute radicular syndrome
- Bilateral acute radicular syndrome
- Unilateral chronic radicular syndrome
- Bilateral chronic radicular syndrome

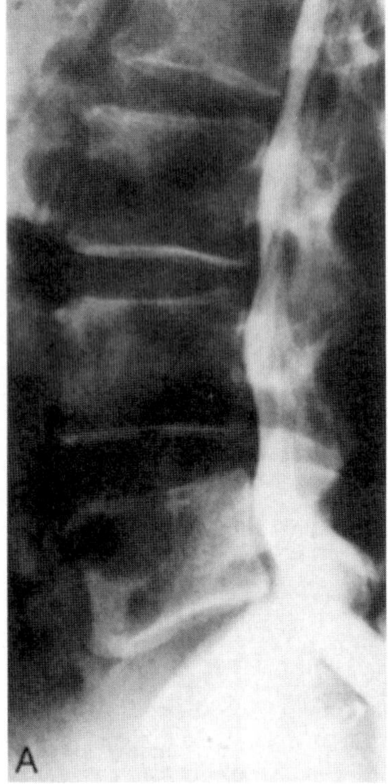

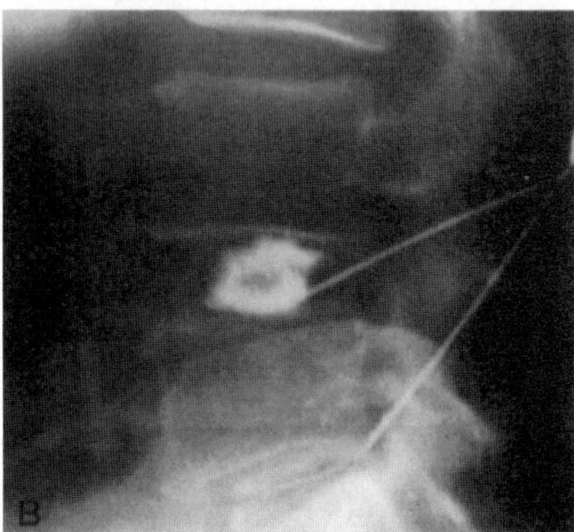

FIGURE 17-9 ● **A:** A lateral myelogram, with a slight "bulge" at L4–L5. **B:** Subsequent normal discogram at L4–L5 and a degenerative disc at L5–S1.

ENTRAPMENT OF A NERVE ROOT AT MORE THAN ONE SITE

This error will be avoided if the mobility of the root is assessed after the apparent source of compression is removed. It should be possible to displace a normal or completely decompressed nerve root at least 1 cm medially. The S1 root can normally be displaced to the midline.

INVOLVEMENT OF MORE THAN ONE ROOT

Incomplete decompression may result when more than one root is involved in an apparently unisegmental degenerative stenosis. This source of failure emphasizes the need for complete preoperative evaluation of the roots involved. The surgeon must know what roots to explore.

OVERLOOKED APOPHYSEAL STENOSIS

A decompression laminectomy for spinal stenosis is always started by the removal of a portion or the whole of one or more laminae. If this is technically difficult because of shingling or overgrowth of the laminae, it is understandable that the surgeon confine his/her attention to a midline decompression. Even though a very complete midline decompression is performed, the patient will not be helped if, as is commonly the case, he or she is suffering from both canal stenosis and concomitant lateral zone stenosis giving rise to root compression. This error is more likely to occur if the lateral zone stenosis is at a different segment from the canal stenosis.

Here again, an accurate preoperative assessment followed by a preoperative design of the procedure required will avoid this only too frequent source of error.

INCOMPLETE MIDLINE COMPRESSION

Sometimes a midline decompression is incomplete. It must be remembered that this operation is most frequently performed on older patients with the surgeon being understandably reluctant to carry out extensive surgery. The operation is frequently tedious, hemorrhagic, time consuming, and apparently destructive. Despite the temptation to short-circuit the operative procedure, when the patient's symptoms superficially appear to stem from laminar compression at one or two segments only, decompression must occur at the appropriate levels.

FORAMINAL DISC

Macnab's landmark article on "Negative Disc Exploration" (20) described the foraminal disc. If you are in the canal looking for a foraminal disc there is a good chance you will miss it, and the patient will wake with identical leg pain.

CONJOINT NERVE ROOT

A small disc herniation compressing a conjoint root can not only produce a lot of sciatica, it can be a very difficult fragment to retrieve. This combination of events occurs most often at L5–S1 and requires a wide decompression, without sacrificing the facet joint, and removal of the fragment under the axilla of the root.

COMPLICATIONS RELATED TO THE SURGICAL PROCEDURE

Classification

Complications to any surgical procedure can be classified into (a) general or local, (b) early (immediate) or late (delayed), and (c) specific or nonspecific.

Complication Rate

Most surgeons rarely have complications! Better stated, most surgeons do not remember (or subconsciously forget) their complications until they complete a follow-up study. Their understanding of adverse effects is even clearer if that follow-up study is completed by an independent observer. Many studies (21,29,30,35) have appeared in the literature describing complication rates; they are listed in Table 17-5.

Complications

Immediate general complications such as intraoperative anesthetic complications, hypotensive complications, and delayed general complications, such as postoperative thrombophlebitis (6, 9) pulmonary embolism, atelectasis, and urinary retention are part of everyone's surgical practice. Readers are referred to other texts for a discussion of these general adverse events.

Early complications to lumbar disc surgery (excluding lumbar fusion) have been artificially divided into local specific and nonspecific complications.

TABLE 17-5

Complication Rates (%) from the Literature

Complication	Spangfort (35) Literature Search	Spangfort (35) Series (2,504 Operations)	Mayfield (21) Series (1,408 Operations)	Ramirez and Thirstad (29) Series (28,395 Operations)
Mortality	0.3	0.1	0.4	0.06
Thrombophlebitis	N/S	1.0	N/S	N/S
Pulmonary embolus	1.7	1.0	0.2	0.2
Cauda equina syndrome	N/S	0.2	0.07	0.08
Wound infection	2.9	3.8	1.0	0.3
Root damage	N/S	0.5	0.1	0.2
Dural tear	N/S	1.6	0.7	0.1

N/S, not specified in the data presented

Local nonspecific complications. Local nonspecific complications are those that can occur in association with any lumbar disc operation. They include (a) major vessel or visceral injury, (b) cauda equina injury, (c) foreign body retention, and (d) pressure complications secondary to positioning on table.

Local specific complications. Local specific complications are those that can occur in association with any lumbar disc operation but are more likely to occur as a surgeon is learning the technique of microsurgery. They include (a) wrong level exposure, (b) missed pathology, (c) intraoperative bleeding obscuring the visual field, (d) dural injury, (e) root injury, and (f) disc space infection.

***Major vessel or visceral injury* (5,7,12,15,34).** Major vessel or visceral injury occurs when an instrument penetrates the anterior annulus. Figure 17-10 demonstrates how this occurs. If you are a surgeon who believes that all of the discal material possible should be removed (36), then this is a complication that must be prevented. The instrument that does the damage is usually a pituitary rongeur or curette, and the complication occurs when either instrument is inserted too deeply into the disc space. Anterior approaches entail a risk of direct injury to the great vessels and their branches, bowels, and bladder.

Cauda equina injury. The term cauda equina syndrome (CES) denotes the postoperative appearance of a compressive neuropathy involving multiple lumbar and sacral roots. The involvement of the roots from S2 caudally, with bladder and bowel dysfunction, is the hallmark of a CES. Associated, usually, are varying degrees of motor and sensory deficits in the lower extremities. Compression of the cauda equina may have occurred during the surgery, from excessive retraction on the dural sheath, but more often is a delayed complication (hours or days) caused by a growing extradural hematoma.

CLINICAL PRESENTATION

Most CES starts in the recovery room or soon after the patient arrives back on the floor. Less commonly they will evolve slowly over the first few postoperative days (32).

The features are (a) numbness in the perineum; (b) urinary retention or incontinence; (c) decreased rectal tone; (d) progressive motor weakness, starting in the feet and ankles; (e) decreased sensation starting in the perineum, sacral strips, and the feet; and (f) progression of the motor and sensory dysfunction. Often enough, the postoperative presentation of the CES is absent leg pain, so do not get lulled into thinking the absence of leg pain post-decompression rules out the CES.

McLaren and Bailey (23) have pointed out that this complication is more prone to occur when a limited laminectomy, through a standard incision, is done in the presence of a stenotic spinal canal. The cornerstones of treatment of this complication are early recognition and immediate evacuation of the hematoma with a wider decompression of any residual stenotic segments.

Foreign body retention. Everyone is aware of a patient who, after persisting postoperative symptoms, was found at surgery (reoperation) to have a retained cottonoid or other foreign mate-

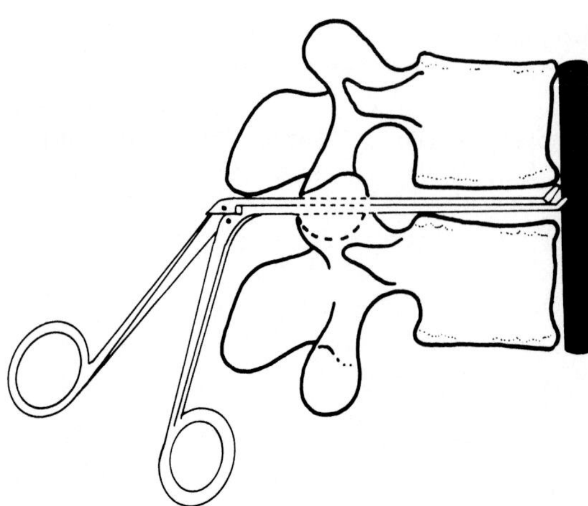

FIGURE 17-10 ● Perforation of the anterior annulus with a sharp instrument may damage the aorta. (Redrawn from Crock HV. *A Short Practice of Spinal Surgery.* New York: Springer-Verlag; 1993.)

rial pressuring the nerve root. Every surgeon can only insist on time-honored nursing protocols, at the time of closure, to prevent this complication.

Complications secondary to positioning on the operating room table. Most surgeons use a variation of the kneeling position for lumbar disc surgery. This is an interesting phenomenon because most reports on the lateral position report fewer complications from positioning on the operating room (OR) table. Almost all of the complications from improper positioning of a patient, under general anesthesia, are related to prolonged pressure on neurologic structures. These include (a) brachial plexus stretch, (b) radial nerve palsy, (c) ulnar nerve palsy, and (d) peroneal nerve palsy.

The most serious of all of these neurologic complications is stretching of the brachial plexus, which is prone to occur in the heavy-set, muscular man with arthritic changes in the neck. In these patients in particular, and all patients in general, the neck should be place in a position of slight flexion (in particular: no extension). The shoulders are to be in no more than 90 degrees of abduction and should be in some flexion.

Other neurologic structures prone to pressure palsies are the ulnar nerve, peroneal nerve, and radial nerve (listed in order of frequency). Careful padding of the relative pressure points will prevent injury to the nerves. Other areas that may be pressure damaged in the kneeling position are the eyes, breasts and chest cage, and the prepatellar region. Careful padding is necessary to prevent their occurrence. There have been reports of perioperative posterior ischemic optic neuropathy that implicate prone positioning and hypotension as risk factors (4).

Dural injury. It is not possible to perform a large volume of spine surgery, especially through a limited surgical exposure, and not cause injury to the dura. Hopefully, it is infrequent! It is not necessary that this include injury to the nerve root but it may be an associated complication. Fortunately, it appears that the incidence of significant long-term sequelae is low (17).

Concern with Dural Tears. Obviously, dural tears are not desired, but they do occur. They are of concern because:

1. They result in a loss of cerebrospinal fluid (CSF) that results in postoperative low-pressure headaches.
2. They represent a potential entry route for infection.
3. They can lead to immediate postoperative leaks of CSF through a fistulous tract in the wound.
4. If undiscovered and unrepaired, they may form pseudocysts (pseudomeningocele) in the region of the nerve root, entrapping nerve roots or producing symptoms by mass effect.

The appearance of nonbloody (clear) fluid in the wound should alert the surgeon to the possibility of a dural tear being present. There are other possibilities for the appearance of this clear fluid, including a CSF leak from yesterday's myelogram, synovial fluid from a synovial cyst, and the scrub nurse handing you wet tools.

These three situations are self-limiting flows of fluid. In the case of the synovial cyst, the fluid has a yellowish tinge. The persistent flow of clear fluid, especially with respiratory inspiration is the signal that a dural tear is present and must be found. The principles of repair of dural tears are as follows (8):

1. Recognize the tear, its extent, and the necessity for immediate repair. Under the microscope, dural leaks are being viewed with 5 to 10 times magnification. A small puncture, not much larger than a needle puncture rent in the dura, does not need to be repaired. Any dural injury that has length to it—that is, can be closed with one or more 6-0 to 7-0 sutures—must be repaired.
2. Ensure that the exposure is wide enough and the field dry enough that an adequate repair can be accomplished. This may mean extending the microsurgical incision and bony decompression.
3. The author's preferred method of repair is direct suture, using a thin fat graft to ensure a watertight repair (Fig. 17-11). Larger defects that cannot be closed in a direct fashion as in Figure 17-11 can be closed with a fascial graft.
4. Once the repair is completed, the integrity of the repair should be tested with a Valsalva maneuver.

Probably, the most important step to prevent late complications is to suture the muscle tightly down on the laminar defect overlying the repair (Fig. 17-12) and complete a watertight closure at every level of suture.

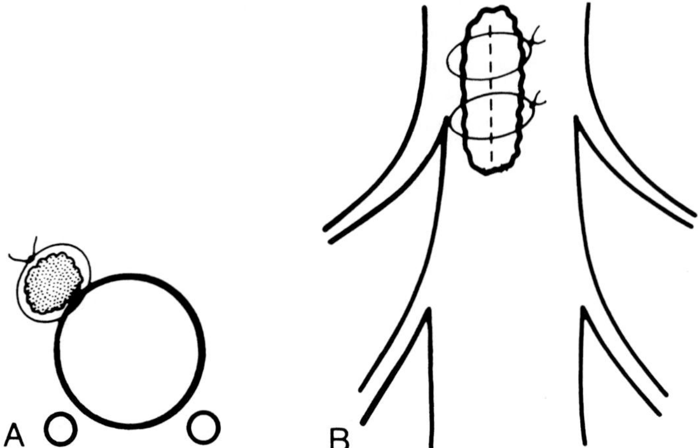

FIGURE 17-11 ● **A** and **B:** Dural repair in two steps: direct repair of defect and oversewn fat graft.

Other methods of dural repair such as a Gelfoam patch, muscle patch, and gels have been tried without success. Newer products such as Gelfilm and fibrin glue are showing promise (14,27,43). Ignoring the dural rent (except for pin holes) and keeping the patient in bed postoperatively are also unlikely to be successful.

Postoperatively, the patient without spinal headaches may need to be kept in bed for 1 to 2 days to facilitate sealing of the repair. For a low-pressure headache, a period of bed rest up to 7 days and a subarachnoid drain may be necessary (43). Limit the hourly CSF drainage to 10–15cc to avoid tonsilar herniation at the foramen magnum. Persistent leakage may require surgical re-exploration.

Root damage. Root damage at the time of microsurgery is almost always associated with dural injury. It is difficult, but possible, to damage the root in the foramen and not have a dural tear. It is more likely that the root injury is proximal to the ganglion and that the appearance of clear CSF is the first indication of trouble. When searching for the source of the CSF, the appearance of severed rootlets is proof of the root damage. Root damage can also occur without a dural tear, as the result of excessive traction.

Factors leading to root damage are (a) poor instrumentation; (b) aggressive surgical technique; (c) inadequate exposure before retraction of the root; (d) distortion of normal root location by the pathology; (e) excessive retraction, especially if adhesions are present or a very large axillary disc is present; and (f) anomalous roots.

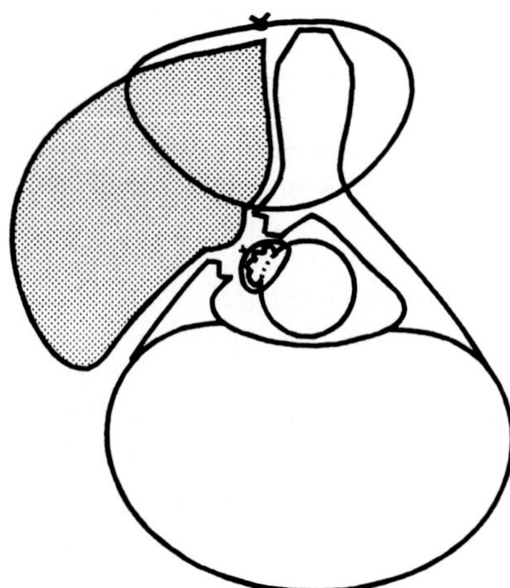

FIGURE 17-12 ● After the dural tear has been repaired, use a couple of large sutures through the interspinous ligament to suture the paraspinal muscles down on the repair.

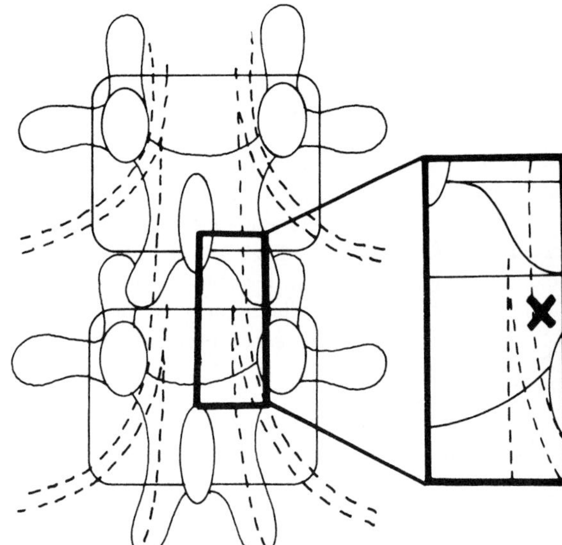

FIGURE 17-13 • X marks the spot where root damage occurs. The usual combination is an inadequate exposure of the lateral edge of the nerve root and discal displacement of the root in the area marked with X.

The instrument that does the damage is usually the Kerrison rongeur, used in an aggressive manner. The injury occurs close to the takeoff of the root (Fig. 17-13) and occurs because of failure to obey one cardinal rule of spine surgery: Before placing a sharp instrument in the spinal canal and before retracting the root, clearly define the lateral border of the nerve root.

Treatment. There is nothing one can do to lacerated rootlets except to place them back within the dural sheath if possible. Repairing the laceration in the dural nerve root sheath is not only impossible but inadvisable because you will cause isolated root stenosis and recurrent postoperative leg pain symptoms. Fortunately, the damage of a few rootlets results in limited neurologic dysfunction because of multiple sources of innervation for most lower extremity motor and sensory function.

POSTOPERATIVE FAILURES

DISC SPACE INFECTION

The incidence of disc space infection in microsurgery is approximately 1% (16,47). The incidence of disc space infection for standard laminectomy/discectomy is approximately 0.5% across the literature (21,28). It is thought that there is a higher incidence of disc space infection in microsurgery because the microscope is over top of the open wound, introducing the possibility of manipulating the exposed, unsterile eye pieces by the surgeon or art assistant.

To prevent this, make all microscope adjustments before draping the microscope and moving it over the patient. Also, position the microscope for the ligamentum flavum incision and then limit future manipulations of the microscope during the case. To adjust the focus on the microscope during the case, either raise or lower the OR table (and thus the patient) or raise and lower the microscope with a floor-operated control. In this fashion, one can avoid touching the microscope after it is placed in its correct position and thus reduce the possibility of contamination coming off the microscope and entering the surgical field.

PROPHYLACTIC ANTIBIOTICS

Most surgeons would agree that surgery involving the use of implants (e.g., total hip) requires the use of prophylactic antibiotics. The use of prophylactic antibiotics in a microsurgical spinal operation is more controversial (39). With an approximate rate of disc space infection of 0.5% to 1% it would require a prospective, multicentered trial of 2,000 to 3,000 patients to determine the effectiveness of prophylactic antibiotics. The use of prophylactic antibiotics in lumbar microsurgery is empirical but employed by most surgeons. The authors use one intravenous (IV) dose of an appropriate first-generation cephalosporin at the beginning of the surgical procedure. If a foreign body is implanted (e.g., instrumentation), a course of antibiotics is used postoperatively for 24 hours.

ARACHNOIDITIS (SPINAL)

Arachnoiditis, by definition, is an inflammation of the pia-arachnoid membrane, resulting in adhesions between nerve roots and between the pia mater and the arachnoid membrane.

There are two arachnoid membranes in the spinal canal (Fig. 17-14): the pia-arachnoid (a rich vascular membrane closely adherent to the spinal cord and cauda equina nerve roots) and the arachnoid membrane (an avascular membrane composed of fibrous and elastic tissue, more closely related geographically to the dura mater). Between the pia mater and the arachnoid membrane lies the subarachnoid space, where CSF normally flows.

Etiology

There does not appear to be one single cause of arachnoiditis. In any series of patients with arachnoiditis, there is a common thread of one or more of the following factors.

1. Prior lumbar spine surgery.
2. Prior myelogram with oil-based or ionic water-soluble contrast agents.
3. Prior spinal injury, usually a herniated nucleus pulposus (HNP) or spinal stenosis and, on occasion, blunt spine trauma.
4. Direct dural injury, especially if blood enters the dural space, can cause dural and arachnoid scarring.

Postoperative epidural scar formation is a natural consequence of any spinal operation and, more often than not, is asymptomatic. It is not to be used interchangeably or confused with spinal (adhesive) arachnoiditis.

Other etiologic agents causative of arachnoiditis include a subarachnoid hemorrhage, meningitis, spinal anesthesia, and intrathecal chymopapain injection. Recently, Nelson (26) has called attention to the obvious danger of intrathecal methylprednisolone acetate and the potential danger of epidural cortisone injections as a causative factor in arachnoiditis.

Clinical Presentation

Arachnoiditis has a slow, insidious onset at varying intervals after the etiologic insult. Initially, the patient may complain of leg pain in a single root distribution, but eventually there is a complaint of back pain (100%) and various degrees and types of bilateral leg symptoms (75%). The symptoms are strikingly aggravated by activity and, surprisingly, unrelieved by rest. Other symptoms may include nighttime leg cramps, paresthesia, dysesthesia, motor weakness, and sphincter dysfunction (25%). Most men are impotent as a result of arachnoiditis.

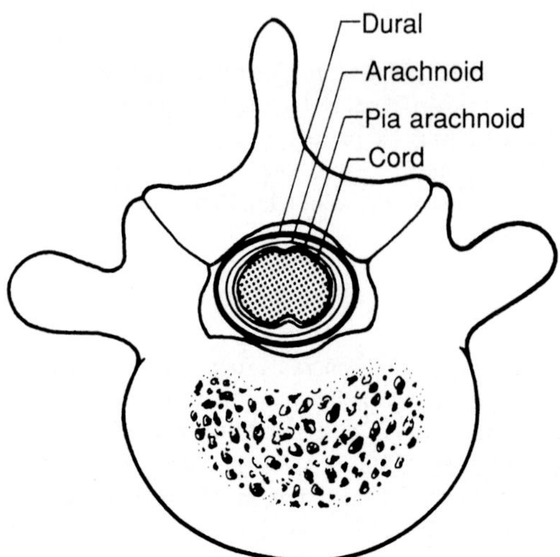

FIGURE 17-14 ● The arachnoid membranes within the dural sheath.

The characteristic physical findings, if any, are multiple root involvement on motor and sensory examination and mild SLR reduction.

Stages of Arachnoiditis

Staging of arachnoiditis has been developed on myelography [more recently on magnetic resonance imaging (MRI)] and at surgery:

Stage 1 Radicular stage, during which the pathology is confined to a single or a few roots. At this stage, the roots are obviously inflamed and swollen.

Stage 2 Arachnoiditis stage in which roots clump together because of the fibrinous exudate but still occupy the central subarachnoid space.

Stage 3 Adhesive arachnoiditis in which roots are densely adherent to the periphery of the spinal dural canal, leaving an empty central cauda equina canal. At this stage, the roots are atrophic and scarred.

Investigation

Until recently, the standard of investigation for arachnoiditis has been myelography. Myelographic changes early in the disease include root sleeve cutoff and clumping of roots (Fig. 17-15) and homogeneous contrast pattern without root shadows. Later, the contrast column takes on the appearance of candle drippings and/or loss of fine root detail at multiple levels (Fig. 17-16), with varying degrees of filling defects and CSF or contrast-filled cysts. These changes extend over a few to many lumbar spinal levels. Occasionally, they are confined to a single level in the form of a complete block, although many of these so-called arachnoiditis patients turn out to have spinal stenosis without arachnoiditis.

Ross et al. (31) have described the MRI appearance of arachnoiditis based on the examination of MRIs and myelograms in 12 confirmed patients (Fig. 17-16). They described three types of changes:

Type 1: Roots are adherent and clumped centrally.

Type 2: Roots are clumped peripherally and the meninges are thickened. There is the appearance of the empty dural sac.

Type 3: No roots are seen because they are one amorphous mass with the dura and CSF. These patients have a complete block on myelography.

Treatment

Unfortunately, there is little one can offer the patient with arachnoiditis. Various surgical procedures have been proposed, such as neurolysis, with or without the dura sewn open, with or without the intrathecal administration of lysing agents. None of these proposals have stood the test of timely follow-up of the patient.

The various conservative treatment measures used in chronic pain centers seem to be of limited use.

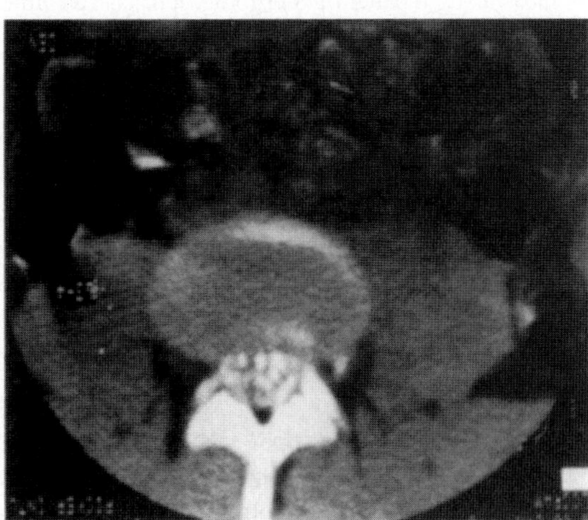

FIGURE 17-15 • Arachnoiditis: root clumping on CT.

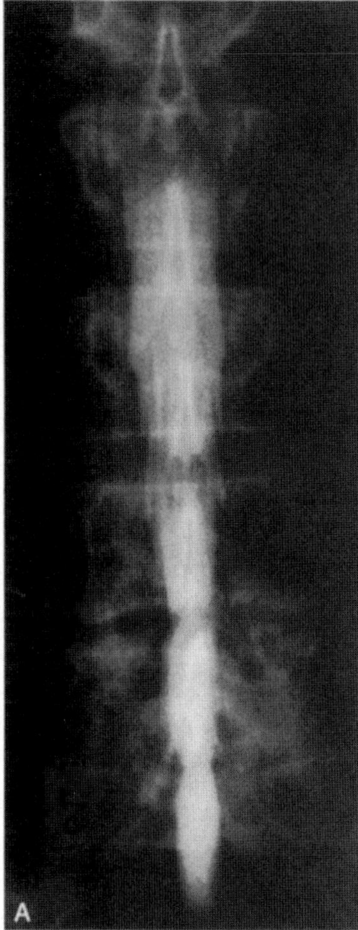

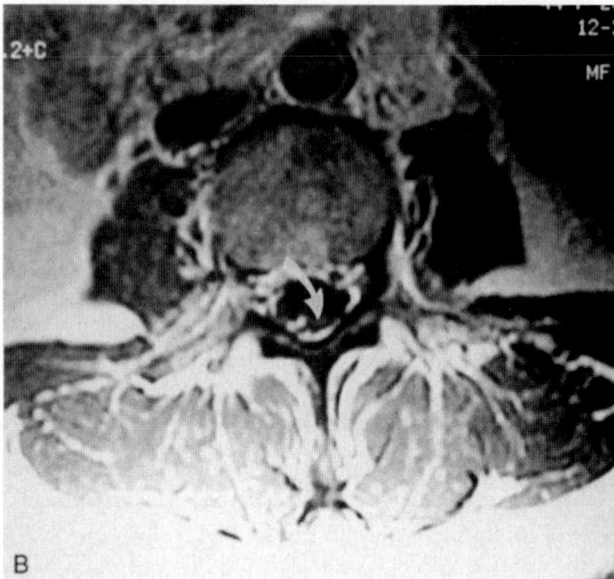

FIGURE 17-16 ● **A:** Severe arachnoiditis: loss of root detail and root cutoff at multiple levels. **B:** An axial T1 MRI with arachnoiditis: note the irregular outline of the common dural sac, clumping of the roots *(arrow),* and increased signal from fatty degeneration in the roots.

CHANGE OF SYMPTOMS OR RECURRENCE OF SYMPTOMS

It is almost impossible to separate "change" from "recurrence" of symptoms without an overlapping classification. To present a symptom-based approach to this group of failed spine surgical patients, we have divided the patients into two groups: those undergoing encroachment surgery and those undergoing stabilization surgery.

Obviously, a patient undergoing both encroachment and stabilization surgery could have failures from either group.

Failures After Encroachment Surgery

The reason for the original surgery in this group of patients obviously was based on the diagnosis of radicular pain from various causes. Failure of the surgery to cure the disease can arise from one of four scenarios.

1. The patient wakes with identical leg pain.
2. The patient reports relief of leg pain and notices increased back pain.
3. The patient notices a change in leg pain postoperatively.
4. The patient reports relief of leg pain for varying lengths of time and then notices recurrence of leg pain.

Patient Wakes with Identical Leg Pain

When the patient wakes with identical leg pain, a re-evaluation must be made. Ensure that surgery has been performed at the appropriate level. Incomplete surgery may have been done at the right level or the root may have been excessively retracted during the procedure. Less often, the reason for persistent leg pain is an erroneous operating diagnosis, such as a missed conus tumor, extrapelvic conditions, or other diagnoses listed in Table 17-3.

Relief of Leg Pain/Increased Back Pain

The sciatic pain may be relieved, but the patient may be plagued by continuing back pain. In many of these patients, if you go back over their initial history you will find that their story was one of recurrent episodes of backache of increasing severity, duration, and frequency, culminating in an attack of incapacitating sciatic pain that necessitated operative intervention. These patients have been suffering for a long period of time from segmental instability giving rise to low back pain. The disc rupture, even though it precipitated the operative intervention, is only one part of the mechanical insufficiency of the spine. Removal of the disc alone in these patients will leave them with the same type of back pain of which they complained in the past. This is the group of patients who should be treated initially by combining disc with fusion, when this is feasible.

If the laminectomy involves destruction of the posterior joints, it may well lead to subsequent back pain, particularly if the involved segment is very mobile; indeed, if decompression requires a total excision of one or both posterior joints, then a segmental fusion is mandatory.

When operating on a listhetic segment, be it a spondylolytic or degenerative spondylolisthesis, it is essential to avoid removing the disc at the slip level at all costs. Obviously, no symptom-producing pathology can be left behind, but all too often there is no real symptom-producing pathology present in the disc at the slip level, yet it is "decompressed" anyway. This removes one of the few soft tissue stabilizers left and may result in an increased slip postoperatively. If a fusion was not done at the time of disc excision, increasing back pain postoperatively will make a fusion necessary in many of these patients.

Change in Leg Pain

When the patient notices a change of leg pain postoperatively, one of the problems that may arise after laminectomy is subsequent peridural and periradicular fibrosis (21). This unfortunate sequel is much more likely to occur in the extensive laminectomy required for decompression of the cauda equina and the emerging nerve roots in a patient suffering from multisegmental spinal stenosis. Some surgeons prefer to use a thin fat graft, as an interposition membrane placed between the dura and the sacrospinales, but there is no uniform agreement among spine surgeons regarding fat grafts.

The patient with root scarring notices some relief of leg pain postoperatively only to notice the gradual recurrence of leg pain in the same preoperative distribution. This time around, the pain is more constant in its presence and although aggravated by activity, it is not totally relieved by rest. The pain usually has a dysesthetic component to it.

Unfortunately, little can be done surgically for this complication, with palliative conservative measures offering some hope of control.

Recurrent Leg Pain

Compared with the patients with acute and chronic unilateral radicular syndromes, patients with a recurrent HNP or lateral zone stenosis differ in one major way—they have had previous surgery. Otherwise, they present with dominant radicular symptoms, clear evidence of nerve root tension (SLR reduction), and varying degrees of neurologic involvement.

A recurrent HNP almost always occurs at the location of the previous surgical exercise (same level/same side).

Patients who have recurrent HNP do have a difference in neurologic presentation. Because of the scar tissue tacking the dural sheath and its contents to the back of the disc space, a small disc herniation is capable of causing significant pain and neurologic changes. Unusual neurologic patterns may also occur and may include double root involvement that is more common than in a virgin HNP; for example, because of scar tissue fixing the dura to the L4–L5 disc space, a recurrent L4–L5 HNP, same level same side as the previous HNP, may cause both fifth and first root involvement.

Nature and site of recurrent pathology. Recurrent HNP most often occurs at the same level/same side (80%–90%) (44). The next most frequent site of a recurrent HNP is a different level (10%), and a recurrent HNP, same level, opposite side, has an incidence of occurrence of 5% at most.

Recurrent pathology caused by lateral zone stenosis usually occurs at the same level as previous surgery and may occur on one or both sides. The pathology is usually facet subluxation into the foramen, due to developing instability after the prior surgical procedure. The patient with a recurrent HNP same level/opposite side or different level than previous surgery can be treated as a virgin HNP with no hesitation to plan a microsurgical procedure. It is these patients who can be handled with a well-planned microsurgical procedure.

Investigation of the patient with recurrent herniated nucleus pulposus. There is a tendency for clinicians and radiologists to get lost in the minutiae of investigating a patient with recurrent HNP. Tests that are of little value in documenting the structural lesion in recurrent pathology include myelography, myelogram/computed tomography (CT), plain CT, electromyography, and discography.

All of the previously listed tests lack both sensitivity and specificity in documenting the occurrence of a disc herniation at a previously operated level. Specifically, myelography (2), with or without postinjection CT scan, cannot distinguish scar from a recurrent HNP. Teplick et al. (40) have attempted to distinguish scar from recurrent HNP on plain CT scan by the shape of the defect, the deformity of the dural sac, and other parameters. Like myelography, these distinctions are not sensitive or specific enough to be used with any authority to document the presence or absence of a recurrent HNP.

Tests Useful in Documenting the Structural Lesion in Recurrent Pathology

Magnetic resonance imaging. Because MRI is capable of showing biochemical changes as well as morphologic characteristics of tissues, it has become the investigative procedure of choice for recurrent HNP (3).

In the immediate postoperative period, the MRI changes, due to the hemorrhage and edema of wound healing, produce dramatic changes (Fig. 17-17). These changes preclude a useful study until wound healing is completed and scar tissue begins to mature (6–12 weeks). Beyond this time, MRI changes of epidural scar versus recurrent HNP are viewed according to the following criteria: (a) location of the mass in the epidural space, (b) signal intensity, (c) mass effect, and (d) gadolinium enhancement (Fig. 17-18). Some authors have advocated contrast enhanced CT scanning (33), but this is used infrequently compared to MRI with gadolinium.

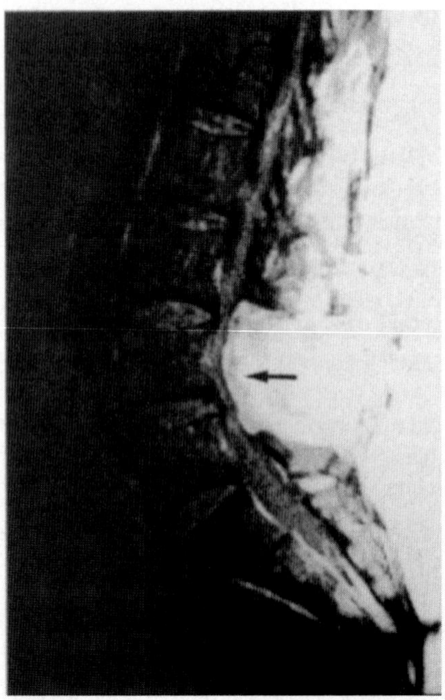

FIGURE 17-17 ● A postoperative complication. A massive hematoma *(arrow)* (high-signal intensity) causing cauda equina compression (10 days postoperatively).

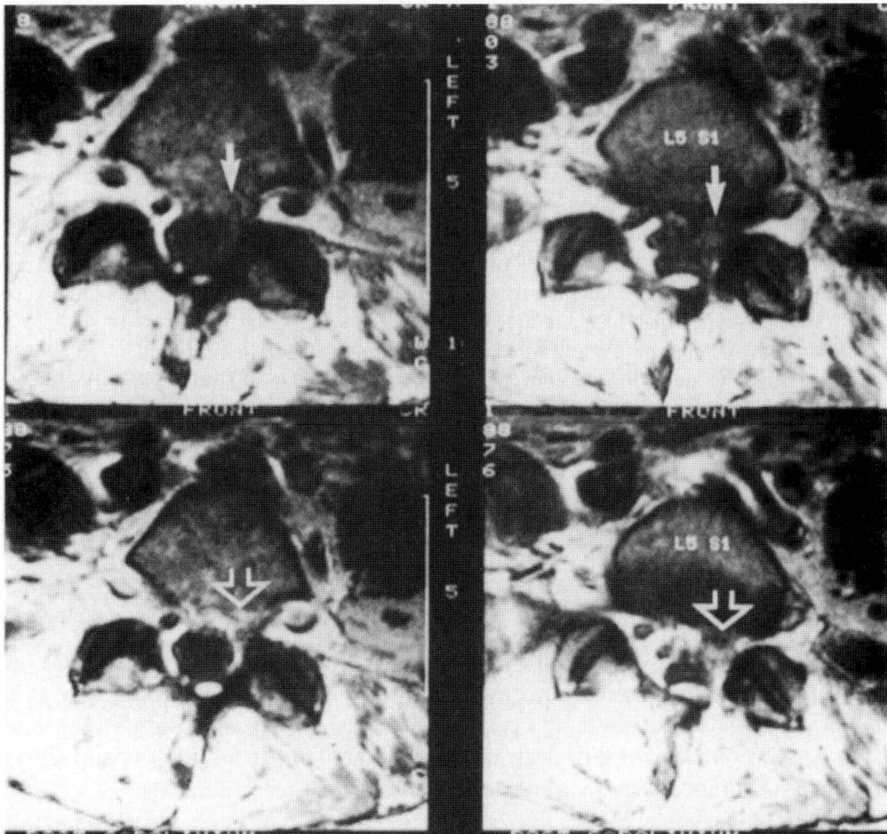

FIGURE 17-18 ● **Top row:** A patient with recurrent left leg pain and a mass (T1 axial MRI) at a site of previous surgery. **Bottom row:** Post-gadolinium injection shows no recurrent fragment (left bottom), but a very definite recurrent disc herniation in T1 axial MRI [bottom right *(arrow)*].

Treatment of recurrent herniated nucleus pulposus. Although all patients with sciatica, recurrent or not, deserve a trial of conservative care, there is reasonable expectation that patients with a recurrent HNP will persist with their symptoms and require surgical intervention. (44). Conventional surgical dictum is that repeat surgery, anywhere in the body, is best done through a wide exposure. Those familiar with the use of the microscope disagree (16,46). If there is any indication for the use of the microscope in lumbar spine surgery: this is it. The illumination and magnification better show the difference between scar and neurologic tissues, making it a safer operation.

FAILURES AFTER SPINAL FUSION

Failures after spinal fusion may be considered under the headings of (a) pain derived from the grafted area, (b) pain derived from the spine above the graft, and (c) donor site pain.

Pain Derived from the Fused Areas

When Dr. Macnab wrote the first edition of this book, spinal instrumentation was seldom used in lumbar spine fusion. Since the introduction of spinal (pedicle) instrumentation systems (37), a large number of lumbar fusions are augmented by instrumentation. Needless to say this advance has been associated with a whole new set of complications and strategies for revision (18,22,24). The more frequent use of interbody fusion has added a further level of complexity to the situation (38). When you set out to achieve a fusion (for back pain) and fail to obtain a solid arthrodesis, you have the number one complication of spinal fusion.

PSEUDARTHROSIS

Radiologically, a pseudarthrosis may be difficult to demonstrate. Moreover, a pseudarthrosis can be present without pain and the mere demonstration of the lesion does not necessarily mean that the source of the patient's continuing disability has been found (49). Increasing work tolerance after infiltration of the pseudarthrosis with local anesthetic tends to indict the lesion as the source of pain, although it must be remembered that an injection of this nature is a powerful hypnotic suggestion. To arrive at any valid conclusion, it is necessary to assess the suggestibility of the patient first by observing the result of injection of normal saline. Discography may well prove to be the best diagnostic tool. Discography in the presence of a solid fusion, although demonstrating an irregular pattern, is generally painless. If there is a pseudarthrosis, discography is painful at the involved segment. Dr. Macnab opined that this technique carries with it an accuracy rate of about 80%; we have broad doubts about discography and limited experience in this specific problem.

Other investigative steps often used to try and demonstrate a pseudarthrosis are flexion/extension films and three-dimensional CT reconstruction. The problem with all of these investigations is the high level of false-positive and false-negative outcomes. This has lead to the opinion of many spine surgeons that the only consistent way to prove or disprove a pseudarthrosis is surgical re-exploration of the fusion mass, looking for a pseudarthrosis and/or detecting movement of vertebral segments within the fusion mass.

In the surgical management of a pseudarthrosis, the failure rate of refusion has been alarmingly high. This probably arises from the fact that it is difficult to obtain, in the fusion area, a good vascular bed with a potent source of osteoblasts capable of revascularizing and reossifying the graft. It is best to reoperate on the spine in an area in which there has been no previous interference. If the previous fusion was midline, an intertransverse fusion is the best approach for repair. If the previous fusion was intertransverse, then the fusion bed should be along the spinous processes. If the previous fusion was a combination of an intertransverse and posterior fusion, the so-called Cowl fusion, then an anterior interbody fusion is the only feasible method of salvage. There are studies supporting the use of pedicle instrumentation for posterior revision surgery (41).

Root Compression

The patient may develop symptoms and signs of root compression that may be due to a rupture of an intervertebral disc underneath the fusion or it may be due to an iatrogenic spinal stenosis. A ruptured disc very rarely occurs under a solid spinal fusion; it is much more likely to occur in the presence of a pseudarthrosis. In those instances in which there is a ruptured disc under a fusion that is irrefutably solid, in all probability it was present at the time the fusion was performed.

Whereas the symptoms resulting from a recent disc rupture are fairly rapid in onset, the symptoms resulting from an iatrogenic spinal stenosis are slow in developing. The clinical picture is clear-cut. A patient with a solid spinal fusion, usually intertransverse and incorporating the L4–L5 segment, which before operation had radiologic evidence of interlaminar narrowing, slowly develops the claudicant type of sciatic pain that one associates with root compression secondary to spinal stenosis. On examination, these patients frequently present evidence of impairment of root conduction at more than one segment.

Pain Derived from the Spine above the Graft

Adjacent level degeneration. In follow-up studies from between 5 and 30 years post-fusion, the rate of adjacent level degeneration has varied between 30% and 50% (13). However, radiographic changes have not necessarily correlated with the clinical picture.

Spondylolysis acquisita. A spondylolysis may develop at the segment above the spinal fusion. Spondylolysis acquisita is probably much more common than previously acknowledged because it may well be missed on a routine lateral view taken for the postoperative assessment of the stability of a spinal fusion. It is probably advisable in all patients who have undergone a spinal fusion and subsequently suffer from persisting discomfort to take oblique views of the spine to show the pars interarticularis of the segment above the lesion.

The exact etiology of the lesion is not known. It may be a stress fracture. The development of a stress fracture may be predisposed to by dissection of the muscle masses away from the lamina at the segment above a spinal fusion. A dissection such as this would interfere to a fairly marked degree with the venous drainage of the lamina, giving rise to partial death of bone in this area. If, subsequently, extra stresses are placed on such a bone by the placement of a graft below it, then the pars interarticularis may break and spondylolysis develop.

The lesion is not seen in patients in whom an intertransverse fusion has been carried out. Theoretically, spondylolysis acquisita should not occur with an intertransverse fusion because the site of the lesion is supported by the uppermost portion of the graft.

Lumbodorsal strain. The significance of a chronic lumbodorsal strain after a lumbosacral fusion has not been sufficiently recognized. When the lumbosacral segment is fused, extra mechanical stresses are placed on the lumbodorsal junction and a previously asymptomatic degenerative change at this level may, after lumbosacral fusion, produce pain referred to both buttocks and down as low as the great trochanters.

Here again, treatment is prophylactic, recognizing the possibility and investigating the probability in every patient considered for spinal fusion. If the lesion does occur, there is no reason why a localized segmental fusion should not be undertaken.

COMPLICATIONS RELATED TO USE OF INSTRUMENTATION SYSTEMS

There are three ways to try to immobilize a spine with instrumentation: (a) hold onto the pedicle, (b) hold onto the lamina, and (c) stabilize the interbody space. By far, the most popular of these methods are those systems that hold onto the pedicles. Complications attendant on the use of these systems include (a) infection; (b) root irritation or injury; (c) vascular injury; (d) screw/plate, rod breakage or disengagement; (e) degenerative changes at the motion segment above the fusion; and (f) painful hardware.

Pseudarthrosis with Instrumentation

The instrumentation systems have enjoyed wide support amongst spine surgeons because they decrease the pseudarthrosis rate (37). It is still possible to end up with a pseudarthrosis in an instrumented fusion. It may be very hard to demonstrate on investigation and require re-exploration of the fusion mass.

DONOR SITE PAIN

Continuing pain may be derived from the donor site. The superficial gluteal nerve (cluneal nerves) crosses the iliac crest approximately the breadth of four fingers away from the midline (Fig. 17-19). If an incision over the iliac crest is used to obtain the graft, the superficial gluteal nerve may be di-

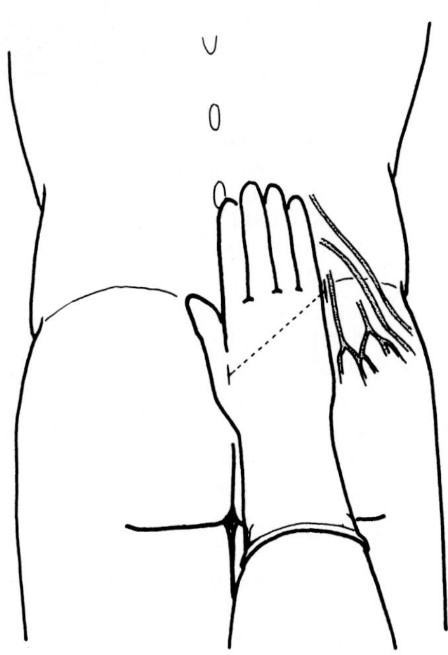

FIGURE 17-19 ● The superficial gluteal nerve crosses the iliac crest approximately the breadth of four fingers away from the midline.

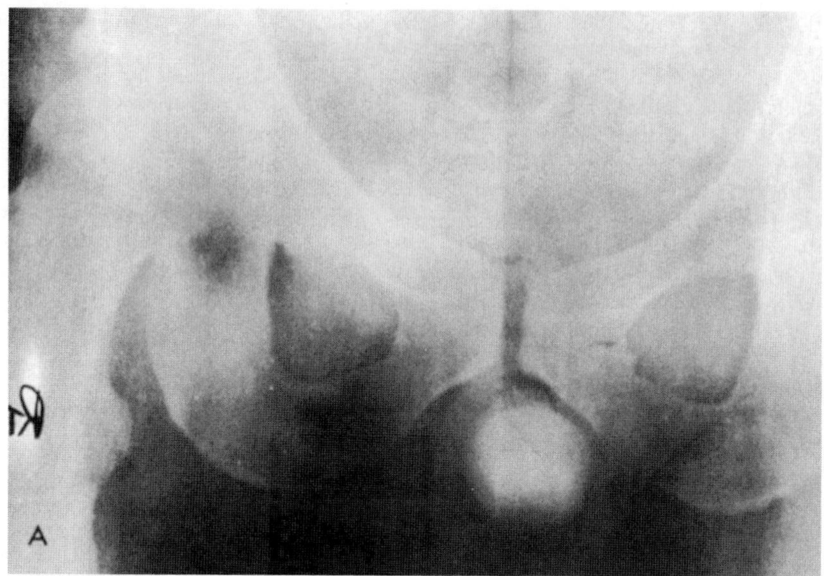

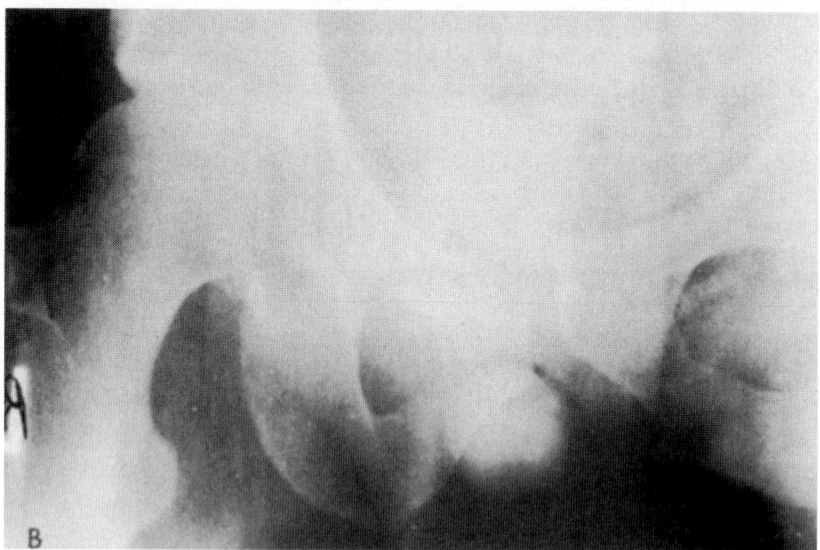

FIGURE 17-20 ● Instability of the symphysis pubis associated with sacroiliac instability. This patient had instability of the left sacroiliac joint. In the first radiograph **(A),** the patient is standing on his right leg, and in the second radiograph **(B),** he is taking full weight on his left leg. Note the gross excursion of the symphysis pubis that is demonstrated when the patient takes his weight on the left leg.

vided and trapped in the scar and become a source of pain. It is preferable to curve the lower end of the midline incision to expose the posterior superior iliac spine and obtain bone from this site.

The treatment of neuroma pain is very ungratifying and all efforts must be made to avoid cutting these nerves. If the patient had unilateral leg pain before surgery, it is wise to make the donor site incision on the opposite iliac crest so that residual postoperative symptoms due to root pathology are not confused by the potential for neuroma formation.

Sacroiliac Pain

Sacroiliac instability may occur if the donor site encroaches markedly on the sacroiliac joint, particularly if the iliolumbar ligament is divided. This is probably the most important of all the stabilizing ligaments of the sacroiliac joint. In cadavers, if this ligament is divided, the sacroiliac joint can be opened up easily, like the two halves of a book. Patients with sacroiliac instability will present with pain over the sacroiliac joint and the pain will radiate down the lateral aspect of the great trochanter onto the front of the thigh. Weight-bearing on the involved extremity increases the pain, and the patients tend to limp with a combined Trendelenburg and antalgic gait. The pain is reproduced by straining the sacroiliac joints by resisted abduction of the hip and is temporarily relieved by infiltration of the involved sacroiliac joint with local anesthetic. With gross instability, movement at the symphysis pubis may be observed when the radiographs are taken with the patient standing first on one leg, then on the other (Fig. 17-20).

Some of these patients may even require a sacroiliac fusion to get rid of this troublesome, residual, significant disability.

DIAGNOSES OF QUESTIONABLE SIGNIFICANCE

On occasion, failed low back pain patients reach an intolerable state symptomatically and, with the failure of accepted medical treatment, they reach for anything that offers hope. They fall into the hands of unscrupulous practitioners with legitimate and not so legitimate backgrounds; they are "awakened to new hope" with fancy-sounding diagnoses of questionable significance. Such diagnoses include fat nodule entrapment, neuroma formation, and various tendinitis and bursitis conditions. Before following this direction, these patients should be encouraged to attend the many fine chronic pain clinics or rehabilitation centers specializing in these problems. Readers are referred to Wilkinson's (45) book for further reading about this most difficult group of patients.

CONCLUSION

The intention of every surgeon is to make an accurate diagnosis as to the cause of symptoms and try, with a skillful surgical procedure, to relieve the symptoms. Surgeons are not perfect, and sometimes the outcome of surgery falls short of expectations of the patient and the surgeon. In today's legal climate in the United States, this failure of the surgeon to achieve a good result is called a complication and is grounds for a malpractice action. Surgeons, in this unchecked environment, are being forced into the role of guarantors, a godlike position many are finding difficult to sustain. Whether an unanticipated result to spine surgery is a complication, an adverse effect, iatrogenic, or act of God is not at issue in this chapter. The situations described represent occurrences that direct the result of surgery away from the goal the patient and the surgeon are trying to achieve. For centuries, surgeons have recognized these happenings as either complications, the results of their misadventures and technical errors, or acts of God, but all leading to a less-than-acceptable result of the surgical exercise. Less-than-acceptable results in surgery for lumbar disc disease do occur.

Unfortunately, these patients fall victim to the misconception that failed back surgery can only be cured by more surgery by the same surgeon. In the end, they appear in the clinics for patients with failed back surgery after multiple surgeries and multiple investigations. Most of these patients end up abusing narcotics and becoming psychologically destroyed. If there ever is a place for preventative medicine, this is it.

REFERENCES

1. Bertagnoli R, Zigler J, Karg A, Voight S. Complications and strategies for revision surgery in total disc replacement. *Orthop Clin North Am.* 2005;36:389–395.
2. Braun IF, Horfman MD, Davis PC, et al. Contrast enhancement in CT differentiation between recurrent disc herniation and postoperative scar: prospective study. *AJNR.* 1985;6:607–612.
3. Bundschuh CV, Modic MT, Ross JS, et al. Epidural fibrosis and recurrent disk herniation in the lumbar spine: MR imaging assessment. *AJNR.* 1988;9:169–178.
4. Buono LM, Foroozan R. Perioperative posterior ischemic optic neuropathy: review of the literature. *Surv Ophthalmol.* 2005;50:15–26.
5. Capana AH, Williams RW, Austin DC, et al. Lumbar discectomy—percentage of disc removal and detection of anterior annulus perforation. *Spine.* 1981;6:610–614.
6. Dearborn JT, Hu SS, Tribus CB, Bradford DS. Thromboembolic complications after major thoracolumbar spine surgery. *Spine.* 1999;24:1471–1476.
7. DeSaussure RL. Vascular injury coincident to disc surgery. *J Neurosurg.* 1959;16:222–229.

8. Eismont FJ, Wiesel SW, Rothman RH. Treatment of dural tears associated with spinal surgery. *J Bone Joint Surg Am.* 1981;63:1132–1136.
9. Ferree BA. Deep venous thrombosis following lumbar laminotomy and laminectomy. *Orthopedics.* 1994;17: 35–38.
10. Glassman SD, Anagnost SC, Parker A, et al. The effects of cigarette smoking and smoking cessation on spinal fusion. *Spine.* 2000;15:2608–2615.
11. Greene K. *Preoperative nutritional status of total joint patients: relationship to postoperative wound complications.* Presented at American Academy of Orthopaedic Surgeons Annual Meeting. Las Vegas, Nevada; February 1989.
12. Harbison EC. Major vascular complications of intervertebral disc surgery. *Ann Surg.* 1954;140:342–348.
13. Hilibrand AS, Robbins M. Adjacent segment degeneration and adjacent segment disease: the consequences of spinal fusion? *Spine J.* 2004;4:190S–194S.
14. Hodges SD, Humphreys SC, Eck JC, Covington LA. Management of incidental durotomy without mandatory bed rest. A retrospective review of 20 cases. *Spine.* 1999;24:2062–2064.
15. Holscher EC. Vascular and visceral injuries during lumbar disc surgery. *J Bone Joint Surg Am.* 1968;50:383–393.
16. Hudgins WR. The role of microdiscectomy. *Orthop Clin North Am.* 1983;14:589–603.
17. Jones AA, Stambough JL, Balderston RA, et al. Long-term results of lumbar spine surgery complicated by unintended incidental durotomy. *Spine.* 1989;14:443–446.
18. Kostuik J. Surgical treatment of failures of laminectomy and spinal fusion. *Lumbar Spinal Stenosis.* St. Louis: Mosby Yearbook; 1992:425–470.
19. Long DM, Filtzer DL, BenDebba M, Hendler NH. Clinical features of the failed-back syndrome. *J Neurosurg.* 1988;69:61–71.
20. Macnab I. Negative disc exploration. *J Bone Joint Surg Am.* 1971;53:891–903.
21. Mayfield FH. Complications of laminectomy. *Clin Neurosurg.* 1976;23:435–439.
22. McAfee PC, Cunningham BW, Lee GA, et al. Revision strategies for salvaging or improving failed cylindrical cages. *Spine.* 1999;24:2147–2153.
23. McLaren AC, Bailey SI. Cauda equina syndrome: complication of lumbar discectomy. *Clin Orthop.* 1986;204: 143–149.
24. Mueller WM, Larson SJ. Complications of spinal instrumentation. In: Tarlov EC, ed. *Complications of Spinal Surgery. Neurosurgical Topics.* Park Ridge, IL: American Association of Neurological Surgeons; 1991:15–21.
25. Nachemson A. Advances in low-back pain. *Clin Orthop.* 1985;200:266–278.
26. Nelson DA. Dangers from methylprednisolone acetate therapy by intraspinal injection. *Arch Neurol.* 1988;45:804–806.
27. Patel MR, Louie W, Rachlin J. Postoperative cerebrospinal fluid leaks of the lumbosacral spine: management with percutaneous fibrin glue. *AJNR.* 1996;17:495–500.
28. Pheasant HC. Sources of failure in laminectomies. *Orthop Clin North Am.* 1975;6:319–329.
29. Ramirez LF, Thisted R. Complication and demographic characteristics of patients undergoing lumbar discectomy in community hospitals. *Neurosurgery.* 1989;25:226–231.
30. Rish BL. A critique of the surgical management of lumbar disc disease in a private neurological practice. *Spine.* 1984;9:500–504.
31. Ross JS, Masaryk TJ, Modic MT, et al. MR imaging of lumbar arachnoiditis. *AJR.* 1987;149:1025–1032.
32. Rydevik B, Brown MD, Lundborg G. The pathoanatomy and pathophysiology of nerve root compression. *Spine.* 1984;9:7–15.
33. Schubiger O, Valavanis A. CT differentiation between disc herniation and postoperative scar formation. The value of contrast enhancement. *Neuroradiology.* 1980;22:251–254.
34. Smith RA, Estridge MN. Bowel perforation following lumbar disc surgery. *J Bone Joint Surg Am.* 1964;46: 826–828.
35. Spangfort EV. The lumbar disc herniation. A computer aided analysis of 2,504 operations. *Acta Orthop Scand.* 1972;142(suppl):1–95.
36. Spengler DM. Lumbar discectomy: results with limited disc excision and selective foraminotomy. *Spine.* 1982;7:604–607.
37. Steffee AD, Biscup RS, Sitkowski DJ. Segmental spine plates with pedicle screw fixation: a new internal fixation device for disorders of the lumbar and thoracolumbar spine. *Clin Orthop.* 1986;203:45–53.
38. Stromberg L, Toohey JS, Neidre A, et al. Complications and surgical considerations in posterior lumbar interbody fusion with carbon fiber interbody ages and Steffee pedicle screws and plates. *Orthopedics.* 2003;26:1039–1043.
39. Tenney JH, Vlahov D, Salcman M, Ducker TB. Wide variation in risk of wound infection following clean neurosurgery. *J Neurosurg.* 1985;62:243–247.
40. Teplick JG, Teplick SK, Haskin ME. The postoperative lumbar spine. In: Yost MJD, ed. *Computed Tomography of the Spine.* Baltimore: Williams & Wilkins; 1984.
41. Thalgott J, et al. Reconstruction of failed lumbar surgery with narrow A-O DCP plates for spinal arthrodesis. *Spine.* 1991;16:5170–5175.
42. van Ooij A, Oner FC Verbout AJ. Complications of artificial disc replacement: a report of 27 patients with the SB Charite disc. *J Spinal Disord Tech.* 2003;16:369–383.
43. Wang JC, Bohlman HH, Riew KD. Dural tears secondary to operations on the lumbar spine. Management and results after a two year minimum follow-up of eighty-eight patients. *J Bone Joint Surg Am.* 1998;80:1728–1732.
44. Weir BKA, Jacobs GA. Reoperation rate following lumbar discectomy. An analysis of 662 lumbar discectomies. *Spine.* 1980;5:366–370.1.

45. Wilkinson HA. *The Failed Back Syndrome, Etiology and Therapy.* Philadelphia: Harper & Row; 1983.
46. Williams RW. Microlumbardiscectomy: a 12-year statistical review. *Spine.* 1986;11:851–852.
47. Wilson DH, Harbaugh R. Microsurgical and standard removal of the protruded lumbar disc: a comparative study. *Neurosurgery.* 1981;8:422–427.
48. Wong D, Mayer T, Watters W et al. *Sign Mark and X-Ray (SMaX): A NASS Patient Safety Program.* LaGrange, IL: North American Spine Society; 2001.
49. Zucherman J, Schofferman J. Pathology of failed back surgery syndrome. In: White AH, ed. *Failed Back Surgery Syndrome,* Vol. 1, No. 1. Philadelphia: Hanley & Belfus; 1986:1–12.

Index

Page numbers in *italics* denote figures; those followed by *t* denote tables.

B

T

U

V

W

X

Y

Z